# Basic Statistics and Pharmaceutical Statistical Applications

## Second Edition

## Biostatistics: A Series of References and Textbooks

Series Editor

**Shein-Chung Chow, Ph.D.**

*Professor*

*Department of Biostatistics and Bioinformatics*

*Duke University School of Medicine*

*Durham, NC, U.S.A.*

1. *Design and Analysis of Animal Studies in Pharmaceutical Development,* Shein-Chung Chow and Jen-pei Liu
2. *Basic Statistics and Pharmaceutical Statistical Applications,* James E. De Muth
3. *Design and Analysis of Bioavailability and Bioequivalence Studies, Second Edition, Revised and Expanded,* Shein-Chung Chow and Jen-pei Liu
4. *Meta-Analysis in Medicine and Health Policy,* Dalene K. Stangl and Donald A. Berry
5. *Generalized Linear Models: A Bayesian Perspective,* Dipak K. Dey, Sujit K. Ghosh, and Bani K. Mallick
6. *Difference Equations with Public Health Applications,* Lemuel A. Moyé and Asha Seth Kapadia
7. *Medical Biostatistics,* Abhaya Indrayan and Sanjeev B. Sarmukaddam
8. *Statistical Methods for Clinical Trials,* Mark X. Norleans
9. *Causal Analysis in Biomedicine and Epidemiology: Based on Minimal Sufficient Causation,* Mikel Aickin
10. *Statistics in Drug Research: Methodologies and Recent Developments,* Shein-Chung Chow and Jun Shao
11. *Sample Size Calculations in Clinical Research,* Shein-Chung Chow, Jun Shao, and Hansheng Wang
12. *Applied Statistical Design for the Researcher,* Daryl S. Paulson
13. *Advances in Clinical Trial Biostatistics,* Nancy L. Geller
14. *Statistics in the Pharmaceutical Industry, 3rd Edition,* Ralph Buncher and Jia-Yeong Tsay
15. *DNA Microarrays and Related Genomics Techniques: Design, Analysis, and Interpretation of Experiments,* David B. Allsion, Grier P. Page, T. Mark Beasley, and Jode W. Edwards
16. *Basic Statistics and Pharmaceutical Statistical Applications, Second Edition,* James E. De Muth

# Basic Statistics and Pharmaceutical Statistical Applications

## Second Edition

**James E. De Muth**

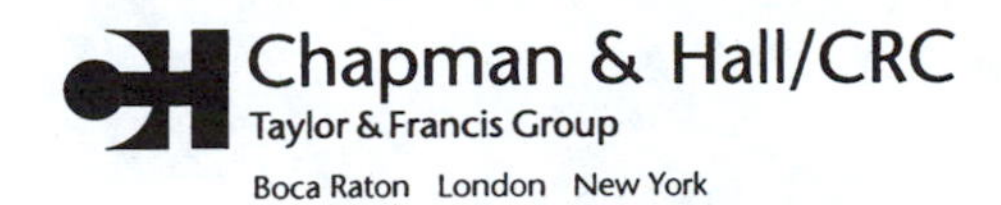

Chapman & Hall/CRC
Taylor & Francis Group
Boca Raton London New York

Chapman & Hall/CRC is an imprint of the
Taylor & Francis Group, an informa business

Published in 2006 by
Chapman & Hall/CRC
Taylor & Francis Group
6000 Broken Sound Parkway NW, Suite 300
Boca Raton, FL 33487-2742


Printed in the United States of America on acid-free paper
10 9 8 7 6 5 4 3 2 1

International Standard Book Number-10: 0-8493-3799-2
International Standard Book Number-13: 978-0-8493-3799-4



**Library of Congress Cataloging-in-Publication Data**

Catalog record is available from the Library of Congress

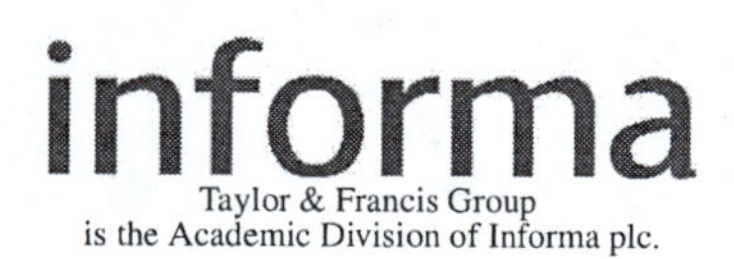


**Visit the Taylor & Francis Web site at**
**http://www.taylorandfrancis.com**

**and the CRC Press Web site at**
**http://www.crcpress.com**

**To Judy,
Jenny and Betsy**

# Preface

The first edition of this book, published seven years ago, was a fairly successful attempt to provide a practical, easy-to-read, basic statistics book for two primary audiences, those in the pharmaceutical industry and those in pharmacy practice. Reviewing the contents and current uses, several shortcomings were identified and hopefully corrected. This second edition represents not only an update of the previous edition, but a considerable expansion on topics relevant to both intended audiences. As described in a later section of this preface, most of the expanded information is in the area of biostatistics and how it relates to professional practice experiences, thus making it more appropriate for undergraduate statistics courses for Pharm.D. students. However, those in the industry have not been completely ignored. New sections address their specific statistical issues and are presented in the second edition.

The author has been fortunate to have taught an additional 68 short courses since the 1999 release of the first edition. Valuable input through the learners attending these classes and new examples from these individuals have been helpful in identifying missing materials in the previous edition. In addition, the author had the opportunity to work closely with a variety of excellent statisticians while serving as the Chair of the USP Biostatistics Expert Committee (2000-2005). Both of these activities have helped contribute to the updating and expansion of this book.

### A Book for Non-Statisticians

As stated in the preface of the first edition, statistics provide useful methods to analyze the world around us, evaluate the findings and hopefully make beneficial decisions. These various tests provide a methodology for answering questions faced by pharmacists and members of the pharmaceutical industry. A popular phrase in the profession has been "outcome measurements." Statistics provide a means for summarizing data and making constructive decisions about the observed outcomes and their potential impact. This organized approach to evaluating observed data helps us avoid jumping to conclusions and making choices that may be unwise or even dangerous to individuals served by our profession.

Unfortunately, many individuals fear, even hate, statistics. Why? There appear to be two major reasons for this dislike. The first is the naive belief that statistics is associated with higher mathematics and therefore difficult to learn. On the contrary, as seen in the following pages, most basic statistical tests involve four-function math

(+, -, x, ÷), with a few square roots thrown in for good measure. By avoiding "heavy-duty" mathematics, hopefully even the mathematically challenged learner will benefit and increase his or her confidence using these procedures. The second major reason for disliking this area of mathematics is the association with unpleasant past experiences with statistics. In many cases, undergraduate and graduate courses are taught by individuals who are deeply concerned and interested in how statistical formulae work and the rationale behind the manipulation of the data. Unfortunately they may spend too much time on the derivation of the statistical tests, rather than focusing on practical day-to-day uses for these tools and successful interpretation of their results. One of the primary goals of this book is to dispel some of the fear and anxiety associated with the basic statistical tests used in the pharmacy profession and to assist individuals using statistical computer software to help them interpret their results correctly.

**Purpose of This Book**

The primary purpose of this book is to serve as an introduction to statistics for undergraduate and graduate students in pharmacy, as well as a reference guide for individuals in various pharmacy settings, including the pharmaceutical industry. It is designed for individuals desiring a brief introduction to the field of statistics, as well as those in need of a quick reference for statistical problem solving. It is a handbook, a guide and reference for researchers in need of methods to statistically analyze data. It does not deal with the theoretical basis or derivation of most of the formulae presented; rather, it serves as a quick and practical tool for the application of the most commonly employed statistical tests.

A greater knowledge of statistics can assist pharmacy students, pharmacists and individuals working in the pharmaceutical industry in at least four ways:

1. When reading articles in a refereed journal we assume that the material has been thoroughly checked and the information presented is accurate. Unfortunately, reviews of the medical literature have found numerous errors and these will be discussed in Chapter 24. It is important to be cognizant of possible statistical mistakes when reading the literature.
2. Pharmacists and pharmacy decision makers are constantly gathering data to improve or justify their professional services, or are involved in clinical trials to help identify more effective therapies for their patient clientele. Appropriate interpretation of data can assist in supporting new programs or expanded services. However, we must be careful to use appropriate statistical tests and avoid errors that could eventually come back to haunt us.
3. Scientists working in the pharmaceutical industry are constantly presented with data and knowledge of the use of both descriptive and inferential statistics can be helpful for preparing reports, regulatory documentation, or other problem-solving activities.
4. For pharmacists, the Board of Pharmaceutical Specialties has developed board certification for pharmacotherapy with the designation "Board

Certified Pharmacotherapy Specialist." Certification requires the candidate to pass a rigorous examination that includes therapeutics, research design, basic data analysis and biostatistics, clinical pharmacokinetics and knowledge of physical examination findings. An increased comfort level with statistics and greater understanding of the appropriate tests can assist with this endeavor.

**How is This Book Similar to the First Edition?**

The approach to presenting the topic of statistics has not changed. This edition is still divided into three major sections: 1) the underpinnings required to understand inferential statistical tests; 2) inferential statistics to help in problem solving; and 3) supportive materials in the form of flow charts and tables.

Using the analogy from the preface in the first edition, let us imagine for a moment a heavy object suspended in midair, held in place by a rope. By definition a rope is a flexible line composed of fibers twisted together to give tensile strength to the line. The strength of a rope is based on the interwoven nature of this series of fibers. The individual fibers by themselves can support very little weight, but combined and wrapped with other fibers can form a product capable of supporting a great deal of weight. Statistics can be thought of in similar terms. A very useful and powerful device, a statistical test is based on a number of unique interwoven areas, such as types of variables, random sampling, probability, measures of central tendency and hypothesis testing. In order to understand how statistical tests work, it is necessary to have a general understanding of how these individual areas (fibers) work together to make the test (rope) a strong and effective procedure. At the same time a poorly knotted rope will eventually weaken and untie. Similarly, poorly designed experiments and/or inappropriate statistical tests will eventually fail, producing erroneous results. Therefore, the first section of this book will briefly explore some of the basic fibers involved in strengthening this rope we call statistics. The later chapters will focus on: 1) the most commonly used tests; 2) when these tests should be used; 3) conditions that are required for their correct use; and 4) how to properly interpret the results. The incorrect use of statistics (through their inappropriate application) or misinterpretation of the results of the statistical test can be as dangerous as using faulty or biased data to reach the decision. Our statistical rope could quickly fray and the object come crashing to the ground.

The second section presents the various statistical tests commonly found in pharmacy and the pharmaceutical literature. A cursory view of today's literature indicates that these same tests are still commonly used. Each chapter includes example problems and their answers. The problems are derived from the areas of pharmacy, analytical chemistry, and clinical drug trials.

Designed to serve as both a teaching aid and reference manual, each chapter is divided into two major sections. The first is a description of each statistical test or related subject matter. Most statistical tests are discussed briefly with respect to their appropriate use, applications, limitations and specific mathematical formulae. With each procedure, decision-making models are specified (hypotheses, decision rules, abbreviated tables of critical values and interpretation of the findings). The second section consists of a series of example problems. The best approach to learning statistics is through examples, thus most statistical tests will have at least one example problem to aid the learner in observing the practical applications of each test and the interpretation of the results. The problems in this book attempt to illustrate practical examples found in a variety of pharmacy settings and contain the full mathematical computations and interpretation of the test results.

The last section of the book includes tables of critical values needed to make appropriate decisions from the statistical tests. Also included is a series of flow charts to assist the user to identify the most appropriate inferential statistic, given the type of data being analyzed.

Unfortunately, something needed to be reduced in order to maintain a book of reasonable volume, avoiding an excessive increase in the number of pages. To accomplish this, the number of problems and worked out solutions presented at the end of most chapters has been decreased. They are still present to help learners who wish to do the calculations and check their answers, but the number of such problems is smaller in this second edition of the book.

**How Does This Book Represent an Improvement over the First Edition?**

Is the subtitle of this book "updated and expanded" correct? Virtually every chapter has new information either in the form of additional paragraphs or entirely new sections. Most of the first eight chapters (presented as seven chapters in the first edition) have remained the same with minor additions throughout and new sections including a description of the trimmed mean (Chapter 5), various forms of data transformations to create normal distributions (Chapter 6) and measures of the propagation of random error (Chapter 8). The majority of the new information is presented during the discussion of the inferential statistical tests in Chapters 9 though 23.

Chapter 11 on multiple comparison tests is a greatly expanded version of the previous chapter titled "post hoc procedures." Where the original 1999 chapter presented only three tests, this expanded version describes nine multiple comparison techniques and references several others. This expansion in the number of comparisons should cover all the results normally reported by various computer software packages.

The chapter introducing factorial designs (Chapter 12) has been expanded to discuss post hoc procedures for two-way ANOVAs, repeated measures designs and Latin Square designs. Chapter 13 surveys additional types of bivariate correlations and discusses various assessments for independence and randomness. The chapter on linear regression (Chapter 14) now includes information on inverse prediction, handling of multiple data points at different levels of the independent variable and assessment of parallelism of slopes for two samples. Chapter 15 has a new section addressing power and sample size determination for two-sample Z-tests of proportions.

The original two chapters on chi square in the first edition have been reformatted and expanded into four new chapters (16 through 19). Much of the new material will be discussed in the following paragraph, but Chapter 17 deserves special note. This chapter is new and presents measures of association, primarily with nominal and ordinal data. Over 15 tests are presented and others as references, many of which appear in software packages and can assist the researcher in determining which one(s) are appropriated under given situations. Chapter 21 presents an increased number of nonparametric tests including new information on *post hoc* comparisons for a significant Kruskal-Wallis test, the Kolmogorov-Smirnov goodness-of-fit test, the Anderson-Darling test, and various runs and range tests. Appendix B presents eight new tables that are required for the interpretation of some of the new inferential statistics.

The majority of the new information could be described as "biostatistics" and of benefit to those pharmacists and researchers involved with clinical trials. Chapter 18 on odds ratios and relative risk ratios is new and provides valuable information for dealing with probability, odds and risk. Chapter 19 introduces the topic of evidence-based practice with discussions of sensitivity and specificity, predictive values and likelihood ratios. Chapter 20 is an entirely new chapter dealing with survival statistics including not only actuarial analysis and Kaplan-Meier procedure, but comparison of different curves, hazard ratio analysis and an introduction to multiple regression with survival data using proportional hazards regression. Finally a new section in Chapter 22 addresses clinical equivalence and noninferiority studies.

At the same time, industrial pharmacists and scientist have not been overlooked. Of particular note are new sections on process capability (Chapter 7), tolerance limits (Chapter 7) and methods for assessing repeatability and reproducibility (Chapter 12).

Hopefully the readers and researchers using the second edition of this book will find this new and expanded information helpful for their daily problem solving activities and reporting of their findings.

## Acknowledgments

As noted in the first edition of this book, many people have contributed directly or indirectly to the completion of both editions of the book. Thanks to all the participants in the 60-plus short courses since the first edition of this book. Through their excellent questions and my sometimes response of "I'm not sure"; they have stimulated problem-solving activities that have resulted in many of the new sections in this edition. Without their insightful and challenging questions, there would not have been a need for a second edition.

As mentioned in the opening paragraph, serving as Chair of the USP Expert Committee on Biostatistics from 2000 to 2005 was a fantastic learning experience. The members of this Committee were extremely professional and volunteered their expertise not only for the improvement of public standards for pharmaceuticals, but helped educate the Committee Chair. I have missed working with these individuals and publicly thank Robert Capen (Merck), Bob Dillard (Takeda), Clare Gnecco (CBER/FDA), Heyward Hull, III (ICAgen), Jacks Lee (Aventis Pasteur), Don Schuirmann (CDER/FDA), Charles Tan (Merck), Lynn Torbeck (Torbeck and

Associates), Dan Weiner (Pharsight), Doris Weisman (Lilly) and Edith Zang (Institute for Cancer Prevention) for their patience and assistance over the five-year tenure of this Committee. Also, thanks to the three USP staff liaisons who supported the activities of the Committee and provided guidance for the Chair: Will Brown, Tahseen Mirza and Horacio Pappa.

Involvement with USP also provided the opportunity for me to meet and work with Walter Hauck, Professor and Head of the Biostatistics Section for the Division of Clinical Pharmacology at Thomas Jefferson University, who in addition to his other responsibilities serves as a consultant to USP. Walter continually served as a source for clarifying statistical issues and has an amazing ability to express clearly explained statistical concepts through the written word.

Although a friend and long-term teaching partner prior to our work at USP, thanks to Lynn Torbeck of Torbeck Associates in Evansville, IL, for his constant input into my statistical growth. When a complex issue arises and the literature fails me, he always serves as a valuable source of information. His help, support of teaching activities and friendship are greatly appreciated. The knowledge and insight brought to the table by Lynn, Walter and the USP Committee members are examples of why I classify myself as a "statistical hobbyist" and not a professional statistician!

Thanks to Russell Dekker, former Chief Publishing Officer for Marcel Dekker, Inc. (publishers of the first edition of this book). Russell suggested and encouraged (even hassled) me into preparing both editions of this book. Although the current publisher has been very helpful, the experience of working with Russell on this book was sorely missing during the last 18 months of this project.

As with the first edition of this book, the accomplishment of completing the following materials is directly attributable to the love and support of my family. A very special thank you to my wife Judy and to our daughters, Jenny and Betsy, for their continued patience and encouragement. Although he provided no direct encouragement, our Chocolate Labrador, Dodger, also helped by providing company and keeping my feet warm in the basement during the development of this edition.

*James E. De Muth*

# Contents

## Contents

# Symbols

| | |
|---|---|
| $\alpha$ (alpha) | type I error; probability used in statistical tables, $p$ |
| $\alpha'$ | Bonferroni adjusted type I error, Sidák test statistic |
| $\alpha_{ew}$ | experimentwise error rate = $1 - (1 - \alpha)^C$ |
| $\beta$ (beta) | type II error; population slope |
| $1 - \beta$ | power |
| $\beta_1, \beta_2, \beta_3$ | regression coefficients (beta weights) |
| $\Gamma$ (gamma) | Goodman-Kruskal's gamma statistic |
| $\delta$ (delta) | difference |
| $\eta$ (eta) | correlation ratio |
| $\theta$ (theta) | equivalence interval |
| $\kappa$ (kappa) | Cohen's kappa statistic |
| $\mu$ (mu) | population mean |
| $\mu_0$ | target mean in control charts |
| $\mu_d$ | population mean difference (matched-pair t-test) |
| $\mu_{\overline{X}}$ | mean of the sampling distribution of $\overline{X}$ |
| $\nu$ (nu) | degrees of freedom in analysis of variance |
| $\rho$ (rho) | Spearman rank correlation coefficient; population correlation coefficient |
| $\rho_\alpha$ | Cronbach's alpha statistic |
| $\rho_{KR20}, \rho_{KR21}$ | Kuder-Richardson test statistics |
| $\sigma$ (sigma) | population standard deviation |
| $\sigma^2$ | population variance |
| $\sigma_{\overline{X}}$ | standard deviation of the sampling distribution of $\overline{X}$ |
| $\tau_b$ (tau) | Kendall's tau-b statistic |
| $\tau_c$ | Kendall's tau-c statistic |
| $\phi$ (phi) | phi coefficient, phi statistic |
| $\chi^2$ (chi) | chi square coefficient |
| $\chi^2_{CMH}$ | Cochran-Mantel-Haenszel chi square test statistic |
| $\chi^2_{corrected}$ | Yate's correction for continuity statistic |
| $\chi^2_{McNemar}$ | McNemar test statistic |
| $\chi^2_{MH}$ | Mantel-Haenszel chi square test statistic |
| $\chi^2_r$ | Friedman two-way analysis of variance test statistic |
| $\psi_I$ (psi) | estimator for Scheffé's procedure |
| $\varpi^2$ (omega) | coefficient of determination for nonlinearity |

# Symbols

|  |  |
|---|---|
| $a$ | y-intercept, intercept of a sample regression line |
| $A_n^2$ | Anderson-Darling test statistic |
| $AD_i$ | absolute deviation |
| $ARR$ | absolute risk reduction |
| $b$ | sample slope, slope of a sample regression line |
| $c$ or $C$ | number of columns in a contingency table; number of possible comparison with two levels; Cochran's C test statistic; Pearson's C statistic, contingency coefficient |
| $C^*$ | Sakoda's adjusted Pearson's C statistic |
| $cf$ | cumulative frequency |
| $CI$ | confidence interval |
| $CEO$ | control event odds |
| $CER$ | control event rate |
| $C_p$, $C_{pk}$, $C_{pm}$ | process capability indexes |
| $CV$ | coefficient of variation |
| $d$ | difference between pairs of values or ranks; Durbin-Watson coefficient |
| $D$ | Komogorov-Smirnov goodness-of-fit test statistic |
| $\overline{d}$ | sample mean difference (matched-pair t-test) |
| $df$ | degrees of freedom |
| $d_{xy}$, $d_{yx}$ | Somers' D statistic |
| e | 2.7183, the base of natural logarithms |
| $E$ | event or expected frequency with chi square |
| $E^2$ | coefficient of nonlinear correlation |
| $E(T)$ | expected total value for Wilcoxon matched-pairs test |
| $E(x)$ | expected value |
| $EEO$ | experimental event odds |
| $EER$ | experimental event rate |
| $f$ | frequency, frequency count |
| $F$ | analysis of variance coefficient, test statistic |
| $F_{max}$ | Hartley's F-max test statistic |
| $FN$ | false-negative results |
| $FP$ | false-positive results |
| $H$ | Kruskal-Wallis test statistic |
| $H'$ | Kruskal-Wallis test statistic corrected for ties |
| $H_0$ | null hypothesis, hypothesis under test |
| $H_1$ | alternate hypothesis, research hypothesis |
| $\hat{h}(t_i)$ | hazard rate |
| $K_{intervals}$ | number of class intervals in a histogram |
| $L$ | Lord's range test statistic |
| $LCL$ | lower control line in a control chart |
| $LSL$ | lower specification limit for capability indices |
| $LTL$ | lower tolerance limit |
| $LR^+$, $LR^-$ | likelihood ratio |

## Symbols

| | |
|---|---|
| $Log$ | logarithm to the base 10 |
| $M$ | median, huge rule outlier test statistic |
| $MS_B$ | mean square between |
| $MS_E$ | mean squared error |
| $MS_R$ | mean squared residual |
| $MS_{Rx}$ | mean squared treatment effect |
| $MS_W$ | mean square within |
| $n$ | number of values or data points in a sample |
| $N$ | number of values in a population, total number of observations |
| $n!$ | factorial |
| $\binom{n}{x}$ | combination statement |
| $NNT$ | number needed to treat |
| $O$ | observed frequency with chi square |
| $OR$ | odds ratio |
| $p$ | probability, level of significance, type I error; Fisher's exact test statistic; median test statistic |
| $p(E)$ | probability of event $E$ |
| $p(x)$ | probability of outcome $x$ |
| $p(E_1 \text{ and } E_2)$ | probability that both events $E_1$ and $E_2$ will occur |
| $p(E_1 \cap E_2)$ | probability that both events $E_1$ and $E_2$ will occur |
| $p(E_1 \text{ or } E_2)$ | probability that either events $E_1$ or $E_2$ will occur |
| $p(E_1 \cup E_2)$ | probability that either events $E_1$ or $E_2$ will occur |
| $p(E_1 \mid E_2)$ | probability that event $E_1$ will occur given $E_2$ has occurred |
| ${}_nP_x$ | permutation notation |
| $PVN$ | predicted value negative |
| $PVP$ | predicted value positive |
| $q$ | studentized range statistic |
| $Q$ | Cochran's Q test statistic; Yule's Q statistic |
| $Q_1$ | 25th percentile |
| $Q_3$ | 75th percentile |
| $r$ | correlation coefficient, Pearson's correlation |
| $r$ or $R$ | number of rows in a contingency table |
| $R$ | range |
| $r^2$ | coefficient of determination |
| $R^2$ | coefficient of multiple determination |
| $r_{xy}$ | reliability coefficient, correlation statistic |
| $R_1, R_2$ | sum of ranks for samples of $n_1$, $n_2$ in Mann-Whitney U test |
| $rf$ | relative frequency |
| $RR$ | relative risk |
| $RR_{MH}$ | Mantel-Haenszel relative risk ratio |
| $RRR$ | relative risk reduction |
| $RSD$ | relative standard deviation |
| $S$ or $SD$ | sample standard deviation |

| | |
|---|---|
| $S^2$ | sample variance or Scheffé's value |
| $S_p$ | pooled standard deviation |
| $S_p^2$ | pooled variance |
| $S_{y/x}$ | standard error of the estimate for linear regression |
| $S_r$ | residual standard deviation |
| $\hat{S}_i$ | survival function estimate |
| $SE$ | standard error term |
| $SEM$ | standard error of the mean, standard error |
| $SE(\hat{h}_i)$ | standard error of the hazard rate |
| $SE(\hat{S}_i)$ | standard error of the survival function estimate |
| $SIQR$ | semi-interquartile range |
| $t$ | t-test statistic |
| $T$ | Wilcoxon signed rank test statistic; Tshuprow's T statistic; extreme studentized deviate test statistic, Grubbs test statistic |
| $TN$ | true-negative results |
| $TP$ | true-positive results |
| $U$ | Mann-Whitney U test statistic |
| $UC$ | Theil's uncertainty coefficient |
| $UCL$ | upper control line in a control chart |
| $USL$ | upper specification limit for capability indices |
| $UTL$ | upper tolerance limit |
| $V$ | Cramer's V statistic |
| $x$ | variable used to predict $y$ in regression model |
| $x_i$ | any data point or value |
| $x'_i$ | transformed data point |
| $\overline{X}$ | sample mean |
| $\overline{X}_G$ | geometric mean; grand mean |
| w | width of a class interval |
| $W$ | Shapiro-Wilk's W test statistic; Kendall's coefficient of concordance |
| $y$ | variable used to predict $x$ in regression model |
| $Y$ | Yule's Y statistic |
| $z$ | z-test statistic |
| $Z_0$ | reliability coefficient for repeatability and reproducibility |
| $z_x$ | standardized score for an abscissa |
| $z_y$ | standardized score for an ordinate |

# 1

# Introduction

Statistics can be simply defined as the acquisition of knowledge through the process of observation. We observe information or data about a particular phenomena and from these observations we attempt to increase our understanding of the event that data represents. According to Conover (1999), it provides a means to measure the amount of subjectivity that goes into researcher's conclusions, separating "science" from "opinion." Physical reality provides the data for this knowledge and statistical tests provide the tools by which decisions can be made.

## Types of Statistics

As noted by Daniel (1978) "...statistics is a field of study concerned with (1) the organization and summarization of data, and (2) the drawing of inferences about a body of data when only a part of the data are observed." All statistical procedures can be divided into two general categories: descriptive or inferential. **Descriptive statistics**, as the name implies, describe data that we collect or observe (**empirical data**). They represent all of the procedures that can be used to organize, summarize, display, and categorize data collected for a certain experiment or event. Examples include: the frequencies and associated percentages; the average or range of outcomes; and pie charts, bar graphs or other visual representations for data. These types of statistics communicate information, they provide organization and summary for data, or afford a visual display. Such statistics must: 1) provide an accurate representation of the observed outcomes; 2) be presented as clear and understandable as possible; and 3) be as efficient and effective as possible.

**Inferential statistics** represent a wide range of procedures that are traditionally thought of as statistical tests (i.e., t-test, analysis of variance, or chi square test). These statistics infer or make predictions about a large body of information based on a sample (a small subunit) from that body. It is important to realize that the performance of an inferential statistical test involves more than simple mathematical manipulation. The reason for using these statistical tests is to solve a problem or answer a question. Therefore, inferential statistics actually involves a series of steps: 1) establishing a research question; 2) formulating a hypothesis that will be tested; 3) selecting the most appropriate test based on the type of data collected; 4) selecting the data correctly; 5) collecting the required data or observations; 6) performing the statistical test; and 7) making a decision based on the result of the test. This last step, the decision making, will result in either the rejection of or failure to reject the hypothesis being tested and will ultimately answer the research question posed in the first step of the process. These seven steps will be discussed in more detail at the end of this chapter.

The first sections of this book will deal mainly with descriptive statistics, including presentation modes (Chapter 4) and with data distribution and measures of central tendency (Chapters 5 and 6). These measured characteristics of the observed data have implications for the inferential tests that follow. Chapter 8 on hypothesis testing will give guidance toward the development of statements that will be selected by the decisions reached through the inferential statistics. The information beginning with Chapter 9 covers specific inferential statistical tests that can be used to make decisions about an entire set of data based on the small subset of information selected.

In fact, statistics deal with both the known and unknown. As researchers, we collect data from experiments and then we present these initial findings in concise and accurate compilations (known as descriptive statistics). However, in most cases the data that we collect is only a small portion (a **sample**) of a larger set of information (a **population**) for which we desire information. Through a series of mathematical manipulations the researcher will make certain guesses (unknown, inferential statements) about this larger population.

## Parameters and Statistics

As mentioned, statistical data usually involve a relatively small portion of an entire population, and through numerical manipulation, decisions and interpretations (inferences) are made about that population. To illustrate the use of statistics and some of the terms presented later in this chapter, consider the following example:

> A pharmaceutical manufacturing company produces a specific dosage form of a drug in batches (lots) of 50,000 tablets. In other words, one complete production cycle is represented by 50,000 tablets.

**Parameters** are characteristics of populations. In this particular case the population would be composed of one lot of 50,000 units. To define one of the population's parameters, we could weigh each of the 50,000 tablets and then be able to: 1) calculate the average weight for the entire lot; and 2) determine the range of weights within this one particular batch, by looking at the extreme weights (both lightest and heaviest tablet). This would give us the exact weight parameters for the total batch; however, it would be a very time-consuming process. An even more extreme situation would be to use a Stokes or Strong-Cobb Hardness Tester to measure the hardness of each tablet. We could then determine the average hardness of the total batch, but in the process we would destroy all 50,000 tables. This is obviously not a good manufacturing procedure.

In most cases, calculating an exact population parameter may be either impractical or impossible (due to required destructive testing as shown in the second example). Therefore, we sample from a given population, perform a statistical analysis of this information, and make a statement (inference) regarding the population. **Statistics** are characteristics of samples, they represent summary measures computed on observed sample values. For the above example, it would be more practical to periodically withdraw 20 tablets during the manufacturing process, then perform weight and hardness tests, and assume these sample statistics are representative of the entire population of 50,000 units.

Continuing with our manufacturing example, assume that we are interested in the average weight for each tablet (the research question). We assume there is some variability, however small, in the weights of the tablets. Using a process described in Chapter 3, we will sample 20 tablets that are representative of the 50,000 tablets in the lot and these will become our best "guess" of the true average weight. These 20 tablets are weighed and their weights are averaged to produce an average sample weight. With some statistical manipulation (discussed in Chapter 7) we can make an educated guess about the actual average weight for the entire population of 50,000 tablets. As explained in Chapter 7, we would create a confidence interval and make a statement such as "with 95% certainty, the true average weight for the tablets in this lot is somewhere between 156.3 and 158.4 milligrams." Statistical inference involves the degree of confidence we can place on the accuracy of the measurements to represent the population parameter.

It is important to note (and will be further discussed in Chapter 8) that if we are careful and accurate about our sample collection and summary, then our descriptive statistic should be 100% accurate. However, when we make inferences or statements about a larger population from which we have sampled, because it is an educated guess, we must accept a percentage of chance that this inference may be wrong. Therefore, descriptive statistics can be considered accurate, but inferential statistics are always associated with a certain (hopefully small) chance of error (Figure 1.1).

For consistency in this book, parameters or population values are represented by Greek symbols (for example $\mu$, $\sigma$, $\psi$) and sample descriptive statistics are denoted by letters (for example $\overline{X}$, $S^2$, $r$).

Samples, which we have noted are only a small subset of a much larger population, are used for nearly all statistical tests. Through the use of formulas these descriptive sample results are manipulated to make predictions (inferences) about the population from which they were sampled.

## Sampling and Independent Observations

One of the underlying assumptions for any inferential test is that the data obtained from a population is collected through some random **sampling** process. As discussed in Chapter 3, in a completely random sample, each individual member or observation in the population has an equal chance of being selected for the sample. In the above example, sampling was conducted in such a matter that theoretically each

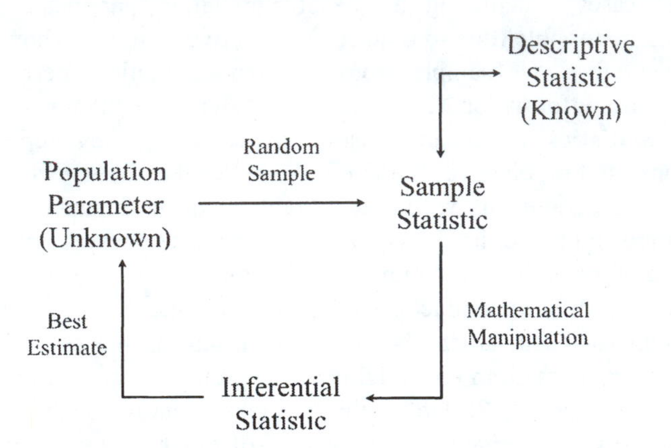


**Figure 1.1** Descriptive and inferential statistics.

of the 50,000 tablets has an equal chance of being selected.

The second required assumption for any inferential statistical test is that the observations be measured independently of each other. Therefore, no member of the sample should affect the outcome of any other member of the sample. The simplest example of this type of **independence** would be the proctoring of an examination to insure that students do not cheat, thereby assuring independent performance by each person being tested. In the case of laboratory analysis, equipment should be properly cleaned and calibrated, so that the seventh sample assayed is not influenced by the sixth sample and the seventh sample does not affect any remaining assays. In other words, an independent observation or result must represent an outcome not dependent on the result of any other observation, either past or future. Formulas used in this book assume that there is independence among observations in the sample.

**Types of Variables**

A **variable** is any attribute, characteristic, or measurable property that can vary from one observation to another. Any observation could have an infinite number of variables, such as height, weight, color, or density. For example, consider pharmacy students in a specific graduating class (at the moment the degree is awarded) and just a few of the numerous variables that could be associated with each student:

sex
height
weight
marital status
class rank
previous undergraduate degree (yes/no)
systolic blood pressure

blood type (A,B,AB,O)
blood glucose level
employed/unemployed
accepted into graduate school (yes/no)
final examination score in physical pharmacy

The number of possible variables is limited only by our imagination. Also, the fact that we can measure a certain characteristic implies that students will differ with respect to that characteristic, and thus the characteristic becomes a variable. Variables may be either discrete or continuous. The determination of whether a variable is discrete or continuous is critical in selecting the appropriate test required for statistical analysis.

A **discrete variable** is characterized by gaps or interruptions. These types of variables are also referred to as "qualitative," "category," or "nominal" (from the Latin word *nominalis* meaning "of a name"). These variables involve placing observations into a specific, finite number of categories or classifications. Examples include distinct colors, dosage form (tablets vs. capsules), and passage or failure of a specific assay criteria. Discrete variables can represent predetermined blocks of data, such as above and below a midpoint in a distribution. With relationship to the population, discrete variables for a sample must be both exhaustive and mutually exclusive. Levels of a discrete variable are **exhaustive** when the categories of that variable account for all possible outcomes. For example, males and females are exhaustive for the population of human beings based on gender; whereas age groups 0-20, 21-40, 41-60, and 61-80 are not exhaustive because there are humans over 80 years old. Similarly, levels of a discrete variable must be set to be **mutually exclusive** where categories do not have members in common with each other. Age groupings 0-20, 20-40, 40-60, and 60-80 are not mutually exclusive because ages 20, 40, and 60 are each included in two of the discrete groups. To represent a mutually exclusive and exhaustive set of categories, the age groupings should be as follows: 20 years or less, 21-40 years, 41-60 years, or 61 and older. A second example might be a predetermined dissolution criteria for tablets. In this case the outcomes are represented by two mutually exclusive and exhaustive results; either the tablet passes or fails the specified criteria. From the above list of possible variables for pharmacy graduates, discrete variables include:

sex
marital status
previous undergraduate degree (yes/no)
blood type (A,B,AB,O)
employed/unemployed
accepted into graduate school (yes/no)

In contrast, a **continuous variable** has no gaps or interruptions. Also referred to as "quantitative" variables, they are probably the most commonly encountered variables in pharmacy research. Where discrete variables usually imply some form of counting, continuous variables involve measurements. Examples include age, weight, viscosity, or blood glucose levels. In the case of our pharmacy graduates, continuous variables would include:

height
weight
class rank
systolic blood pressure
blood glucose level
final examination score in physical pharmacy

With a discrete variable, outcomes or measures are clearly separated from one another (i.e., males and females). With continuous variables it is possible to imagine more possible values between them. Theoretically, no matter how close two measures are together, a difference could be found if a more precise instrument were used. Consider age, which is a continuous variable; it can be measured by years, months, days, hours, minutes, seconds, or even fractions of a second. Therefore, any measurement result for a continuous variable actually represents a range of possible outcomes and in theory, any value for a continuous variable is considered to occupy a distance or interval from half a unit below to half a unit above the value. These numbers ("real limits") are useful in providing an accurate interpretation of statistical tests using interval or ratio scales, which are discussed below. To illustrate this, assume the most precise analytical balance in a laboratory measures the weight of a sample to be 247 mg. If we could use a more exact balance we might find that the sample actually weighs 247.2 mg. An even more precise instrument could identify the weight in micrograms. Therefore, our original weight of 247 mg actually represents an infinite range of weights from the real limits 246.5 to 247.5 mg. The major limitation in measuring a continuous variable is the sensitivity of the instrumentation used with that value.

Occasionally, a continuous variable is presented on a **rating scale** or modified into a discrete variable. For example, study results may be: 1) dichotomized into either above or below the midpoint, 2) arbitrarily classified as high, medium, or low results, or 3) measured on a continuum that either "passes" or "fails" a predefined level. Even though each of these examples represent the results of a continuous measurement, by placing them *a priori* (before the test) on a rating scale they can be handled as discrete variables.

Parallel nomenclature for measurements of a variable could be in terms of types of scales, with a **scale of measurement** implying a set of numbers. As mentioned, discrete variables would involve the simplest type. Also called a **nominal scale,** observations are qualitatively classified based on a characteristic that was being measured. They differ only in kind and cannot be arranged in any meaningful order (i.e., largest to smallest). Examples of nominal scale measurements would be male vs. female, a tablet vs. a capsule vs. a solution, or survival vs. death.

The second type of measure scale is the **ordinal scale**, in which quantitative observations are related to each other or some predetermined criteria. There is a hierarchy to the levels of the scale with some type of rank order. We are not concerned here with the amount of difference between two observations, but their relative position (for example, if the second observation is less than, equal to or greater than the first observation). Ordinal scales may be used when it is not possible to make more precise measurements. For example, seen below is a scale for measuring the state of cognitive impairment in Alzheimer's patients using a seven-point scale.

| Cognitive Performance Scale | Description |
|---|---|
| 0 | Intact |
| 1 | Borderline Intact |
| 2 | Mild Impairment |
| 3 | Moderate Impairment |
| 4 | Moderate-Severe Impairment |
| 5 | Severe Impairment |
| 6 | Very Severe Mild Impairment |

The numbers are attached simply to show the arranged order, not the degree of difference between the various measures. With ordinal scales, even though order exists among categories, the magnitude of the difference between two adjacent levels is not the same throughout the scale. For example, is the magnitude of difference between mild and moderate impairment (previous scale), the same as the magnitude between severe and very severe impairment? Ordinal scales are extremely important in nonparametric statistical procedures (Chapter 21). Both nominal and ordinal scales are sometimes referred to as **nonmetric scales**. Also, for both of these nonmetric scales it is possible to have only two possible levels. These are termed **dichotomous** or **binary** variables. If there are no relative positions (i.e. males vs. females) it is a dichotomous nominal variable. If there is a relative position (i.e., passing or failing a criteria) the variable is a dichotomous ordinal scale.

The third type of measurement scale is the **interval scale**, where the difference between each level of the scale is equal. The scales represent a quantitative variable with equal difference between scale values; however, ratios between the scale values have no meaning because of an arbitrary zero. For example the ratio between 40°C and 20°C does not imply that the former measure is twice as hot as the second.

If a genuine zero is within an interval scale it becomes a **ratio scale**; for example, measures of weight or height. If an object weights 500 mg and a second object weights 250 mg, the first object is twice the weight of the second. Other examples of ratio scales would include percentage scales and frequency counts. With interval and ratio scales most arithmetic operations (i.e., addition and subtraction) are permissible with these numbers. Ratio and interval scales are sometimes referred to as **metric scales**.

## Independent and Dependent Variables

In addition to a variable being defined as continuous or discrete, it may also be considered independent or dependent. Most statistical tests require at least one **independent variable** that is established in advance and controlled by the researcher. Also called a **predictor variable**, the independent variable allows us to control some of the research environment. At least one or more **dependent variables** are then measured against their independent counterparts. These **response** or **criterion variables** are beyond our control and dependent on the levels of the independent variable used in the study. Independent variables are usually qualitative (nominal) variables but also may be continuous or ordinal. For example, subjects in a clinical trial are assigned to a new drug therapy or control group, their selection is made before the study and this becomes the independent variable (treatment vs. control). The therapeutic outcomes (i.e., decreased blood pressure, pharmacokinetic data, length of hospitalization) are variables dependent on the group to which they were assigned. A second example is a measure of the amount of active ingredient in the core tablet portion of an enteric coated tablet for the same medication, using the same process, at three different manufacturing facilities (New Jersey, United Kingdom, and Puerto Rico). The independent variable is the facility location (a discrete variable with three levels) and the dependent variable would be the average content (amount of active ingredient) of the drug at each facility. Note in the second example that only three facilities are used in the study and each sample must come from one of these sites and cannot come from two different locations at the same time; thus representing mutually exclusive and exhaustive observations that fulfill the requirements for a discrete variable. It is assumed that samples were selected appropriately (through some random process, discussed in Chapter 3) and content is measured using the same apparatus and using the same procedures and conducted in such a manner that each result is independent of any other sample.

In designing any research study, the investigator must control or remove as many variables as possible, measure the outcome of only the dependent variable, and compare these results based on the different levels or categories of the independent variable(s). The extraneous factors that might influence the dependent variable's results are known as **confounding** or **nuisance variables**. In the previous example, using different instruments to measure the contents at different sites may produce different results even though the tablets are the same at all three sites.

## Selection of the Appropriate Statistical Test

In order to select the correct inferential test procedure, it is essential that as researchers, we understand the variables involved with our data. Which variables are involved for a specific statistical test? Which variable or variables are under the researcher's control (independent) and which are not (dependent)? Is the independent variable discrete or continuous? Is the dependent variable continuous or discrete? As seen in Appendix A, answering these questions automatically gives direction toward the correct statistical procedure to use in a given situation. All the statistical procedures listed in the flow chart in Appendix A will be discussed in Chapters 9 through 23. To illustrate the use of this Appendix, consider the previous example on clinical trials (measure of therapeutic outcomes based on assignment to the treatment or control group). Starting in the box in the upper left corner of Panel A in Appendix A, the first question would be: Is there an independent, researcher-controlled variable? The answer is yes, we assign volunteers to either the experimental or control groups. Therefore, we would proceed down the panel to the next box: is the independent variable continuous or discrete? It is discrete, because we have two nominal levels that are mutually exclusive and exhaustive. Continuing down Panel A, are the results reported as a percentage or proportion of a certain outcome? Assuming that our results are length of hospital stay in days, the answer would be no and we again continue down the page to the next decision box. Is the dependent variable continuous or discrete? Obviously number of days is a continuous measure; therefore we proceed to Panel B. The first question in Panel B asks the number of discrete independent variables. In this example there is only one, whether the volunteer received the study drug or control. Moving down Panel B, what is the number of levels (categories) within the independent variable? There are only two, therefore we continue down this panel. The next decision will be explained in Chapter 9, but for the moment we will accept the fact that the data is not paired and move down once again to the last box on the left side of Panel B. Similarly, for the point of our current discussion we will assume that the population variance is unknown and that our sample is from a population in which the dependent variable is normally distributed and that both levels produce a similar distribution of values (these will be explained in Chapter 6). Thus, we continue to the right and then down to the last point on the right side of the panel and find that the most appropriate inferential statistical test for our clinical trial would be a two-sample t-test.

### Procedures for Inferential Statistical Tests

Most individuals envision statistics as a labyrinth of numerical machinations. Thus, they are fearful of exploring the subject. As mentioned in the preface, the statistics in this book rely primarily on the four basic arithmetic functions and an occasional square root. The effective use of statistics requires more than knowledge of the mathematical required formulas. This is especially true today, when personal computers can quickly analyze sample data. There are several important parts to completing an appropriate statistical test.

1. **Establish a research question**. It is impossible to acquire new knowledge and to conduct research without a clear idea of what you wish to explore. For example, we would like to know if three batches of a specific drug are the same regarding their content uniformity. Simply stated: are these three batches equal?

2. **Formulate a hypothesis**. Although covered in a later chapter, we should formulate a hypothesis that will be either rejected or not rejected

based on the results of the statistical test. In this case, the hypothesis that is being tested is that Batch A equals Batch B equals Batch C. The only alternative to this hypothesis is that the batches are not all equal to each other.

3. **Select an appropriate test**. Using information about the data (identifying the dependent and independent variables) the correct test is selected based on whether these variables are discrete or continuous. For example, batches A, B, and C represent an independent variable with three discrete levels and the assay results for the drug's contents is a continuous variable dependent upon the batch from which it was selected. Therefore, the most appropriate statistical test would be one that can handle a continuous dependent variable to a discrete independent variable with three categories. If we once again proceeded through Appendix A we would conclude that the "analysis of variance" test would be most appropriate (assuming normality and homogeneity of variance, terms discussed later in this book). A common mistake is to collect the data first, without consideration of these first three requirements for statistical tests, only to realize a that statistical judgment cannot be made because of the arbitrary format of the data.

4. **Sample correctly**. The sample should be randomly selected from each batch (Chapter 3). An appropriate sample size should be selected to provide the most accurate results (Chapter 8).

5. **Collect data**. The collection should insure that each observed result is independent of any other assay.

6. **Perform test**. Only this portion of the statistical process actually involves the number crunching associated with statistical analysis. Many commercially available computer packages are available to save us the tedium of detailed mathematical manipulations.

7. **Make a decision**. Based on the data collected and statistically manipulated from the samples, a statement (inference) is made regarding the entire population from which the sample was drawn. In our example, based on the results of the test statistics, the hypothesis that all three batches are equal (based on content uniformity), is either rejected or the sample does not provide enough information to reject the hypothesis. As discussed in Chapter 8, the initial hypothesis can be rejected, but never proven true.

To comprehend the principles underlying many of the inferential statistical tests it is necessary that we have a general understanding of probability theory and the role that probability plays in statistical decision making. The next chapter focuses on this particular area.

## References

Conover, W.J. (1999). *Practical Nonparametric Statistics*, John Wiley and Sons, New York, p. 2.

Daniel, W.W. (1999). *Biostatistics: A Foundation for Analysis in the Health Sciences*, Seventh edition, John Wiley and Sons, New York, p. 1.

## Suggested Supplemental Readings

Bolton, S. (1997). *Pharmaceutical Statistics: Practical and Clinical Applications*, Third edition, Marcel Dekker, Inc., New York, pp. 538-541.

Zar, J.H. (1999). *Biostatistical Analysis*, Fourth edition, Prentice-Hall, Englewood Cliffs, NJ, pp. 1-5, 16-19.

## Example Problems

1. Which of the following selected variables, associated with clinical trials of a drug, are discrete variables and which are continuous?

    Experimental vs. controls (placebo)
    Dosage form – table/capsule/other
    Bioavailability measurements ($C_{max}$, $T_{max}$, AUC)
    Test drug vs. reference standard
    Fed vs. fasted state (before/after meals)
    Prolactin levels (ng/l)
    Manufacturer (generic vs. brand)
    Male vs. female subjects
    Age (in years)
    Smoking history (cigarettes per day)
    "Normal" vs. geriatric population

2. Which of the following selected variables associated with a random sample of 50,000 tablets, mentioned earlier in this chapter, are discrete variables and which are continuous?

    Amount of active ingredient (content uniformity)
    Dissolution test – pass or fail criteria
    Disintegration rate
    Change in manufacturing process – old process vs. new
    Friability – pass or fail criteria
    Hardness
    Impurities – present or absent
    Size – thickness/diameter

Tablet weight
Immediate release or sustained release
Formulation A, B, or C

3. The ability to identify independent and dependent variables, and determine if these variables are discrete or continuous is critical to statistical testing. In the examples listed below, identify the following:

   Is there an independent variable? Is this independent variable continuous or discrete? What is the dependent variable? Is this dependent variable continuous or discrete?

   a. During a clinical trial, volunteers were randomly divided into two groups and administered either: 1) the Innovators antipsychotic medication or 2) Acme Chemical generic equivalent of the same drug. Listed below are the results of the trial ($C_{max}$). Is there any difference between the two manufacturers' drugs based on this one pharmacokinetic property?

Result of Clinical Trial for $C_{max}$ (ng/ml)

| | Innovator | Acme Chemical |
|---|---|---|
| Mean | 289.7 | 281.6 |
| S.D. | 18.1 | 20.8 |
| n | 24 | 23 |

   b. During a cholera outbreak in a war-devastated country, records for one hospital were examined for the survival of children contracting the disease. These records also reported the children's nutritional status. Was there a significant relationship between their nutrition and survival rate?

| | Nutritional Status | |
|---|---|---|
| | Poor ($N_1$) | Good ($N_2$) |
| Survived ($S_1$) | 72 | 79 |
| Died ($S_2$) | 87 | 32 |

   c. Samples were taken from a specific batch of drug and randomly divided into two groups of tablets. One group was assayed by the manufacturer's own quality control laboratories. The second group of tablets was sent to a contract laboratory for identical analysis.

Percentage of Labeled Amount of Drug

| Manufacturer | | Contract Lab | |
|---|---|---|---|
| 101.1 | 98.8 | 97.5 | 99.1 |
| 100.6 | 99.0 | 101.1 | 98.7 |
| 100.8 | 98.7 | 97.8 | 99.5 |

d. An instrument manufacturer ran a series of tests to compare the pass/fail rate of a new piece of disintegration equipment. Samples were taken from a single batch of uncoated tablets. Two different temperatures were used and tested for compendia recommended times. Success was defined as all six tablets disintegrating in the disintegration equipment.

| | Success | Failure | |
|---|---|---|---|
| 39°C | 96 | 4 | 100 |
| 35°C | 88 | 12 | 100 |
| | 184 | 16 | 200 |

e. Three physicians were selected for a study to evaluate the length of stay for patients undergoing a major surgical procedure. All these procedures occurred in the same hospital and were without complications. Eight records were randomly selected from patients treated over the past twelve months. Was there a significant difference, by physician, in the length of stay for these surgical patients?

Days in the Hospital

| Physician A | Physician B | Physician C |
|---|---|---|
| 9 | 10 | 8 |
| 12 | 6 | 9 |
| 10 | 7 | 12 |
| 7 | 10 | 10 |
| 11 | 11 | 14 |
| 13 | 9 | 10 |
| 8 | 9 | 8 |
| 13 | 11 | 15 |

f. Acme Chemical and Dye received from the same raw material supplier three batches of oil from three different production sites. Samples were drawn from drums at each location and compared to determine if the viscosity was the same for each batch.

| Batch A | Batch B | Batch C |
|---|---|---|
| 10.23 | 10.24 | 10.25 |
| 10.33 | 10.28 | 10.20 |
| 10.28 | 10.20 | 10.21 |
| 10.27 | 10.21 | 10.18 |
| 10.30 | 10.26 | 10.22 |

g. Two different scales were used to measure patient anxiety levels upon admission to a hospital. Method A was an established test instrument, while Method B (which had been developed by the researchers) was quicker and an easier instrument to administer. Was there a correlation between the two measures?

| Method A | Method B | Method A | Method B |
|---|---|---|---|
| 55 | 90 | 52 | 97 |
| 66 | 117 | 36 | 78 |
| 46 | 94 | 44 | 84 |
| 77 | 124 | 55 | 112 |
| 57 | 105 | 53 | 102 |
| 59 | 115 | 67 | 112 |
| 70 | 125 | 72 | 130 |
| 57 | 97 | | |

**Answers to Problems**

1. Discrete variables:

   Experimental vs. controls (placebo)
   Dosage form – table/capsule/other
   Test drug vs. reference standard
   Fed vs. fasted state (before/after meals)
   Manufacturer (generic vs. brand)
   Male vs. female subjects
   "Normal" vs. geriatric population

   Continuous variables:

   Bioavailability measurements ($C_{max}$, $T_{max}$, AUC)
   Prolactin levels (ng/l)
   Age (in years)
   Smoking history (cigarettes per day)

2. Discrete variables:

   Dissolution – pass or fail criteria
   Friability – pass or fail criteria
   Impurities – present or absent

   Change in manufacturing process – old process vs. new
   Immediate release or sustained release
   Formulation A, B, or C

   Continuous variables:

   Amount of active ingredient (content uniformity)
   Disintegration rate
   Hardness
   Size – thickness/diameter
   Tablet weight

3. a. Independent variable: Two manufacturers (Innovator vs. Acme)
Discrete

Dependent variable: Pharmacokinetic measure ($C_{max}$)
Continuous

b. Independent variable: Nutritional status (poor vs. good)
Discrete

Dependent variable: Survival (lived vs. died)
Discrete

c. Independent variable: Laboratory (manufacturer vs. contract lab)
Discrete

Dependent variable: Assay results (% labeled amount of drug)
Continuous

d. Independent variable: Temperature (39°C vs. 35°C)
Discrete

Dependent variable: Disintegration results (pass vs. fail)
Discrete

e. Independent variable: Physician (A vs. B vs. C)
Discrete

Dependent variable: Length of stay in hospital (days)
Continuous

f. Independent variable: Batch of raw material (batch A vs. B vs. C)
Discrete

Dependent variable: Viscosity
Continuous

g. Independent variable: Method A (gold standard)
Continuous

Dependent variable: Method B
Continuous

# 2

# Probability

As mentioned in the previous chapter, statistics involve more than simply the gathering and tabulating of data. Inferential statistics are concerned with the interpretation and evaluation of data and making statements about larger populations. The development of the theories of probability have resulted in an increased scope of statistical applications. Probability can be considered the "essential thread" that runs throughout all statistical inference (Kachigan, 1991).

## Classic Probability

Statistical concepts covered in this book are essentially derived from probability theory. Thus, it would be only logical to begin our discussion of statistics by reviewing some of the fundamentals of probability. The **probability** of an event [$p(E)$] is the likelihood of that occurrence. It is associated with discrete variables. The probability of any event is the number of times or ways an event can occur ($m$) divided by the total number of possible associated events ($N$):

$$p(E) = \frac{m}{N} \qquad \text{Eq. 2.1}$$

In other words, probability is the fraction of time in which the event will occur, given many opportunities for its occurrence. For example, if we toss a fair coin, there are only two possible outcomes (a head or a tail). The likelihood that one event, for example a tail, is 1/2 or $p(T_{ail}) = 0.5$.

$$p(T_{ail}) = \frac{1}{2} = 0.50$$

A synonym for probability is **proportion**. If the decimal point is moved two numbers to the right, the probability can be expressed as a percentage. In the previous example, the proportion of tails is 0.5 or there is a 50% chance of tossing a tail or 50% of the time we would expect a tail to result from a toss of a fair coin.

The **universe** ($N$), which represents all possible outcomes, is also referred to as the **outcome space** or **sample space**. Note that the outcomes forming this sample space are mutually exclusive and exhaustive. The outcomes that fulfill these two requirements are called **simple outcomes**. Other common examples of probabilities can be associated with a normal deck of playing cards. What is the probability of drawing a red card from a deck of playing cards? There are 52 cards in a deck, of which 26 are red; therefore, the probability of drawing a red card is

$$p(Red)=\frac{26}{52}=\frac{1}{2}=0.50$$

Note that cards must be red or black, and cannot be both; thus, representing mutually exclusive and exhaustive simple outcomes. What is the probability of drawing a queen from the deck? With four queens per deck the probability is

$$p(Queen)=\frac{4}{52}=\frac{1}{13}=0.077$$

Lastly, what is the probability of drawing a diamond from the deck? There are 13 diamonds per deck with an associated probability of

$$p(Diamond)=\frac{13}{52}=\frac{1}{4}=0.25$$

Does this guarantee that if we draw four cards one will be a diamond? No. Probability is the likelihood of the occurrence of an outcome over the "long run." However, if we draw a card, note its suit, replace the card, and continue to do this 100, 1000, or 10,000 times we will see the results close to if not equal to 25% diamonds.

There are three general rules regarding all probabilities. The first is that a probability cannot be negative. Even an impossible outcome would have $p(E) = 0$. Second, the sum of probabilities of all mutually exclusive outcomes for a discrete variable is equal to one. For example, with the tossing of a coin, the probability of a head equals 0.50, the probability of a tail also equals 0.50 and the sum of both outcomes equals 1.0. Thus the probability of an outcome cannot be less than 0 or more than 1.

$$0 \leq p(E) \leq 1$$

A probability equal to zero indicates that it is impossible for that event to occur. For example, what is the probability of drawing a "blue" card from a standard deck of playing cards? Such an outcome would be impossible and have a probability of zero. This is sometime referred to as an **empty set**. In contrast, a probability of 1.0 means that particular event will occur with utter certainty or a **sure event**.

At times our primary interest may not be in a single outcome, but with a group of simple outcomes. Such a collection is referred to as a **composite outcome**. Because of the **addition theorem**, the likelihood of two or more mutually exclusive outcomes equals the sum of their individual probabilities.

$$p(E_i \text{ or } E_j) = p(E_i) + p(E_j) \qquad \text{Eq. 2.2}$$

For example, the probability of a composite outcome of drawing a face card (jack, queen, or king) would equal the sum of their probabilities.

$$p(F_{ace\ card}) = p(K_{ing}) + p(Q_{ueen}) + p(J_{ack}) = \frac{1}{13} + \frac{1}{13} + \frac{1}{13} = \frac{3}{13} = 0.231$$

For any outcome *E*, there is a complementary event ($\overline{E}$), which can be considered "not *E*" or "*E* not." Since either *E* or $\overline{E}$ must occur, but cannot occur at the same time then $P(E) + P(\overline{E}) = 1$ or written for the complement

$$p(\overline{E}) = 1 - p(E) \qquad \text{Eq. 2.3}$$

The complement is equal to all possible outcomes minus the event under consideration. For example, in one of the previous examples, it was determined that the probability of drawing a queen from a deck of cards is 0.077. The complimentary probability, or the probability of "not a queen" is

$$p(\overline{Q}_{ueen}) = 1 - p(Q_{ueen}) = 1 - 0.077 = 0.923$$

Our deck of cards could be considered a universe or a population of well-defined objects. Probabilities can then be visualized using simple schematics as illustrated in Figure 2.1. Figure 2.1-A illustrates the previous example of the likelihood of selecting a queen or a card that is not a queen. Note that the two outcomes are visually mutually exclusive and exhaustive. This type of figure can be helpful when more than one variable is involved.

Probabilities can be either theoretical or empirical. The previous examples with a deck of cards can be considered **theoretical probabilities** because we can base our decision on formal or logical grounds. In contrast, **empirical probabilities** are based on prior experience or observation of prior behavior. For example, the likelihood of a 25 year-old female dying of lung cancer cannot be based on any formal or logical considerations. Instead, probabilities associated with risk factors and previous mortalities would contribute to such an empirical probability.

A visual method for identifying all of the possible outcomes in a probability exercise is the **tree diagram**. Branches from the tree correspond to the possible results. Figure 2.2 displays the possible outcome from tossing three fair coins.

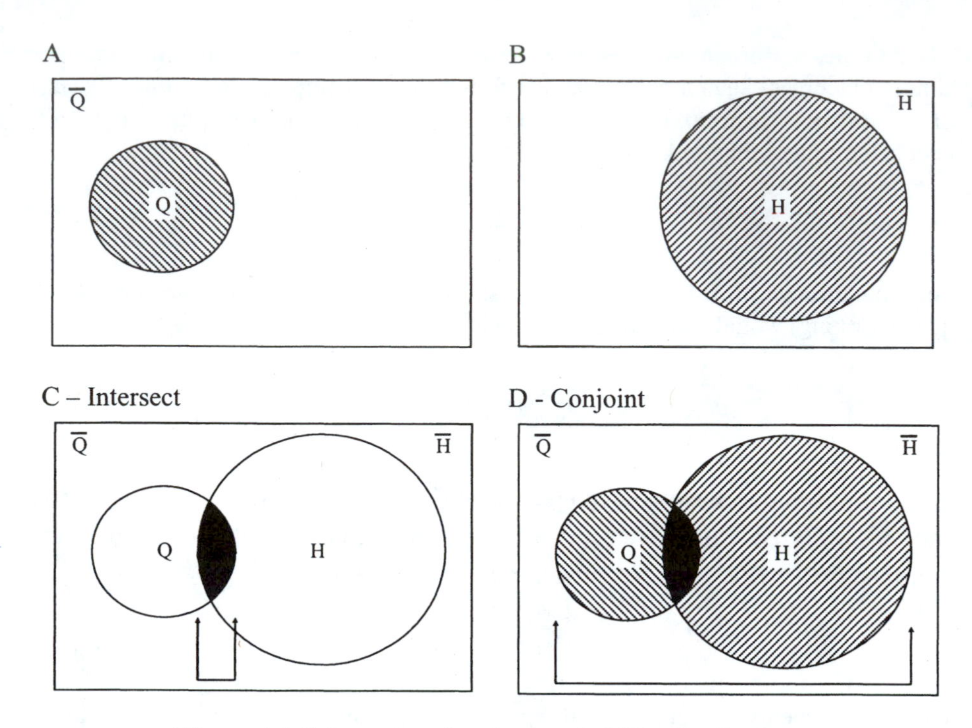


**Figure 2.1** Schematics of various probability distributions.

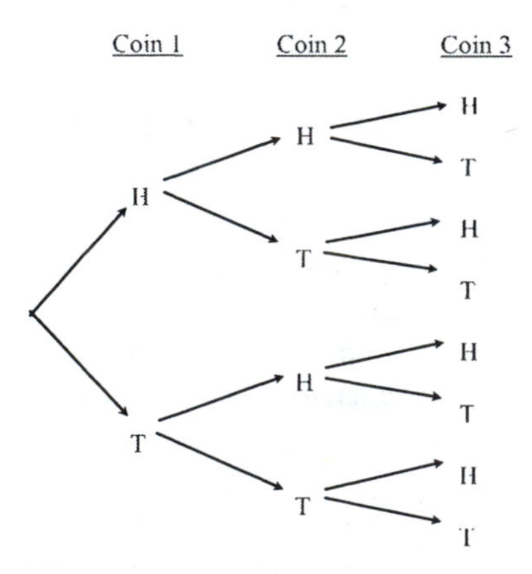


**Figure 2.2** Tree diagram of the result of tossing three fair coins.

**Probability Involving Two Variables**

In the case of two different variables (i.e., playing card suit and card value), it is necessary to consider the likelihood of both variables occurring, *p(A)* and *p(B)*, which are not mutually exclusive. A **conjoint** or **union** $(A \cup B)$ is used when calculating the probability of <u>either</u> *A* <u>or</u> *B* occurring. An **intersect** $(A \cap B)$ or **joint probability** is employed when calculating the probability of <u>both</u> *A* <u>and</u> *B* occurring at the same time. The probability of an intersect is either given, or in the case of theoretical probabilities, easily determined using the **multiplication theorem**, in which $p(A \cap B) = p(A) \times p(B)$ if *A* and *B* are independent of each other.

$$p(A \text{ and } B) = p(A) \times p(B) \qquad \text{Eq. 2.4}$$

For example what is the probability of drawing a card that is both a queen and a heart (Figure 2.1-C)?

$$p(\text{queen and heart}) = p(Q \cap H) = 1/52$$

$$p(\text{queen and heart}) = p(\text{queen}) \times p(\text{heart}) = 1/13 \times 1/4 = 1/52$$

In this case there is obviously only one queen of hearts in a deck of cards. What is the probability of drawing either a queen or a red card from the deck? Looking at Figure 2.1-D it is possible to see that using the addition theorem the probability of queen and the probability of a heart could be added together. However, the intersect represents an overlapping of the two probabilities or the p(*A* or *B*) equals the sum of the two probabilities minus the probability associated with the intersect.

$$p(A \cup B) = p(A) + p(B) - p(A \cap B) \qquad \text{Eq. 2.5}$$

Therefore, if we subtract one of the two intercept areas seen in Figure 2.1.C we can compute the conjoint:

$$p(\text{queen or heart}) = p(Q \cup H) = p(Q) + p(H) - p(Q \cap H)$$

$$p(\text{queen or heart}) = 4/52 + 13/52 - 1/52 = 16/52$$

Here there are 13 heart cards and four queens for a total of 17, but one of the queens is also a heart, thus the 16 possible outcomes. The conjoint is sometimes referred to as the additive rule for two events that are not mutually exclusive.

To illustrate these points further, consider the following example using empirical probability data. In a national survey, conducted in the early 1990s, on the availability of various types of hardware required to utilize different methods of programming for continuing pharmaceutical education, it was found that out of the 807 respondents: 419 had access to a personal computer capable of downloading external software; 572 had cable television in their homes; and 292 had both personal computers and cable television. Assuming that this sample is representative of all pharmacists nationally, what was the probability (at that point in time) of selecting a pharmacist at random and finding that this individual had access to a personal computer?

$$p(PC) = \frac{m(PC)}{N} = \frac{419}{807} = 0.519$$

What is the probability of selecting a pharmacist at random and finding that this individual had cable television?

$$p(TV) = \frac{m(TV)}{N} = \frac{572}{807} = 0.709$$

What is the probability of selecting a pharmacist at random and finding that this individual <u>did not</u> have cable television?

$$p(noTV) = \frac{m(noTV)}{N} = \frac{(807 - 572)}{807} = 0.291$$

or considering $p(noTV)$ as a compliment

$$p(noTV) = 1 - p(TV) = 1 - 0.709 = 0.291$$

Note that the sum of all possible outcomes for cable television equals 1.

$$Total\ p(cable\,TV) = p(TV) + p(noTV) = 0.709 + 0.291 = 1.000$$

What is the probability of selecting a pharmacist at random who had both access to a personal computer and cable television?

$$p(PC \cap TV) = \frac{m(PC \cap TV)}{N} = \frac{292}{807} = 0.362$$

**Conditional Probability**

Many times it is necessary to calculate the probability of an outcome, given that a certain value is already known for a second variable. For example, what is the probability of event $A$ occurring given the fact that only a certain level (or outcome) of a second variable ($B$) is considered.

$$p(A)\ given\ B = p(A \mid B) = \frac{p(A \cap B)}{p(B)} \qquad \text{Eq. 2.6}$$

For example, what is the probability of drawing a queen from a stack of cards containing only the red cards from a single deck?

$$p(queen \mid heart) = \frac{p(Q \cap H)}{p(H)} = \frac{1/52}{13/52} = 1/13$$

In this example, if all the hearts are removed from a deck of cards, 1/13 is the probability of selecting a queen from the extracted hearts.

Another way to consider the **multiplication theorem** in probability for two events that are not mutually exclusive is based on conditional probabilities. The probability of the joint occurrence $(A \cap B)$ is equal to the product of the conditional probability of $A$ given $B$ times the probability of $B$ (if $p(B) > 0$):

$$p(A \cap B) = p(A \mid B)\, p(B) \qquad \text{Eq. 2.7}$$

From the previous example, if a selected pharmacist had a personal computer, what is the probability that this same individual also had cable television?

$$p(TV \mid PC) = \frac{p(PC \cap TV)}{p(PC)} = \frac{(0.362)}{(0.519)} = 0.697$$

If the selected pharmacist had cable television, what is the probability that this same individual also had access to a personal computer?

$$p(PC \mid TV) = \frac{p(PC \cap TV)}{p(TV)} = \frac{(0.362)}{(0.709)} = 0.511$$

Conditional probability can be extremely useful in determining if two variables are independent of each other or if some type of interaction occurs. For example, consider the above example of pharmacists with cable television and/or personal computers. The data could be arranged as follows, with those pharmacists having both cable television and personal computers counted in the upper left box.

| | Cable TV | No Cable TV |
|---|---|---|
| Computer | | |
| No Computer | | |

Assume for the moment that only 300 pharmacists were involved in the sample and by chance 50% of these pharmacists had personal computers:

| | Cable TV | No Cable TV | |
|---|---|---|---|
| Computer | | | 150 |
| No Computer | | | 150 |
| | 200 | 100 | 300 |

If there is no relationship between cable TV and personal computer ownership (independence) then we would expect the same proportion of computer owners and those not owning computers to have cable TV service (100 and 100 in each of the left boxes) and the same proportion of individuals not receiving cable:

| | Cable TV ( $A$ ) | No Cable TV ( $\bar{A}$ ) | |
|---|---|---|---|
| Computer (B) | 100 | 50 | 150 |
| No Computer ( $\bar{B}$ ) | 100 | 50 | 150 |
| | 200 | 100 | 300 |

In this example:

$$p(Cable\ TV \mid Computer) = p(Cable\ TV \mid No\ Computer) = p(Cable\ TV)$$

Thus, $p(A \cap B)$ will equal $p(A)$ if the outcomes for $A$ and $B$ are independent of each other. This aspect of conditional probability is extremely important when discussing the Chi Square Test of Independence in Chapter 16.

**Probability Distribution**

A **discrete random variable** is any discrete variable with levels that have associated probabilities and these associated probabilities can be displayed as a distribution. Many times a graph or table can be used to illustrate the outcomes for these discrete random variables. For example, consider the rolling of two fair dice. There is only one possible way to roll a two: a one (on die 1) and a one (on die 2). Two outcomes could produce a three: a one (on die 1) and a two (on die 2); or a two (on die 1) and a one (on die 2). Table 2.1 represents all the possible outcomes from rolling two dice.

Knowing the frequency of each possible outcome and the total number of possible events ($N$), it is possible to calculate the probability of any given outcome (Eq. 2.1). If fair dice are used the probability of rolling a two is:

$$p(2) = \frac{1}{36} = 0.0278$$

Whereas the probability of a three is:

$$p(3) = \frac{2}{36} = 0.0556$$

Therefore it is possible to construct a table of probabilities for all outcomes for this given event (rolling two dice). As seen in Table 2.2, the first column represents the outcome, and the second and third columns indicate the associated frequency and probability for each outcome, respectively. The fourth column is the accumulation of

**Table 2.1** Outcomes Expected from Rolling Two Dice

| Outcome | Die 1 | Die 2 | Freq. | Outcome | Die 1 | Die 2 | Freq. |
|---|---|---|---|---|---|---|---|
| 2 | 1 | 1 | 1 | 8 | 2 | 6 | 5 |
| | | | | | 3 | 5 | |
| 3 | 1 | 2 | 2 | | 4 | 4 | |
| | 2 | 1 | | | 5 | 3 | |
| | | | | | 6 | 2 | |
| 4 | 1 | 3 | 3 | | | | |
| | 2 | 2 | | 9 | 3 | 6 | 4 |
| | 3 | 1 | | | 4 | 5 | |
| | | | | | 5 | 4 | |
| 5 | 1 | 4 | 4 | | 6 | 3 | |
| | 2 | 3 | | | | | |
| | 3 | 2 | | 10 | 4 | 6 | 3 |
| | 4 | 1 | | | 5 | 5 | |
| | | | | | 6 | 4 | |
| 6 | 1 | 5 | 5 | | | | |
| | 2 | 4 | | 11 | 5 | 6 | 2 |
| | 3 | 3 | | | 6 | 5 | |
| | 4 | 2 | | | | | |
| | 5 | 1 | | 12 | 6 | 6 | 1 |
| 7 | 1 | 6 | 6 | | | | |
| | 2 | 5 | | | | | |
| | 3 | 4 | | Total possible ways = 36 | | | |
| | 4 | 3 | | | | | |
| | 5 | 2 | | | | | |
| | 6 | 1 | | | | | |

probabilities from smallest to largest outcome. For example, the cumulative probability for four or less is the sum of the probabilities of one, two, three, and four (Eq. 2.2). Obviously the probabilities for any discrete probability distribution when added together should add up to 1.0 (except for rounding errors) since it represents all possible outcomes and serves as a quick check to determine that all possible outcomes have been considered. In order to prepare a probability table, two criteria are necessary: 1) each outcome probability must be equal to or greater than zero and less than or equal to one; and 2) the sum of all the individual probabilities must equal 1.00. Note once again that these are mutually exclusive and exhaustive outcomes. If two dice are rolled on a hard flat surface there are only 11 possible outcomes (3.5, 6.7, or 11.1 are impossible outcomes). Also, two different results cannot occur at the same time.

Many of the founders of probability were extremely interested in games of chance and in some cases were compulsive gamblers (Bernstein, 1996). Therefore,

**Table 2.2** Probability of Outcomes Expected from Rolling Two Dice

| Outcome | Frequency | Probability | Cumulative Probability |
|---|---|---|---|
| 2 | 1 | 0.0278 | 0.0278 |
| 3 | 2 | 0.0556 | 0.0834 |
| 4 | 3 | 0.0833 | 0.1667 |
| 5 | 4 | 0.1111 | 0.2778 |
| 6 | 5 | 0.1389 | 0.4167 |
| 7 | 6 | 0.1666 | 0.5833 |
| 8 | 5 | 0.1389 | 0.7222 |
| 9 | 4 | 0.1111 | 0.8333 |
| 10 | 3 | 0.0833 | 0.9166 |
| 11 | 2 | 0.0556 | 0.9722 |
| 12 | 1 | 0.0278 | 1.0000 |
| $\Sigma =$ | 36 | 1.0000 | |

for those readers interested in vacationing or attending conventions in Las Vegas or Atlantic City, Table 2.3 presents a summary of the possible hands one could be dealt during a poker game. Notice these also represent mutually exclusive and exhaustive events. Half the time you will get a hand with nothing, only 7.6% of the time will you receive two pairs or better (1-0.9238). Note also that we are dealt only one hand at a time. Each hand that is dealt should be independent of the previous hand, assuming we have an honest dealer and that numerous individual decks are combined to produce the dealer's deck. Therefore, the cards received on the tenth deal should

**Table 2.3** Probabilities of Various Poker Hands

| Possible Hands | Ways to Make | p |
|---|---|---|
| Royal flush (ace through ten, same suit) | 4 | .000002 |
| Straight flush (five cards in sequence, same suit) | 40 | .000015 |
| Four of a kind | 624 | .00024 |
| Full house (three of a kind and a pair) | 3,744 | .0014 |
| Flush (five cards, same suit) | 5,108 | .0020 |
| Straight (five cards in sequence) | 10,200 | .0039 |
| Three of a kind | 54,912 | .0211 |
| Two pairs | 123,552 | .0475 |
| One pair | 1,098,240 | .4226 |
| Nothing | 1,302,540 | .5012 |
| Totals | 2,598,964 | .99996 |

Modified from: Kimble, G.A. (1978). *How to Use (and Misuse) Statistics*. Prentice-Hall, Englewood Cliffs, NJ, p. 91.

not be influenced by the ninth hand. This fact dispels the **gambler's fallacy** that eventually the cards will improve if one plays long enough. As a parallel, assume that a fair coin is tossed ten times and the results are all heads. The likelihood of this occurring is 0.1%, which will be proven later. Would it not be wise to call tails on the eleventh toss? Not really, if the coin is fair you still have a 50/50 chance of seeing a head on the eleventh throw, even though there have been ten previous heads.

## Counting Techniques

With the previous example, it is relatively easy to calculate the number of possible outcomes of rolling two dice. However, larger sets of information become more difficult and time consuming. The use of various counting techniques can assist with these calculations.

**Factorials** are used in counting techniques. Written as $n!$, a factorial is the product of all whole numbers from $1$ to $n$.

$$n! = n(n-1)(n-2)(n-3)\ldots(1) \qquad \text{Eq. 2.8}$$

For example:

$$8! = 8 \cdot 7 \cdot 6 \cdot 5 \cdot 4 \cdot 3 \cdot 2 \cdot 1 = 40{,}320$$

Because it is beyond the scope of this book, we will accept by definition that:

$$0! = 1.0 \qquad \text{Eq. 2.9}$$

**Permutations** represent the number of possible ways objects can be arranged where *order is important*. For example, how many different orders (arrangements) can be assigned to five sample tablets in a row (tablets A,B,C,D, and E)? First let us consider the possible arrangements if tablet A is selected first (Figure 2.3). Thus, if A is first, there are 24 possible ways to arrange the remaining tablets. Similar results would occur if Tablets B, C, D, or E are taken first. The resultant number of permutations being:

$$24 \cdot 5 = 120 \text{ possible arrangements}$$

This is identical to a five-factorial arrangement:

$$5! = 5 \cdot 4 \cdot 3 \cdot 2 \cdot 1 = 120$$

Thus, when order is important, a permutation for $n$ objects is $n!$. In other words, there are $n!$ possible ways to arrange $n$ distinguishable objects.

If the permutation involves less than the total $n$, a factorial adjustment is easily calculated. In the above example how many possible ways could three of the five

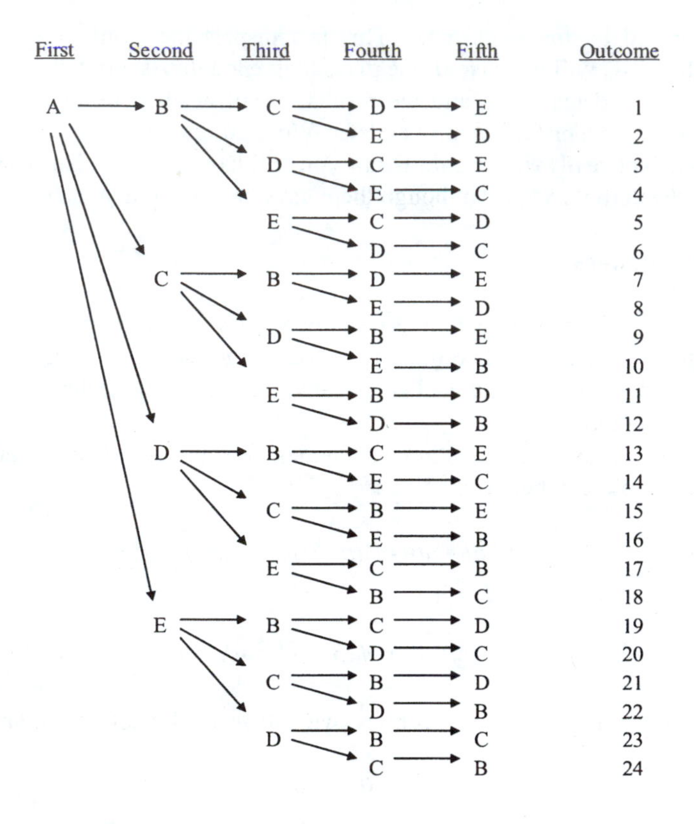


**Figure 2.3** Possible ways to arrange five tablets with tablet "A" first.

tablets can be arranged? Once again, let us look at the possibilities if tablet A is selected first (Figure 2.4). In this case, there are 12 possible ways to arrange the tablets when A is assayed first. Thus, the total possible ways to assay 3 out of 5 tablets is:

$$12 \cdot 5 = 60 \text{ ways}$$

An easier way to calculate these permutations is to use the formula:

$$_nP_x = \frac{n!}{(n-x)!} \qquad \text{Eq. 2.10}$$

where $n$ is the total number of possible objects and $x$ is the number in the arrangement. In the example cited above, the possible number of arrangements for selecting five tablets, three at a time, is:

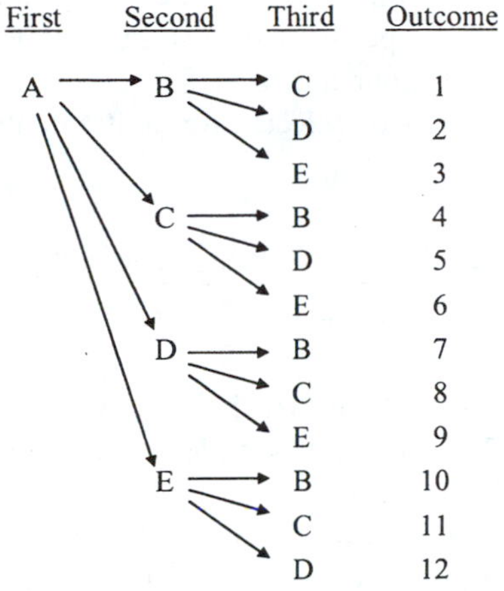

| First | Second | Third | Outcome |
|---|---|---|---|
| A | B | C | 1 |
| | | D | 2 |
| | | E | 3 |
| | C | B | 4 |
| | | D | 5 |
| | | E | 6 |
| | D | B | 7 |
| | | C | 8 |
| | | E | 9 |
| | E | B | 10 |
| | | C | 11 |
| | | D | 12 |

**Figure 2.4** Possible ways to arrange three out of five tablets with tablet "A" first.

$$_5P_3 = \frac{n!}{(n-x)!} = \frac{5!}{2!} = \frac{5 \times 4 \times 3 \times 2 \times 1}{2 \times 1} = 60$$

**Combinations** are used when the order of the observations is <u>not</u> important. For example, assume we want to assay three of the five tablets described above instead of arranging them in a row. The important feature is which three are selected, not the order in which they are chosen. As discussed in the previous chapter, independence is critical to any statistical analysis. Therefore, the order in which they are selected is irrelevant.

In the above example of five sample tablets, the results of the assay of three out of five tablets is the important aspect, not the order in which the tablets were assayed. Orders A-B-C (*1* in Figure 2.4), B-C-A, C-A-B, B-A-C, A-C-B (*4* in Figure 2.4), and C-B-A would yield the same results. Thus the total possible combinations, regardless of order, can be reduced from 60 to only ten possibilities. Using factorials for calculating larger combinations, the formula would be as follows:

$$\binom{n}{x} = \frac{n!}{x!(n-x)!} \qquad \text{Eq. 2.11}$$

Once again, $n$ is the total number of possible objects and $x$ is the number of objects selected for the combination. In the example previously cited:

$$\binom{n}{x} = \frac{n!}{x!(n-x)!} = \frac{5!}{3!2!} = \frac{5 \times 4 \times 3 \times 2 \times 1}{(3 \times 2 \times 1)(2 \times 1)} = 10$$

Consider the following example. During the production of a parenteral agent, the manufacturer samples 25 vials per hour for use in various quality control tests. Five of these vials sampled each hour are used for tests of contamination. How many possible ways could these vials be selected for contamination testing for one specific hour?

$$\binom{25}{5} = \frac{25!}{20!\,5!} = \frac{25 \times 24 \times 23 \times 22 \times 21 \times 20!}{5 \times 4 \times 3 \times 2 \times 1 \times 20!} = 53{,}130$$

In this particular case, the order with which the samples are evaluated is unimportant and therefore produces 53,130 possible sample combinations.

In a second example involving a dose proportionality study, 60 volunteers are randomly assigned to ten groups of six subjects each for the various segments (or legs) of a study. The first group receives the lowest dose, the second group receives the second lowest dose, up to the last group which receives the largest dose. At the last minute the sponsor of the study decides to reduce the maximum dose and will require only the first six segments of the study. How many ways can the assigned groups be selected for this abbreviated study?

$${}_6P_{10} = \frac{10!}{10-6!} = \frac{10 \times 9 \times 8 \times 7 \times 6 \times 5 \times 4!}{4!} = 151{,}200$$

With the groupings of subjects, order is important since each group will receive progressively larger dosages of the drug. With the order being important, there are 151,200 different way of selecting six of the ten groups of volunteers.

## Binomial Distribution

The binomial distribution is one of the most commonly encountered probability distributions. It consists of two mutually exclusive outcomes, sometimes referred to as **Bernoulli trials**. The distribution was developed by the Swiss mathematician Jakob Bernoulli in the 1600s (Dawson and Trapp, 2001, p. 74). The simplest example would be a coin toss, where the probability of tossing a head is .50 and a tail is .50. If we toss two fair coins the possible results are displayed in the upper half of Figure 2.5. Note that these probabilities are excellent examples of the multiplication theorem. The first example is an example of two mutually exclusive outcomes (heads on the first coin and heads on the second coin).

$$p(H_1 \cap H_2) = p(H_1)p(H_2) = (0.50)(0.50) = 0.25$$

This is identical to the third possible outcome of zero heads, as seen in Figure 2.5. In the case of one head, we see a conditional probability.

Two Coins

| Coin 1 | Coin 2 | Outcome | Probability |
|---|---|---|---|
| H | H | 1/4 | 0.25 of 2 heads |
| H | T | 1/2 | 0.50 of 1 head |
| T | H | | |
| T | T | 1/4 | 0.25 of 0 heads |

Three Coins

| Coin 1 | Coin 2 | Coin 3 | Outcome | Probability |
|---|---|---|---|---|
| H | H | H | 1/8 | 0.125 of 3 heads |
| H | H | T | 3/8 | 0.375 of 2 heads |
| H | T | H | | |
| T | H | H | | |
| H | T | T | 3/8 | 0.375 of 1 head |
| T | H | T | | |
| T | T | H | | |
| T | T | T | 1/8 | 0.125 of 0 heads |

**Figure 2.5** Probability of outcomes from tossing two or three coins.

$$p(H_2 | H_1) = \frac{p(H_2 \cap H_1)}{p(H_1)} = \frac{0.25}{0.50} = 0.50$$

The total outcomes for two coins are three combinations and four permutations. If we increase the number of fair coins to three we see the results in the bottom of Figure 2.5, where there are four combinations and eight permutations.

Obviously, the possible combinations and permutations become more difficult to define as the number of coins or observations increase. In 1303 Chu Shih-chieh, a Chinese mathematician, created what he called the "precious mirror of the four elements" (Bernstein, 1996, p. 64). This later became known as **Pascal's Triangle** and provides a method for calculating outcomes associated with events where the likelihood of success is 50% and failure is 50%. Figure 2.6 illustrates this triangle, the numbers in the upper portion represent frequency counts and the lower half show proportions or probability. With respect to the frequencies, the two numbers in the top line of the bolded triangles are summed to create the third lower point of the triangle. The total of all the frequencies for each row is summed in the far right column. To create the lower triangle in Figure 2.6, each frequency is divided by the sum of frequencies for that row. The result is a matrix that gives the probability of various outcomes (given a 50% chance of success). Notice the second and third rows in the probability matrix are identical to the results reported in Figure 2.5 for two and three coin tosses.

For example, assume we toss a coin six times, what is the probability that we will get two heads? Referring to Figure 2.6, we would go down the sixth row of the

Frequency Matrix

| n | | | | | | | | | f |
|---|---|---|---|---|---|---|---|---|---|
| | 1 | | | | | | | | |
| 1 | 1 | 1 | | | | | | | 2 |
| 2 | **1** | **2** | 1 | | | | | | 4 |
| 3 | 1 | **3** | 3 | 1 | | | | | 8 |
| 4 | 1 | 4 | 6 | 4 | 1 | | | | 16 |
| 5 | 1 | 5 | 10 | 10 | 5 | 1 | | | 32 |
| 6 | 1 | 6 | 15 | 20 | **15** | **6** | 1 | | 64 |
| 7 | 1 | 7 | 21 | 35 | 35 | **21** | 7 | 1 | 128 |

Probability Matrix

| n | | | | | | | | | p |
|---|---|---|---|---|---|---|---|---|---|
| 1 | .5000 | .5000 | | | | | | | 1.00 |
| 2 | .2500 | .5000 | .2500 | | | | | | 1.00 |
| 3 | .1250 | .3750 | .3750 | .1250 | | | | | 1.00 |
| 4 | .0625 | .2500 | .3750 | .2500 | .0625 | | | | 1.00 |
| 5 | .0313 | .1562 | .3125 | .3125 | .1562 | .0313 | | | 1.00 |
| 6 | .0156 | .0938 | .2344 | .3125 | .2344 | .0938 | .0156 | | 1.00 |
| 7 | .0078 | .0547 | .1641 | .2734 | .2734 | .1641 | .0547 | .0078 | 1.00 |

**Figure 2.6** Pascal's triangle.

probability matrix. The first probability (.0156) is associated with no heads, the second (.0938) only one head, the third (.2344) for two heads, and so on to the last probability (.0156) associated with all six tosses being heads. Thus, if we toss a fair coin six times, we would expect two heads approximately 23% of the time.

Unfortunately Pascal's Triangle works only for dichotomous outcomes, which represent a 50/50 chance of occurring (each outcome has a probability of .50). The binomial equation, which follows Pascal's Triangle, is based on the experiments of Jacob Bernoulli in the late 1600s (Bernstein, 1996, p.123). This can be used to calculate the likelihood associated with any number of successful outcomes regardless of the probability associated with that success, providing the probabilities of the independent events are known. The probability for each individual outcome can be calculated using the following formula:

$$p(x) = \binom{n}{x} p^x q^{n-x} \qquad \text{Eq. 2.12}$$

where $n$ is the number of possible outcomes, $x$ is number of successful outcomes, $p$ is probability of success and $q$ is the probability of failure (or not success, $1 - p$). For example, what is the probability of having 2 heads out of 6 coin tosses?

$$p(x) = \binom{n}{x} p^x q^{n-x} = p(2) = \binom{6}{2} (.5)^2 (.5)^{6-2}$$

$$p(2) = \frac{6!}{2!4!} (.5)^2 (.5)^4 = 15(0.25)(0.0625) = 0.2344$$

Here we produce the exact same results as seen with Pascal's Triangle.

Four conditions must be met in order to calculate a binomial equation: 1) there must be a fixed number of trials ($n$); 2) each trial can result in only one of two possible outcomes that are defined as a success or failure; 3) the probability of success ($p$) is constant; and 4) each of the trials produce independent results, unaffected by any previous trial.

Using the binomial equation we can create a probability table to represent the associated probabilities. Again, let us use the example of coin tossing. The possible outcomes for heads based on ten tosses of a fair coin (or tossing ten separate fair coins at one time) would result in the distribution presented in Table 2.4. Using a binomial table it is possible to answer all types of probability questions by referring to the individual probabilities or the cumulative probabilities. For example, what is the probability of one head in ten tosses of a fair coin?

$$p(1) = 0.010$$

What is the probability of less than three heads in ten tosses?

$$p(0,1,2) = p(0) + p(1) + p(2) = 0.001 + 0.010 + 0.044 = 0.055$$

Because of the addition theorem we can sum all the probabilities for events less than three heads. Alternatively, we could read the results off the cumulative table, $p(<3)$ = 0.055. What is the probability of seven or more heads in ten tosses?

$$p(7,8,9,10) = 0.117 + 0.044 + 0.010 + 0.001 = 0.172$$

Or, to read off the cumulative table for $1 - p(<7)$ = 1 - 0.828 = 0.172. What is the probability of four to six heads in ten tosses?

$$p(6\ or\ less) - p(<4) = 0.828 - 0.172 = 0.656$$

$$p(4,5,6) = 0.205 + 0.246 + 0.205 = 0.656$$

**Table 2.4** Possible Results from Tossing a Fair Coin Ten Times

| Outcome - f(x) (number of heads) | p(f(x)) | Cumulative p(f(x)) |
|---|---|---|
| 0 | 0.001 | 0.001 |
| 1 | 0.010 | 0.011 |
| 2 | 0.044 | 0.055 |
| 3 | 0.117 | 0.172 |
| 4 | 0.205 | 0.377 |
| 5 | 0.246 | 0.623 |
| 6 | 0.205 | 0.828 |
| 7 | 0.117 | 0.945 |
| 8 | 0.044 | 0.989 |
| 9 | 0.010 | 0.999 |
| 10 | 0.001 | 1.000 |

The binomial distribution can be applied to much of the data that is encountered in pharmacy research. For example:

- LD50 determination (animals live or die after dosing; used to determine the dose that kills 50% of the animals).
- ED50 determination (drug is effective or not effective; used to determine the dose that is effective in 50% of the animals).
- Sampling for defects (in quality control; product is sampled for defects and tablets are acceptable or unacceptable).
- Clinical trials (treatment is successful or not successful).
- Formulation modification (palpability preference for old and new formulation) (Bolton, 1984).

## Poisson Distribution

Another discrete probability distribution is the Poisson distribution. As will be discussed in Chapter 6, the binomial distribution tends to be bell-shaped as $n$ increases for any fixed value of $p$. However, dichotomous outcomes in which one of the two results has a very small probability of occurrence (i.e., 0.02 or 0.05), the binomial distribution will more than likely not produce a desired bell-shaped distribution. The Poisson process can be used to calculate probabilities associated with various events when $p$ is relatively small:

$$p(x) = \frac{\mu^x}{x!} e^{(-\mu)} \qquad \text{Eq. 2.13}$$

where $e$ is the constant 2.7183, the base of natural logarithms. In this case the best estimate of $\mu$ is $np$ (the symbol $\mu$ will be discussed later in Chapter 5). Therefore, the formula can be rewritten:

$$p(x) = \frac{(np)^x}{x!} e^{(-np)} \quad \text{Eq. 2.14}$$

It can be shown, for every $x$, that $p(x)$ is equal to or greater than zero and that the sum of all the p(x) equals 1.0, thus satisfying the requirements for a probability distribution. This produces a slightly more conservative distribution, with larger *p*-values associated with 0 and smaller numbers of outcomes. Because the two events of the Poisson distribution are mutually exclusive they can be summed similar to our discussion of a probability distribution.

For example, during production of a dosage form, the pharmaceutical company normally expects to have 2% of the tablets in a batch to have less than 95% of the labeled amount of a drug. These are defined as defective tablets. If 20 tablets are randomly sampled from a batch, what is the probability of finding three defective tablets? In this example: $p = .02$, the probability of a defect; $n$ is 20 for the total sample size and $x$ is 3 for the outcome of interest:

$$p(3) = \frac{[(20)(.02)]^3}{3!} e^{(-0.4)} = (.01)(.6703) = .0067$$

There is less than a 1% likelihood of randomly sampling and finding three defective tablets out of 20. What is the probability of finding one defective tablet:

$$p(1) = \frac{[(20)(.02)]^1}{1!} e^{(-0.4)} = (.4)(.6703) = .2681$$

Listed below is a comparison of the difference between results using the binomial and Poisson processes:

| Number of defective tablets | Poisson p(f(x)) | Binomial p(f(x)) |
|---|---|---|
| 0 | 0.6703 | 0.6676 |
| 1 | 0.2681 | 0.2725 |
| 2 | 0.0536 | 0.0528 |
| 3 | 0.0067 | 0.0065 |
| 4 | 0.0007 | 0.0005 |

It is possible to take this one step further and create a binomial distribution table for the probability of defective tablets and criteria for batch acceptance or rejection. Based on a sample of 20 tablets:

| Defective tablets | Poisson p(f(x)) | Cumulative p(f(x)) |
|---|---|---|
| 0 | 0.6703 | 0.6703 |
| 1 | 0.2681 | 0.9384 |
| 2 | 0.0536 | 0.9920 |
| 3 | 0.0067 | 0.9987 |
| 4 | 0.0005 | 0.9992 |

Thus, there is a 94% chance (0.9384) of finding one or no defective tablets in 20 samples if there is an expected 2% defect rate. Finding more than one defect is a rare occurrence and can serve as a basis for rejecting a production batch, depending upon the manufacturer's specifications.

### References

Bernstein, P.L. (1996). *Against the Gods: The Remarkable Story of Risk*, John Wiley and Sons, New York.

Bolton, S. (1984). *Pharmaceutical Statistics: Practical and Clinical Applications*, Marcel Dekker, Inc., New York, p. 82.

Dawson, B. and Trapp, R.G. (2001), *Basic and Clinical Biostatistics*, Third edition, Lange Medical Books, New York, p. 74.

Kachigan, S.A. (1991). *Multivariate Statistical Analysis*, Second edition, Radius Press, New York, p. 59.

### Suggested Supplemental Readings

Daniel, W.W. (1999). *Biostatistics: A Foundation for Analysis in the Health Sciences*, Seventh edition, John Wiley and Sons, New York, pp. 57-76.

Forthofer, R.N. and Lee, E.S. (1995). *Introduction to Biostatistics: A Guide to Design, Analysis and Discovery*, Academic Press, San Diego, pp. 93-102, 125-141.

### Example Problems

1. A total of 150 healthy females volunteered to take part in a multicenter study of a new urine testing kit to determine pregnancy. One-half of the volunteers were pregnant, in their first trimester. Urinary pHs were recorded and 62 of the volunteers were found to have a urine pH less than 7.0 (acidic) at the time of the study. Also, 36 of these women with acidic urine were also pregnant.

   If one volunteer is selected at random:

a. What is the probability that the person is pregnant?

b. What is the probability that the person has urine that is acidic (less than pH 7)?

c. What is the probability that the person has a urine that is basic (pH equal to or greater than 7)?

d. What is the probability that the person is both pregnant <u>and</u> has urine that is acidic (less than pH 7)?

e. What is the probability that the person is either pregnant <u>or</u> has urine that is acidic (or less than pH 7)?

f. If one volunteer is selected at random from only those women with acidic urinary pHs, what is the probability that the person is also pregnant?

g. If one volunteer is selected at random from only the pregnant women, what is the probability that the person has a urine pH of 7.0 or greater?

2. Three laboratory technicians work in a quality control laboratory with five different pieces of analytical equipment. Each technician is qualified to operate each piece of equipment. How many different ways can each piece of the equipment be assigned to each technician?

3. Ten tablets are available for analysis, but because of time restrictions the scientist will only be able to sample five tablets. How many possible ways can these tablets be sampled?

4. With early detection, the probability of surviving a certain type of cancer is .60. During a mass screening effort eight individuals were diagnosed to have early manifestations of this cancer.

   a. What is the probability that all eight patients will survive their cancer?

   b. What is the probability that half will die of the cancer?

5. Calculate the following:

   a. $\binom{6}{2}$    b. $\binom{9}{5}$    c. $\binom{30}{3}$

**Answers to Problems**

1. 150 healthy female volunteers in a multicenter study for a new pregnancy test. The probability of randomly selecting one volunteer:

a. Who is pregnant

$$p(PG) = \frac{m(PG)}{N} = \frac{75}{150} = 0.500$$

b. Who has acidic urine

$$p(pH\downarrow) = \frac{m(pH\downarrow)}{N} = \frac{62}{150} = 0.413$$

c. Who has nonacidic urine

$$p(pH\uparrow) = 1 - p(pH\downarrow) = 1 - 0.413 = 0.587$$

d. Who is both pregnant <u>and</u> has acidic urine

$$p(PG \cap pH\downarrow) = \frac{m(PG \cap pH\downarrow)}{N} = \frac{36}{150} = 0.240$$

e. Who is either pregnant <u>or</u> has acidic urine

$$p(PG \cup pH\downarrow) = p(PG) + p(pH\downarrow) - p(PG \cap pH\downarrow)$$

$$p(PG \cup pH\downarrow) = 0.500 + 0.413 - 0.240 = 0.673$$

f. Who is pregnant from those women with acidic urine

$$p(PG \mid pH\downarrow) = \frac{p(PG \cap pH\downarrow)}{p(pH\downarrow)} = \frac{0.24}{0.413} = 0.581$$

g. Who has nonacidic urine from those women who are pregnant

$$p(pH\uparrow \mid PG) = \frac{p(PG \cap pH\uparrow)}{p(PG)} = \frac{0.260}{0.500} = 0.520$$

2. The ways of assigning three laboratory technicians to five pieces of equipment:

$$\binom{n}{x} = \frac{n!}{x!(n-x)!} = \binom{5}{3} = \frac{5!}{3!2!} = \frac{5 \cdot 4 \cdot 3 \cdot 2 \cdot 1}{(3 \cdot 2 \cdot 1)(2 \cdot 1)} = 10$$

3. The possible ways to sample five out of ten tablets:

$$\binom{n}{x} = \frac{n!}{x!(n-x)!} = \binom{10}{5} = \frac{10!}{5!5!} = \frac{10 \cdot 9 \cdot 8 \cdot 7 \cdot 6 \cdot 5!}{(5 \cdot 4 \cdot 3 \cdot 2 \cdot 1)(5!)} = 252$$

4. The outcomes for eight patients where the survival rate is 0.60:

   a. That all eight patients will survive:

$$p(8) = \binom{8}{0}(0.60)^8(0.40)^0 = (1)(0.0168)(1) = 0.017$$

   b. That half will die:

$$p(4) = \binom{8}{4}(0.60)^4(0.40)^4 = (70)(0.1296)(0.0256) = 0.232$$

5. Calculate the following:

   a.

$$\binom{6}{2} = \frac{6!}{2!\,4!} = \frac{6 \times 5 \times 4!}{2 \times 1 \times 4!} = \frac{30}{2} = 15$$

   b.

$$\binom{9}{5} = \frac{9!}{5!\,4!} = \frac{9 \times 8 \times 7 \times 6 \times 5!}{4 \times 3 \times 2 \times 1 \times 5!} = 126$$

   c.

$$\binom{30}{3} = \frac{30!}{3!\,27!} = \frac{30 \times 29 \times 28 \times 27!}{3 \times 2 \times 1 \times 27!} = 4060$$

# 3

# Sampling

Samples from a population represent the best estimate we have of the true parameters of that population. Two underlining assumptions for all statistical tests are that: 1) the samples are randomly selected or assigned at random to the different levels of the independent variable and 2) observations are measured independently of each other. Therefore, insuring that samples are randomly selected from the study population is critical for all statistical procedures.

The **target population** is that population about which the researcher desires information. However, the population from which actual information is extracted is the **sampled population**. For example, assume the Phase III study is being designed to assess the effects of a new drug on patients with congestive heart failure (the study protocol will identify inclusion and exclusion criteria to carefully define "congestive heart failure"). It would be impossible to sample for all the people in the world meeting that meet the definition and make up the target population. Instead the researchers focus on a multicenter, worldwide study where local principle investigators recruit volunteers who meet the criteria for the study. This sample population (which has the similar to the target population, at least with respect to the characteristics under investigation) is then tested with the drug. Based on the design of the study, the volunteers may be further divided into two groups; the first receiving the new drug for CHF, the second group received the current gold standard for treating CHF. The decision of which therapy is received would be based on simple random assignment of the volunteers to one of the two therapies.

The best representation of a given target population comes from a **probability sample** of either the target population or the sampled population. Examples of a probability sample include a simple random sample, as well as systematic, stratified, and cluster samples that will be discussed in this chapter. Other nonprobability sampling plans include a convenience sample or a quota sample, A **sample of convenience** is a collection of data points or observation that is easy to obtain. Unfortunately, it is not possible to accurately estimate population characteristics of the population using such samples. A **quota sample** is a second nonprobability-based where a prespecified number of observations are collected that may represent the most accessible elements though they might not be representative of the population. It is similar to convenience sampling and widely used in opinion polling and market research. For example, in a certain marketing study by a pharmaceutical manufacturer, people are interviewed who fulfill a certain quota for females, native Americans, certain strata on a socioeconomic scale.

**Random Sampling**

As mentioned in Chapter 1, as researchers we will be interested in identifying characteristics of a population (parameters). In most cases it will not be possible to obtain all the information about that particular characteristic. Instead, a sample will be obtained that will hopefully represent a suitably selected subset of the population. The probability theories presented in Chapter 2, and upon which statistics is based, require randomness.

In order to be a random sample, all elements of the population must have an equal chance (probability) of being included in the sample. In other words, each of the 50,000 tablets coming off a scale-up production run should have an equal likelihood of being selected for analysis. If the manufacturer in the above example sampled tablets only at the beginning or the end of the production run, the results may not be representative of all the tablets. A procedure should be developed to ensure periodic sampling; for example, every 30 minutes during the production run.

**Simple random sampling** may be accomplished for a smaller number of units by using a random numbers table or by numbers generated at random using a calculator or computer. For example, assume that we are in a quality control department and want to analyze a batch of ointments. Samples have been collected during the production run and 250 tubes are available in the quality control department (these tubes are numbered in order from the first sample to the 250th tube). Because of time and expense, we are only able to analyze 10 tubes. The ten samples would be our best guess of the target population (the production) represented by the 250 tubes of ointment (the sampling population).

The best way to select the ten ointment tubes is through the use of a **random numbers table** (Table B1, Appendix B). Random numbers tables, usually generated by computers, are such that each digit (1, 2, 3, etc.) has the probability of occurring (.10) and theoretically each pair of numbers (21, 22, 23, etc.) or triplicate (111, 112, 113, etc.) would have the same probability of occurrence, .01 and .001, respectively. We would begin using a random numbers table by dropping a pencil or pen point on the table to find an arbitrary starting point. To illustrate the use of this table, assume the pencil lands at the beginning of the sixth column, eighth row, in our Table B1:

23616

We have decided *a priori* (before the fact; before the dropping of the pencil point) to select numbers moving to the right of the point. We could have also decided to move to the left, up or down the table. Because we are sampling tubes between 001 and 250, the number would be selected in groupings of three digits.

$\underline{236}16$

Thus, the first number would be 236 or the 236th ointment sample would be selected. The next grouping of three digits to the right would include the last two digits of this column and the first digit of the next column to the right.

23616 45170

The 164th ointment tube would be the second sample. Note there is nothing significant about the placements of the vertical and horizontal breaks in Table B1, they are simply included to make the table easier to read and use. The third set of three digits (517) exceeds the largest number (250) and would be ignored. Continuing to the right in groups of three digits, the third sample would be the 78th tube.

23616 45170 78646

To this point the first three samples would be ointment tubes 236, 164, and 078. The next three groupings all exceed 250 and would be ignored.

23616 45170 78646 77552 01582
23616 45170 78646 77552 01582
23616 45170 78646 77552 01582

The next sample that can be selected from this row is 158. The fourth sample is the 158th ointment tube.

23616 45170 78646 77552 01582

The researcher has decided to continue down the page (the individual could have used the same procedure moving up the page). Therefore, the last digit in the eighth row is combined with the first two digits in the ninth row to create the next sampling possibility.

......... 23616 45170 78646 77552 01582
11004 06949 40228 ....

With the 211th tube as the fifth sample, the remaining samples are selected moving across the row and ignoring numbers in excess of 250.

11004 06949 40228 95804 06583 10471 83884 27164 50516 89635
11004 06949 40228 95804 06583 10471 83884 27164 50516 89635
11004 06949 40228 95804 06583 10471 83884 27164 50516 89635
11004 06949 40228 95804 06583 10471 83884 27164 50516 89635
11004 06949 40228 95804 06583 10471 83884 27164 50516 89635

If any of the three digit number combinations had already been selected, it would also be ignored and the researcher would continue to the right until ten numbers were randomly selected. In this particular random sampling example, the ten tubes selected to be analyzed were:

| Tubes | |
|---|---|
| 004 | 078 |
| 022 | 158 |
| 047 | 164 |
| 065 | 211 |
| 069 | 236 |

Dropping the pencil at another location would have created an entirely different set of numbers. Thus, using this procedure, all of the ointment tubes have an equal likelihood of being selected.

## Other Probability Sampling Procedures

Other types of **selective sampling** are often used because they are convenient, relatively easy to accomplish, and often more realistic than pure random sampling. Selective sampling offers a practical means for producing a sample that is representative of all the units in the population. A sample is biased when it is not representative and every attempt should be made to avoid this situation. There are three alternative techniques: systematic, selective, and cluster sampling.

**Systematic sampling** is a process by which every *nth* object is selected. Consider a mailing list for a survey. The list is too large for us to mail to everyone in this population. Therefore, we select every 6th or 10th name from the list to reduce the size of the mailing while still sampling across the entire list (A-Z). The limitation is that certain combinations may be eliminated as possible samples (i.e., spouses or identical twins with the same last names); therefore, producing a situation where everyone on the mailing does not have an equal chance of being selected. In the pharmaceutical industry this might be done during a production run of a certain tablet where at selected time periods (every 30 or 60 minutes) tablets are randomly selected as they come off the tablet press and weighed to ensure the process is within control specifications. In this production example, the time selected during the hour can be randomly chosen in an attempt to detect any periodicity (regular pattern) in the production run.

In **stratified sampling** the population is divided into groups (strata) with similar characteristics and then individuals or objects can be randomly selected from each group. For example, in another study we may wish to insure a certain percentage of smokers (25%) are represented in both the control and experimental groups in a clinical trial (n=100 per group). First the volunteers are stratified into smokers and nonsmokers. Then, 25 smokers are randomly selected for the experimental group and an additional 25 smokers are randomly selected as controls. Similarly two groups of 75 nonsmoking volunteers are randomly selected to complete the study design. Stratified sampling is recommended when the strata are very different from each other and all of the objects or individuals within each stratum are similar.

Also known as "multistage" sampling, **cluster sampling** is employed when there are many individual "primary" units that are clustered together in "secondary", larger units that can be subsampled. For example, individual tablets (primary) are contained in bottles (secondary) sampled at the end of a production run. Assume that 150 containers of a bulk powder chemical arrive at a pharmaceutical manufacturer and the quality control laboratory needs to sample these for the accuracy of the chemical or lack of contaminants. Rather than sampling each container they randomly select ten containers. Then within each of the ten containers they further extract random samples (from the top, middle, or bottom) to be assayed.

In the final analysis, the selective sampling procedure that is chosen by the investigator depends on the experimental situation. There are several factors to be considered when choosing a sampling technique. They include: 1) cost of sampling, both associated expense and labor; 2) practicality, using a random number table for one million tablets during a production run would be unrealistic if not impossible to accomplish; 3) the nature of the population the sample is taken from: periodicity, unique strata or clustering of smaller units within larger ones; and 4) the desired accuracy and precision of the sample.

## Precision, Accuracy, and Bias

As mentioned, it is desirable that sample data be representative of the true population from which it is sampled and every effort should be made to ensure this is accomplished.

**Precision** refers to how closely data are grouped together or the compactness of the sample data. Illustrated in Figure 3.1 are data where there is less scatter, or closely clustered data, which have greater precision (Samples A and C). Also included is Sample B with a great deal of scatter and which does not have great precision. Precision measures the variability of a group of measurements. A precise set of measurements is compact and, as discussed in Chapter 5, is reflected by a small standard deviation or a small relative standard deviation.

However, assume that the smaller box within Samples A, B, and C represent the true value for the population from which the samples were taken. In this example, even though Samples A and C have good precision, Sample C provided the only accurate as a predictor of the population. **Accuracy** is concerned with "correctness" of the results and refers to how closely the sample data represents the true value of the population. It is desirable to have data that is both accurate and precise.

An analogy for precision and accuracy is to consider Figure 3.1 as an example of target shooting with the smaller box representing the bull's-eye. Sample C is desired because all of the shots are compacted near or within the bull's-eye of the target. Sample B is less precise, yet some shots reach the center of the target. Sample A is probably the most precise, but it lacks accuracy. This lack of accuracy is bias. **Bias** can be thought of as **systematic error** that causes some type of constant error in the measurement or idiosyncrasy with the measurement system. In the example of target shooting, the system error might be improper adjustment of the aiming apparatus or failure to account for wind velocity, either of which would cause a constant error. In a laboratory environment, systematic errors could be caused by contamination, calibration errors, losses or degradation of the product, sampling errors, unsuitable methods, or through operator incompetence. Ideally, investigators should use random sampling to avoid "selection

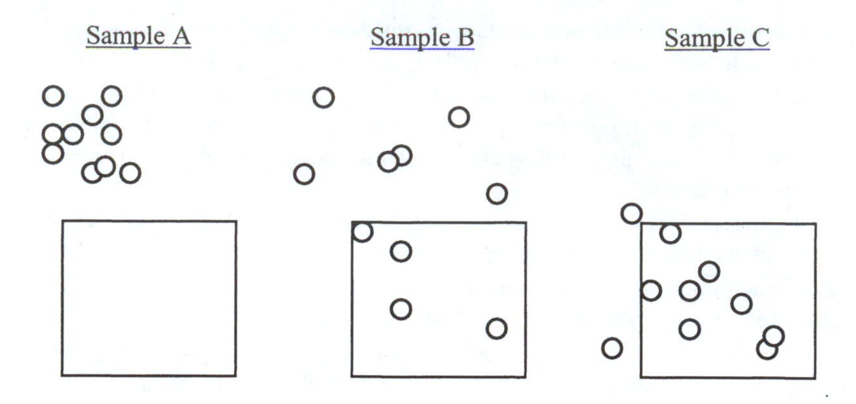


**Figure 3.1** Samples comparing precision and accuracy.

bias." **Selection bias** occurs when certain characteristics make potential observations more (or less) likely to be included in the study. For example, always sampling from the top of storage drums may bias the results based on particle size, assuming smaller particles settle to the lower regions of the drums. Bias can result from an incorrect sampling, inappropriate experimental design, inadequate blinding, or mistakes (blunders) in observing or recording the data.

Even random samples of the same pool of objects (i.e., tablets of a particular batch) are very unlikely to be exactly the same. For example, the average weight of ten tablets will vary from sample to sample. Multiple samples from the same pool or population will result in a distribution of possible outcomes, which is called the sampling distribution (Chapter 6). All data points in a set of data are subject to two different types of error: systematic and random errors. **Random errors**, or chance errors, are unpredictable and will vary in sign (+ or –) and magnitude; but systematic errors always have the same sign and magnitude, and produce biases.

## Reliability and Validity

Closely related to the accuracy of the sample data is its reliability and validity. **Reliability** is a collection of factors and judgments that, when taken together, are a measure of reproducibility. Reliability is the consistency of measures and deals with the amount of error associated with the measured values. In order for data to be reliable, all sources of error and their magnitude should be known, including both constant errors (bias) and random (chance) errors. With respect to this measure of reproducibility, if subjects are tested twice and there is a strong relationship between successive measurements (correlation, Chapter 13) this is referred to as **test-retest reliability**. It is a method of pairing the scores on the first test and the retest to determine the reliability. A second type of reliability measure, in the case of a knowledge test, is to divide the test into two portions: one score on the odd items and one score on the even items (or first half and second half of the test). If there is a strong relationship between the scores on the two halves it is called **split-half reliability**. Reliability is basic to every measurement situation and interpretation that we place on our sample data (see Chapter 17).

**Validity** refers to the fact that the data represents a true measurement. A valid piece of data describes or measures what it is supposed to represent. It is possible for a sample to be reliable without being valid, but it cannot be valid without being reliable. Therefore, the degree of validity for a set of measurements is limited by its degree of reliability. Also, if randomness is removed from the sampling technique used to collect data, it potentially removes the validity of our estimation of a population parameter.

## Suggested Supplemental Readings

Bolton, S. (1997). *Pharmaceutical Statistics: Practical and Clinical Applications*, Third edition, Marcel Dekker, New York, pp. 102-109.

Forthofer, R.N. and Lee, E.S. (1995). *Introduction to Biostatistics: A Guide to Design, Analysis and Discovery*, Academic Press, San Diego, pp. 23-35.

## Example Problems

1. Using the random numbers table presented as Table B1 in Appendix B, randomly sample three tablets from Table 3.1. Calculate the average for the three values obtained by the sample (add the three numbers and divide by three).

2. Repeat the above sampling exercise five times and record the average for each sample. Are these averages identical?

3. From the discussion in Chapter 2, how many possible samples (n = 3) could be randomly selected from the data in Table 3.1?

**Table 3.1** Results of Weights for Fifteen Tablets (mg)

| Sample | Weight | Sample | Weight | Sample | Weight | Sample | Weight |
|---|---|---|---|---|---|---|---|
| 1 | 649 | 14 | 653 | 27 | 645 | 40 | 650 |
| 2 | 654 | 15 | 646 | 28 | 650 | 41 | 651 |
| 3 | 644 | 16 | 644 | 29 | 656 | 42 | 639 |
| 4 | 648 | 17 | 649 | 30 | 649 | 43 | 648 |
| 5 | 650 | 18 | 647 | 31 | 649 | 44 | 652 |
| 6 | 636 | 19 | 650 | 32 | 657 | 45 | 648 |
| 7 | 652 | 20 | 652 | 33 | 643 | 46 | 669 |
| 8 | 662 | 21 | 646 | 34 | 653 | 47 | 647 |
| 9 | 646 | 22 | 648 | 35 | 645 | 48 | 664 |
| 10 | 650 | 23 | 655 | 36 | 650 | 49 | 649 |
| 11 | 648 | 24 | 651 | 37 | 647 | 50 | 653 |
| 12 | 651 | 25 | 642 | 38 | 651 | | |
| 13 | 660 | 26 | 647 | 39 | 654 | | |

**Answers to Problems**

1. Answers will vary based on the sample.

2. Chances are the five samples will all be different and the averages could vary from 639 to 665 mg depending on which three samples are selected. The most common results will be near the center (650 mg) for all 50 measurements. The reason for this will be explained in Chapter 6 where sample distributions are discussed.

3. There are 19,600 possible samples:

$$\binom{n}{x} = \frac{n!}{x!(n-x)!} = \frac{50!}{3!(50-3)!} = \frac{50 \cdot 49 \cdot 48 \cdot 47!}{(3 \cdot 2 \cdot 1)(47!)} = 19{,}600$$

# 4

# Presentation Modes

Data can be communicated in one of four different methods: 1) verbal; 2) written descriptions; 3) tables; or 4) graphic presentations. This chapter will focus on the latter two methods for presenting descriptive statistics. Often the graphic representation of data may be beneficial for describing and/or explaining research data. The main purpose in using a graph is to present a visual representation of the data and the distribution of observations.

The old adage "a picture is worth a thousand words" can be especially appropriate with respect to graphic representation of statistical data. Visualizing data can be useful when reviewing preliminary data, for interpreting the results of inferential statistics, and for detecting possible extreme or erroneous data (outliers). A variety of graphic displays exist and a few of the most common are presented in this chapter.

## Tabulation of Data

The simplest and least informative way to present experimental results is to list the observations (raw scores). For example, working in a quality control laboratory we are requested to sample 30 tetracycline capsules during a production run and to report to the supervisor the results of this sample. Assume the information in Table 4.1 represents the assay results for the random sample of 30 capsules. Data presented in this format is relatively useless other than to merely provide the individual results.

We could arrange the results of the 30 samples in order from the smallest assay result to the largest (Table 4.2). With this ordinal ranking of the data we begin to see certain characteristics of our data: 1) most of the observations cluster near the middle of the distribution (i.e., 250 mg) and 2) the spread of outcomes varies from as small as 245 mg to as large as 254 mg.

The purpose of descriptive statistics is to organize and summarize information; therefore, tables and graphics can be used to present this data in a more useful format. What we are doing is called the process of **data reduction**; trying to take data and reduce it down to more manageable information. The assay results seen in Tables 4.1 and 4.2 represent a continuous variable (mg of drug present); however, as

**Table 4.1** Results from the Assay of 30 Tetracycline Capsules

| Capsule # | mg | Capsule # | mg | Capsule # | mg |
|---|---|---|---|---|---|
| 1 | 251 | 11 | 250 | 21 | 250 |
| 2 | 250 | 12 | 253 | 22 | 254 |
| 3 | 253 | 13 | 251 | 23 | 248 |
| 4 | 249 | 14 | 250 | 24 | 252 |
| 5 | 250 | 15 | 249 | 25 | 251 |
| 6 | 252 | 16 | 252 | 26 | 248 |
| 7 | 247 | 17 | 251 | 27 | 250 |
| 8 | 248 | 18 | 249 | 28 | 247 |
| 9 | 254 | 19 | 246 | 29 | 251 |
| 10 | 245 | 20 | 250 | 30 | 249 |

**Table 4.2** Rank Ordering from Smallest to Largest

| Rank | mg | Rank | mg | Rank | mg |
|---|---|---|---|---|---|
| 1 | 245 | 11 | 249 | 21 | 251 |
| 2 | 246 | 12 | 250 | 22 | 251 |
| 3 | 247 | 13 | 250 | 23 | 251 |
| 4 | 247 | 14 | 250 | 24 | 252 |
| 5 | 248 | 15 | 250 | 25 | 252 |
| 6 | 248 | 16 | 250 | 26 | 252 |
| 7 | 248 | 17 | 250 | 27 | 253 |
| 8 | 249 | 18 | 250 | 28 | 253 |
| 9 | 249 | 19 | 251 | 29 | 254 |
| 10 | 249 | 20 | 251 | 30 | 254 |

mentioned in Chapter 1, continuous data can be grouped together to form categories and then handled as a discrete variable. Assume that the desired amount (labeled amount) of tetracycline is 250 mg per capsule. The data can be summarized to report results: 1) focusing on those which capsules meet or exceed the labeled amount:

| Outcome | n | % |
|---|---|---|
| <250 mg | 11 | 36.7 |
| ≥250 mg | 19 | 63.3 |
| Total | 30 | 100.0 |

(*n* representing the number of occurrences in a given level of this now discrete variable); 2) showing capsules that do not exceed the labeled amount:

| Outcome | f | % |
|---|---|---|
| ≤250 mg | 18 | 60.0 |
| >250 mg | 12 | 40.0 |
| Total | 30 | 100.0 |

(the number of occurrences can also be listed as *f* or the frequency of the outcomes,); or 3) listing those capsules that exactly meet the label claim and those which fall above or below the desired amount:

| Outcome | f | cf | % | cum.% |
|---|---|---|---|---|
| <250 mg | 11 | 11 | 36.7 | 36.7 |
| =250 mg | 7 | 18 | 23.3 | 60.0 |
| >250 mg | 12 | 30 | 40.0 | 100.0 |

Notice in this last table that the cumulative frequencies (*cf*) and cumulative percentages (*cum.%*) are reported, in addition to the frequency and percentage. The **frequency** or number of observations for each discrete level appears in the second column. The third column represents the **cumulative frequency,** which is obtained by summing the frequencies for the level of interest plus each preceding discrete level. The last two columns report the percentages associated with each level of the discrete variable. The fourth column, also called the **relative frequency** (*rf*), is the frequency converted to the percentage of the total number of observations. The last column shows the cumulative outcomes expressed as **cumulative percent** or proportion of the observations. One of the problems associated with converting a continuous, quantitative variable into a categorical, discrete variable is a loss of information. Notice in the last table that 10 different values (ranging from 245 to 254 mg) have been collapsed into only three discrete intervals. Also notice that the last table represents three mutually exclusive and exhaustive categories.

### Visual Displays for Discrete Variables

Often simple data, such as the previous example, can be presented in a graphic form. **Bar graphs** are appropriate for visualizing the frequencies associated with different levels of a discrete variable. Also referred to as **block diagrams**, they are drawn with spaces between the bars symbolizing the discontinuity among the levels of the discrete variable (this is in contrast to histograms for continuous data that will be discussed later). In Figure 4.1, information is presented using the three mutually exclusive and exhaustive levels created for the data in Table 4.2. In preparing bar graphs, the horizontal plane (x-axis or **abscissa**) usually represents observed values or the discrete levels of the variable (in this case <250, =250, or >250 mg.). The vertical axis (y-axis or **ordinate**) represents the frequency or proportion of observations (in this case the frequency).

A **line chart** is similar to a bar chart except that thin lines, instead of thicker

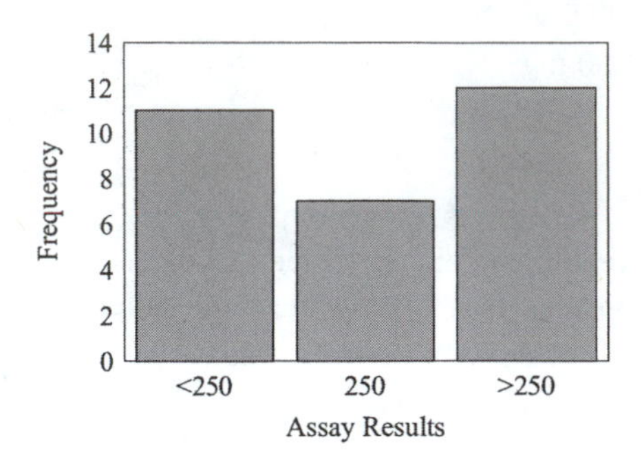


**Figure 4.1** Example of a bar graph.

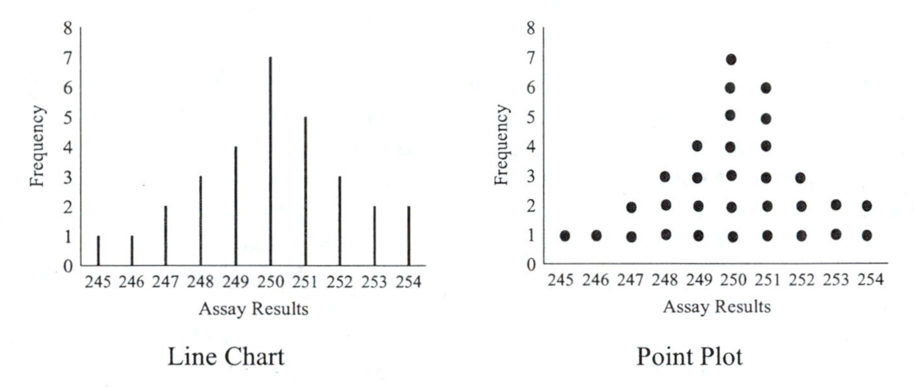


**Figure 4.2** Examples of a line chart and point plot.

bars, are used to represent the frequency associated with each level of the discrete variable. **Point plots** are identical to line charts; however, instead of a line a number of points or dots equivalent to the frequency are stacked vertically for each value of the horizontal axis. Also referred to as **dot diagram**, point plots are useful for small data sets. Using the data presented in Table 4.2, a corresponding line chart and dot diagram are presented in Figure 4.2.

**Pictograms** are similar to bar charts. They present the same type of information, but the bars are replaced with a representative number of icons. This type of presentation for descriptive statistics dates back to the beginning of civilization when pictorial images were used to record numbers of people, animals, or objects (Figure 4.3).

**Pie charts** provide a method for viewing and comparing levels of a discrete variable in relationship to that variable as a whole. Whenever a data set can be divided into parts, a pie chart may provide the most convenient and effective method for presenting the data (Figure 4.4).

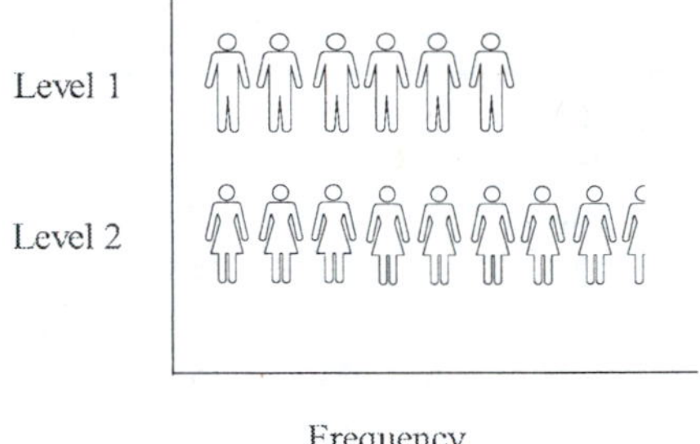


**Figure 4.3** Example of a pictogram.

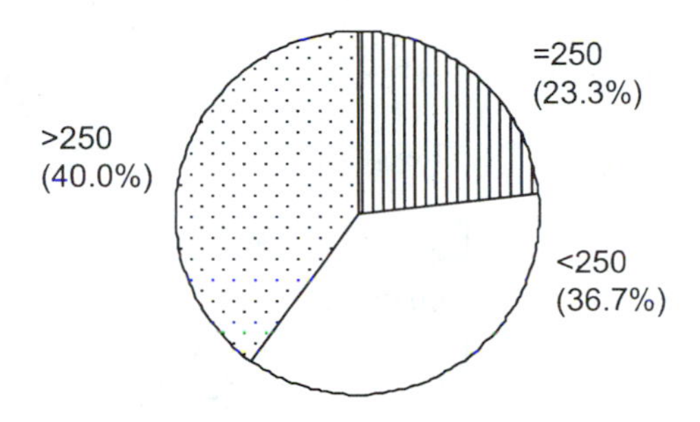


**Figure 4.4** Example of a pie chart.

### Visual Displays for Continuous Variables

The **stem-and-leaf plot** is a visual presentation for continuous data. Also referred to as a **stemplot**, it was developed by John Tukey in the 1960s and contains features common to both the frequency distribution and dot diagrams. Digits, instead of bars are used to illustrate the spread and shape of the distribution. Each piece of data is divided into "leading" and "trailing" digits. For example, based on the range of data points, the observation *125* could be divided into the either *12* and *5*, or *1* and *25*, as the leading and trailing digits. All the leading digits are sorted from lowest to highest and listed to the left of a vertical line. These digits become the stem. The trailing digits are then written in the appropriate row to the right of the vertical line. These become the leaves. The frequency or "depth" of the number of leaves at each value in the lead digit of the stem are listed on the left side and can be used to calculate the median, quartiles, or percentiles. An *M* and *Q* are placed on the vertical line to identify the **median** and **quartiles**. These measures of central tendency will be discussed in the next chapter. For the present, the median represents that value below which 50% of the observations fall. The quartiles are the values below which 25% and 75% of the data would be located, respectively. For example, the data presented for 125 patients in Table 4.3 can be graphically represented by the stemplot in Figure 4.5. The appearance of the stemplot is similar to a horizontal bar graph (rotated 90 degrees from the previous example of a bar graph); however, individual data values

Table 4.3 $C_{max}$ Calculations for Bigomycin in Micrograms (mcg)

| | | | | | | | | | | | |
|---|---|---|---|---|---|---|---|---|---|---|---|
| 739 | 775 | 765 | 751 | 761 | 738 | 759 | 761 | 764 | 765 | 749 | 767 |
| 764 | 743 | 739 | 759 | 752 | 762 | 730 | 734 | 759 | 745 | 743 | 745 |
| 751 | 760 | 768 | 766 | 756 | 741 | 741 | 774 | 756 | 749 | 760 | 765 |
| 743 | 752 | 729 | 735 | 725 | 750 | 745 | 745 | 738 | 763 | 752 | 737 |
| 706 | 769 | 760 | 755 | 767 | 750 | 728 | 778 | 740 | 741 | 771 | 752 |
| 756 | 746 | 788 | 743 | 725 | 765 | 754 | 766 | 755 | 772 | 758 | 763 |
| 734 | 728 | 755 | 778 | 785 | 718 | 730 | 731 | 714 | 752 | 770 | 732 |
| 770 | 755 | 720 | 754 | 764 | 731 | 790 | 793 | 753 | 780 | 732 | 751 |
| 766 | 751 | 762 | 734 | 755 | 761 | 740 | 767 | 775 | 755 | 766 | 736 |
| 755 | 755 | 770 | 741 | 751 | 774 | 780 | 724 | 720 | 746 | 754 | 766 |
| 743 | 743 | 775 | 732 | 762 | | | | | | | |

| Frequency | Stem | | Leaves |
|---|---|---|---|
| 1 | 70 | | 6 |
| 2 | 71 | | 48 |
| 8 | 72 | | 00455889 |
| 18 | 73 | | 001122244456788999 |
| 19 | 74 | Q | 0011113333355556699 |
| 31 | 75 | M | 0011111222223444555555556668999 |
| 28 | 76 | Q | 0001112222334445555666677789 |
| 12 | 77 | | 000124455588 |
| 4 | 78 | | 0058 |
| 2 | 79 | | 03 |
| 125 | | | |

**Figure 4.5** Example of a stem-and-leaf plot.

are retained. Also shown are the maximum and minimum scores, and also the range (distance from the largest to smallest observation) can be easily calculated. The stem-and-leaf plot also could be expanded to provide more information about the distribution. In the above example, if each stem unit was divided into halves (upper and lower), then the leaves would be established for 70.0-70.4, 70.5-70.9, 80.0-80.4, etc.

A **back-to-back stemplot** could be used to visually compare two sets of data. For example the information in Table 4.4 is plotted in Figure 4.6. Visually the data obtained for the two formulations appear to be different. In Chapter 9, we will reevaluate this data to determine if there is a statistically significant difference or if the difference could be due to some type of random difference.

Similar to the back-to-back stemplot, the **cross diagram** is a simple graphic representation for two or more levels of a discrete independent variable and a dependent continuous variable. The values for the dependent variable are represented on a horizontal or vertical line (Figure 4.7). Data are plotted on each side of the line

**Table 4.4** $C_{max}$ Values for Two Formulations of the Same Drug

| Formulation A | | | | | | Formulation B | | | | | |
|---|---|---|---|---|---|---|---|---|---|---|---|
| 125 | 130 | 135 | 126 | 140 | 135 | 130 | 128 | 127 | 149 | 151 | 130 |
| 128 | 121 | 123 | 126 | 121 | 133 | 141 | 145 | 132 | 132 | 141 | 129 |
| 131 | 129 | 120 | 117 | 126 | 127 | 133 | 136 | 138 | 142 | 130 | 122 |
| 119 | 133 | 125 | 120 | 136 | 122 | 129 | 150 | 148 | 136 | 138 | 140 |

| Formulation A | | Formulation B |
|---:|:---:|:---|
| 97 | 11 | |
| 98766655321100 | 12 | 27899 |
| 6553310 | 13 | 0002236688 |
| 0 | 14 | 0112589 |
| | 15 | 01 |

**Figure 4.6** Example of a back-to-back stem-and-leaf plot.

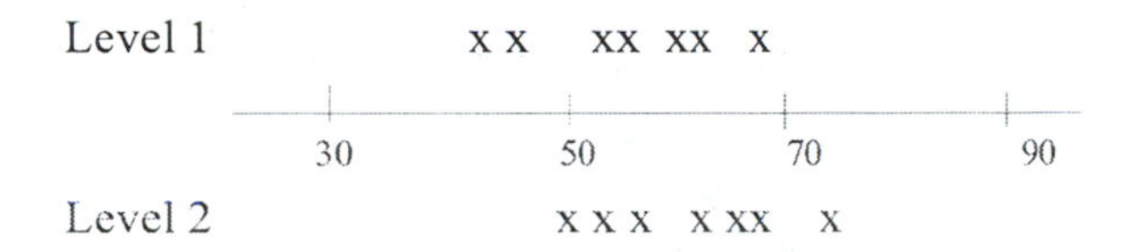


**Figure 4.7** Example of a cross diagram.

based on which level of the independent variable they represent.

One simple plot that displays a great deal of information about a continuous variable is the **box-and-whisker plot** (Figure 4.8). The box plot illustrates the bulk of the data as a rectangular box in which the upper and lower lines represent the third quartile (75% of observations below $Q_3$) and first quartile (25% of observations below $Q_1$), respectively. The second quartile (50% of the observations below this point) is depicted as a horizontal line through the box. The arithmetic average may or may not be shown as an *x*. Vertical lines (whiskers) extend from the top and bottom lines of the box to an upper and lower **adjacent value**. The adjacent values equal three **semi-interquartile ranges** (SIQR) above and below the median. The SIQR is the distance between the upper or lower quartile and the median, or:

$$SIQR = \frac{(Q_3 - Q_1)}{2} \qquad \text{Eq. 4.1}$$

Observations that fall above or below the adjacent values can be identified as potential outliers (Chapter 23).

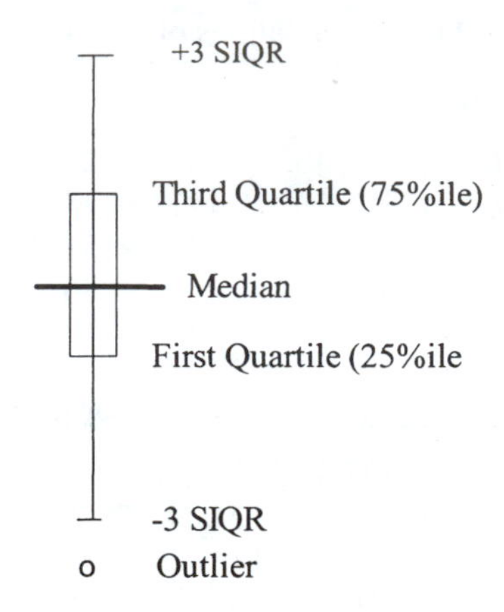


**Figure 4.8** Example of a box and whisker plot.

Similar to bar charts and point plots, **histograms** are useful for displaying the distribution for a continuous variable, especially as sample sizes become larger or if it becomes impractical to plot each of the different values observed in the data. The vertical bars are connected and reflect the continuous nature of the observed values. Each bar represents a single value or a range of values within the width of that bar. For example, a histogram representing the 30 tetracycline capsules listed in Table 4.1 is presented in Figure 4.9. Each value represents a continuous variable and the equipment used had precision to measure to only the whole mg (i.e., 248 or 251 mg). If more exact instruments were available, the measurements might be in tenths or hundredths of a milligram. Therefore, the value of 248 really represents an infinite number of possible outcomes between 0.5 mg below and 0.5 mg above that particular measure (247.5 to 248.5 mg). Similarly, the value 250 represents all possible results between 249.5 and 250.5 mg. The histogram representing this continuum is presented in Figure 4.10.

Both the stem-and-leaf plots and the box-and-whisker plots are examples of **exploratory data analysis techniques**. These techniques were developed by John Tukey (Tukey, 1977) and colleagues. They provide the researcher with a visual method for identifying trends, relationships, or unexpected patterns in sample data.

The data in Figure 4.10 represent an **ungrouped frequency distribution**, which is a visual representation of each possible outcome and its associated frequency. Such a distribution shows the extremes of the outcomes, as well as how they are distributed and if they tend to concentrate in the center or to one end of the scale. Unfortunately, with large data sets or where there is increased precision in the measurement, ungrouped frequency distributions may become cumbersome and produce a histogram with many points on the abscissa with frequency counts of only one or two per level. A more practical approach would be to group observed values or outcomes into **class intervals**. In a **grouped frequency distribution**: 1) all class intervals must be the same width, or size; 2) the intervals are mutually exclusive and exhaustive;

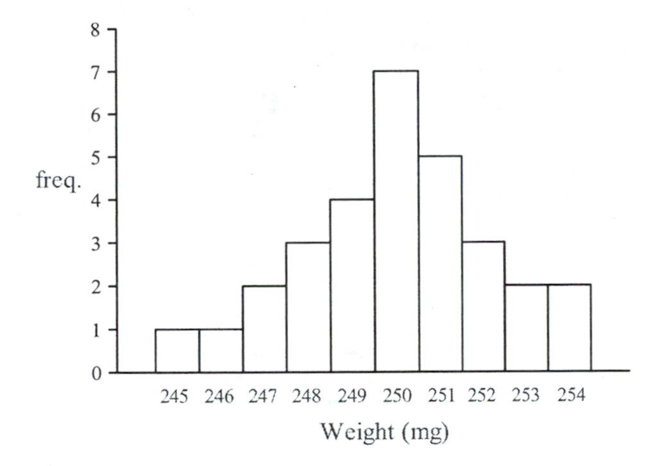


**Figure 4.9** Example of a histogram.

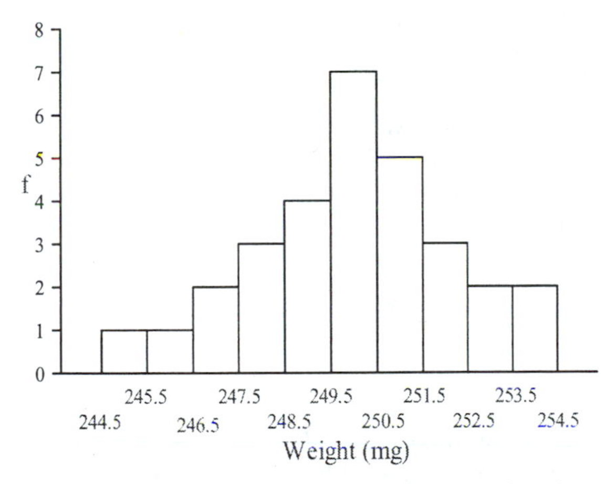


**Figure 4.10** Example of a histogram with correction for continuity.

and 3) the interval widths should be assigned so the lowest interval includes the smallest observed outcome and the top interval includes the largest observed outcome. The number of class intervals and their size (boundaries) must be specified. Two questions exist regarding these intervals: how many intervals should be used and what should be the width for each interval? To illustrate this process, consider the pharmacokinetic data presented in Table 4.3, representing a sample of patients (n=125) receiving the fictitious drug bigomycin. As mentioned previously, the range is the difference between the largest and smallest value in a set of observations and represents the simplest method for presenting the dispersion of the data. In this example the largest observation is 792 mcg and the smallest is 706 mcg. The difference represents the **range** of the observations:

Table 4.5 Number of Intervals for Various Sample Sizes Using Sturges' Rule

| Sample Size | K Intervals |
|---|---|
| 23-45 | 6 |
| 46-90 | 7 |
| 91-181 | 8 |
| 182-363 | 9 |
| 364-726 | 10 |
| 727-1454 | 11 |
| 1455-2909 | 12 |

$$792\ mcg - 706\ mcg = 86\ mcg$$

But into how many class intervals should this data be divided? Some authors provide approximations such as ten to 20 (Snedecor and Cochran, 1989), eight to 12 (Bolton, 1984), or five to 15 intervals (Forthofer and Lee, 1995). However, **Sturges' rule** (Sturges, 1926) provides a less arbitrary guide to determine the number of intervals based on the sample size (*n*):

$$K_{intervals} = 1 + 3.32 \log_{10}(n) \qquad \text{Eq. 4.2}$$

A quick reference on the number of intervals for various sample sizes based on Sturges' rule is presented in Table 4.5. The interval width is found by dividing the range by the prescribed number of intervals:

$$width\ (w) = \frac{range}{K} \qquad \text{Eq. 4.3}$$

In our current example, for a sample size of 125 and a range of 86, the number of intervals and width of those intervals would be:

$$K = 1 + 3.32 \log_{10}(125) = 1 + 3.32(2.10) = 7.97 \approx 8\ intervals$$

$$w = \frac{range}{K} = \frac{86}{8} = 10.75 \approx 11\ mcg$$

Thus, the most representative histogram would consist of 8 intervals, each with a width of 11. In order to include the smallest and largest values the sections of the histogram would be divided as seen in the first column of Table 4.6. However, the values represent a continuous variable; therefore, correcting for continuity, the true boundaries (**interval boundary values**) of each interval of the histogram and their associated frequencies would be the second column of Table 4.6.

**Table 4.6** Example of Intervals Created Using Sturges' Rule

| Interval | Interval Boundary values | Frequency |
|---|---|---|
| 706-716 | 705.5-716.5 | 2 |
| 717-727 | 716.5-727.5 | 6 |
| 728-738 | 727.5-738.5 | 18 |
| 739-749 | 738.5-749.5 | 22 |
| 750-760 | 749.5-760.5 | 35 |
| 761-771 | 760.5-771.5 | 28 |
| 772-782 | 771.5-782.5 | 10 |
| 783-793 | 782.5-793.5 | 4 |

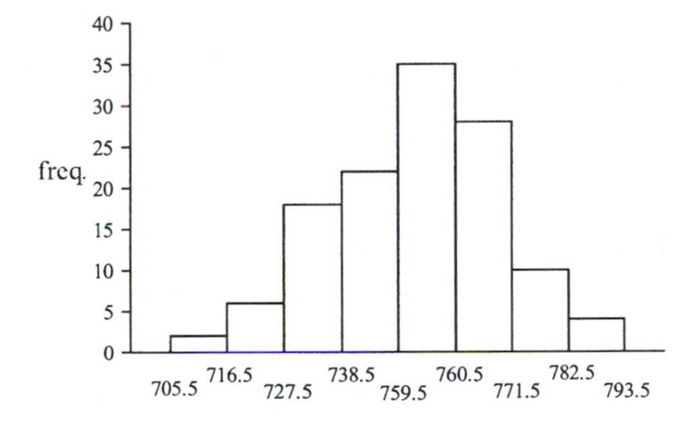


**Figure 4.11** Histogram for data presented in Table 4.3.

Note that the distribution represents eight intervals that are mutually exclusive and exhaust all possible outcomes. The histogram would appear as presented in Figure 4.11. The center of this distribution can be calculated, as well as a measure of dispersion and these will be discussed in the following chapter.

A **frequency polygon** can be constructed by placing a dot at the midpoint for each class interval in the histogram and then these dots are connected by straight lines. This frequency polygon gives a better concept of the shape of the distribution. The **class interval midpoint** for a section in a histogram is calculated as follows:

$$Midpoint = \frac{highest + lowest\ point}{2} \qquad \text{Eq. 4.4}$$

For class interval 705.5 to 716.6 the midpoint would be:

$$Midpoint = \frac{highest + lowest\ point}{2} = \frac{705.5 + 716.5}{2} = 711$$

The midpoints for the above histogram are:

| Class Interval | Midpoint ($m_i$) | Frequency ($f_i$) |
|---|---|---|
| 705.5-716.5 | 711 | 2 |
| 716.5-727.5 | 722 | 6 |
| 727.5-738.5 | 733 | 18 |
| 738.5-749.5 | 744 | 22 |
| 749.5-760.5 | 755 | 35 |
| 760.5-771.5 | 766 | 28 |
| 771.5-782.5 | 777 | 10 |
| 782.5-793.5 | 788 | 4 |
| | Total = | 125 |

The frequency polygon is then created by listing the midpoints on the x-axis, frequencies on the y-axis, and drawing lines to connect the midpoints for each interval as presented in Figure 4.12 for the previous data. The midpoint of the class interval represents all the values within that interval and will be used in drawing frequency polygons and in the calculation of measures of central tendency (Chapter 5). Unfortunately there is some loss of precision with grouped frequency distribution because only one value (the midpoint) represents all the various data points within the class interval.

At times it may be desirable to prepare graphs that show how the values accumulate from lowest class intervals to highest. These **cumulative frequency polygons** display the frequency or percentage of the observed values falling below each interval. By using such a drawing it is possible to establish certain percentiles. Figure 4.13 shows a cumulative frequency polygon for the same data presented in the above frequency polygon (data from Table 4.3). Note that lines are drawn from the 25th (*Q1*), 50th (*Q2*), and 75th (*Q3*) percentile on the y-axis (point at which 25, 50, and 75% of the results fall below) and where they cross the polygon is the approximation of each percentile. If the population from which the sample approximates a normal or bell-shaped distribution, the cumulative distribution is usually S-shaped or **ogive**.

If there were an infinite number of midpoints (the interval width in both the histogram and frequency polygon approaches zero), it would be represented by a smooth curve. The skewness of a distribution describes the direction of the stringing out of the tail of the curve (Figure 4.14). In a **positively skewed distribution** most of the values in the frequency distribution are at the left end of the distribution with a few high values causing a tapering of the curve to the right side of the distribution. In contrast, a **negatively skewed distribution** has most of the values at the right side of the distribution with a few low values causing a tapering of the curve to the left side of the distribution. Another way to think of skewness is the amount of tilt or lack of tilt in a distribution.

If a sample were normally distributed it would not be skewed to the left or right and would be symmetrical in shape. The normal distribution and its

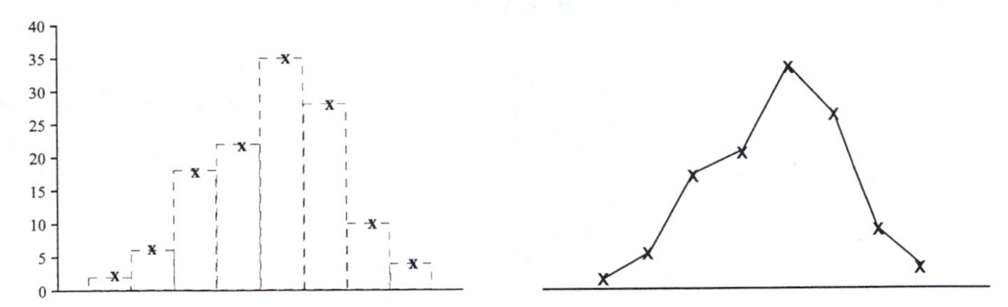


**Figure 4.12** Example of a frequency polygon.

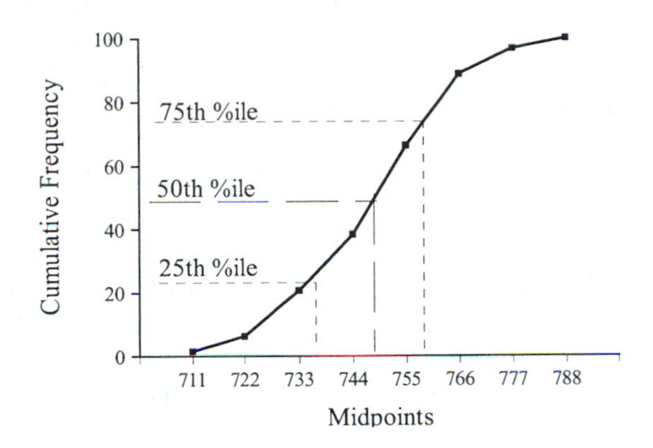


**Figure 4.13** Example of a cumulative frequency polygon.

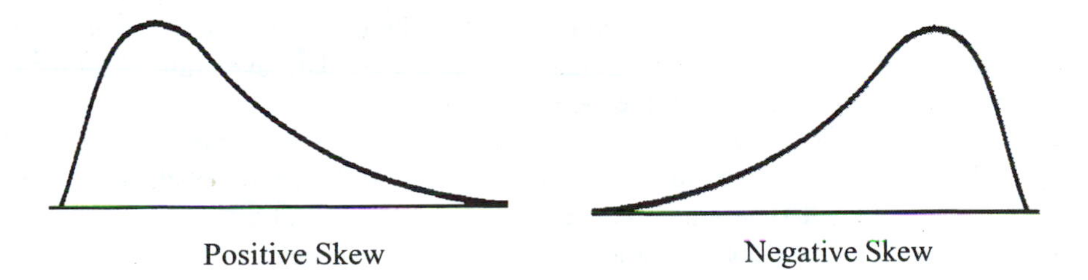


**Figure 4.14** Examples of skewed distributions.

characteristics will be discussed at great length in Chapter 6.

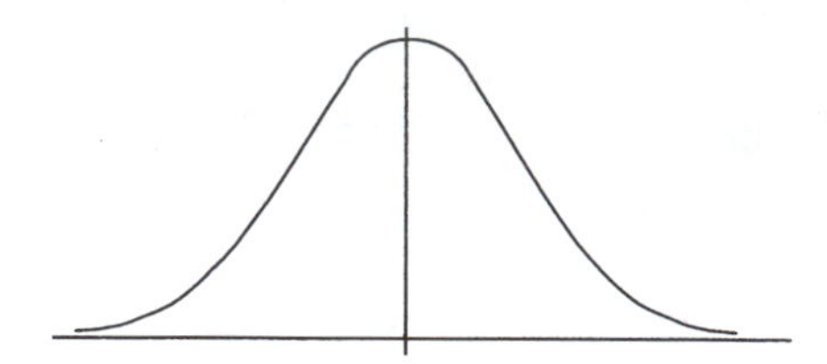

**Kurtosis** is a property associated with a frequency distribution and refers to the shape of the distribution of values regarding its relative flatness and peakedness. **Mesokurtic** is a frequency distribution that has the characterists of a normal bell-shaped distribution. If the normal distribution is more peaked than a traditional bell-shaped curve is it termed **leptokurtic** and **platykurtic** refers to a shape that is less peaked or flatter than the normal bell-shaped curve.

## Visual Displays for Two or More Continuous Variables

A **scatter diagram** or **scatter plot** is an extremely useful graphic presentation for showing the relationship between two continuous variables. The two-dimensional plot has both horizontal and vertical axes that cover the ranges of the two variables. Plotted data points represent paired observations for both the $x$ and $y$ variable (Figure 4.15). These types of plots are valuable for correlation and regression inferential tests (Chapters 13 and 14).

A **sequence plot** is a plot where the horizontal axis represents a logical or physical sequencing of data. An example might be a measurement of successive lots of a particular product, where the vertical axis is a continuous variable and the horizontal axis represents the first lot, followed by the second, then the third, etc. If time is considered, then data is arranged chronologically on the horizontal axis. This **time series graph** is a visual representation of changes in data over time, in which the dependent variable is placed on the y-axis (Figure 4.16).

Further data reduction techniques for continuous data will be presented in the next chapter where we will explore methods for defining the center of distributions and how data distributed around that center. However, visual/graphic techniques should be considered as a possible alternative to obtain a "feel" for the shape of the statistical descriptive data.

## References

Snedecor, G.W. and Cochran, W.G. (1989). *Statistical Methods*. Iowa State University Press, Ames, p. 18.

Bolton, S. (1997). *Pharmaceutical Statistics: Practical and Clinical Applications*. Third edition, Marcel Dekker, Inc., New York, p. 43.

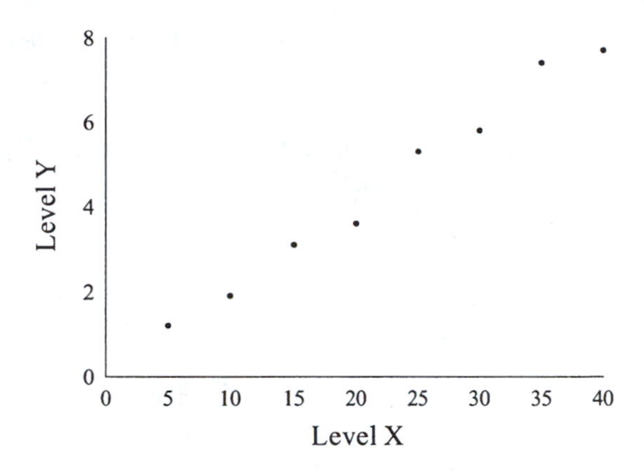


**Figure 4.15** Example of a scatter diagram.

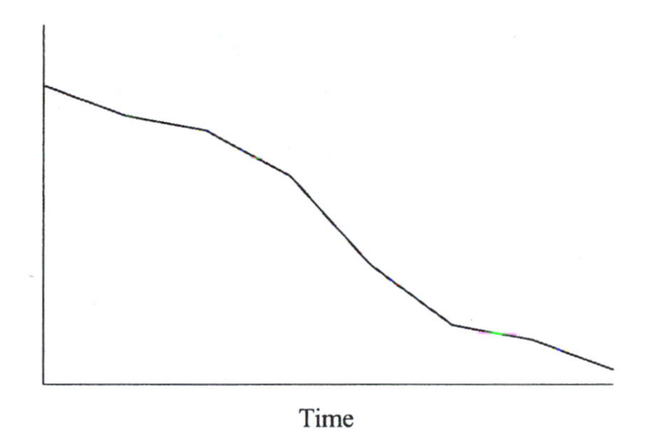


**Figure 4.16** Example of a sequence plot.

Forthofer, R.N. and Lee, E.S. (1995). *Introduction to Biostatistics*. Academic Press, San Diego, p. 52.

Sturges, H.A. (1926). "The choice of a class interval," *Journal of the American Statistical Association* 21:65-66.

**Suggested Supplemental readings**

Daniel, W.W. (1999). *Biostatistics: A Foundation for Analysis in the Health Sciences*, Seventh edition, John Wiley and Sons, New York, pp. 16-27.

Mason, R.L., Gunst, R.F., and Hess, J.L. (1989). *Statistical Design and Analysis of Experiments*, John Wiley and Sons, New York, pp. 44-62.

Fisher, L.D. and van Belle, G. (1993). *Biostatistics: A Methodology for the Health Sciences*, John Wiley and Sons, New York, pp. 35-52.

Tukey, J.W. (1977). *Exploratory Data Analysis*, Addison-Wesley, Reading, PA.

**Example Problems**

1. During clinical trials, observed adverse effects are often classified by the following scale:

| | |
|---|---|
| Mild: | Experience was trivial and did not cause any real problem. |
| Moderate: | Experience was a problem but did not interfere significantly with patient's daily activities or clinical status. |
| Severe: | Experience interfered significantly with the normal daily activities or clinical status. |

   Based on 1109 patients involved in the Phase I and II clinical trials for bigomycin, it was observed that 810 experienced no adverse effects, while 215, 72, and 12 subjects suffered from mild, moderate, and severe adverse effects, respectively. Prepare visual and tabular presentations for this data.

2. The following assay results (percentage of label claim) were observed in 50 random samples during a production run.

| | | | | | | | | | |
|---|---|---|---|---|---|---|---|---|---|
| 102 | 100 | 96 | 99 | 101 | 102 | 100 | 105 | 97 | 100 |
| 92 | 103 | 101 | 100 | 99 | 102 | 96 | 100 | 101 | 98 |
| 107 | 95 | 98 | 100 | 100 | 99 | 97 | 104 | 101 | 103 |
| 98 | 101 | 100 | 105 | 99 | 101 | 102 | 100 | 87 | 98 |
| 101 | 103 | 93 | 99 | 101 | 97 | 100 | 102 | 99 | 104 |

   Report these results as a box-and-whisker plot, stemplot, and histogram.

3. During a study of particle sizes for a blended powder mixture, the results of percent of powder retained on the various sites were 50.1%, 27.2%, 10.4%, 6.0%, and 5.1% in sieve mesh sizes of 425, 180, 150, 90, and 75 μM, respectively. Only 1.2% was captured on the pan (<75 μM). Prepare a visual and tabular presentation for this data.

4. Comparison of two methods for measuring anxiety in patients is listed below:

| Method A | Method B | Method A | Method B |
|---|---|---|---|
| 55 | 90 | 52 | 97 |
| 66 | 117 | 61 | 110 |
| 46 | 94 | 44 | 84 |
| 63 | 124 | 55 | 112 |
| 57 | 105 | 53 | 102 |
| 59 | 115 | 67 | 112 |
| 70 | 125 | 72 | 130 |
| 57 | 97 | | |

Prepare a scatter plot to display the relationship between these two variables.

## Answers to Problems

1. Incidence of reported adverse drug effects:

   a. Tabular results

Severity of Adverse Effects

| Severity | n | % | Cum. % |
|---|---|---|---|
| none | 810 | 73.0 | 73.0 |
| mild | 215 | 19.4 | 92.4 |
| moderate | 72 | 6.5 | 98.9 |
| severe | 12 | 1.1 | 100.0 |
| | 1109 | 100.0 | |

   b. Bar graph

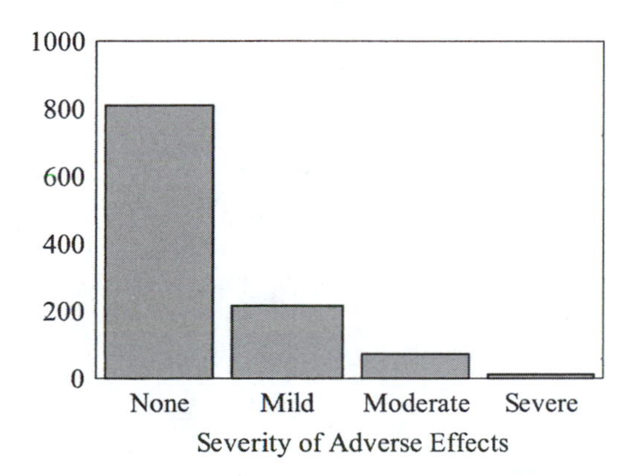

c. Pie chart

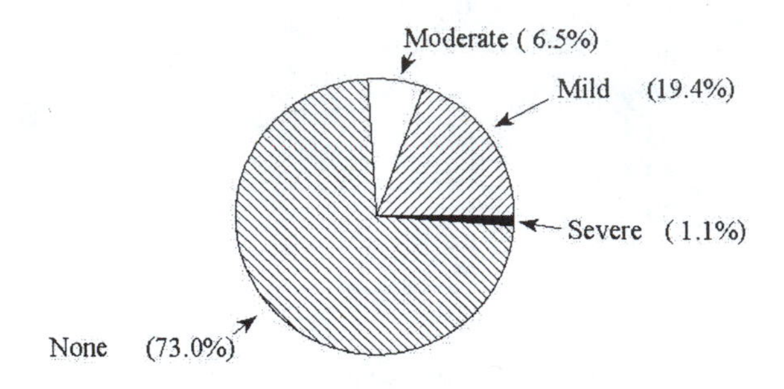


2. Distribution of assay results:

a. Box-and-whisker plot

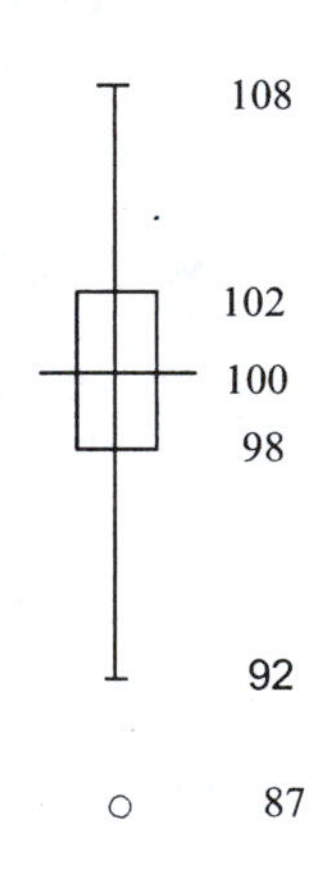


b. Stemplot

| Frequency | Stem | | Leaves |
|---|---|---|---|
| 0 | 8 | | |
| 1 | | | 7 |
| 2 | 9 | | 23 |
| 16 | | Q | 5667778888999999 |
| 28 | 10 | MQ | 0000000000111111112222233344 |
| 3 | | | 557 |
| 50 | | | |

b. Histogram

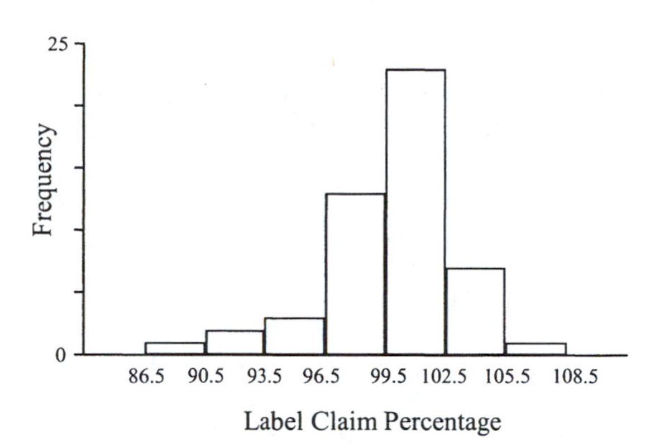


3. Particle size determination:

a. Tabular results

Percent of Particles Retained on Various Sieve Screens

| Mesh Size (μM) | % Retained | Cum. % Retained |
|---|---|---|
| 425 | 50.1 | 50.1 |
| 180 | 27.2 | 77.3 |
| 150 | 10.4 | 87.7 |
| 90 | 6.0 | 93.7 |
| 75 | 5.1 | 98.8 |
| pan (<75) | 1.2 | 100.0 |
| | 100.0 | |

c. Pie chart

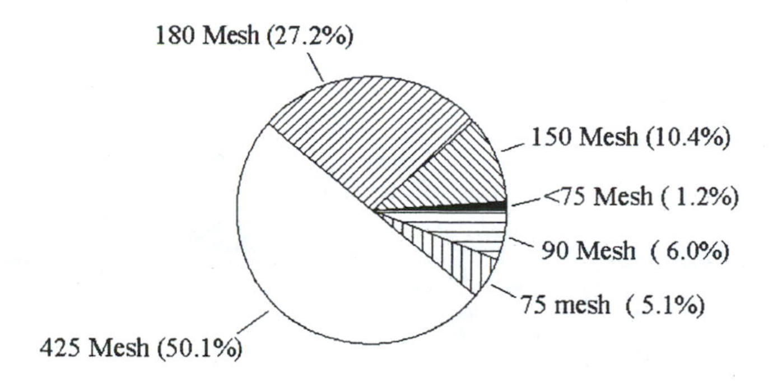

d. Bar chart

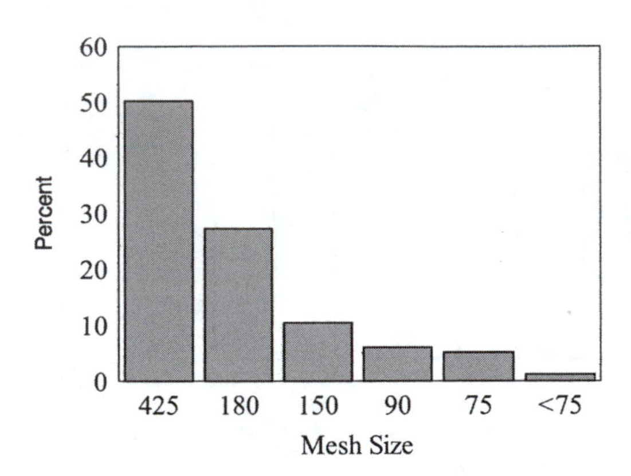


e. Scatter plot

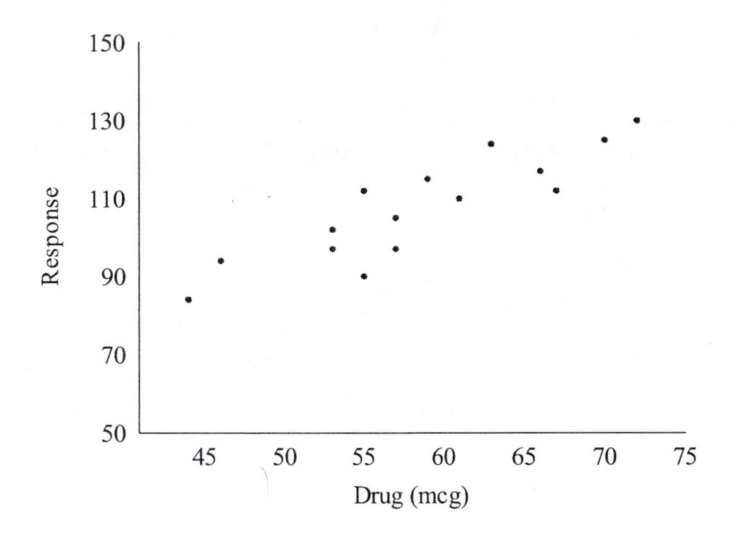

# 5

# Measures of Central Tendency

Central tendency involves description statistics for the observed results of a continuous variable and takes into consideration two important aspects: 1) the center of that distribution and 2) how the observations are dispersed within the distribution. Three points are associated with the center (mode, median, and mean) and three other measures are concerned with the dispersion (range, variance, and standard deviation).

Measures of central tendency can be used when dealing with ordinal, interval, or ratio scales. It would seem logical, with any of these continuous scales, to be interested in where the center of the distribution is located and how observations tend to cluster around or disperse from this center. Many inferential statistical tests involve continuous variables (see Appendix A) and all require information about the central tendency of associated sample data.

## Centers of a Continuous Distribution

The **sample mode** is simply that value with the greatest frequency of occurrence. In other words, the value that is most "popular" in a continuous distribution of scores. For example, what is the mode for the following group of observations?

2,6,7,5,3,8,7,6,5,3,2,5,4,6,8,3,4,4,7,6,5,1,5

Graphically the distribution would look as presented in Figure 5.1. In this distribution of observations, the **modal value** is 5 because it has the greatest frequency. The mode is the simplest, but least useful measure of the center for a distribution. The mode is most useful when continuous data has been divided into categories (i.e., a histogram) or where it represents the category with the greatest frequency.

A distribution may be multimodal and have several different values that have the same greatest relative frequency. Such a distribution may have several peaks. An example of a **bimodal distribution** appears below with slow and fast metabolizers of isoniazid (Figure 5.2). The first peak (to the left) represents a central point for the rapid metabolizers (a lower concentration of drug after six hours) and the second peak depicts the slow metabolizers where higher concentrations are seen at the same

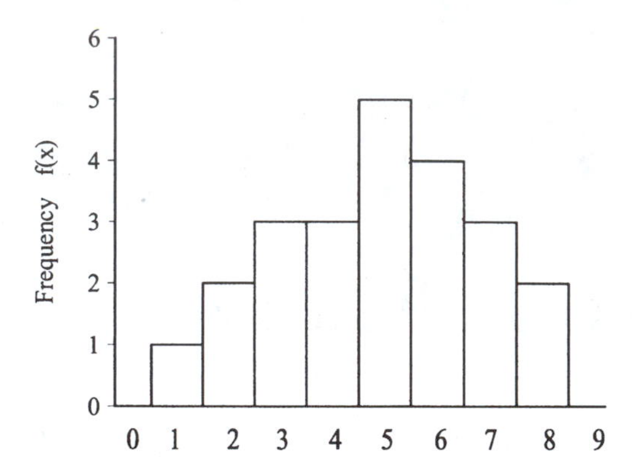


**Figure 5.1** Histogram of sample data.

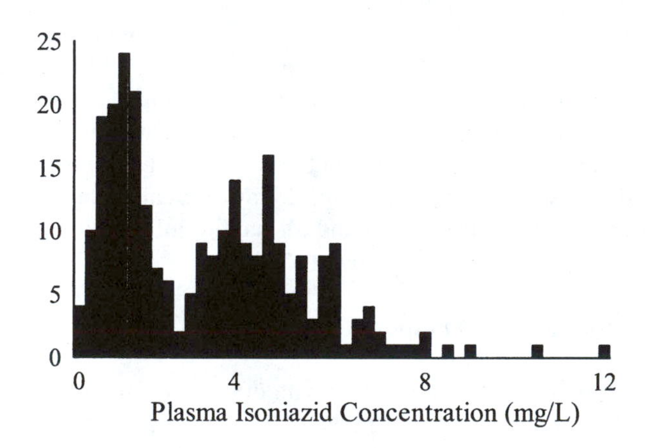


**Figure 5.2** Bimodal distribution (Evans, 1960).

point in time.

The **sample median** is the center point for any distribution of scores. It represents that value below which 50% of all scores are located. The median (from the Latin word *medianus* or "middle") divides the distribution into two equal parts (the 50th **percentile**). For example, using the same data as the previous example for the mode, a rank ordering of the scores from lowest to highest would produce the following:

Example 5A: 1,2,2,3,3,3,4,4,4,5,5, <u>5</u>, 5,5,6,6,6,6,7,7,7,8,8

In this case 5 is the median, which is the value that falls in the exact center of the distribution. If there is an even number of observations, the 50th percentile is between the two most central values and the median would be the average of those two central scores. For example, in the following set of numbers the median (represented by a underlined area) is located between the two center values (ten data points are above and ten data points are below this center):

Example 5B: 20,22,23,24,24,24,25,25,25,25, __ 26,26,26,27,27,28,28,28,29,30

The calculation of the median would be:

$$\frac{25+26}{2}=25.5$$

The **median value** is a better estimate of the center of a distribution than the mode. However, it is neither affected by, nor representative, of extreme values in the sample distribution. For example, consider the following two samples:

| | | |
|---|---|---|
| Example 5C | Sample 1 | 36,45,48,50, 50, 51,51,53,54 |
| Table weights in mg: | Sample 2 | 47,48,49,50, 50, 51,52,57,68 |

Even though both samples have the same median (50 mg), Sample 1 appears to have more observations that are relatively small and Sample 2 has more samples that are large. The two samples appear to be different, yet both produce the same median. If possible, a measure of the center for a given distribution should consider all extreme data points (i.e., 36 and 68). However, at the same time, this inability to be affected by extreme values also represents one of the advantages of using the median as a measure of the center. The median is a robust statistic and not affected by any one observation. As will be seen in Chapter 23, an outlier or atypical data point, can strongly affect the arithmetic center of the distribution, especially in small sample sizes. The median is insensitive to these extreme values.

The median is a relative measure, in that it is defined by its position in relation to the other ordered values for a set of data points. In certain cases it may be desirable to describe a particular value with respect to its position related to other values. The most effective way to do this is in terms of its **percentile location** (the percent of observations that the data point exceeds):

$$percentile=\frac{number\ of\ values\ less\ than\ the\ given\ value}{total\ number\ of\ values}\ x\ 100 \qquad \text{Eq. 5.1}$$

For example consider Table 4.2 where 30 tetracycline capsules were placed in ranked order from smallest to largest. If one were interested in the percentile for 252 mg (the 24th largest value) the calculation would be

$$percentile=\frac{23}{30}\ x\ 100=77\ percentile$$

Thus, 252 mg represents the 77th percentile for the data presented in Table 4.2. At the same time, when using percentiles, it is possible to calculate variability in a distribution, especially a distribution that is skewed in one direction. In this case, the measure would be the **interquartile range** or **interrange** (the distance between the 25th and the 75th percentiles).

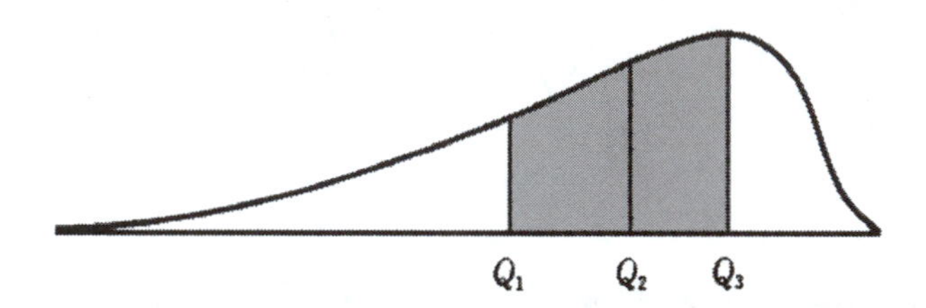


The **sample mean** is what is commonly referred to as the **average**. It is the weighted center point of a distribution, and is computed by summing up all the observations or scores and dividing by the total number of observations.

$$\overline{X} = \frac{x_1 + x_2 + x_3 + \ldots + x_n}{n}$$

The character $\overline{X}$ (*x*-bar) will be used to symbolize the sample mean. The observed values of a given variable are designated with the same letter (usually *x*) and each individual value is distinguished with a subscript number or letter. For example $x_i$ indicates the *i*th observation in a set of data. The symbol sigma ($\Sigma$) indicates the addition (summation) of all variable observations. Also referred to as the **arithmetic mean**, the formula for this equation is written as follows:

$$\overline{X} = \frac{\sum_{i=1}^{n} x_i}{n} \qquad \text{Eq. 5.2}$$

In this equation, all observations ($x_i$) for variable *x* are added together from the first (*i*=1) to the last (*n*) observation and divided by the total number of sample observations (*n*). Equation 5.2 can be simplified as follows:

$$\overline{X} = \frac{\sum x}{n}$$

The advantage in using the mean over the other measures of central tendency is that it takes into consideration how far each observation differs from the center and allows for extreme scores to impact this measure of center. Other measures do not account for this consideration. The mean can be thought of as a balancing point or center of gravity for our distribution. For the above Example 5A the mean would be:

$$\bar{X} = \frac{2+6+7+...5}{23} = 4.9$$

We typically calculate a mean (and other measures of central tendency) to one decimal point beyond the precision of the observed data. In this case the precison of the data in Example 5A is to the whole number, thus the mean is expressed in tenths. Other authors have established more definitive rules for rounding and significant figures (Torbeck, 2004).

The relative positioning of the three measures of a continuous variable's center can give a quick, rough estimate of the shape of the distribution. As will be discussed in the next chapter, in a normal (bell-shaped) distribution the mode = median = mean; in the case of a positively skewed distribution the mode < median < mean and for a negatively skewed distribution the mode > median > mean.

If data is normally distributed, or the sample is assumed to be drawn from a normally distributed population, the mean and standard deviation are the best measures of central tendency. The median is the preferred measure of central tendency in skewed distributions where there are a few extreme values (either small or large). In such cases the interquartile range is the appropriate measure of dispersion.

In the third example (Example 5C – tablet weights), the two medians were identical, and the means for the two samples differ because the extreme measures (i.e., 36 and 68 mg) were considered in this weighted measure of central tendency:

$$\text{Sample 1:} \quad \bar{X}_1 = 48.7 \text{ mg}$$
$$\text{Sample 2:} \quad \bar{X}_2 = 52.4 \text{ mg}$$

## Dispersion within a Continuous Distribution

The mean is only one dimension in the measure of central tendency, namely, the weighted middle of the sampling distribution. Seen in Figure 5.3 are two distributions that have the exact same median (5) and the same mean (4.9). However, the dispersions of data around the center of these two distributions are considerably different. Thus, measures of central tendency should also be concerned with the spread or concentration of data points around the center of the distribution.

The **sample range** is the simplest method for reporting a distribution of observations and represents the difference between the largest and smallest value in a set of outcomes. In Example 5A the largest observation is 8 and the smallest is 1. The range for these observations is 7. Similarly, the ranges for the two sample batches of tablet weights in Example 5C are:

Sample 1: 54-36 = 18 mg
Sample 2: 68-47 = 21 mg

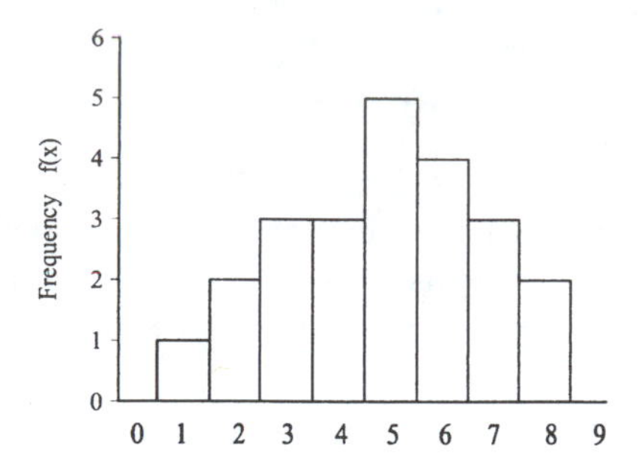


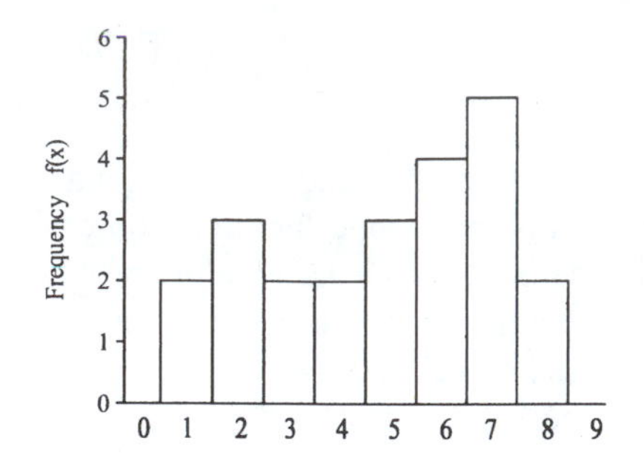


**Figure 5.3** Example of distributions with the same mean and median.

Some texts and statisticians prefer to correct for continuity (due to the fact that the continuous variable actually extends to one decimal smaller and larger than the measure). In Sample 1 listed above, 54 to 36, would be 54 to 36 inclusive or 54.5 to 35.5. In this case the range would be:

$$R = (largest\ observation\ -\ smallest\ observation) + 1$$

$$R = 54 - 36 + 1 = 19\ mg$$

If the range were measured in tenths, then 0.1 would be added; if the range is in hundredths, then add an additional 0.01, and so on.

A second measure of dispersion already discussed is the interquartile range. Even though the range and interquartile range are quick and easy measures of dispersion, they possess a limitation similar to the median; specifically they do not account for the actual numerical value of every individual observation. Much like the mean, a measure is needed to account for how *each* observation varies from the center of the distribution.

One possible measure would be to determine the distance between each value and the center (Figure 5.4). Unfortunately, because the distances to the left and to the right of the mean are equal (since the mean is the weighted center), the sum of all the individual differences ($\Sigma x_i - \overline{X}$) equals zero and provides no useful information. Therefore, the sum of all the squared differences between the individual observations and the mean is computed, and divided by the number of degrees of freedom (n – 1). This average of the squared deviations produces an intermediate measure known as the **sample variance**:

$$S^2 = \frac{(x_1 - \overline{X})^2 + (x_2 - \overline{X})^2 + (x_3 - \overline{X})^2 + \ldots + (x_n - \overline{X})^2}{n - 1}$$

**Degrees of freedom** (*df*) is used to correct for bias in the results that would occur if just the number of observations (*n*) was used in the denominator. If the **average squared deviation** is calculated by dividing the summed squared differences by *n*

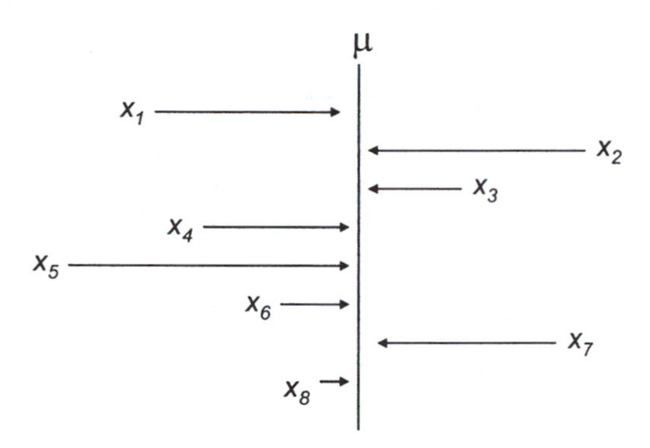


**Figure 5.4** Distribution of observations around the mean.

observations, it tends to underestimate the variance. The term "degrees of freedom" is best examined by considering the example where the sum of all the deviations ($x_i - \overline{X}$) equals zero. All but one number has the "freedom" to vary. Once we know all but the last data point ($n - 1$), we can predict the last value because the sum of all the deviations must equal zero. Therefore, to prevent bias, most statistical analyses involve degrees of freedom ($n - 1$) rather than the total sample size ($n$). The sample variance formula can be written:

$$S^2 = \frac{\Sigma(x_i - \overline{X})^2}{n-1} \quad \text{Eq. 5.3}$$

Obviously as the size of our sample of data increases, the effect of dividing by $n$ or $n$-1 becomes negligible. However, for theoretical purposes, degrees of freedom will continually appear in descriptive as well as inferential equations.

The variance, using the data from Example 5A (with a mean of 4.9), is calculated as follows:

$$S^2 = \frac{(2-4.9)^2 + (6-4.9)^2 + (7-4.9)^2 + \ldots(5-4.9)^2}{23-1} = 3.8$$

An easier method for calculating the variance would be as follows:

$$S^2 = \frac{n(\Sigma x^2) - (\Sigma x)^2}{n(n-1)} \quad \text{Eq. 5.4}$$

where each observation is squared and both the sum of the observation and the sum of the observations squared are entered into the formula. Algebraically, this produces the exact same results as the original variance formula (Eq. 5.3). Once again, using data from Example 5A, this method produces the same variance:

| $x_i$ | $x_i^2$ |
|---|---|
| 2 | 4 |
| 6 | 36 |
| ... | ... |
| 5 | 25 |
| 112 | 628 |

$$S^2 = \frac{n(\Sigma x^2) - (\Sigma x)^2}{n(n-1)} = \frac{23(628) - (112)^2}{23(22)}$$

$$S^2 = \frac{14444 - 12544}{506} = \frac{1900}{506} = 3.8$$

Variance is only an intermediate measure of dispersion. Each difference ($x_i - \overline{X}$) was squared to produce the variance term. The square root of the variance is needed to return the results to the same measurement scale used for the mean (for example, if the mean is expressed in mg, then this new measure (called the standard deviation will also be expressed as mg).

The **sample standard deviation** (*S* or *SD*) is the square root of the variance. It also measures variability about the mean and is most commonly used term to express the dispersion of the observations.

$$S = \sqrt{S^2} \qquad \text{Eq. 5.5}$$

Using the previous set of data as an example:

$$S = \sqrt{3.8} = 1.9$$

It is important to note that the variance has no relevant term of measurement, but the standard deviation is expressed in the same units as the mean. For the sake of illustration, consider the observations for the two samples of tablet weights in Example 5C:

| | $\overline{X}$ | $S^2$ | $S$ | $n$ |
|---|---|---|---|---|
| Sample 1 | 48.7 | 29.5 | 5.4 | 9 |
| Sample 2 | 54.4 | 42.3 | 6.5 | 9 |

In this case the average weights of the tablets in Sample 1 would be 48.7 mg with a standard deviation of 5.4 mg. The variance is simply 29.5, not 29.5 mg or mg squared.

**Table 5.1**. Data for Samples of Bottles of Cough Syrup

| Original Samples (volume in ml) | | | | Samples Ordered Smallest to Largest | |
|---|---|---|---|---|---|
| Sample | Volume | Sample | Volume | | |
| 1 | 120.7 | 16 | 119.0 | 118.3 | 120.1 |
| 2 | 120.2 | 17 | 121.1 | 118.5 | 120.1 |
| 3 | 119.6 | 18 | 121.7 | 118.9 | 120.1 |
| 4 | 120.1 | 19 | 119.2 | 119.0 | 120.2 |
| 5 | 121.3 | 20 | 120.0 | 119.0 | 120.2 |
| 6 | 120.7 | 21 | 120.8 | 119.2 | 120.4 |
| 7 | 121.0 | 22 | 119.9 | 119.6 | 120.5 |
| 8 | 119.7 | 23 | 119.8 | 119.7 | 120.7 |
| 9 | 118.3 | 24 | 119.9 | 119.7 | 120.7 |
| 10 | 118.9 | 25 | 120.2 | 119.8 | 120.8 |
| 11 | 120.5 | 26 | 120.0 | 119.8 | 121.0 |
| 12 | 121.4 | 27 | 120.1 | 119.9 | 121.1 |
| 13 | 120.4 | 28 | 119.0 | 119.9 | 121.3 |
| 14 | 118.5 | 29 | 120.1 | 120.0 | 121.4 |
| 15 | 119.8 | 30 | 119.7 | 120.0 | 121.7 |

To illustrate the use of central tendency measures, thirty bottles of a cough syrup are randomly sampled from a production line and the results are reported in Table 5.1. The descriptive statistics reporting the measures of central tendency for the sample would be:

Mode: 120.1 ml (largest frequency of 3 outcomes)

Median: the average of the center two values (15th and 16th ranks)

$$\frac{120.0+120.1}{2}=120.05\ ml$$

Mean: weighted average of all 30 samples

$$\overline{X}=\frac{120.7+120.2+...119.7}{30}=120.05\ ml$$

Range: 121.7 – 118.3 = 3.4 ml

Variance:

$$S^2=\frac{(120.7-120.05\,)^2+...(119.7-120.05\,)^2}{30(29)}=0.70$$

**Table 5.2** Symbols Used for Sample and Population Measures of Central Tendency

| | Sample Statistic | Population Parameter |
|---|---|---|
| Mean | $\overline{X}$ | $\mu$ |
| Variance | $S^2$ | $\sigma^2$ |
| Standard deviation | $S$ | $\sigma$ |
| Number of observations | $n$ | $N$ |

Standard deviation:

$$S = \sqrt{0.70} = 0.84\ ml$$

Lastly, since the standard deviation can be thought of as the square root of the mean of the squared deviations, some textbooks refer to variance as the **root mean square**, or **RMS** value.

**Population versus Sample Measures of Central Tendency**

The statistics presented thus far have represented means, variances, and standard deviations calculated for sample data and not an entire population. The major reason for conducting a statistical analysis is to use sample data as an estimate of the parameters for the entire population of events. For example; it is impractical, and impossible if destructive methods are used, to sample all the tablets in a particular batch. Therefore, compendia or in-house standards for content uniformity testing might consist of a sample of 30 tablets randomly selected from a batch of many thousands of tablets.

**Parameters** are to populations as **statistics** are to samples. As seen in Table 5.2, the observed statistics (mean and standard deviation from the sample) are the best estimates of the true population parameters (the population mean and population standard deviation). Note in Table 5.2 that the Greek symbols $\mu$ (mu) and $\sigma$ (sigma) are used to represent the population mean and population standard deviation, respectively. Also, in the formulas that follow, $N$ replaces $n$ for the total observations in a population. These symbols will be used throughout the book with Greek symbols referring to population parameters.

The **population mean** is calculated using a formula identical to the sample mean:

$$\mu = \frac{\sum_{i=1}^{N} X_i}{N} \qquad \text{Eq. 5.6}$$

The formula for the **population variance** is similar to that of the sample estimate, except that the numerator is divided by the number of all observations ($N$). If all the data is known about the population, it is not necessary to use degrees of freedom to correct for bias.

$$\sigma^2 = \frac{\sum_{i=1}^{N}(x_i - \mu)^2}{N} \qquad \text{Eq. 5.7}$$

Similar to the sample standard deviation, the **population standard deviation** is the square root of the population variance.

$$\sigma = \sqrt{\sigma^2} \qquad \text{Eq. 5.8}$$

One should be cautious using scientific or programmable calculators when computing the standard deviation. Some calculators may compute the population standard deviation, some the sample standard deviations and others can display both measures. It is important to know which measure of dispersion is calculated by your calculator, especially when dealing with smaller sample sizes. A quick and simple check to determine the type of standard deviation(s) displayed on a calculator is to enter the three values 1, 2, and 3. The mean is obviously 2.0. If a sample standard deviation ($S$) is calculated the result will be 1.0; whereas the population standard deviation ($\sigma$) is 0.8165.

**Measurements Related to the Sample Standard Deviation**

The variability of data may often be better described as a relative variation rather than as an absolute variation (i.e., the standard deviation). This can be accomplished by calculating the **coefficient of variation** ($CV$) that is the ratio of the standard deviation to the mean.

$$CV = \frac{\text{standard deviation}}{\text{mean}} \qquad \text{Eq. 5.9}$$

The $CV$ is usually expressed as a percentage (**relative standard deviation** or ***RSD***) and can be useful in many instances because it places variability in perspective to the distribution center.

$$RSD = CV \times 100 \text{ (percent)} \qquad \text{Eq. 5.10}$$

In the previous Example 5A ($CV = 1.94/4.87 = 0.398$ and $RSD = 0.398 \times 100 = 39.8$), the standard deviation is 40% of the mean. In the previous example of the liquid volumes (Table 5.1), the coefficient of variation and $RSD$ would be:

**Table 5.3** Examples with Relative Standard Deviations

| | Assayed Amount of Drug | | | % Labeled Claim |
|---|---|---|---|---|
| | 9.96 | 99.6 | 996 | 99.6 |
| | 10.05 | 100.5 | 1005 | 100.5 |
| | 9.92 | 99.2 | 992 | 99.2 |
| | 9.92 | 99.2 | 992 | 99.2 |
| | 9.86 | 98.6 | 986 | 98.6 |
| | 9.85 | 98.5 | 985 | 98.5 |
| | 10.01 | 100.1 | 1001 | 100.1 |
| | 9.90 | 99.0 | 990 | 99.0 |
| | 9.96 | 99.6 | 996 | 99.6 |
| | 9.86 | 98.6 | 986 | 98.6 |
| Mean = | 9.929 | 99.29 | 992.9 | 99.29 |
| S.D. = | 0.067 | 0.666 | 6.657 | 0.666 |
| RSD = | 0.67% | 0.67% | 0.67% | 0.67% |

$$CV = \frac{0.835}{120.05} = 0.007$$

$$RSD = 0.007 \times 100 = 0.7\%$$

Thus, relative standard deviations present an additional method of expressing this variability, which takes into account its relative magnitude (expressed as the ratio of the standard deviation to the mean). Table 5.3 illustrates the amount of assayed drug and the second and third columns represent 10- and 100-fold increases in the original values. These increases also result in a 10- and 100-fold increase in both the mean and standard deviation, but the relative standard deviation remains constant. In the pharmaceutical industry, this can be used as a measure of precision between various batches of a drug, if measures are based on percent label claim (column 4 in Table 5.3).

A second example illustrating the relative standard deviation would be the peak area on an HPLC reading:

| | HPLC Peak ($x$) | $x^2$ |
|---|---|---|
| Run 1 | 59.45 | 3534.30 |
| Run 2 | 59.50 | 3540.25 |
| Run 3 | 58.70 | 3445.69 |
| Run 4 | 59.25 | 3510.56 |
| | 236.90 | 14030.80 |

Measures of central tendency are as follows:

Mean:

$$\overline{X} = \frac{236.9}{4} = 59.23\ ml$$

Variance:

$$S^2 = \frac{4(14030.8) - (236.9)^2}{4(3)} = 0.13$$

Standard deviation:

$$S = \sqrt{0.13} = 0.36\ ml$$

Coefficient of variation:

$$C.V. = \frac{0.36}{59.23} = 0.0061$$

Relative standard deviation:

$$RSD = 0.0061\ x\ 100 = 0.61\%$$

**Trimmed Mean**

In certain software statistical packages a trimmed mean is reported in the descriptive results along with the algebraic mean. This measure represents the weighted center for the majority of the data, but "trims" the extreme values, usually 5%, from each end of the distribution. The remaining 90% of the data is then used to compute the mean. This offers two advantages over the traditional mean: 1) it eliminated outliers (Chapter 23); and 2) for positively or negatively skewer distributions it approximates the median and gives a better estimate of center. The disadvantages are that it could greatly decrease the variance for the sample data and may eliminate important information provided by outliers. In the case of a normal, bell-shaped distribution (Chapter 6), removal of 5% of the upper end of the distribution and removal of 5% of the lower end will not affect the mean because of the symmetry of the distribution. To illustrate this, consider three distributions (Figure 5.5) each representing a sample of 200 observations: 1) *A* is approximately normally distributed; 2) *B* is positively skewed; and 3) *C* is negatively skewed. Measures of center would be as follows:

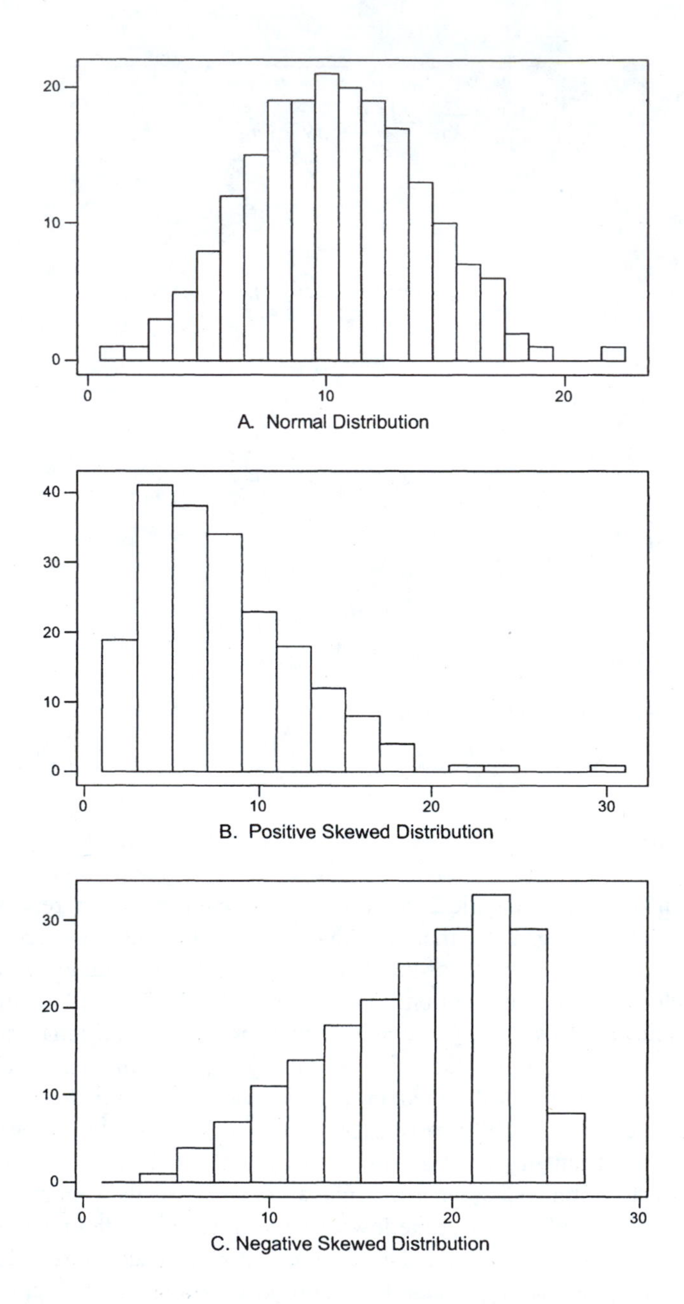


**Figure 5.5** Various distributions prior to trimming the mean.

| Distribution | Mean | Trimmed Mean | Median |
|---|---|---|---|
| A. Normal distribution | 10.37 | 10.35 | 10.0 |
| B. Positive skew | 7.470 | 7.144 | 7.0 |
| C. Negative skew | 17.545 | 17.767 | 18.0 |

The problem rests with the reduced spread when the data is trimmed:

| | Standard Deviation | |
|---|---|---|
| Distribution | Untrimmed | Trimmed |
| A. Normal distribution | 3.665 | 2.963 |
| B. Positive skew | 4.527 | 3.472 |
| C. Negative skew | 5.125 | 4.337 |

As seen in these examples, the standard deviation is decreased from 15.3 to 23.3% by simply removing the extreme 10% of the distribution.

**Alternative Computational Methods for Calculating Central Tendency**

Various other methods can be used to determine sample means and standard deviations. They include calculations from binomial distributions, probability distributions, and frequency distributions.

**Binomial Distribution**. As mentioned in Chapter 2, the binomial distribution is concerned with two mutually exclusive outcomes. If the probability of one of the outcomes is known, the mean (or **expected value**, *E(x)*) and standard deviation for the distribution can be calculated. In this case the measure of central tendency represents the mean and standard deviation of the values taken by the variable in many repeated binomial experiments. For example, if we flipped a fair coin 1000 times, we would expect on the average to have 500 heads (defined as success with $p = 0.50$). The mean is

$$\overline{X} \text{ or } E(x) = n \cdot p \qquad \text{Eq. 5.11}$$

with a variance of

$$S^2 \text{ or } Var(x) = n \cdot p \cdot q \qquad \text{Eq. 5.12}$$

and standard deviation of

$$S = \sqrt{n \cdot p \cdot q} \qquad \text{Eq. 5.13}$$

where $p$ is the probability of success, $q$ the probability of failure ($1.00 - p$) and $n$ is total number of outcomes or observations. The binomial distribution tends to the normal distribution as $n$ increases, however, in small samples the distribution may be noticeably skewed. For that reason, $np$ should be greater than 5 to use this approximation.

As an example, the probability of rolling a six on one toss of the die is 0.1667. If a single die is tossed 50 times what is the expected number of times a six will appear? What is the variability of this expected outcome? In this case $p(6) = 1/6 = 0.1667$; $q(\text{not } 6) = 1 - 0.1667 = 0.8333$; and $n$ is 50 for the sample size.

$$E(x) = np = (50)(0.1667) = 8.3$$

The average number of times six would appear in 50 rolls is 8.3 times. The standard deviation would be:

$$S = \sqrt{npq} = \sqrt{(50)(0.1667)(0.833)} = 2.6$$

**Probability Distribution**. If the probabilities of all possible outcomes are known, the mean and standard deviation for the distribution can be calculated by first creating a table:

| $x$ | $p(x)$ | $x \cdot p(x)$ | $x^2 \cdot p(x)$ |
|---|---|---|---|
| $x_1$ | $p(x_1)$ | $x_1 \cdot p(x_1)$ | $x_1 \cdot x_1 \cdot p(x_1)$ |
| $x_2$ | $p(x_2)$ | $x_2 \cdot p(x_2)$ | $x_2 \cdot x_2 \cdot p(x_2)$ |
| $x_3$ | $p(x_3)$ | $x_3 \cdot p(x_3)$ | $x_3 \cdot x_3 \cdot p(x_3)$ |
| ... | ... | ... | ... |
| $x_n$ | $p(x_n)$ | $x_n \cdot p(x_n)$ | $x_n \cdot x_n \cdot p(x_n)$ |
| $\Sigma =$ | 1.00 | $\Sigma(x \cdot p(x))$ | $\Sigma(x^2 \cdot p(x))$ |

where $x_i$ is the occurrence and $p(x_i)$ is the probability of that occurrence. The mean is represented by the third column:

$$\overline{X} = \Sigma(x \cdot p(x)) \qquad \text{Eq. 5.14}$$

The variance and standard deviations involve the sums of the third and fourth columns:

$$S^2 = [\Sigma(x^2 \cdot p(x))] - [\Sigma(x \cdot p(x))]^2 \qquad \text{Eq. 5.15}$$

$$S = \sqrt{[\Sigma(x^2 \cdot p(x))] - [\Sigma(x \cdot p(x))]^2} \qquad \text{Eq. 5.16}$$

To illustrate the process, what is the mean and standard deviation for the following values and their respective probabilities of occurrence?

| Value | Probability | Value | Probability | Value | Probability |
|---|---|---|---|---|---|
| 0 | 0.07776 | 4 | 0.11646 | 8 | 0.00017 |
| 1 | 0.22680 | 5 | 0.04042 | 9 | 0.00001 |
| 2 | 0.29700 | 6 | 0.00971 | 10 | 0.00000 |
| 3 | 0.22995 | 7 | 0.00150 | | |

| $x$ | $p(x)$ | $x \cdot p(x)$ | $x^2 \cdot p(x)$ |
|---|---|---|---|
| 1 | 0.22680 | 0.22680 | 0.22680 |
| 2 | 0.29700 | 0.59400 | 1.18800 |
| 3 | 0.22995 | 0.68985 | 2.06955 |
| 4 | 0.11646 | 0.46584 | 1.86336 |
| 5 | 0.04042 | 0.20210 | 1.01050 |
| 6 | 0.00971 | 0.05826 | 0.34956 |
| 7 | 0.00150 | 0.01050 | 0.07350 |
| 8 | 0.00017 | 0.00136 | 0.01088 |
| 9 | 0.00001 | 0.00009 | 0.00081 |
| 10 | 0.00000 | 0.00000 | 0.00000 |
| $\Sigma=$ | 1.00000 | 2.24880 | 6.79296 |

$$\overline{X} = \Sigma(x \cdot p(x)) = 2.2488 = 2.25$$

$$S^2 = [\Sigma(x^2 \cdot p(x))] - [\Sigma(x \cdot p(x))]^2$$

$$S^2 = 6.79296 - (2.24880)^2 = 1.74$$

$$S = \sqrt{S^2} = \sqrt{1.74} = 1.32$$

**Frequency Distribution.** If data is presented that reports the frequency of each occurrence (for example, the frequency of response to a Likert-type scale), the mean and standard deviation can be calculated as follows where $x_i$ is the event and $f(x_i)$ is the frequency associated with that event.

| $x$ | $f(x)$ | $x \cdot f(x)$ | $x^2 \cdot f(x)$ |
|---|---|---|---|
| $x_1$ | $f(x_1)$ | $x_1 \cdot f(x_1)$ | $x_1 \cdot x_1 \cdot f(x_1)$ |
| $x_2$ | $f(x_2)$ | $x_2 \cdot f(x_2)$ | $x_2 \cdot x_2 \cdot f(x_2)$ |
| $x_3$ | $f(x_3)$ | $x_3 \cdot f(x_3)$ | $x_3 \cdot x_3 \cdot f(x_3)$ |
| ... | ... | ... | ... |
| $x_n$ | $f(x_n)$ | $x_n \cdot f(x_n)$ | $x_n \cdot x_n \cdot f(x_n)$ |
| $\Sigma=$ | $\Sigma f(x) = N$ | $\Sigma(x \cdot f(x))$ | $\Sigma(x^2 \cdot f(x))$ |

The mean is:

$$\overline{X} = \frac{\Sigma(x \cdot f(x))}{N} \qquad \text{Eq. 5.17}$$

In this case $N$ represents the sum of all the sample frequencies ($n_1 + n_2 ... + n_i$) and not a population $N$. The variance is:

$$S^2 = \frac{N\,[\Sigma(x^2 \cdot f(x))] - [\Sigma(x \cdot f(x))]^2}{N(N-1)} \qquad \text{Eq. 5.18}$$

with a standard deviation of:

$$S = \sqrt{\frac{N[\Sigma(x^2 \cdot f(x))] - [\Sigma(x \cdot f(x))]^2}{N(N-1)}} \qquad \text{Eq. 5.19}$$

For an example using a frequency distribution, a final examination in which 12 pharmacy students scored 10 points, 28 scored 9, 35 scored 8, 26 scored 7, 15 scored 6, 8 scored 5, and one student scored 4. What is the mean and standard deviation on this final examination?

| $x$ | $f(x)$ | $x \cdot f(x)$ | $x^2 \cdot f(x)$ |
|---|---|---|---|
| 10 | 12 | 120 | 1200 |
| 9 | 28 | 252 | 2268 |
| 8 | 35 | 280 | 2240 |
| 7 | 26 | 182 | 1274 |
| 6 | 15 | 90 | 540 |
| 5 | 8 | 40 | 200 |
| 4 | 1 | 4 | 16 |
| $\Sigma=$ | 125 | 968 | 7738 |

$$\overline{X} = \frac{\Sigma(x \cdot f(x))}{N} = \frac{968}{125} = 7.74$$

$$S^2 = \frac{N\,[\Sigma(x^2 \cdot f(x))] - [\Sigma(x \cdot f(x))]^2}{N(N-1)} = \frac{125(7738) - (968)^2}{125(124)} = 1.95$$

$$S = \sqrt{S^2} = \sqrt{1.95} = 1.40$$

**Central Tendency from a Histogram.** An estimate of the mean and standard deviation involves using the frequency distribution and the midpoint of each interval:

$$Midpoint = \frac{highest + lowest\ points}{2} = \frac{705.5 + 716.5}{2} = 711 \qquad \text{Eq. 5.20}$$

A table can be prepared by tabulating the midpoint and their associated frequencies:

| Interval Range | Midpoint ($m_i$) | Frequency ($f_i$) | $m_if_i$ | $m_i^2f_i$ |
|---|---|---|---|---|
| Interval 1 | $m_1$ | $f_1$ | $m_1f_1$ | $m_1^2f_1$ |
| Interval 2 | $m_2$ | $f_2$ | $m_2f_2$ | $m_2^2f_2$ |
| Interval 3 | $m_3$ | $f_3$ | $m_3f_3$ | $m_3^2f_3$ |
| ... | ... | ... | ... | ... |
| Interval n | $m_n$ | $f_n$ | $m_nf_n$ | $m_n^2f_n$ |
| | $\Sigma=$ | $n$ | $\Sigma m_if_i$ | $\Sigma m_i^2f_i$ |

The midpoint of each class interval, $m_i$, was weighted by its corresponding frequency of occurrence, $f_i$. The computation of the mean and standard deviation involves a table similar to that used for frequency distributions discussed under central tendency. With a mean of

$$\overline{X} = \frac{\Sigma m_i f_i}{N} \qquad \text{Eq. 5.21}$$

a variance of

$$S^2 = \frac{n(\Sigma m_i^2 f_i) - (\Sigma m_i f_i)^2}{n(n-1)} \qquad \text{Eq. 5.22}$$

and a standard deviation as the square root of the variance or

$$S = \sqrt{\frac{n(\Sigma m_i^2 f_i) - (\Sigma m_i f_i)^2}{n(n-1)}} \qquad \text{Eq. 5.23}$$

Using the pharmacokinetic example in Chapter 4 (Table 4.3), the mean and standard deviation are calculated below. How accurate is the measure of the mean and standard deviation using Sturge's Rule to create the histogram? The data is presented in Table 5.4 and the calculation of the mean and standard deviation using the above formulas are presented below. The sample statistics for all the observations presented in the original table of $C_{max}$ is: Mean = 752.4 mcg and S.D. = 16.8 mcg. In this particular case, there is less than 5% difference between the means and standard deviations, which were calculated from the raw data and calculated from the

**Table 5.4** Intervals Created Using Sturge's Rule for Table 4.3

| Interval Range | Midpoint | Frequency | $m_if_i$ | $m_i^2f_i$ |
|---|---|---|---|---|
| 705.5-716.5 | 711 | 2 | 1,422 | 1,011,042 |
| 716.5-727.5 | 722 | 6 | 4,332 | 3,127,704 |
| 727.5-738.5 | 733 | 18 | 13,194 | 9,671,202 |
| 738.5-749.5 | 744 | 22 | 16,368 | 12,177,792 |
| 749.5-760.5 | 755 | 35 | 26,425 | 19,950,875 |
| 760.5-771.5 | 766 | 28 | 21,448 | 16,429,168 |
| 771.5-782.5 | 777 | 10 | 7,770 | 6,037,290 |
| 782.5-793.5 | 788 | 4 | 3,152 | 2,483,776 |
| | Σ = | 125 | 94,111 | 70,888,849 |

intervals created by Sturge's Rule.

$$\overline{X} = \frac{94{,}111}{125} = 752.9\ mcg$$

$$S^2 = \frac{125(70{,}888{,}849) - (94{,}111)^2}{125(124)}$$

$$S^2 = \frac{4{,}225.804}{15{,}500} = 272.63$$

$$S = \sqrt{S^2} = \sqrt{272.63} = 16.51\ \ mcg$$

If one were interested in calculating the median for a histogram the following formula could be used:

$$Median = L + w \cdot \left( \frac{\frac{n}{2} - F}{f} \right)$$

where $L$ is the lower limit of the interval that contains the median, $w$ is the width of the class interval for each interval, $n$ is the total sample size, $F$ is the cumulative frequency corresponding to the lower limit of the interval (cumulative frequency for all the intervals in the histrogram below the one containing the median) and $f$ is the number of observations in the interval that contains the median. Using the example in Table 5.4, the interval with the median is 749.5-760.5, because 48 observations fall below 749.5 mcg (38.4%) and 83 observations are below 760.5 mcg (66.4%). With a width of 11 mcg, the median is:

$$Median = 749.5 + 11 \cdot \left( \frac{\frac{125}{2} - 48}{35} \right) = 754.1$$

**References**

Evans, D.A.P., et al. (1960). "Genetic control of isoniazid metabolism in man," *British Medical Journal* 2:489.

Torbeck, L.D. (2004). "Significant digits and rounding," *Pharmacopeial Forum* 30(3):1090-1095.

**Suggested Supplemental Readings**

Daniel, W.W. (1999). *Biostatistics: A Foundation for Analysis in the Health Sciences*, Seventh edition, John Wiley and Sons, New York, pp. 36-43.

Forthofer, R.N. and Lee, E.S. (1995). *Introduction to Biostatistics: A Guide to Design, Analysis and Discovery*, Academic Press, San Diego, pp. 61-67, 71-77.

Snedecor, G.W. and Cochran W.G. (1989). *Statistical Methods*, Iowa State University Press, Ames, IA, pp. 26-36.

**Example Problems**

1. Pharmacy students completing the final examination for a pharmacokinetics course received the following scores. Report the range, median, mean, variance, and standard deviation for these results.

| Student | % | Student | % | Student | % | Student | % |
|---|---|---|---|---|---|---|---|
| 001 | 85 | 009 | 78 | 017 | 77 | 025 | 97 |
| 002 | 79 | 010 | 85 | 018 | 83 | 026 | 76 |
| 003 | 98 | 011 | 77 | 019 | 87 | 027 | 69 |
| 004 | 84 | 012 | 86 | 020 | 78 | 028 | 86 |
| 005 | 72 | 013 | 90 | 021 | 60 | 029 | 80 |
| 006 | 84 | 014 | 84 | 022 | 88 | 030 | 92 |
| 007 | 70 | 015 | 75 | 023 | 87 | 031 | 85 |
| 008 | 90 | 016 | 96 | 024 | 82 | 032 | 80 |

2. Calculate the measures of central tendency for noradrenaline levels (nmol/L) obtained during a clinical trial involving 15 subjects.

| | | | | |
|---|---|---|---|---|
| 2.5 | 2.6 | 2.5 | 2.4 | 2.4 |
| 2.5 | 2.5 | 2.6 | 2.5 | 2.6 |
| 2.3 | 2.7 | 2.3 | 2.8 | 2.2 |

3. Calculate the measures of central tendency for prolactin levels (ng/L) obtained during a clinical trial involving 10 subjects.

| | | | | |
|---|---|---|---|---|
| 9.4 | 7.0 | 7.6 | 6.3 | 6.7 |
| 8.6 | 6.8 | 10.6 | 8.9 | 9.4 |

4. In a study designed to measure the effectiveness of a new analgesic agent, 8 mg of drug was administered to 15 laboratory animals. The animals were subjected to the Randall-Selitto paw pressure test and the following results (in grams) were observed.

| Number | Response | Number | Response | Number | Response |
|---|---|---|---|---|---|
| 1 | 240 | 6 | 260 | 11 | 265 |
| 2 | 295 | 7 | 275 | 12 | 240 |
| 3 | 225 | 8 | 245 | 13 | 260 |
| 4 | 250 | 9 | 225 | 14 | 275 |
| 5 | 245 | 10 | 260 | 15 | 250 |

Calculate the mean, median, variance, and standard deviation for this data.

**Answers to Problems**

1. Final examination results for a pharmacokinetics course (Table 5.5):

   a. Range: Highest to lowest grade = 98 – 60 = 38 percent

   b. Median: Value between 16th and 17th observation = 84 percent

   c. Sample mean

$$\overline{X} = \frac{\sum x}{n} = \frac{85+79+98+\ldots 85+80}{32} = 82.4 \ percent$$

   d. Sample variance

$$S^2 = \frac{(85-82.4)^2+(79-82.4)^2+\ldots(80-82.4)^2}{31} = 67.16$$

**Table 5.5** Examination Results Ranked in Descending Order

| | | | |
|---|---|---|---|
| 98 | 87 | 84 | 77 |
| 96 | 86 | 83 | 77 |
| 95 | 86 | 82 | 76 |
| 92 | 85 | 80 | 75 |
| 90 | 85 | 80 | 72 |
| 90 | 85 | 79 | 70 |
| 88 | 84 | 78 | 69 |
| 87 | 84 | 78 | 60 |

e. Sample standard deviation

$$S = \sqrt{S^2} = \sqrt{67.16} = 8.19 \text{ percent}$$

2. Noradrenaline levels obtained during a clinical trial.

| | $x$ | $x^2$ | |
|---|---|---|---|
| | 2.5 | 6.25 | |
| | 2.5 | 6.25 | |
| | 2.3 | 5.29 | |
| | 2.6 | 6.76 | |
| | 2.5 | 6.25 | |
| | 2.7 | 7.29 | |
| | 2.5 | 6.25 | |
| | 2.6 | 6.76 | |
| | 2.3 | 5.29 | |
| | 2.4 | 5.76 | |
| | 2.5 | 6.25 | |
| | 2.8 | 7.84 | |
| | 2.4 | 5.76 | |
| | 2.6 | 6.76 | |
| | 2.2 | 4.84 | |
| $\sum x =$ | 37.4 | 93.60 | $= \sum x^2$ |

Mean:

$$\overline{X} = \frac{\sum x}{n} = \frac{37.4}{15} = 2.49 \text{ nmol/L}$$

Variance:

$$S^2 = \frac{n(\sum X^2) - (\sum X)^2}{n(n-1)} = \frac{15(93.6) - (37.4)^2}{(15)(14)} = 0.025$$

Standard Deviation:

$$S = \sqrt{S^2} = \sqrt{0.025} = 0.158 \ nmol / L$$

3. Prolactin levels obtained during a clinical trial.

| | x | $x^2$ | |
|---|---|---|---|
| | 9.4 | 88.36 | |
| | 8.6 | 73.96 | |
| | 7.0 | 49.00 | |
| | 6.8 | 46.24 | |
| | 7.6 | 57.76 | |
| | 10.6 | 112.36 | |
| | 6.3 | 39.69 | |
| | 8.9 | 79.21 | |
| | 6.7 | 44.89 | |
| | 9.4 | 88.36 | |
| $\sum x =$ | 81.3 | 679.83 | $= \sum x^2$ |

Mean:

$$\overline{X} = \frac{\sum x}{n} = \frac{81.3}{10} = 8.13 \ ng/L$$

Variance:

$$S^2 = \frac{\sum(x_i - \overline{X})^2}{n-1}$$

$$S^2 = \frac{(9.4 - 8.13)^2 + (8.6 - 8.13)^2 \ldots + (9.4 - 8.13)^2}{9} = 2.096$$

Standard deviation:

$$S = \sqrt{S^2} = \sqrt{2.096} = 1.45 \ ng / L$$

4. Randall-Selitto paw pressure test and the following results (in grams) were observed.

$$\sum x = 3{,}810 \qquad \sum x^2 = 972{,}800 \qquad n = 15$$

Sample mean:

$$\overline{X} = \frac{\sum x}{n} = \frac{3810}{15} = 254 \text{ grams}$$

Sample variance:

$$S^2 = \frac{n(\sum X^2) - (\sum X)^2}{n(n-1)} = \frac{15(972{,}800) - (3{,}810)^2}{15(14)} = 361.4$$

Sample standard deviation:

$$S = \sqrt{S^2} = \sqrt{361.4} = 19.0 \text{ grams}$$

Median = eighth response in rank order = 250 grams

# 6

# The Normal Distribution and Data Transformation

Described as a "bell-shaped" curve, the normal distribution is a symmetrical distribution that is one of the most commonly occurring outcomes in nature and its presence is assumed in several of the most commonly used statistical tests. Properties of the normal distribution have a very important role in the statistical theory of drawing inferences about population parameters (estimating confidence intervals) based on samples drawn from that population.

New since the first edition of this book is an expanded section on ways to transform initial data to produce distributions approximating a normal distribution and a discussion of various graphic and mathematical methods for testing normality.

## The Normal Distribution

The normal distribution is the most important distribution in statistics. This curve is a special frequency distribution that describes the population distribution of many continuously distributed biological traits. The normal distribution is often referred to as the **Gaussian distribution**, after the mathematician Carl Friedreich Gauss, even though it was first discovered by the French mathematician Abraham DeMoivre (Porter, 1986).

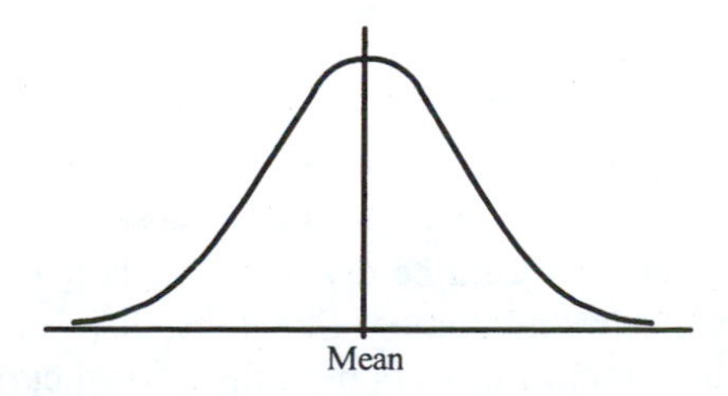


It is critical at this point to realize that we are focusing our initial discussion on the *total population, not a sample*. As mentioned in the previous chapter, in the population, the mean is expressed as $\mu$ and standard deviation as $\sigma$.

The characteristics of a normal distribution are as follows. First, the normal

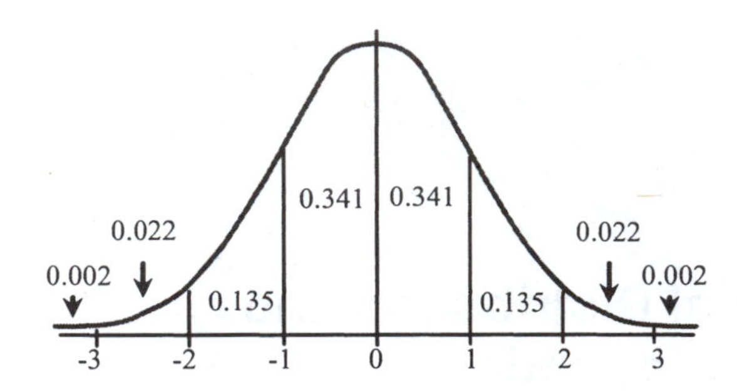


**Figure 6.1** Proportions between various standard deviations under a normal distribution.

distribution is continuous and the curve is symmetrical about the mean. Second, the mode, median, and mean are equal and represent the middle of the distribution. Third, since the mean and median are the same, the 50th percentile is at the mean with an equal amount of area under the curve, above and below the mean. Fourth, the probability of all possible outcomes is equal to 1.0, therefore, the total area under the curve is equal to 1.0. Since the mean is the 50th percentile, the area to left or right of the mean equals 0.5. Fifth, by definition, the area under the curve between one standard deviation above and one standard deviation below the mean contains an area equal to approximately 68% of the total area under the curve. At two standard deviations this area is approximately 95%. Sixth, as distance from the mean (in the positive or negative direction) approaches infinity, the frequency of occurrences approaches zero. This last point illustrates the fact that most observations cluster around the center of the distribution and very few occur at the extremes of the distribution. Also, if the curve is infinite in its bounds we cannot set absolute external limits on the distribution.

The frequency distribution (curve) for a normal distribution is defined as follows:

$$f_i = \frac{1}{\sigma\sqrt{2\pi}} e^{-(x_i-\mu)^2/2\sigma^2} \qquad \text{Eq. 6.1}$$

where: $\pi$ (pi) = 3.14159 and $e$ = 2.71828 (the base of natural logarithms).

In a normal distribution, the area under the curve between the mean and one standard deviation is approximately 34%. Because of the symmetry of the distribution, 68% of the curve would be divided equally above and below the mean. Why 34%? Why not a nice round number like 35%, 30%, or even better, 25%? The standard deviation is that point of inflection on the normal curve where the frequency distribution stops its descent to the baseline and begins to pull parallel with the x-axis. Areas or proportions of the normal distribution associated with various standard deviations are seen in Figure 6.1.

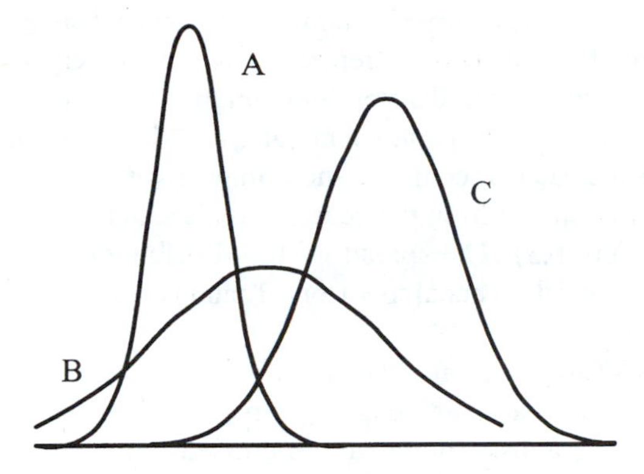


**Figure 6.2** Example of three normal distributions with different means and different standard deviations.

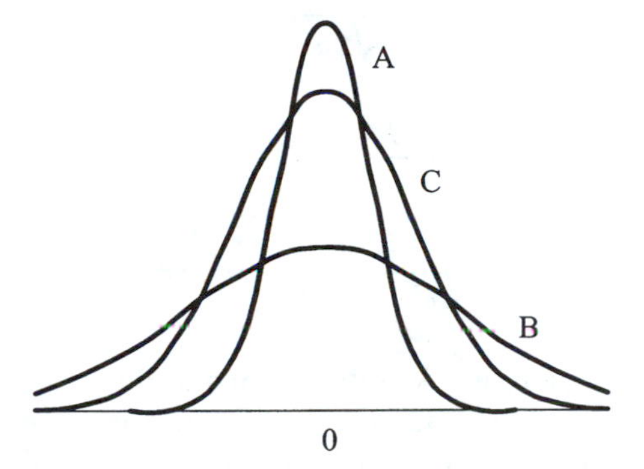


**Figure 6.3** Example of three normal distributions with the same mean and different standard deviations.

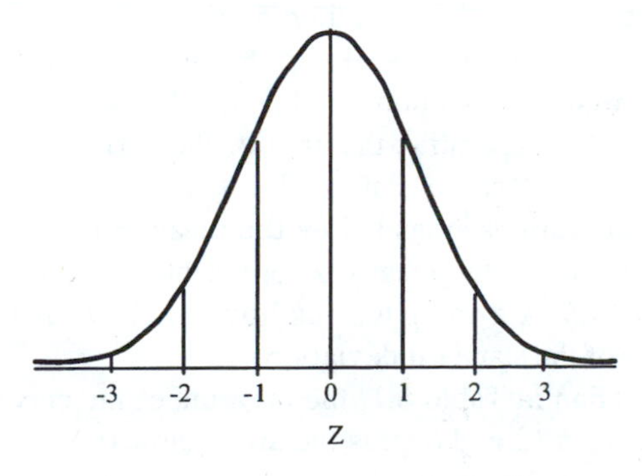


**Figure 6.4** Standard normal distribution.

The term "*the* bell-shaped curve" is a misnomer since there are many bell-shaped curves, ranging from those that are extremely peaked with very small ranges to those that are much flatter with wide distributions (Figure 6.2). A normal distribution is completely dependent on its parameters of $\mu$ and $\sigma$. A standardized normal distribution has been created to compare and compute variations in such a distribution regardless of center or spread from the center. In this standard normal distribution the mean equals 0 (Figure 6.3). The spread of the distribution is also standardized by setting one standard deviation equal to +1 or –1, and two standard deviations equal to +2 or –2 (Figure 6.4).

As seen previously, the area between +2 and –2 is approximately 95%. Additionally, fractions of a standard deviation are calculated and their equivalent areas presented. If such a distribution can be created (with a mean equal to zero and standard deviation equal to one) then the equation for the frequency distribution (Eq. 6.1) can be simplified to:

$$f_i = \frac{1}{\sqrt{2\pi}} e^{-(x_i)^2/2}$$

$$f_i = \frac{1}{2.5066272} 2.71828^{-(x_i)^2/2}$$

$$f_i = 1.084437\Gamma^{(x_i)^2/2} \qquad \text{Eq. 6.2}$$

Table 6.1 is an abbreviation of a **standard normal distribution** (a more complete distribution is presented in Table B2 in Appendix B, where every hundredth of the z-distribution is defined between 0.01 to 3.69). An important feature of the standard normal distribution is that the number of standard deviations away from the population mean can be expressed as a given percent or proportion of the area of the curve. The symbol z, by convention, symbolizes the number of standard deviations away from the population mean. The numbers in these tables represent the area of the curve that falls between the mean (z = 0) and that point on the distribution above the mean (i.e., z = +1.5, would be the point at 1.5 standard deviations above the mean). Since the mean is the 50th percentile, the area of the curve that falls below the mean (or below zero) is .5000. Because a normal distribution is symmetrical, this table could also represent the various areas below the mean. For example, for z = –1.5 (or 1.5 standard deviations below the mean), z represents the same area from 0 to –1.5, as the area from 0 to +1.5. A z-value tells us how far above and below the mean any given score is in units of the standard deviation.

Using the information in Table 6.1, the area under the curve that falls below +2 would be the area between +2 and 0, plus the area below 0.

Area (<+2) = Area (between 0 and +2) + Area (below 0)
Area (<+2) = .4772 + .5000 = .9772

**Table 6.1** Selected Areas of a Normal Standardized Distribution (Proportion of the Curve between 0 and z)

| z | Area | z | Area | z | Area |
|---|---|---|---|---|---|
| .00 | .0000 | 1.00 | .3413 | 2.00 | .4772 |
| .05 | .0199 | 1.05 | .3531 | 2.05 | .4798 |
| .10 | .0398 | 1.10 | .3543 | 2.10 | .4821 |
| .15 | .0596 | 1.15 | .3749 | 2.15 | .4842 |
| .20 | .0793 | 1.20 | .3849 | 2.20 | .4861 |
| .25 | .0987 | 1.25 | .3944 | 2.25 | .4878 |
| .30 | .1179 | 1.30 | .4032 | 2.30 | .4893 |
| .35 | .1368 | 1.35 | .4115 | 2.35 | .4906 |
| .40 | .1554 | 1.40 | .4192 | 2.40 | .4918 |
| .45 | .1736 | 1.45 | .4265 | 2.45 | .4929 |
| .50 | .1915 | 1.50 | .4332 | 2.50 | .4938 |
| .55 | .2088 | 1.55 | .4394 | 2.55 | .4946 |
| .60 | .2257 | 1.60 | .4452 | 2.60 | .4953 |
| .65 | .2422 | 1.65 | .4505 | 2.65 | .4960 |
| .70 | .2580 | 1.70 | .4554 | 2.70 | .4965 |
| .75 | .2734 | 1.75 | .4599 | 2.75 | .4970 |
| .80 | .2881 | 1.80 | .4641 | 2.80 | .4974 |
| .85 | .3023 | 1.85 | .4678 | 2.85 | .4978 |
| .90 | .3159 | 1.90 | .4713 | 2.90 | .4981 |
| .95 | .3289 | 1.95 | .4744 | 2.95 | .4984 |

These probabilities can be summed because of the addition theorem discussed in Chapter 2.

All possible events would fall within this standard normal distribution ($p\Sigma(x)$ = 1.00). Since the probability of all events equals 1.00 and the total area under the curve equals 1.00, then various areas within a normalized standard distribution can also represent probabilities of certain outcomes. In the above example, the area under the curve below two standard deviations (represented as +2) was .9972. This can also be thought of as the probability of an outcome being less than two standard deviations above the mean. Conversely, the probability of being two or more standard deviations above the mean would be 1.0000 – .9772 or .0228.

Between three standard deviations above and below the mean, approximately 99.8% of the observations will occur. Therefore, assuming a normal distribution, a quick method for roughly approximating the standard deviation is to divide the range of the observations by six, since almost all observations will fall within these six intervals. For example, consider the data in Table 4.3. The true standard deviation for this data is 16.8 mcg. The range of 86 mcg, divided by six would give a rough approximation of 14.3 mcg.

It is possible to calculate the probability of any particular outcome within a normal distribution. The areas within specified portions of our curve represent the probability of the values of interest lying between the vertical lines. To illustrate this, consider a large container of tablets (representing a total population) that is expected to be normally distributed with respect to the tablet weight. What is the probability of randomly sampling a tablet that weighs within 1.5 standard deviations of the mean?

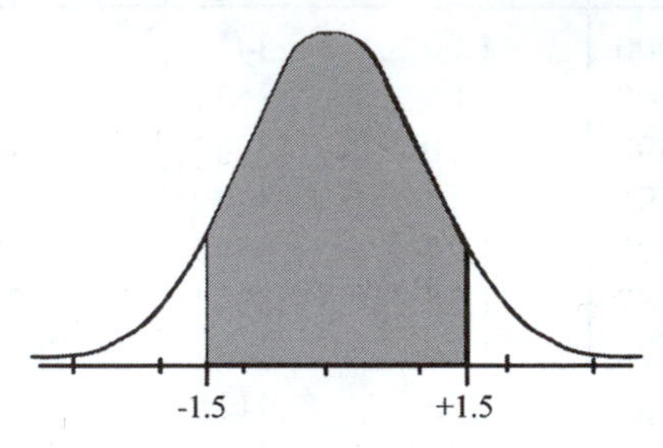


Because weight is a continuous variable, we are concerned with p(>–1.5 or <+1.5). From Table 6.1:

$$
\begin{array}{lr}
p(z<+1.5) = \text{Area between 0 and } +1.5 = & .4332 \\
p(z>-1.5) = \text{Area between 0 and } -1.5 = & \underline{.4332} \\
p(z\ -1.5 \text{ to } +1.5) = & .8664
\end{array}
$$

There is a probability of .8664 (or 87% chance) of sampling a tablet within 1.5 standard deviations of the mean. What is the probability of sampling a tablet greater than 2.25 standard deviations above the mean?

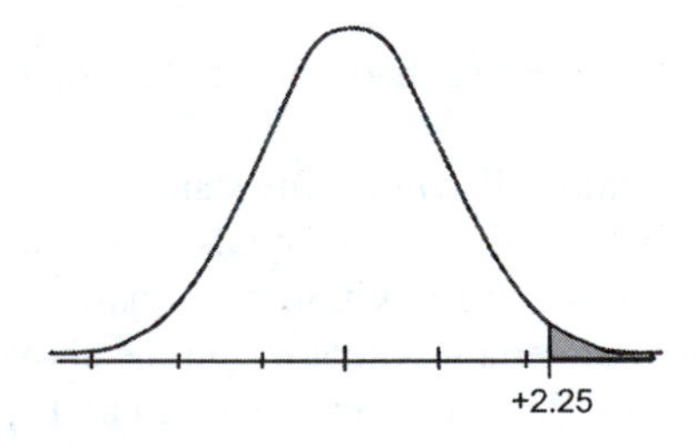


First, we know that the total area above the mean is .5000. By reading Table 6.1, the area between 2.25 standard deviations (z = 2.25) and the mean is .4878 (the area between 0 and +2.25). Therefore the probability of sampling a tablet weighing more than 2.25 standard deviations above the mean weight is:

$$p(z>+2.25) = .5000 - .4878 = .0122$$

If we wish to know the probability of a tablet being less than 2.25 standard deviations above the mean, the complement probability of being less than a z-value of +2.25 is:

$$p(z<+2.25) = 1 - p(z>+2.25) = 1.000 - .0122 = .9878$$

Also calculated as:

$$p(z<+2.25) = p(z<0) + p(z<2.25) = .5000 + .4878 = .9878$$

If the mean and standard deviation of a population are known, the exact location (z above or below the mean) for any observation can be calculated using the following formula:

$$z = \frac{x - \mu}{\sigma} \qquad \text{Eq. 6.3}$$

Because values in a normal distribution are on a continuous scale and are handled as continuous variables, we must correct for continuity. Values for *x* would be as follows:

Likelihood of being: greater then 185 mg = $p(>185.5)$;
less than 200 mg = $p(<199.5)$;
200 mg or greater = $p(>199.5)$; and
between and including 185 and 200 mg = $p(>184.5 \text{ and } <200.5)$.

To examine this, consider a sample from a known population with expected population parameters (previous estimates of the population mean and standard deviation, for example based on prior production runs). With an expected population mean assay of 750 mg and a population standard deviation of 60 mg, what is the probability of sampling a capsule with an assay greater than 850 mg?

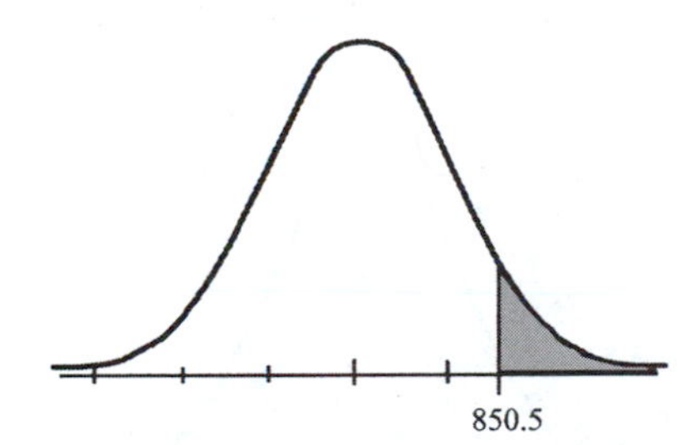


As a continuous variable, the $p(>850 \text{ mg})$ is actually $p(>850.5 \text{ mg})$ when corrected for continuity.

$$z = \frac{x - \mu}{\sigma} = \frac{850.5 - 750}{60} = \frac{100.5}{60} = +1.68$$

$$p(z>+1.68) = .5000 - p(z<1.68)$$
$$= .5000 - .4535 = .0465$$

Given the same population as above, what is the probability of randomly sampling a capsule with an assay between 700 and 825 mg?

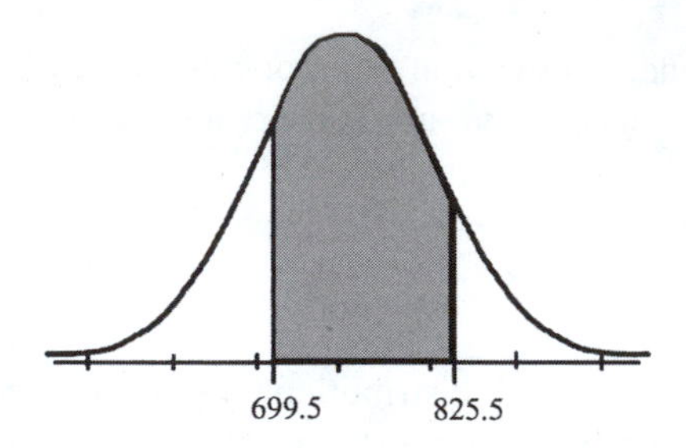


Once again correcting for continuity, p(<825 mg) is rewritten as p(<825.5 mg) and p(>700 mg) is really p(>699.5 mg).

$$z = \frac{x - \mu}{\sigma} = \frac{825.5 - 750}{60} = \frac{75.5}{60} = +1.26$$

$$z = \frac{x - \mu}{\sigma} = \frac{699.5 - 750}{60} = \frac{-50.5}{60} = -0.84$$

$$\begin{aligned} \text{p(between 699.5 and 825.5)} &= p(z<+1.26) + p(z>-0.84) \\ &= .3962 + .2995 = .6957 \end{aligned}$$

Given the same population, what is the probability of randomly sampling a capsule with an assay less than 600 mg?

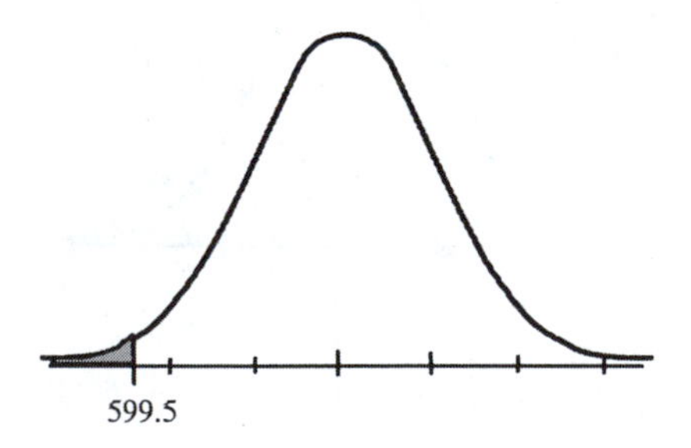


As a continuous variable, p(<600 mg) is p(>599.5 mg):

$$z = \frac{x - \mu}{\sigma} = \frac{599.5 - 750}{60} = \frac{-150.5}{60} = -2.5$$

$$\begin{aligned} p(z<-2.5) &= .5000 - p(z<2.5) \\ &= .5000 - .4938 = .0062 \end{aligned}$$

Thus, in these examples with the given population mean and standard deviation, the likelihood of randomly sampling a capsule greater than 850 mg is approximately 5%, a capsule less than 600 mg is less than 1%, and a capsule between 700 and 825 mg is almost 70%.

Lastly, the probability of obtaining any one particular value is zero, but we can determine probabilities for specific ranges. Correcting for continuity, the value 750 (the mean) actually represents an infinite number of possible values between 749.5 and 750.5 mg. The area under the curve between the center and the upper limit would be

$$z = \frac{x-\mu}{\sigma} = \frac{750.5-750}{60} = \frac{0.5}{60} = +0.01$$

$$p(z<0.01) = .004$$

Since there would be an identical area between 749.5 and the mean, the total proportion associated with 750 mg would be

$$p(750\ mg) = .008$$

In the previous examples we knew both the population mean ($\mu$) and the population standard deviation ($\sigma$). However, in most statistical investigations this information is not available and formulas must be employed that use estimates of these parameters based on the sample results.

Important z-values related to other areas under the curve for a normal distribution include:

$$90\%\ -1.64 < z < +1.64$$
$$95\%\ -1.96 < z < +1.96$$
$$99\%\ -2.57 < z < +2.57$$

## Determining if the Distribution is Normal

The sample used in a study is our best guess of the characteristics of the population: the center, the dispersion, and the shape of the distribution. Therefore, the appearance of the sample is our best estimate if the population is normally distributed. In the absence of any information that would disprove normality, it is assumed that a normal distribution exists (i.e., initial sample does not look extremely skewed or bimodal).

One quick method to determine if the population is normally distributed is to determine if the sample mean and median are approximately equal. If they are about the same (similar in value) then the population probably has a normal distribution. If the mean is substantially greater than the median, the population is probably positively skewed and if the mean is substantially less than the median, a negatively skewed population probably exists.

Normality can be estimated visually by looking at a histogram or box plot of the sample data, or by plotting data on graph paper or probability paper. Using a **box-and-whisker plot** (described in Chapter 4), it would reflect a normally distributed population if the top and bottom lines of the box plot (25th and 75th percentiles) were approximately equidistant from the center line (the median). Visually inspecting a **histogram** can indicate if the distribution for sample data is approximately normal, with most of the result clustering near the center and few observations at each end of the distribution. A **scatter plot** (also described in Chapter 4) can use sample data to plot a theoretical cumulative distribution functions (cdf) on the x-axis against actual cumulative distribution functions on the y-axis. If normality exists a straight line will be produced. Finally a scatter plot reflecting a **quantile-by-quantile plot,** with the expected cumulative distributions by quintiles for a normal distribution on one axis and of the quantiles for the observed sample data on the other axis, should create a 45° line. The quantile-by-quantile plot could be used in a similar manner for other well-defined distributions.

Two other similar visual methods to determine if sample data is consistent with expectations for a normal distribution are to plot a **cumulative frequency curve** using normal graph paper or a **normal probability plot** use special graph paper known as **probability paper.** In a cumulative frequency curve, data is arranged in order of increasing size and plotted on normal graph paper:

$$\%\,cumulative\ frequency = \frac{cumulative\ frequency}{n} \, x\, 100$$

If the data came from a normally distributed population, the result will be an S-shaped curve.

Probability paper (i.e., National #12-083 or Keuffel and Esser #46-8000) has a unique nonlinear scale on the cumulative frequency axis that will convert the S-shaped curve to a straight line. The normal probability plot or P-P plot will produce a 45° straight line can be drawn through the percent cumulative frequency data points if the estimated population is normally distributed. If the curvilinearly relationship exists, the population distribution is skewed. Using the distribution presented in Table 6.2, Figure 6.5 illustrates the data presented as a: a) box-and-whisker plot; b) histogram; 3) cumulative frequency curve; and 4) probability plot.

As mentioned in Chapter 4, **kurtosis** is the characteristic of a frequency distribution that refers to the shape of the distribution of values regarding its relative flatness and peakedness. It indicates the extent to which a distribution is more peaked or flat-topped than a normal distribution. For the normal distribution, the theoretical kurtosis value equals zero and the distribution is described as mesokurtic. If the distribution has long tails (relatively larger tails), the statistic will be greater than zero and called leptokurtic. The kurtosis value can be estimated using sample data:

**Table 6.2.** Assay Results for 100 Randomly Sampled Tablets

| Tablet Assay | f | cf |
|---|---|---|
| 112 | 1 | 1 |
| 116 | 1 | 2 |
| 117 | 2 | 4 |
| 118 | 2 | 6 |
| 119 | 4 | 10 |
| 120 | 5 | 15 |
| 121 | 7 | 22 |
| 122 | 8 | 30 |
| 123 | 8 | 38 |
| 124 | 10 | 48 |
| 125 | 11 | 59 |
| 126 | 7 | 66 |
| 127 | 8 | 74 |
| 128 | 6 | 80 |
| 129 | 6 | 86 |
| 130 | 3 | 89 |
| 131 | 3 | 92 |
| 132 | 2 | 94 |
| 133 | 2 | 96 |
| 134 | 1 | 97 |
| 135 | 1 | 98 |
| 137 | 1 | 99 |
| 140 | 1 | 100 |

$$Kurtosis = \frac{\sum (x - \overline{X})^4}{nS^4} - 3 \qquad \text{Eq. 6.4}$$

A rule-of-thumb kurtosis should be within the +3 to −3 range when the data are normally distributed. Negative kurtosis means there are too many cases in the tails of the distribution; where as a positive kurtosis reflects too few cases in the tails. Using the data presented in Table 6.2, the mean is 124.95 with a standard deviation of 4.63, the kurtosis is:

$$Kurtosis = \frac{(112 - 124.95)^4 + (116 - 124.95)^4 \ldots + (140 - 124.95)^4}{100(4.63)^4} - 3$$

$$Kurtosis = \frac{168{,}534.58}{45954.07} - 3 = 0.67$$

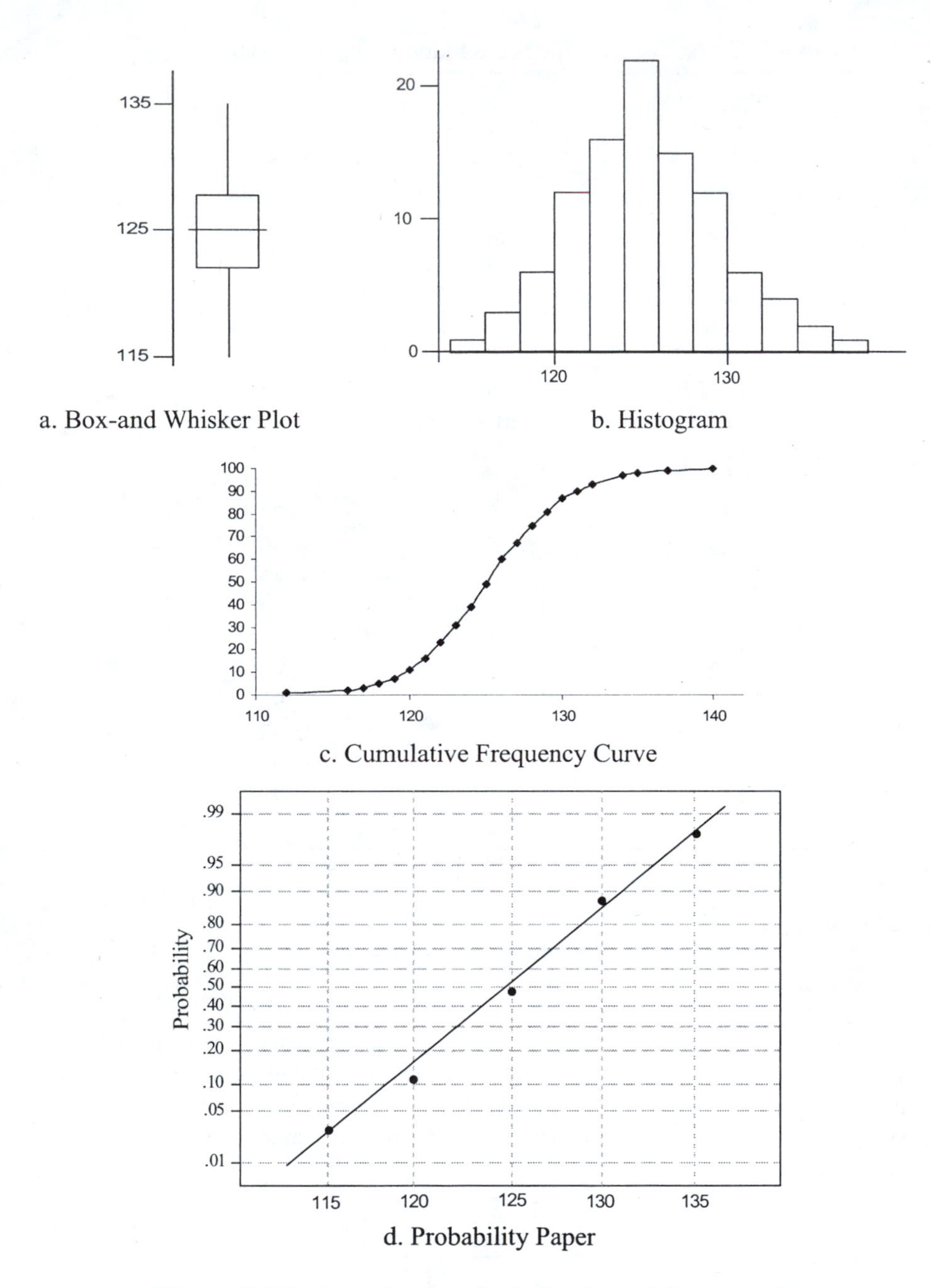


a. Box-and Whisker Plot

b. Histogram

c. Cumulative Frequency Curve

d. Probability Paper

**Figure 6.5** Various visual methods for determining normality.

The result is well below a +3 and one can assume normality, which is similar to the visual results observed in Figure 6.5.

Several statistical procedures exist to test for population normality based on sample data. These tests include: 1) chi-square goodness-of-fit test; 2) the Kolmogorov-Smirnov D test; 4) Anderson-Darling test; 5) the Lilliefors test and 6) Shapiro-Wilk's W test. Both the **chi-square goodness-of-fit test** and **Kolmogorov-Smirnov test** will be described in Chapters 16 and 21, respectively, with fully worked out examples.

Both the **Anderson-Darling test** and **Lilliefors test** are modifications of the K-S test and the latter is sometimes referred to as the **Kolmogorov-Smirnov Lilliefors test**. Without the Lilliefors correction, the Kolmogorov-Smirnov test (K-S test) is more conservative (greater likelihood of a rejecting normality). The Anderson-Darling test gives more weight to the talkies of the distribution than the K-S test. When sample size is large, one should be cautious because even small deviations from normality can be significant with the K-S test or chi-square goodness-of-fit tests. Information about these tests can be found in D'Agostino and Stephens (1986).

The **Shapiro-Wilk's W test** is another standard test for normality and is recommended for smaller sample sized (2000 or less). It is conducted by regressing the quantiles of the observed data against that of the best-fit for the normal distribution. The Shapiro-Wilk's W-statistics is calculated as follows.

$$W = \frac{\left(\sum a_i x_i\right)^2}{\sum\left(x_i - \overline{X}\right)^2} \qquad \text{Eq. 6.5}$$

where the $x_i$ are the ordered sample values ($x_{(1)}$ is the smallest) and the $a_i$'s are coefficients from a table, based on the means and variances of the ordered statistics of a sample from a normal distribution (Shapiro and Wilk, 1965). The resultant W-statistic (ranging from 0 to 1) is then compared to a table of critical values. Computer software computes the W-statistic and corresponding p-value. A significant statistic (small values for W, with corresponding p-value $<0.05$) would result in the reject the assumption that the sample comes from a normally distributed population.

All of the previously mentioned tests are classified as **empirical distribution function** statistics or EDF tests. They involve making a good guess of the "true distribution function" (in this case a normal distribution) and by using the observed results from a random sample. Graphs can be constructed, where the empirical distribution function, *S(x)*, is always a step function and each step has a height *1/n*. These graphs and/or the above statistics computed to determine the amount of discrepancy there is between the theoretical, *F(x)* distribution and the experimental (empirical) results.

**Data Transformations: An Overview**

A normal distribution is defined by its mean ($\mu$) and its standard deviation ($\sigma$). When a sample is taken from a normal distribution population, $\overline{X}$ and $s$ summarize all of the information available in the sample about the parent distribution. Unfortunately, the ability to use $\overline{X}$ and $s$ as summary statistics does not apply to nonnormal distributions. Certain inferential statistics, such as confidence intervals (Chapter 7), cannot be applied, and if applied, intervals tend to be wider and tests of hypothesis (Chapter 8) have less power. Also, as will be seen in future chapters, inferential statistical tests are based on assumptions and the validity of results obtained from these tests will depend on how well these assumptions were met. One assumption for several commonly used tests (i.e., t-test, F-test, correlation) is that the data is sampled from a normally distributed population. As seen in the previous section it is possible graphically or through statistical procedures to determine if the population (via sample results) is normally distributed. What if the population is assumed to be nonnormal in its distribution? Through the use of various transformation procedures, nonnormally distributed data can be altered to create a new distribution that approximates the symmetric bell-shaped curve of a normal distribution. We have already seen an example of data transformation when we created a standard normal distribution where a normal distribution was created with a mean of 0 and a standard deviation of 1. Distributions were standardized by changing the original data points to standard scores (z-scores) using Eq. 6.3.

**Lognormal Transformation and the Geometric Mean**

The most commonly encountered transformations are involved with populations that appear to be positively skewed. In this case, **logarithmic** or **lognormal transformations** are used to when most of the values are to the left of the distribution (near zero) and few values are in the right side of the curve. This process involves converting each number to its logarithmic form:

$$x_i' = log(x_i) \qquad \text{Eq. 6.6}$$

Logarithms in base 10 are usually used, but any base would be satisfactory. Use of data transformations should make theoretical sense. Note that as the log of zero is undefined and will leads to error messages. If zeros are present in the sample, one can pick an arbitrary small value (i.e., 0.0001) and replace all zeros with that value. Some statisticians prefer the following equation based on theoretical grounds and is preferred when dealing with small number of observations. Also, this equation removes the problem of dealing with zeros:

$$x_i' = log(x_i + 1) \qquad \text{Eq. 6.7}$$

Either transformation can be used if the variable effects are multiplicative rather than additive.

For calculating the center of the logarithmic transformation of data, the **geometric mean** is reported. Because of the few extreme values to the right of the curve, the arithmetic mean ($\overline{X}$) would be "pulled" to the right. Performing a logarithmic transformation would produce a distribution that is approximately a normal distribution and the final mean will be more to the "left" and thus closer to the

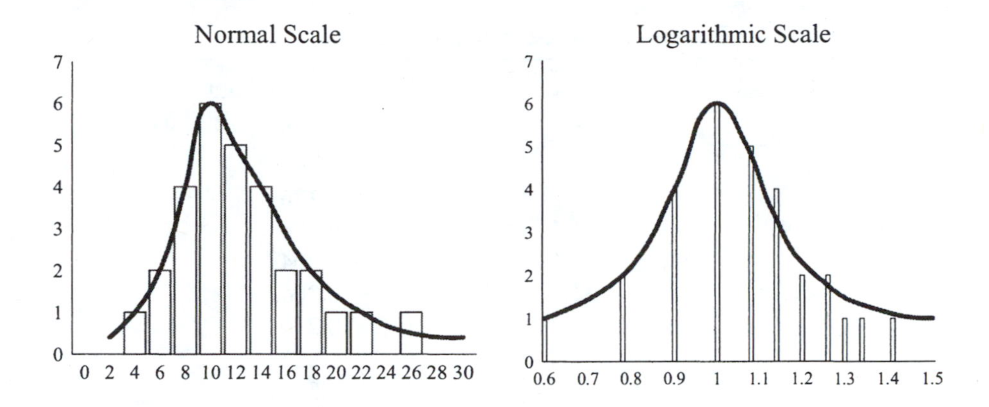


**Figure 6.6** Comparisons of data on a normal and logarithmic scale.

median of the original distribution.

This process involves converting each number to its logarithmic form (Eq. 6.6 or Eq. 6.7). These values are summed and divided by the total number of observations to produce an average logarithmic value. This value is then converted back to real numbers by taking the antilog, which represents the geometric mean.

$$\overline{X}_G = antilog\left(\frac{\sum log(x_i)}{n}\right) \qquad \text{Eq. 6.8}$$

Illustrated below are two sets of identical data, with the left on a normal scale and the right using a logarithmic scale. Notice the dotted line on the normal scale appears to be skewed while the logarithmic scale appears to be more bell-shaped. A positively skewed distribution, as seen above, is often referred to as a **log-normal distribution** (Figure 6.6).

To illustrate this process, consider the $T_{max}$ data observed in 12 health volunteers, which appears in Table 6.3. The arithmetic mean ($\overline{X}$) is 2.33 and the median is 1.65. The few extreme scores in this skewed distribution have pulled the mean to the right of the median. The conversion to a logarithmic transformation of scores is seen in the last column of Table 6.3. The mean for the logarithmic transformed scores is:

$$Average\ log = \frac{0.079 + 0.146 + \ldots 0.857}{12} = 0.304$$

Converted back to the antilog, the geometric mean is:

$$\overline{X}_G = antilog\ (0.304) = 2.01$$

**Table 6.3** $T_{max}$ Results in Ascending Order

| Subject | $T_{max}$ | Log Transformation |
|---|---|---|
| 3 | 1.2 | 0.079 |
| 5 | 1.4 | 0.146 |
| 9 | 1.5 | 0.176 |
| 10 | 1.5 | 0.176 |
| 12 | 1.6 | 0.204 |
| 1 | 1.6 | 0.204 |
| 6 | 1.7 | 0.230 |
| 2 | 1.8 | 0.255 |
| 8 | 2.1 | 0.322 |
| 4 | 2.6 | 0.415 |
| 11 | 3.8 | 0.580 |
| 7 | 7.2 | 0.857 |
| Σ = | 28.0 | 3.644 |

If Eq. 6.7 were used to calculate the log values the geometric mean would be reported as the antilog of the mean minus one. Notice that the geometric mean is much closer to the median of the original distribution of $T_{max}$ data. An alternate formula for calculating the geometric mean is to take the *nth* root of the product of all the observations:

$$\overline{X}_G = \sqrt[n]{product\ of\ all\ data} \qquad \text{Eq. 6.9}$$

This gives the same result as the logarithmic transformation.

$$\overline{X}_G = \sqrt[12]{1.2 \times 1.4 \times 1.5 \times ... 7.2} = 2.01$$

If Eq. 6.8 were used, one would be added to each value and one subtracted from the final result.

## Other Types of Transformations

The **square-root transformation** is similar to the lognormal transformation and useful for more positively skewed data. The transformed data is the square-root of each original measurement and is used when the data consist of counts.

$$x_i' = \sqrt{x_i} \qquad \text{Eq. 6.10}$$

or

$$x_i' = \sqrt{x_i + 0.5} \qquad \text{Eq. 6.11}$$

The square-root transformation is useful when the sample means are approximately proportional to the variances of the samples. Using the second equation (Eq. 6.11) avoids potential problems with zeros in the data and is useful for small data sets. This can be helpful for Poisson distributions, for example, counts associated with rare events such as number of defects in a production run.

The **reciprocal transformation** is also for positively skewed data. Also called **inverse transformation**, this can be used when standard deviation is proportional to the square root of the mean and data is clustering near zero:

$$x_i' = \frac{1}{x_i} \qquad \text{Eq. 6.12}$$

or

$$x_i' = \frac{1}{x_i + 1} \qquad \text{Eq. 6.13}$$

For example, a few patients may take a very long time to respond to a given therapy and cause a skewed distribution. The reciprocal transformation helps make this type of data more symmetrical. Thus, there are three transformation that can be used to normalize positively skewed data (logarithmic, square root, and reciprocal transformations). The inverse (reciprocal) transformation can be used for the most extreme cases of positive skewing. For less severely skewed data the recommended transformation is logarithmic and the square root for the least positively skewed distribution. For Poisson distributions it is recommended to normalize the distribution using the square root transformation.

Theoretically, proportions for binomial distribution are approximately normally distributed when $p$ is near 0.50. However, as $p$ goes to extremes (0 to 20% and 80 to 100%), normality is lost. If the square root of each proportion in a binomial distribution is transformed to its arcsine, the resultant proportions $p'$ will have a distribution that is approximately normal.

$$p' = arcsin\sqrt{p} \qquad \text{Eq. 6.14}$$

This transformation is referred to as the **arcsine transformation, arcsine square root transformation, angular transformation,** or **inverse sine tranformation**. This transformation is used only when the data are proportions or percents.

For data that is negatively skewed data (tailing to the left), subtract each data point from the largest data point and add one to each resulting value. This will result in a positively skewed distribution. This positively skewed distribution, based on the severity of the skew, can be transformed using square root, logarithmic, or inverse transforms. If the data is negatively skewed for proportional data ($0 \leq p \leq 1$) a different log transformation equation can be employed:

$$x_i' = log\left(\frac{x}{1-x}\right) \qquad \text{Eq. 6.15}$$

If transformations are used to modify the data to produce data that assumes the shape of a normal distribution, then mathematical manipulations for the subsequent statistical test are performed on the transformed data, not the original data.

## References

D'Agostino, R. and Stephens, M. (1986). *Goodness-of-Fit Techniques*. Marcel Dekker, New York, pp. 102-184, 372-373.

Kachigan, S.K. (1991). *Multivariate Statistical Analysis*, Second edition, Radius Press, New York, pp. 89-90.

Porter, T.M. (1986). *The Rise of Statistical Thinking*, Princeton University Press, Princeton, NJ, p. 93.

Shapiro, S.S. and Wilk, M.B. (1965). "An analysis of variance test for normality (complete samples)," *Biometrika* 52 (3 and 4): 591-611.

## Suggested Supplemental Readings

Box, G.E.P. and Cox, D.R. (1964)."An analysis of transformations," *Journal of the Royal Statistical Society*, B 26: 211-234.

Natrella, M.G. "The use of transformations," *Experimental Statistics*, National Bureau of Standards Handbook 9, U.S. Department of Commerce, Washington, DC, 1963, pp. 20.1-20.13.

Stephens, M.A. (1974). "EDF statistics for goodness of fit and some comparisons," *Journal of the American Statistical Association* 69(347): 730-737.

## Example Problems

1. Listed in Table 6.4 are the times to maximum concentration observed during a clinical trial. It is believed that the data is positively skewed. Calculate the median, mean, and geometric mean. Based on the sample, does the population appear to be positively skewed?

2. Recalculate the data in Table 6.4 using the square root and reciprocal transformation methods. Calculate the transformed mean and then transform the mean back into the original units of measure.

**Table 6.4** Clinical Trial Results - $T_{max}$ (in hours)

| Subject | $t_{max}$ | Subject | $t_{max}$ | Subject | $t_{max}$ |
|---|---|---|---|---|---|
| A | 1.41 | F | 1.96 | K | 1.62 |
| B | 1.81 | G | 0.78 | L | 1.15 |
| C | 3.25 | H | 1.51 | M | 2.03 |
| D | 1.37 | I | 1.18 | N | 2.21 |
| E | 1.09 | J | 2.56 | O | 0.91 |

**Table 6.5** $t_{max}$ Results in Ascending Order

| Subject | $t_{max}$ | Subject | $t_{max}$ |
|---|---|---|---|
| G | 0.78 | K | 1.62 |
| O | 0.91 | B | 1.81 |
| E | 1.09 | F | 1.96 |
| L | 1.15 | M | 2.03 |
| I | 1.18 | N | 2.21 |
| D | 1.37 | J | 2.56 |
| A | 1.41 | C | 3.25 |
| H | 1.51 | $\Sigma =$ | 24.84 |

**Answers to Problems**

1. Clinical trials data with possible skewed data (Table 6.5):

   a. Median = 1.51 hours

   b. Arithmetic mean

$$\overline{X} = \frac{\Sigma x}{n} = \frac{24.84}{15} = 1.66 \text{ hours}$$

   c. Geometric mean

$$\overline{X}_G = \sqrt[n]{\text{product of all data}}$$

$$\overline{X}_G = \sqrt[15]{0.78 \times 0.91 \times 1.09 \times \ldots 3.25} = 1.54$$

It can be assumed that the distribution is positively skewed, because the mean is larger than the median (pulled to the right) and the geometric mean is much closer to the median.

**Table 6.6** Clinical Trial Results – $T_{max}$ (Square-root and Reciprocal Tranformations)

| Subject | $t_{max}$ | Square root | Reciprocal |
|---|---|---|---|
| A | 1.41 | 1.187 | 0.709 |
| B | 1.81 | 1.345 | 0.552 |
| C | 3.25 | 1.803 | 0.308 |
| D | 1.37 | 1.170 | 0.730 |
| E | 1.09 | 1.044 | 0.917 |
| F | 1.96 | 1.400 | 0.510 |
| G | 0.78 | 0.883 | 1.282 |
| H | 1.51 | 1.229 | 0.662 |
| I | 1.18 | 1.086 | 0.847 |
| J | 2.56 | 1.600 | 0.391 |
| K | 1.62 | 1.273 | 0.617 |
| L | 1.15 | 1.072 | 0.870 |
| M | 2.03 | 1.425 | 0.493 |
| N | 2.21 | 1.487 | 0.452 |
| O | 0.91 | 0.954 | 1.099 |

2. Clinical trials data with possible skewed data, values for alternative transformations appear in Table 6.6:

   a. Mean based on the square-root transformation

$$\overline{X}_{transformed} = \frac{\sum x_i'}{n} = \frac{18.96}{15} = 2.37$$

$$\overline{X} = (\overline{X}_{transformed})^2 = (2.37)^2 = 5.62 \text{ hours}$$

   Note, since there were no zeros in the responses Eq. 6.10 was used in the transformation. If Eq. 6.11 were used the result would be 6.92. The lognormal transformation would be preferable because the transformed mean is closest to the median.

   b. Mean based on the reciprocal transformation

$$\overline{X}_{transformed} = \frac{\sum x_i'}{n} = \frac{10.44}{15} = 1.31$$

$$\overline{X} = \frac{1}{\overline{X}_{transformed}} = \frac{1}{1.31} = 0.766 \text{ hours}$$

Note, since there were no zeros in the responses Eq. 6.12 was used in the transformation. If Eq. 6.13 were used the result would be 0.34. The lognormal transformation would be preferable because the transformed mean is closest to the median.

Notice that the reciprocal transformation creates the greatest change in the mean (intended for the extremely positive skewed data) and the square root the last change in the mean (intended to lesser positively skewed distributions).

# 7

# Confidence Intervals and Tolerance Limits

Intervals can be created to estimate population characteristics based on sample data. Confidence intervals estimate the true population mean based on the best estimator available, the sample means. Although we will never know the exact population mean we can create a range of possible values for the mean and know that the population mean is located within that interval. Similarly, we can use tolerance limits to once again use the sample mean and sample standard deviation to estimate range within which we would expect to find a certain percentage of the observations. In both cases, we can never be 100% certain of our results, but can assume we are correct with a certain amount of confidence in the intervals we create.

## Sampling Distribution

If we have a population and withdraw a random sample of observations from that population, we could calculate a sample mean and a sample standard deviation. As mentioned previously, this information would be our best estimate of the true population parameters.

$$\bar{X}_{\text{sample}} \approx \mu_{\text{population}}$$
$$S_{\text{sample}} \approx \sigma_{\text{population}}$$

The characteristics of dispersion or variability are not unique to samples alone. Individual samples can also vary around the population mean. Just by chance, or luck, we could have sampled from the upper or lower ends of the population distribution and calculated a sample mean that was too high or too low. Through no fault of our own, our estimate of the population mean would be erroneous.

To illustrate this point, let us return to the pharmacokinetic data used in Chapter 4. From this example, we will assume that the data in Table 4.3 represented the *entire population* of pharmacokinetic studies ever conducted on this drug. Due to budgetary restraints or time, we were only able to analyze five samples from this population.

How many possible ways could five samples be randomly selected from this data? Based on the combination formula (Eq. 2.11) there would be

$$\binom{125}{5} = \frac{125!}{5!\,120!} = 234{,}531{,}275$$

possible ways. Thus, it is possible to sample these 125 values in over 234 million different ways and because they are sampled at random, each possible combination has an equal likelihood of being selected. Therefore, by chance alone we could sample the smallest five values in our population (Sample A) or the largest five (Sample D) or any combination in between these extremes (Table 7.1). Samples B and C were generated using the Random Numbers Table B1 in Appendix B.

The mean is a more efficient estimate of the center, because with repeated samples of the same size from a given population, the mean will show less variation than either the mode or the median. Statisticians have defined this outcome as the central limit theorem and its derivation is beyond the scope of this book. However, there are three important characteristics that will be utilized in future statistical tests.

1. The mean of all possible sample means is equal to the mean of the original population from which they were sampled.

$$\overline{X}_{\overline{X}} = \mu \qquad \text{Eq. 7.1}$$

   If we averaged all 234,531,275 possible sample means, this grand mean or **mean of the mean** would equal the population mean ($\mu$ = 752.4 mcg for N = 125) from which they were sampled.

2. The standard deviation for all possible sample means is equal to the population standard deviation divided by the square root of the sample size.

$$\sigma_{\overline{X}} = \frac{\sigma}{\sqrt{n}} \qquad \text{Eq. 7.2}$$

   Similar to the mean of the sample means, the standard deviation for all the possible means would equal the population standard deviation divided by the square root of the sample size. The standard deviation for the means is referred to as the **standard error of the mean** or **SEM**.

3. Regardless of whether the population is normally distributed or skewed, if we plot all the possible sample means, the frequency distribution will approximate that of a normal distribution, based on the **central limit theorem**. This theorem is critical to many

**Table 7.1** Possible Samples from Population Presented as Table 4.3

| | Sample A | Sample B | Sample C | Sample D |
|---|---|---|---|---|
| | 706 | 731 | 724 | 778 |
| | 714 | 760 | 752 | 785 |
| | 718 | 752 | 762 | 788 |
| | 720 | 736 | 734 | 790 |
| | 724 | 785 | 775 | 793 |
| Mean = | 716.4 | 752.8 | 749.4 | 786.8 |
| S.D. = | 6.8 | 21.5 | 20.6 | 5.7 |

statistical formulas because it justifies the assumption of normality. This will approximate a normal distribution, regardless of the distribution of the original population, when the sample size is relatively large. However, a sample size as small as n=30 will often result in a near-normal sampling distribution (Kachigan, 1991).

If all 234,531,275 possible means were plotted, they would produce a frequency distribution that is normally distributed. Because the sample means are normally distributed, values in the normal standardized distribution (z distribution) will also apply to the distribution of sample means. For example, of all the possible sample means:

68% fall within + or – 1.00 SEM
90% fall within + or – 1.64 SEM
95% fall within + or – 1.96 SEM
99% fall within + or – 2.57 SEM

The distribution of the mean will be a probability distribution, consisting of various values and their associated probabilities, and if we sample from any population, the resultant means will be distributed on a normal bell-shaped curve. Most will be near the center and 5% will be outside 1.96 standard deviations of the distribution.

**Standard Error of the Mean versus the Standard Deviation**

As seen in the previous section, in a sampling distribution, the overall mean of the means would be equal to the population mean and the dispersion would depend on the amount of variance in the population. Obviously, the more we know about our population (the larger the sample size), the better our estimate of the population center. The best estimate of the population standard deviation is the sample standard deviation, which can be used to replace the $\sigma$ in Eq. 7.2 to produce a standard error of the mean based on sample data:

$$S_{\bar{x}} = \frac{S}{\sqrt{n}} = SEM \qquad \text{Eq. 7.3}$$

The standard deviation (S or SD) describes the variability within a sample; whereas, the standard error of the mean (SEM) represents the possible variability of the mean itself. The SEM is sometimes referred to as the **standard error** (SE) and describes the variation of all possible sample means and equals the SD of the sample data divided by the square root of the sample size. As can be seen by the formula, the distribution of sample means (the standard error of the mean) will always be smaller than the dispersion of the sample (the standard deviation).

Authors may erroneously present the distribution of sample results by using the SEM to represent information because there appears to be less variability. This may be misleading since the SEM has a different meaning than the SD. The SEM is smaller than the SD and the intentional presentation of the SEM instead of the larger SD is a manipulation to make data look more precise. The SEM is extremely important in the estimation of a true population mean, based on sample results. However, because it is disproportionately low, it should never be used as a measure of the distribution of sample results. For example, the SEM from our previous example of liquid fill volumes (Table 5.1) is much smaller (by a factor of almost six) than the calculated standard deviation:

$$SEM = \frac{0.835}{\sqrt{30}} = 0.152$$

By convention, the term standard error refers to the variability of a sampling distribution. However, authors still use the standard error of the mean to present sample distributions, because the SEM is much smaller than the SD and presents a much smaller variation of the results. An even more troublesome occurrence is the failure of authors to indicate in reports or publications whether a result represents an SD or an SEM. For example, poster or report simply states "456.1 ± 1.3" with no indication of what the term to the right of the ± sign represents. Is this a very tight SD? Is it the SEM? Could it even be the RSD? Without proper labeling, the reader would never know what the dispersion term represents.

Standard error of the mean can be considered as a measure of precision. Obviously, the smaller the SEM, the more confident we can be that our sample mean is closer to the true population mean. However, at the same time, large increases in sample size produce relatively small changes in this measure of precision. For example, using a constant sample SD of 21.5 for sample B, presented above, the measure of SEM changes very little as sample sizes increase past 30 (Figure 7.1). A general rule of thumb is that with samples of 30 or more observations, it is safe to use the sample standard deviation as an estimate of population standard deviation.

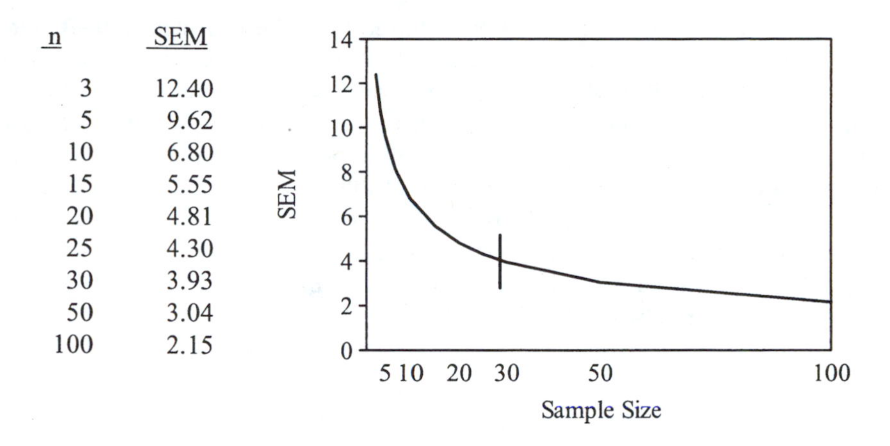

| n | SEM |
|---|---|
| 3 | 12.40 |
| 5 | 9.62 |
| 10 | 6.80 |
| 15 | 5.55 |
| 20 | 4.81 |
| 25 | 4.30 |
| 30 | 3.93 |
| 50 | 3.04 |
| 100 | 2.15 |



**Figure 7.1** Variation in standard error of the means by sample size.

## Confidence Intervals

As discussed in Chapter 5, using a random sample and independent measures, one can calculate measures of central tendency ($\bar{X}$ and $S$). The result represents only one sample that belongs to a distribution of many possible sample means. Because we are dealing with a sample and in most cases do not know the true population parameters, we often must make a statistical "guess" at these parameters. For example, the previous samples A through D (Table 7.1) all have calculated means, any of which could be the true mean for the population from which they were randomly sampled. In order to define the true population mean, we need to allow for a range of possible means based on our estimate:

$$\begin{matrix}\textit{Population} \\ \textit{Mean}\end{matrix} = \begin{matrix}\textit{Estimate} \\ \textit{Sample Mean}\end{matrix} \pm \begin{matrix}\textit{"Fudge"} \\ \textit{Factor}\end{matrix}$$

This single estimate of the population mean (based on the sample) can be referred to as a **point estimate**. The result is a range of possible outcomes defined as **boundary values**, **interval estimators**, or **confidence limits**. At the same time, we would like to have a certain amount of confidence in our statement that the population mean falls within these boundary values. For example, we may want to be 95% certain that we are correct, or 99% certain. Note again that because it is a sample, not an entire population, we cannot be 100% certain of our prediction. The only way to be 100% certain would be to measure every item in the population and in most cases that is either impractical or impossible to accomplish. Therefore, in order to have a certain confidence in our decision (i.e., 95% or 99% certain) we need to add to our equation a factor to allow us this confidence:

$$\begin{matrix}\textit{Population} \\ \textit{Mean}\end{matrix} = \begin{matrix}\textit{Estimate} \\ \textit{Sample Mean}\end{matrix} \pm \begin{matrix}\textit{Reliability} \\ \textit{Coefficient}\end{matrix} \; x \; \begin{matrix}\textit{Standard} \\ \textit{Error}\end{matrix} \qquad \text{Eq. 7.4}$$

This reliability coefficient (sometime referred to as the **confidence coefficient**) can be obtained from the normal standardized distribution. For example if we want to be certain 95% of the time, we will allow an error 5% of the time. We could err on the high side or low side and if we wanted our error divided equally between the two extremes, we would allow a 2.5% error too high in our estimation and 2.5% too low in our estimate of the true population mean. In Table B2 of Appendix B we find that 95% of the area under the curve falls between –1.96 z and +1.96 z. This follows the theory of the normal distribution where 95% of the values, or in this case sample means, fall within 1.96 standard deviations of the mean. The actual calculation for the 95% confidence interval would be:

$$\mu = \overline{X} \pm Z_{(1-\alpha/2)} \times \frac{\sigma}{\sqrt{n}} \qquad \text{Eq. 7.5}$$

The symbol $\alpha/2$ will be defined in the next chapter. For the time being, assume $\alpha/2$ is represented by 1.96 for the case of a 95% confidence interval and the equation would be:

$$\mu = \overline{X} \pm (1.96)\frac{\sigma}{\sqrt{n}}$$

The standard error term or standard error of the mean term, is calculated based on the population standard deviation and specific sample size. If the confidence interval were to change to 99% or 90%, the reliability coefficient would change to 2.57 and 1.64, respectively (based on values in Table B1 where 0.99 and 0.90 of the area fall under the curve). In creating a range of possible outcomes instead of one specific measure, “it is better to be approximately correct, than precisely wrong” (Kachigan, 1991, p. 99).

Many of the following chapters will deal with the topic of confidence intervals and tests involved in this area. But at this point let us assume that we know the population standard deviation ($\sigma$), possibly through historical data or previous tests. In the case of the pharmacokinetic data (Table 4.3), the population standard deviation is known to be 16.8, based on the raw data, and was calculated using the formula to calculate a population standard deviation (Eqs. 5.5 and 5.6). Using the four samples in Table 7.1 it is possible to estimate the population mean based on data for each sample. For example, with Sample A:

$$\mu = 716.4 \pm 1.96\frac{16.8}{\sqrt{5}} = 716.4 \pm 14.7$$

$$701.7 < \mu < 731.1 \ mcg$$

The best estimate of the population mean (for the researcher using Sample A) would

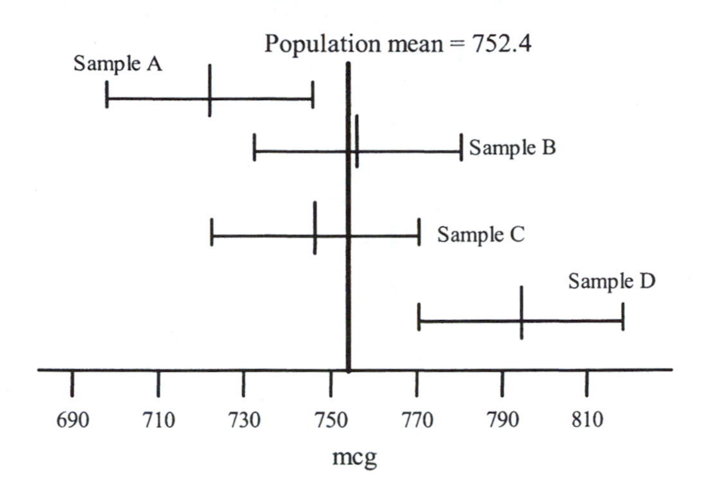


**Figure 7.2** Sample results compared with the population mean.

be between 701.7 and 731.1 mcg. Note that the "fudge factor" would remain the same for all four samples since the reliability coefficient will remain constant (1.96) and the error term (the population standard deviation divided by square root of the sample size) does not change. Therefore the results for the other three samples would be:

Sample B: $\mu = 752.8 \pm 14.7$
$738.1 < \mu < 767.5$ mcg

Sample C: $\mu = 749.4 \pm 14.7$
$734.7 < \mu < 764.1$ mcg

Sample D: $\mu = 786.8 \pm 14.7$
$772.1 < \mu < 801.5$ mcg

From our previous discussion of presentation mode, the true population mean for these 125 data points is a $C_{max}$ of 752.4 mcg. In the case of samples B and C, the true population mean did fall within the 95% confidence interval and we were correct in our prediction of this mean. However, with the extreme samples (A and D), the population mean falls outside the confidence interval (Figure 7.2). With over 234 million possible samples and using the reliability coefficient (95%), almost 12 million possible samples will give us erroneous results.

Adjusting the confidence interval can increase the likelihood of predicting the correct population mean. One more sample was drawn consisting of five outcomes and the calculated mean is 768.4. If a 95% confidence interval is calculated, the population mean falls outside the interval.

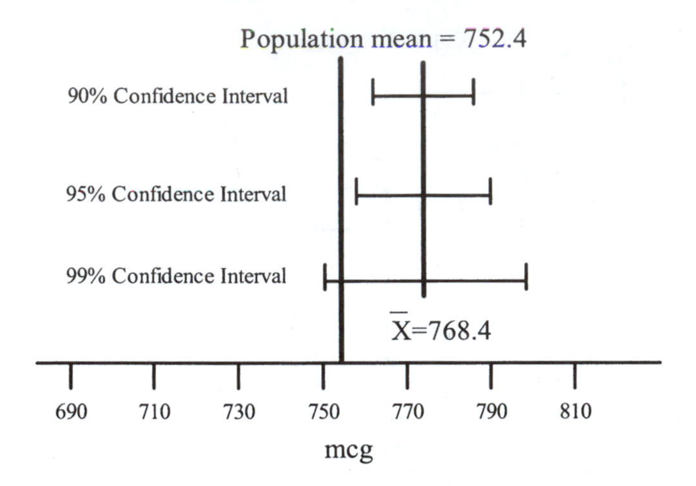


**Figure 7.3** Sample results with different confidence levels compared with the true population mean.

$$\mu = 768.4 \pm 1.96 \frac{16.8}{\sqrt{5}} = 768.4 \pm 14.7$$

$$753.7 < \mu < 783.1 \, mcg$$

However, if we decrease our confidence to 90%, the true population mean ($\mu = 752.4$ mcg) falls even further outside the interval.

$$\mu = 768.4 \pm 1.64 \frac{16.8}{\sqrt{5}} = 768.4 \pm 12.4$$

$$756.0 < \mu < 780.8 \, mcg$$

Similarly, if we increase our confidence to 99%, the true population mean will be found within the predicted limits.

$$\mu = 768.4 \pm 2.57 \frac{16.8}{\sqrt{5}} = 768.4 \pm 19.3$$

$$749.1 < \mu < 787.7 \, mcg$$

As seen in Figure 7.3, as the percentage of confidence increases, the width of the confidence interval increases. Creation and adjustment of the confidence intervals is the basis upon which statistical analysis and hypothesis testing is based.

What we have accomplished is our first inferential statistic; to make a statement about a population parameter (μ) based on a subset of that population ($\overline{X}$). The z-test is the oldest of the statistical tests and was often called the **critical ratio** in early statistical literature. The **interval estimate** is our best guess, with a certain degree of confidence, where the actual parameter exists. We must allow for a certain amount of error (i.e., 5% or 1%) since we do not know the entire population. As shown in Figure 7.3, as our error decreases, the width of our interval estimate will increase. In order to be 100% confident, our estimate of the interval would be from $-\infty$ to $+\infty$ (negative to positive infinity). Also as can be seen in the formula for the confidence interval estimate, with a large sample size, the standard error term will decrease and our interval width will decrease. Relating back to terms defined in Chapter 3, we can relate confidence interval in terms of precision and the confidence level is what we establish as our reliability.

As we shall see in future chapters, a basic assumption for many statistical tests (i.e., student t-test, F-test, correlation) is that populations from which the samples are selected are composed of random outcomes that approximate a normal distribution. If this is true, then we know many characteristics about our population with respect to its mean and standard deviation.

The one troublesome feature of Eq. 7.5 is the fact that it is highly unlikely that we will know a population standard deviation ($\sigma$). An example of an exception might be a quality control situation where a measurement has been repeated many times and is based on historical data. As will be shown in the next section, one could make a reasonable guess of what $\sigma$ should be based on past outcomes. However, in Chapter 8 we will find an alternative test for creating a confidence interval when the population standard deviation is unknown or cannot be approximated.

## Statistical Control Charts

Quality control charts represent an example of the application of confidence intervals using $\sigma$ or an approximation of the population standard deviation. Traditionally, control charts have been used during manufacturing to monitor production runs and insure the quality of the finished product. More recently these charts have been used to monitor the quality of health care systems, along with techniques such as cause-and-effect diagrams, quality-function deployment and process-flow analysis (Laffel, 1989; Wadsworth, 1985). Our discussion of control charts will focus on production issues, but the process could be easily applied to the monitoring of quality performance indicators in the provision of health services.

Statistical quality control is the process of assessing the status of a specific characteristic or characteristics, over a period of time, with respect to some target value or goal. During the production process, control charts provide a visual method for evaluating an intermediate or the final product during the ongoing process. They can be used to identify problems during production and document the history of a specific batch or run.

The use of control charts is one of the most common applications of statistics to the process of pharmaceutical quality control. The design of such charts were originally developed by Walter Shewhart of Bell Telephone Laboratories in 1931 (Shewhart, 1931). Over the years, modifications have been made, but most of the original characteristics of the **Shewhart control chart** continue today. Control charts assess and monitor the variability of a specific characteristic, which is assumed to exist under relatively homogeneous and stable conditions. There are generally two types of control charts: 1) measuring consistency of the production run (**property chart**) around a target value and 2) measuring the variability of the samples (**precision chart**).

To assess and monitor a given characteristic during a production run, we periodically sample items (i.e., tablets, vials) using random or selected sampling and measure the specific variable (i.e., weight, fill rate). The results are plotted on a graph with an x- and y-axis. The x-axis is a "time-ordered" sequence. The outcomes or changes are plotted on the y-axis over this time period to determine if the process is under control.

A **sampling plan** is developed to determine times, at equal intervals, during which samples are selected. In the case of a selected sampling scheme (i.e., every 15 minutes samples are selected from a production line), it is assumed that individual samples are withdrawn at random. How often should a sample be selected? The length of time between samples is dependent on the stability of the process being measured. A relatively stable process (for example, weights of finished tablets in a production run), may require only occasional monitoring, (i.e., every 30 minutes). A more volatile product or one with potential for large deviations from the target outcome may require more frequent sampling. When drawing samples for control charts, the time intervals should be consistent (every 30 minutes, every 60 minutes, etc.) and the sample sizes should be equal. The size and frequency of the sample is dependent on the nature of the control process and desired precision. Sample sizes as small as four or five observations have been recommended (Bolton, 1997, p. 447).

The creation of a quality control chart is a relatively simple procedure. Time intervals are located on the x-axis and outcomes for the variable of interest (or property) is measured on the y-axis. The "property" chart uses either a single measurement (sometime referred to as an **x-chart**) or the mean of several measurements (a **mean chart**) of a selected variable (i.e., capsule weight, tablet hardness, fill volume of a liquid into a bottle). The mean chart ($\overline{X}$ chart) would be preferable to a simple x-chart because it is less sensitive to extreme results because these would offset the remainder of the measures that are averaged. Also, the x-chart consists of a series of single measures and does not provide any information about the variance of outcomes at specific time periods.

Control charts contain a **central line** running through the chart parallel to the x-axis. This central line represents the "target" or "ideal" goal and is often based on historical data from scale up through initial full-scale runs. Also referred to as the **average line**, it defines the target for the variable being plotted. This is seen as the center line in Figure 7.4. In an ideal world, if a process is under control all results should fall on the central line. Unfortunately most outcomes will be observed to fall above or below the line, due to simple random error. The distance from the central line and the actual point measures variability. Thus, in addition to identifying a central line it is important to determine acceptable limits, above and below this line, within which observations should fall.

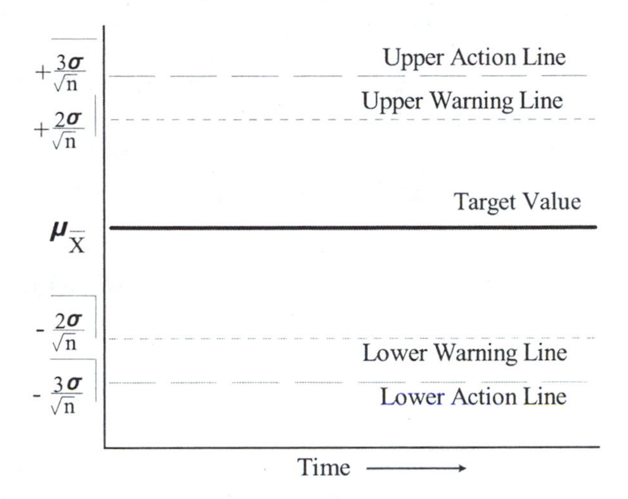


**Figure 7.4** Traditional quality control chart.

There are two types of variability that can be seen in statistical control charts: 1) common cause variability and 2) assignable cause variability. **Common cause variation** is due to random error or normal variability attributed to the sampling process. This type of error is due to natural chance error or error inherent in the process. **Assignable cause variation** is systematic error or bias that occurs in excess of the common-cause variability of the process. Also called **special-cause variation,** it is the responsibility of the person controlling the process to identify the cause of this variation, correct it and maintain a process that is under control. When the control chart shows excessive variation from the ideal outcome the process is said to be "out of statistical control." Thus, the required measures for constructing a statistical quality control chart are: 1) a sampling plan (size and length of time interval); 2) a target value; and 3) an estimate of the random error, which as we shall see is based on either expected standard deviations or ranges.

How much deviation from the central line is acceptable? The original Shewhart format utilized the population standard deviation ($\sigma$) and created **action lines** at three standard deviations above and below the target value. These lines were referred to as the three-sigma limits or the upper and lower control limits (UCL and LCL).

$$UCL = target + \frac{3\sigma}{\sqrt{n}} \qquad \text{Eq. 7.6}$$

$$LCL = target - \frac{3\sigma}{\sqrt{n}} \qquad \text{Eq. 7.7}$$

These are the boundaries within which essentially all of the sample data should fall if the process is under statistical control. In order to create these upper and lower action lines we need to be able to estimate the population standard deviation. This could be based on historical data about a particular product or process, or it can be estimated from previous samples.

One method for estimating $\sigma$ is to calculate an average or "pooled" sample standard deviation. This can be calculated by averaging standard deviations from previous runs:

$$S_p = \frac{S_1 + S_2 + S_3 + \dots S_k}{k} \quad \text{Eq. 7.8}$$

The square of this value is sometimes referred to as the **within-sample estimate of variance** or random error:

$$\sigma^2_{WSE} = \frac{\sum S^2}{k} \quad \text{Eq. 7.9}$$

This pooling the sample variances (or standard deviations) for many subgroups can provide a good estimate of the true population standard deviation.

More recent control charts incorporate additional limits called warning lines. This method involves establishing two sets of lines; warning lines at two sigmas and action lines at three sigmas (see Figure 7.4). Because they only involve two standard deviations above and below the target line, the warning limits are always narrower and do not demand the immediate intervention seen with the action lines. The warning lines would be calculated as follows:

$$\mu_w = \mu_0 \pm \frac{2\sigma}{\sqrt{n}} \quad \text{Eq. 7.10}$$

and the action lines are:

$$\mu_a = \mu_0 \pm \frac{3\sigma}{\sqrt{n}} \quad \text{Eq. 7.11}$$

Some control charting systems even evaluate observations falling outside one standard deviation beyond the central line. As discussed, virtually all samples will fall between ±3-sigma, 95% will be located within ±2-sigma and approximately 2/3 are contained within ±1-sigma. Therefore, deviations outside any of these three parameters can be used to monitor production. Possible indicators of a process becoming "out-of-control" would be two successive samples outside the 2-sigma limit or four successive samples outside the 1-sigma limit or any systematic trends (several samples in the same direction) up or down from the central line (Taylor, 1987, pp. 135-136).

As mentioned previously, two components that can influence a control chart are: 1) the variable or property of interest (systematic or assignable cause variability) and 2) the precision of the measurement (random or common-cause variability). The center, warning and action lines monitor a given property in a quality control chart. However, we are also concerned about the precision or variability of our sample (the random variability). Standard deviations and ranges can be used as a measure of consistency of the samples. Variations in these measures are not seen in a simple Shewhart chart. A **precision chart** measures the amount of random error and consists of a plotting of the sample standard deviation (or the sample range) in parallel with the control chart for the sample means.

In addition to creating a control chart based on the standard deviation, a similar chart can be produced using the easiest of all measures of dispersion, the range. The central line for a range chart is calculated similar to the line used for the property chart. An average range is computed based on past observations.

$$\overline{R} = \frac{R_1 + R_2 + R_3 + \ldots R_k}{k} \qquad \text{Eq. 7.12}$$

Obviously the range is easier to calculate and is as efficient as the standard deviation to measure deviations from the central line if the sample size is greater than five (Mason, 1989, p. 66). Also, to calculate $\overline{R}$, there should be at least eight observations and preferably at least 15 for any given time period (Taylor, 1987, p. 140).

An alternative method for calculating the action lines around the target value utilized $\overline{R}$ and an A-value from Table 7.2.

$$AL = \overline{X} \pm A\overline{R} \qquad \text{Eq. 7.13}$$

Using the above formula will produce action lines almost identical to those created using Eq. 7.11.

To calculate the action lines for variations in the range, as a measure of dispersion, a value similar to the reliability coefficient portion of Eq. 7.5 is selected from Table 7.2. The $D_L$ and $D_U$-values from the table for the lower and upper limits, respectively, are used in the following formulas:

$$\textit{Upper Action Line} = D_U\overline{R} \qquad \text{Eq. 7.14}$$

$$\textit{Lower Action Line} = D_L\overline{R} \qquad \text{Eq. 7.15}$$

Note as more is known about the total population (i.e., larger sample sizes), the values in Table 7.2 become smaller and the action line becomes closer together. Also, based on the values in the table, the lines around the average range will not be symmetrical and the upper action line will always be further from the central, target range. By presenting these two plots in parallel, it is possible to monitor both the variability of the characteristic being measured, as well as the precision of the measurements at each specific time period.

As an example of the use of a quality control chart, consider the intermediate step of producing a core table that will eventually become enteric coated. Periodically

**Table 7.2** Factors for Determining Upper and Lower 3σ Limits for Mean and Range Quality Control Charts

| | | Factors for range chart | |
|---|---|---|---|
| Sample size of subgroup, N | A: Factor for X chart | $D_L$ for lower limit | $D_U$ for upper limit |
| 2 | 1.88 | 0 | 3.27 |
| 3 | 1.02 | 0 | 2.57 |
| 4 | 0.73 | 0 | 2.28 |
| 5 | 0.58 | 0 | 2.11 |
| 6 | 0.48 | 0 | 2.00 |
| 7 | 0.42 | 0.08 | 1.92 |
| 8 | 0.37 | 0.14 | 1.86 |
| 9 | 0.34 | 0.18 | 1.82 |
| 10 | 0.31 | 0.22 | 1.78 |
| 15 | 0.22 | 0.35 | 1.65 |
| 20 | 0.18 | 0.41 | 1.59 |

From: Bolton, S. (1997). *Pharmaceutical Statistics: Practical and Clinical Applications*, Third edition, Marcel Dekker, Inc., New York, p. 658. Reproduced with permission of the publisher.

during the pressing of these core tablets, samples of ten tablets are randomly sampled. The ideal target weight for the individual tablets is 200 mg or a mass weight of 2000 mg for all ten tablets. Based on historical data from previous runs, the expected average range should be 6.2 mg. Using the range as our measure of dispersion, the action lines are determined using the A-values taken from Table 7.2 for n = 10 (A = 0.31):

$$AL = \overline{X} \pm A\overline{R} = 200 \pm 0.31(6.2) = 200 \pm 1.92$$

$$A_U L = 201.92 \qquad A_L L = 198.08$$

The mean range ($\overline{R}$) is 6.2 and using the DU and DL-values from Table 7.2, the following action lines for our measures of precision are:

$$D_U \overline{R} = 1.78(6.2) = 11.04$$

$$D_L \overline{R} = 0.22(6.2) = 1.36$$

During production, with sampling done every thirty minutes, creates the results presented in Table 7.3. Plotting of the results of this run appears in Figure 7.5. Note that there is no significant change in the variability of the samples, as seen in the

**Table 7.3**. Sample Weights (mg) During a Production Run

| Date | Time | Mean | Range |
|---|---|---|---|
| 9/6 | 9:00 | 200.4 | 6.7 |
| | 9:30 | 199.4 | 4.4 |
| | 10:00 | 201.2 | 7.3 |
| | 10:30 | 200.0 | 6.9 |
| | 11:00 | 200.6 | 5.5 |
| | 11:30 | 201.0 | 8.1 |
| | 12:00 | 201.3 | 9.2 |
| | 12:30 | 200.2 | 6.5 |
| | 13:00 | 199.8 | 5.0 |
| | 13:30 | 199.6 | 7.2 |
| | 14:00 | 199.3 | 3.5 |
| | 14:30 | 199.0 | 6.4 |

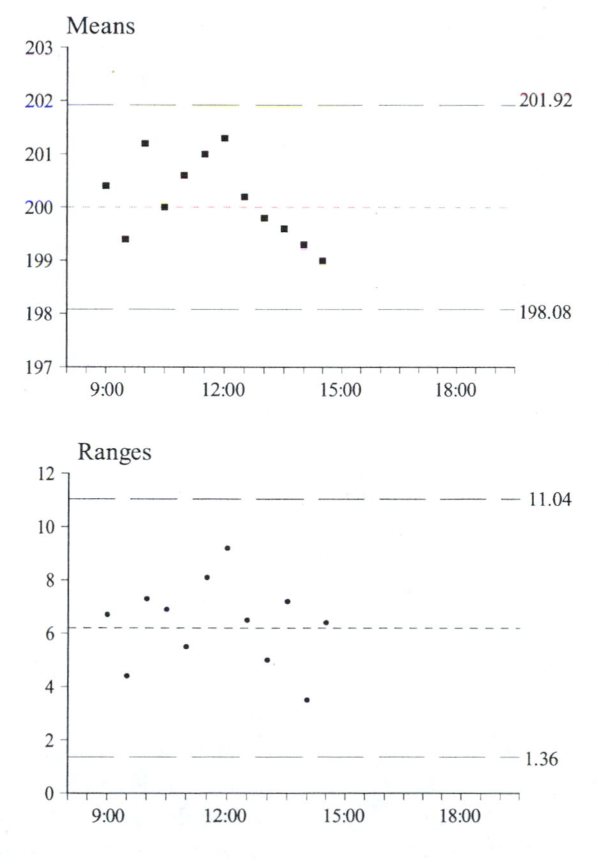


**Figure 7.5** Quality control charts for the means and ranges for the data presented in Table 7.3.

plotting of the ranges. However, there appears to be a downward trend in the mean weights of the tablets and the operator should make adjustments in the process to return the weight back to the target mean.

Sometime **moving averages** and/or **moving ranges** are used for control charts. In these cases, the first two or three samples are averaged and the results used as the point on the control chart. When the next sample is collected, the first value is dropped and a new average is plotted (for both the mean and the range). This process continues, averaging including a new observation and excluding the earliest previous number continued for the whole data set. This yields a series of means and ranges represent the average of multiple consecutive data points.

A second type of control chart is the **cumulative sum** or **CUSUM** charting technique. It is considered more sensitive than Shewhart control charts to modest changes in the characteristic being monitored (Mason, 1989, p. 66). The CuSum charts are more effective in identifying gradual approaches to out-of-control conditions. The name CUSUM is from the fact that successive deviations are accumulated from a fixed reference point in the process. It provides a running, visual summation of deviations, from some preselected reference point. There is evidence of a special-cause variation when the cumulative sum of the deviations is extremely large or extremely small. Further information on CUSUM charts can be found in Mason's book (Mason, 1989, pp. 67-70).

## Process Capability Indices

Process capability is a measure of the inherent variability of a process removing any undesirable special causes that might increase variability. It is the smallest variability due solely to common causes. In manufacturing it is a measurement of the degree to which the process is meeting the manufacturing requirements. It is the repeatability and consistency of that process and is relative to the customer requirements in terms of specification limits for the product.

Possible special causes of variability include different production sites, different equipment, and different operators running that equipment. One way to eliminate these special causes is to collect data using the same operator on the same machine, measuring the same batch of materials.

Studies of process capability are designed to determine what the process is "capable" of doing under controlled conditions (removing any special causes for variability). Another benefit of studying the process capability is to determine the stability of the process by comparing the output of a stable process with the process specifications or by comparing the normal variability of a stable process with the process specification limits.

Process capability compares the process outcome that is "in control" with the specification limits by measures called **capacity indices**. This comparison is a ratio of the deviation between the process specifications (called the specification width) to the deviation of the process values based on six process standard deviation units (referred to as the process width). A "capable process" is defined as one in which all the measurements fall inside the predetermined specification limits (Figure 7.6).

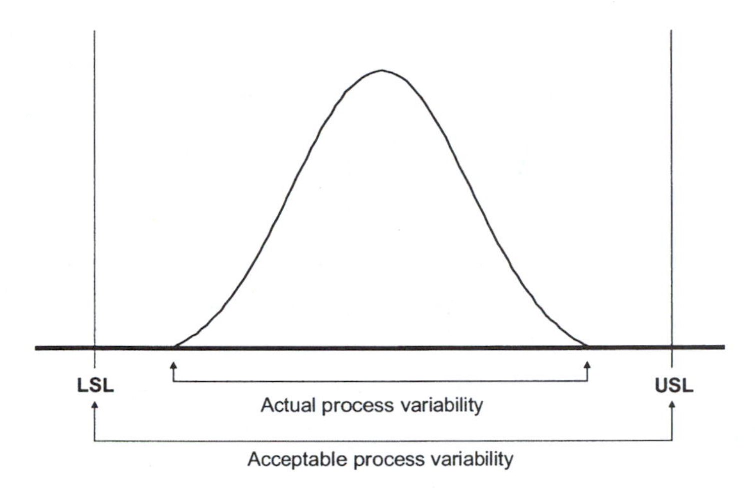


**Figure 7.6** Illustration of a distribution within specification limits.

Capability indices are equations employed to place the distribution from a specific process in relationship to the product specifications. Capability indices are used to determine, given normal variation, if the process is capable of meeting established specifications. Thus, it is assumed that data points are sampled from a normally distributed population. Process capability is expressed as an index and there are three different indices, labeled $C_p$, $C_{pk}$ and $C_{pm}$. These capability indices are valid only when there is a large sample size, usually a minimum of 50 data points. These should be consecutive data points, in at least 10 subgroups, each with five observations.

Several symbols are used in the calculations of the capability indices. $T$ is the target value for the product. The $\mu$ is the process mean and $\sigma$ is the measure of dispersion based on historical experience with the process (often $T$ and $\mu$ are the same value). The $USL$ and $LSL$ are the upper and lower specification limits, respectively. The manufacture sets the specification limits. The specification range is the difference between the $USL$ and $LSL$.

$$Specification\ range = USL - LSL \qquad \text{Eq. 7.16}$$

The specification range is usually from $-3\sigma$ to $+3\sigma$, or a six-sigma spread. As seen in the previous chapter, approximately 99.7% of the area under a normal distribution would be within the plus or minus three sigmas. Thus, the total variability or spread in outcomes should have a total variation of approximately six sigmas.

$C_p$ is a simple index that relates the acceptable variability of the specification limits to the natural variation of the process (expressed as $6\sigma$). It is some times referred to as the **population capability** or **process potential.** The $C_p$ calculated as follows:

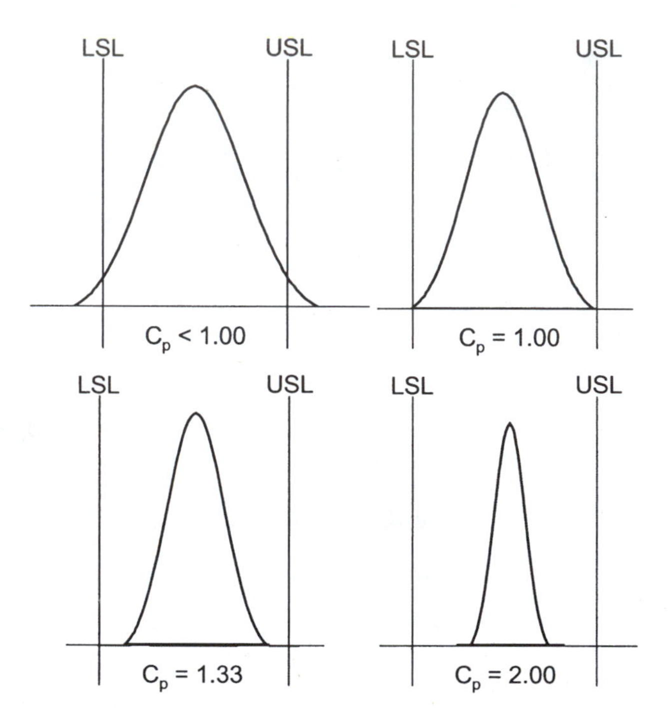


**Figure 7.7** Distributions for various $C_p$ values.

$$C_p = \frac{USL - LSL}{6\sigma} \qquad \text{Eq. 7.17}$$

Various $C_p$ results are illustrated in Figure 7.7. If the $C_p$ is less than one, the process variation exceeds specification, and a significant number of defects may be found. A $C_p$ of less than one indicates that it is not a capable process; not capable of meeting specifications regardless of where the process mean is located. In these cases the process spread is greater than *USL-LSL*.

If the $C_p$ equals one, the process is just meeting specifications and a minimum of 0.3% (100%-99.7%) defects will be detected if the process is centered at the target. This would be when a process is just barely capable; the process variability matches 6 $\sigma$. The $C_p$ evaluates the spread of the process relative to the specification width, it does not provide information on how well the process average, $\mu$, is centered with respect to the target value, *T*. If the process mean shifts slightly to the left or to the right, a significant amount of production output will exceed one of the two specification limits. In this case, the process must be watched closely to identify any shifts from the mean. Control charts are excellent for such monitoring.

If the $C_p$ is greater than one, the process variation is less than the specification limits, but the defect rate might be greater if the process is not centered on the target

**Table 7.4** $C_p$ Values Assuming that the Center of the Distibution is $\mu$

| USL–LSL | $C_p$ | Rejects (parts per million) | % of Specification used |
|---|---|---|---|
| 6σ | 1.000 | 2,700 | 100 |
| 8σ | 1.333 | 64 | 75 |
| 10σ | 1.667 | 0.6 | 60 |
| 12σ | 2.000 | 0.002 | 50 |

value (*T*). Also, the $C_p$ can be highly inaccurate and misleading if the data is not sampled from a normally distributed population. Table 7.4 indicates the expected number of defects for various levels of $C_p$. As seen in Table 7.4 the greater the $C_p$ the more likely the process variability will fall within the specification spread (6 sigma is less than *USL–LSL*). For example, with a $C_p$ of 2.0 indicates a process distribution where 12 sigmas would fit between the USL and LSL. If a manufacturer can tighten its specification limits, they might be able to claim that their product is more consistent or uniform than their competitor. Some pharmaceutical manufacturers are establishing specific process capabilities targets. As a starting point they may require a $C_p$ of 1.33 for supplier qualifications and have a desired goal of 2.0.

A second process capability index is $C_{pk}$ and comparing it to the $C_p$ it is possible to get an indication of the difference between $\mu$ and *T*. The $C_{pk}$ is calculated as follows:

$$C_{pk} = min\left[\frac{USL-\mu}{3\sigma}, \frac{\mu-LSL}{3\sigma}\right] \qquad \text{Eq. 7.18}$$

and the smaller of the two values (*min*) in the parentheses is reported as the $C_{pk}$. If the process approaches a normal distribution and in statistical control, the $C_{pk}$ may be used to estimate the expected percent of defective products, similar to the $C_p$.

An alternative method for estimating the $C_{pk}$ is:

$$C_{pk} = C_p(1-k) \qquad \text{Eq. 7.19}$$

where $k$ is the scaled distance between the midpoint of the specification range $m$ and the process mean, $\mu$. This k-value comes from the Japanese word *katayori*, which means deviation. The specification range is calculated as follows:

$$m = \frac{USL+LSL}{2} \qquad \text{Eq. 7.20}$$

and the $k$ value is derived using the equation

$$k = \frac{|m-\mu|}{\frac{USL-LSL}{2}} \qquad \text{Eq. 7.21}$$

The resultant $k$ must be greater or equal to zero and less than or equal to one. When the $m$ and μ are equal, $k = 0$ in Eq. 7.19 and $C_{pk} = C_p$. The difference between the $C_p$ and $C_{pk}$ is represented by the $k$-value, and indicates how much of the process capability is lost due to poor centering. For example, suppose that $k = 0.25$ and the $C_p = 2.00$, the $C_{pk}$ would be reduced to:

$$C_{pk} = 2.00(1-0.25) = 1.50$$

If the process can be centered, this capability index would increase by 33%. This deviation from the center ($T$) can be calculated as follows:

$$\delta = \frac{C_p}{C_{pk}} x100\% \qquad \text{Eq. 7.22}$$

For this example:

$$\delta = \frac{2.00}{1.50} x100\% = 33.3\%$$

The third capability index is $C_{pm}$; sometimes referred to as the Taguchi capability (named after Genichi Taguchi). This was developed in the late 1980s and the index, similar to the $C_{pk}$, accounts for the proximity of the process mean to a designated target mean, $T$.

$$C_{pm} = \frac{USL-LSL}{6\sqrt{\sigma^2 + (\mu - T)^2}} \qquad \text{Eq. 7.23}$$

If the process mean is centered between the specification limits and the process mean equals the target mean ($T$), then $C_p = C_{pk} = C_{pm.}$ The $C_{pk}$ and $C_{pm}$ are the better indices because that accounts for deviations between the process center and the target center in the distribution.

If the population standard deviation ($\sigma$) is unknown, sample estimates can be used by replacing $\sigma$ with the sample standard deviation ($S$). Slight modifications are made on the previous equations and a hat is added above each index to indicate that it is an estimate based on sample variability:

$$\hat{C}_p = \frac{USL - LSL}{6S} \qquad \text{Eq. 7.24}$$

$$\hat{C}_{pk} = min\left[\frac{USL - \overline{X}}{3S}, \frac{\overline{X} - LSL}{3S}\right] \qquad \text{Eq. 7.25}$$

$$\hat{C}_{pm} = \frac{USL - LSL}{6\sqrt{S^2 + (\overline{X} - T)^2}} \qquad \text{Eq. 7.26}$$

The $k$-deviation can also be calculated based on sample data. The sample mean ($\overline{X}$) is the best estimate of $\mu$ and the sample estimate of $k$ and $C_{pk}$ would be:

$$\hat{k} = \frac{\left|m - \overline{X}\right|}{\frac{USL - LSL}{2}} \qquad \text{Eq. 7.27}$$

and

$$\hat{C}_{pk} = \hat{C}_p(1 - \hat{k}) \qquad \text{Eq. 7.28}$$

If $0 \leq k \leq 1$; then:

$$\hat{C}_{pk} \leq \hat{C}_p \qquad \text{Eq. 7.29}$$

As an example, consider the data presented in Table 7.5 which represent 60 samples randomly selected during the production of a product. The manufacturer has set the specification limits to be within 3% of label claim ($T$ = 100%, $USL$ = 103%, $LSL$ = 97%). From previous production experience with the product the expected mean ($\mu$) and standard deviation ($\sigma$) are 100 and 1%, respectively. However, the sample results are $\overline{X}$ = 100.1 and $S$ = 0.25. The process capability indices are:

$$\hat{C}_p = \frac{USL - LSL}{6S} = \frac{103 - 97}{6(.25)} = 4.00$$

$$\hat{C}_{pk} = min\left[\frac{USL - \overline{X}}{3S}, \frac{\overline{X} - LSL}{3S}\right] = min\left[\frac{103 - 100.1}{3(0.25)}, \frac{100.1 - 97}{3(0.25)}\right]$$

$$\hat{C}_{pk} = min[3.87, 4.13] = 3.87$$

**Table 7.5**. Sample Results During a Production Run

| Time | Sample Results | | | Mean | S.D. | Range |
|---|---|---|---|---|---|---|
| 0:05 | 100.3 | 100.5 | 100.0 | 100.12 | 0.26 | 0.7 |
| | 99.8 | 99.9 | 100.2 | | | |
| 0:20 | 99.9 | 100.2 | 100.4 | 100.07 | 0.27 | 0.7 |
| | 100.3 | 99.7 | 99.9 | | | |
| 0:35 | 100.1 | 100.0 | 100.5 | 100.20 | 0.18 | 0.5 |
| | 100.3 | 100.2 | 100.1 | | | |
| 0:50 | 100.2 | 99.5 | 99.9 | 100.08 | 0.38 | 1.1 |
| | 100.3 | 100.0 | 100.6 | | | |
| 1:05 | 100.2 | 100.3 | 99.8 | 100.08 | 0.17 | 0.5 |
| | 100.0 | 100.1 | 100.1 | | | |
| 1:20 | 100.1 | 100.3 | 99.9 | 100.08 | 0.23 | 0.6 |
| | 100.4 | 99.8 | 100.0 | | | |
| 1:35 | 99.8 | 100.2 | 99.6 | 100.03 | 0.31 | 0.9 |
| | 100.5 | 100.0 | 100.1 | | | |
| 1:50 | 100.2 | 100.3 | 100.0 | 100.13 | 0.20 | 0.5 |
| | 100.4 | 99.9 | 100.0 | | | |
| 2:05 | 100.8 | 100.2 | 99.8 | 100.15 | 0.36 | 1.0 |
| | 100.0 | 99.9 | 100.2 | | | |
| 2:20 | 99.9 | 100.4 | 100.1 | 100.07 | 0.26 | 0.7 |
| | 100.3 | 100.0 | 99.7 | | | |
| | | | Total for all samples: | 100.10 | 0.25 | |

$$\hat{C}_{pm} = \frac{USL - LSL}{6\sqrt{S^2 + (\overline{X} - T)^2}} = \frac{103 - 97}{6\sqrt{(0.25)^2 + (100.1 - 100.0)^2}} = 3.71$$

or as an alternative for $C_{pk}$:

$$m = \frac{USL + LSL}{2} = \frac{103 + 97}{2} = 100$$

$$k = \frac{\left| m - \overline{X} \right|}{\frac{USL - LSL}{2}} = \frac{\left| 100 - 100.1 \right|}{\frac{103 - 97}{2}} = \frac{0.1}{3} = 0.033$$

$$\hat{C}_{pk} = \hat{C}_p(1-\hat{k}) = 4.00(1-0.033) = 4.00(0.967) = 3.87$$

It is possible to do unilateral, or one-sided tests, for determining process capabilities. The previous examples were bilateral, or two-sided cases, and involved both the *USL* and *LSL*. For the unilateral case either the *USL* or *LSL* is used alone:

$$\hat{C}_{pu} = \frac{USL - \overline{X}}{3S} \qquad \text{Eq. 7.30}$$

$$\hat{C}_{pl} = \frac{\overline{X} - LSL}{3S} \qquad \text{Eq. 7.31}$$

and by extension the $C_p$ is:

$$\hat{C}_p = \frac{\hat{C}_{pl} + \hat{C}_{pu}}{2} \qquad \text{Eq. 7.32}$$

and $C_{pk}$ is the smaller value for either $C_{pl}$ or $C_{pu}$:

$$\hat{C}_{pk} = min\left[\hat{C}_{pl}, \hat{C}_{pu}\right] \qquad \text{Eq. 7.33}$$

In addition, estimators can be used replacing $\mu$ and $\sigma$ with $\overline{X}$ and $S$.

It is possible to calculate a confidence interval for the capability indices. Once again, we are assuming a normal distribution population. For the $C_{pk}$ a confidence interval can be calculated using the following equation:

$$C_{pk} = \hat{C}_{pk} \pm z_{1-\alpha/2}\sqrt{\frac{1}{9n} + \frac{\hat{C}_{pk}^2}{2(n-1)}} \qquad \text{Eq. 7.34}$$

Like Eq. 7.4, our best estimate of the true $C_{pk}$ is our sample estimate ($\hat{C}_{pk}$). How confident we are in our decision is controlled by the reliability coefficient ($z_{1-\alpha/2}$) and error term, which in this case in the portion of the equation included in the square root term. This equation is similar to Eq. 7.5 and if we wish to be 95% confident in our decision the reliability coefficient would be 1.96. The resulting confidence interval is evaluated base on its proximity to 1.0, because a capability index of 1.0 just meeting specifications (the ratio of the process specifications to the deviation of the process values is 1.0). The concept of interpreting ratios will be discussed in greater detail in Chapter 18. However, at this point assume that if our confidence interval has value that are all greater than 1.0 that we are 95% confident that we have a capable process. Using our previous example, where $\hat{C}_{pk}$ = 3.87 and $n$ = 60, the confidence interval would be:

$$C_{pk} = 3.87 \pm 1.96\sqrt{\frac{1}{9(60)} + \frac{(3.87)^2}{2(59)}} = 3.87 \pm 0.70$$

$$3.17 < C_{pk} < 4.57$$

Our interpretation is that we are 95% confident that the true $C_{pk}$ is somewhere between 3.17 and 4.57. A value of 1.0 or less cannot possibly fall within this interval there for we have good process capability. Confidence intervals can be calculated of other capability indices, but unfortunately, these intervals involve distributions that will be not be covered until later chapters in this book (the chi-square distribution for $C_p$ and the one-tailed t-distribution for $C_{pu}$ and $C_{pl}$) and are beyond the scope of this book. A reference for calculating these intervals is Bissell (1990).

If sample data comes from a process that does not appear to be normally distributed it is recommended that the data be transformed to create normality or use an nonparametric alternative index ($C_{npk}$), which is based on the median:

$$\hat{C}_{npk} = min\left[\frac{USL - median}{p(.995) - median}, \frac{median - LSL}{median - p(.005)}\right] \qquad \text{Eq. 7.35}$$

where $p(0.995)$ and $p(0.005)$ are the 99.5th and 0.5th percentile of the sample data. More Information about these tests can be found in Johnson and Kotz (1993) or Bothe (1997).

## Tolerance Limits

In the discussion of confidence intervals we employed the process of estimating a range of possible values for the population mean ($\mu$) based on sample data ($\bar{x}$). The result was an interval within which we predicted the true population mean was located. However, sometimes the investigator might be more interested in the approximate range of values for a particular population (i.e., tables being produced during a specific run). In this case, **tolerance limits** indicate the limits (above, or below) that we would expect to find a given proportion of items from the population. It is possible to create both one-sided and two-sided limits. In the case of the two-sided limits tolerance test, with statistical manipulation it is possible to calculate two values (the lower tolerance limit or *LTL* and the upper tolerance limit or *UTL*) between which we have a certain degree of confidence that a given proportion ($p$) of the population will exist. With the one-sided test, we can identify a single value ($X_L$), above which at least a proportion ($p$) will occur with a certain level of confidence.

Suppose we are producing a specific batch of tablets and we know that there is a certain amount of variation in your process. Therefore, over time, the weights of the tablets will vary slightly. Obviously, it is possible to take samples during the production run and calculate the mean ( $\overline{X}$ ) and standard deviation (*S*). But we would like to know lower and upper limits on the tablet weights produced during this specific batch. Therefore we need to use a test that can estimate prescribed extremes in our data, rather than estimate the true center for the population.

In most cases it is impossible to measure the entire population and know the "real world" limits for all tablets produced during a specific run. However, we can determine limits within which we would expect to find 90%, 95%, or 99% of all the tablets produced. If we wanted to know the limits for 99% of all tablets we could create a "tolerance limit for 99% of the population." However as seen previously, we can never be 100% confident in our projection based on sample data, but we can predict with 95% confidence in our decision. Therefore, it should be possible to perform a statistical test to identify a "95% tolerance limits on 99% of the population." This reliability coefficient or confidence coefficient is sometime noted by the Greek letter gamma ($\gamma$).

If it is assumed that the weights of all tablets, when plotted, would produce a bell-shaped curve (data are normally distributed) then we can calculate the tolerance limits using the following formulas:

$$LTL = \overline{X} - KS \qquad \text{Eq. 7.36}$$

$$UTL = \overline{X} + KS \qquad \text{Eq. 7.37}$$

where *K* is a new reliability coefficient. *K*-values for the two-tailed test can be found in Table B3 (Appendix B) and represent the two-tailed test for creating both the upper and lower tolerance limits.

Table B3 is divided into three major columns, each representing our traditional confidence level (1 – α/2). Numbers in the center third of Table B3 would be used if we wish to be 95% confident ($\gamma$) in our decision. Each major section of the table is further divided into the subsections, or columns, that represent the proportion of the population we wish to define. For example, between our tolerance limits we would expect 95%, 99%, or 99.9% of all the population out comes to be located.

Assume we randomly sample 30 tablets during the course of a production run (Table 7.6) and find the sample mean ( $\overline{X}$ ) and standard deviation (*S*) to be 99.96% label claim and 0.286%, respectively. Within what limits would we expect 99% of all the tablets to fall with 95% confidence. Using Table B3 for this example, with 95% certainty, we want to identify the limits within which we would expect 99% of our population. The 95% certainty in found in the center third of the table and 99% of the population is defined by the *K*-value in the sixth column from the left. If our sample size involves 30 tablets, then the *K*-value of 3.350 is found in the sixth column on the row where n = 30. The calculation for the tolerance limits would be as follows:

$$LTL = 99.96 - (3.350)(0.286) = 99.00\%$$
$$UTL = 99.96 + (3.350)(0.286) = 100.92\%$$

**Table 7.6** Tablets Randomly Sampled from a Production Run (% label claim)

| | | | | | |
|---|---|---|---|---|---|
| 100.0 | 100.3 | 99.1 | 100.1 | 99.9 | 99.8 |
| 99.5 | 99.9 | 100.0 | 99.9 | 100.1 | 99.9 |
| 100.4 | 99.8 | 100.2 | 100.3 | 100.0 | 100.1 |
| 100.2 | 100.2 | 100.1 | 100.0 | 99.6 | 100.0 |
| 100.0 | 99.8 | 100.3 | 100.2 | 99.4 | 99.8 |

Thus, with 95% confidence, we would expect 99% of all tablets to contain between 99.0% and 100.9% of the label claim.

The same procedure is used for the one-tailed test, except new K-values are taken from a one-tailed table (Appendix B, Table B4) and a new equation is used to determine a proportion of the population above a given value:

$$X_L = \overline{X} - KS \qquad \text{Eq. 7.38}$$

or below a given point:

$$X_U = \overline{X} + KS \qquad \text{Eq. 7.39}$$

Using the same data presented in Table 7.6, 99% of the population would be above (with $K = 3.064$ for $p = .99$ and $\gamma = 0.95$):

$$X_L = 99.96 - (3.064)(0.286) = 99.08\%$$

with 95% confidence.

The previously calculated tolerance limits assume that the sample is taken from a normal distribution population. If the distribution is not normal, then the true proportion $p$ of the population between the tolerance limits will vary from the intended $p$ depending on the amount of departure from normality. The greater the departure form normality the greater the difference and the tolerance limits obtained tend to be substantially wider than those assuming normality. Natrella (1963) provides guidance for nonnormal conditions and provide statistical tables for such situations.

## References

Bissell, A. F. (1990). "How Reliable is Your Capability Index?" *Applied Statistics* 39:331-340.

Bolton, S. (1997). *Pharmaceutical Statistics: Practical and Clinical Applications*, Third edition, Marcel Dekker, Inc. New York, pp. 444-489.

Bothe, D.R. (1997). *Measuring Process Capability: Techniques and Calculations for Quality and Manufacturing Engineers*, McGraw Hill, New York.

Kachigan, S.K. (1991). *Multivariate Statistical Analysis*, Second edition, Radius Press, New York, pp. 89, 90.

Kotz, S. and Johnson, N. L. (1993). *Process Capability Indices*, Chapman & Hall, New York.

Laffel, G. and Blumenthal, D. (1989). "The case for using industral quality management science in health care organizations," *Journal of the American Medical Association* 262:2869-2873.

Mason, R.L., Gunst, R.F., and Hess, J.L. (1989). *Statistical Design and Analysis of Experiments with Applications to Engineering and Science*, John Wiley and Sons, New York.

Natrella, M.G. "The use of transformations," *Experimental Statistics*, National Bureau of Standards Handbook 9, U.S. Department of Commerce, Washington, DC, 1963, pp. 2-15.

Taylor, J.K. (1987). *Quality Assurance of Chemical Measurements*, Lewis Publications, Chelsea, MI.

Shewhart, W.A. (1931). *Economic Control of Quality of Manufactured Product*. Van Nostrand Reinhold, Princeton, NJ.

Wadsworth, H.M., Stephens, K.S., and Godfrey, A.B. (1986). *Modern Methods for Quality Control and Improvement*, John Wiley and Sons, New York.

**Suggested Supplemental Readings**

Bolton, S. (1997). *Pharmaceutical Statistics: Practical and Clinical Applications*, Third edition, Marcel Dekker, Inc. New York, pp. 444-489.

Cheremisinoff, N.P. (1987). *Practical Statistics for Engineers and Scientists*, Technomic Publishing, Lancaster, PA, pp. 41-50.

Mason, R.L., Gunst, R.F. and Hess, J.L. (1989). *Statistical Design and Analysis of Experiments with Applications to Engineering and Science*, John Wiley and Sons, New York, pp. 62-70.

Taylor, J.K. (1987). *Quality Assurance of Chemical Measurements*, Lewis Publications, Chelsea, MI, pp. 129-146.

**Example Problems**

1. Assume that three assays are selected at random from the following results:

| Tablet Number | Assay (mg) | Tablet Number | Assay (mg) | Tablet Number | Assay (mg) |
|---|---|---|---|---|---|
| 1 | 75 | 11 | 73 | 21 | 80 |
| 2 | 74 | 12 | 77 | 22 | 75 |
| 3 | 72 | 13 | 75 | 23 | 76 |
| 4 | 78 | 14 | 74 | 24 | 73 |
| 5 | 78 | 15 | 72 | 25 | 79 |
| 6 | 74 | 16 | 74 | 26 | 76 |
| 7 | 75 | 17 | 77 | 27 | 73 |
| 8 | 77 | 18 | 76 | 28 | 75 |
| 9 | 76 | 19 | 74 | 29 | 76 |
| 10 | 78 | 20 | 77 | 30 | 75 |

The resultant sample consists of tablets 05, 16, and 27.

a. Based on this one sample and assuming that the population standard deviation ($\sigma$) is known to be 2.01, calculate 95% confidence intervals for the population mean.

b. Again, based on this one sample, calculate the 90% and 99% confidence intervals for the population mean. How do these results compare to the 95% confidence interval for the same sample in the previous example?

c. Assuming the true population mean ($\mu$) is 75.47 for all 30 data points, did our one sample create confidence intervals at the 90%, 95%, and 99% levels, which included the population mean?

2. Assuming the true population mean ($\mu$) is 75.47 and the population standard deviation ($\sigma$) is 2.01 for the question 1, calculate the following:

a. How many different samples of n=3 can be selected from the above population of 30 data points?

b. What would be the grand mean for all the possible samples of n=3?

c. What would be the standard deviation for all the possible samples of n=3?

3. During scale-up and initial production of an intravenous product in a 5-cc vial, it was found that the standard deviation for volume fill was 0.2 cc. Create a Shewhart control chart to monitor the fill rates of the production vials. Monitor

the precision assuming the range is 0.6 cc (6 x σ) and the each sample size is 10 vials.

4. During a production run of an injectable agent, 20 ampules are randomly sampled. Listed below are the volumes contained in each ampule. What are the tolerance limits, by volume, within which we would expect to find 99% of the total ampules in the run and have 99% confidence in our decision?

| | | | |
|---|---|---|---|
| 1.99 | 2.00 | 2.02 | 1.98 |
| 2.01 | 2.01 | 2.01 | 2.02 |
| 2.00 | 1.98 | 1.99 | 2.00 |
| 1.98 | 1.99 | 2.00 | 2.01 |
| 2.03 | 2.00 | 2.00 | 1.99 |

5. Assume that a manufacturer has set the upper and lower specification limits to be within 20% of the target for a given process ($USL$ = 1.20 and $LSL$ = 0.80). A random sample of 100 samples during a production run presents with $\overline{X}$ = 0.93 and $S$ = 0.06. Is this a capable process? Assuming a normally distributed population, use the three difference indices described in the chapter.

**Answers to Problems**

1. Results of different samples will vary based on the random numbers selected off the table. Results can vary from the smallest possible mean outcome of 72.3 to the largest possible mean of 79.0. Assume that our sample results for Sample C were tables 05, 16, and 27. The mean assay result would be:

$$\overline{X} = \frac{78+74+73}{3} = 75\ mg$$

a. The 95% confidence interval would be:

$$\mu = \overline{x} \pm Z_{(1-\alpha/2)} \times \frac{\sigma}{\sqrt{n}}$$

$$\mu = 75 \pm 1.96 \times \frac{2.01}{\sqrt{3}} = 75 \pm 2.27$$

$$72.73 < \mu < 77.27\ mg$$

b. Using the above sample the 90% and 99% confidence intervals for the population mean would be:

$$90\%\ CI: \qquad \mu = 75 \pm 1.64 \times \frac{2.01}{\sqrt{3}}$$

$$73.10 < \mu < 76.90\ mg$$

$$99\%\ CI: \qquad \mu = 75 \pm 2.57 \times \frac{2.01}{\sqrt{3}}$$

$$72.02 < \mu < 77.98\ mg$$

As expected the interval becomes much wider (includes more possible results) when we wish to be 99% certain and becomes smaller as we accept a greater amount of error.

c. Since the true population mean (μ) is 75.47 mg, this would represent the most frequent outcome, but very few samples if any will produce 75.47. Instead we would see a clustering of means around that center point for the population.

2. With $\mu = 75.47$, $\sigma = 2.01$, and $N = 30$

a. There are a possible 4060 different samples of $n = 3$:

$$\binom{n}{x} = \frac{n!}{x!(n-x)!} = \frac{30!}{3!\,27!} = 4060$$

b. The grand mean for all 4060 possible sample means is 75.47 mg:

$$\mu_{\bar{X}} = \mu = 75.47\ mg$$

c. The standard deviation for all 4060 possible sample means is 1.16 mg:

$$\sigma_{\bar{X}} = \frac{\sigma}{\sqrt{n}} = \frac{2.01}{\sqrt{3}} = 1.16\ mg$$

3. Creation of a quality control chart with the target $\mu = 5$ cc, $\sigma = 0.2$ cc, and $n = 10$:

Warning lines (Figure 7.8)

$$\mu_w = \mu_0 \pm \frac{2\sigma}{\sqrt{n}} = 5 \pm \frac{2(0.2)}{\sqrt{10}} = 5 \pm 0.13$$

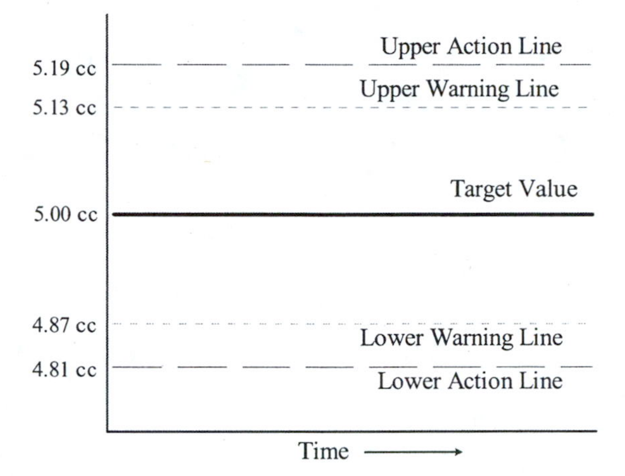


**Figure 7.8.** Warning and action line for question 3.

$$\mu_w = 5.13 \textit{ and } 4.87$$

Action lines (Figure 7.8):

$$\mu_a = \mu_0 \pm \frac{3\sigma}{\sqrt{n}} = 5 \pm \frac{3(0.2)}{\sqrt{10}} = 5 \pm 0.19$$

$$\mu_a = 5.19 \textit{ and } 4.81$$

Action lines using range formulas (Figure 7.9):

$$AL = \overline{X} \pm A\overline{R} = 5 \pm 0.31(0.6) = 5 \pm 0.19$$

$$A_U L = 5.19 \qquad A_L L = 4.81$$

Range action lines:

$$\textit{Upper action line} = D_U \overline{R} = 1.78(0.6) = 1.07$$

$$\textit{Lower action line} = D_L \overline{R} = 0.22(0.6) = 0.13$$

4. Measures of central tendency associated with volumes of the ampules are:

Mean ($\overline{X}$) = 2.000 ml
Standard deviation (S) = 0.014 ml

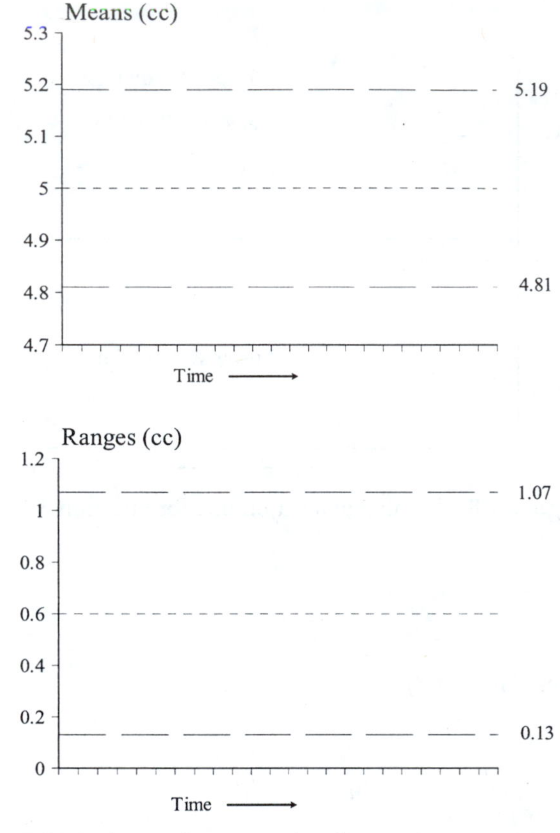


**Figure 7.9**. Action and range action lines using range formulas.

The K-value from Table B3 for 99% confidence ($\gamma$) for 99% of the batch ($p$) is 4.161. The tolerance limits based on n = 20 are:

$$LTL = \overline{X} - KS = 2.000 - (4.161)(0.014) = 1.942\ ml$$

$$UTL = \overline{X} + KS = 2.000 + (4.161)(0.014) = 2.058\ ml$$

Thus, with 99% confidence we would expect 99% of all ampules to have between 1.942 and 2.058 ml of volume.

5. Calculation of capacity indices

$$\hat{C}_p = \frac{USL - LSL}{6S} = \frac{1.20 - 0.80}{6(0.06)} = 1.11$$

$$m = \frac{USL + LSL}{2} = \frac{1.20 + 0.80}{2} = 1.00$$

$$k = \frac{|m - \overline{X}|}{\frac{USL - LSL}{2}} = \frac{|1.00 - 0.95|}{\frac{1.20 - 0..80}{2}} = \frac{0.05}{0.20} = 0.25$$

$$\hat{C}_{pk} = \hat{C}_p(1 - \hat{k}) = 1.11(1 - 0.25) = 1.11(0.75) = 0.83$$

$$\hat{C}_{pm} = \frac{USL - LSL}{6\sqrt{S^2 + (\overline{X} - T)^2}} = \frac{1.20 - 0.80}{6\sqrt{(0.06)^2 + (0.95 - 1.00)^2}} = 0.85$$

The process is capable by the $C_p$ index, but not by the $C_{pk}$ and $C_{pm}$ indices because sample mean is off center from the target.

$$\delta = \frac{C_{pk}}{C_p} = \frac{0.83}{1.11} x100\% = 74.7\%$$

If the sample mean can be shifted back to the center there will be an almost 75% increase in the process capability.

The 95% confidence interval for the $C_{pk}$ is:

$$C_{pk} = \hat{C}_{pk} \pm z_{1-\alpha/2}\sqrt{\frac{1}{9n} + \frac{\hat{C}_{pk}^2}{2(n-1)}}$$

$$C_{pk} = 0.83 \pm 1.96\sqrt{\frac{1}{9(100)} + \frac{(0.83)^2}{2(99)}} = 0.83 \pm 0.13$$

$$0.70 < C_{pk} < 0.96$$

# 8

# Hypothesis Testing

Hypothesis testing is the process of inferring from a sample whether to accept a certain statement about a population or populations. The sample is assumed to be a small representative proportion of the total population. Two errors can occur, rejection of a true hypothesis or failing to reject a false hypothesis.

As mentioned in the beginning of Chapter 1, inferential statistical tests are intended to answer questions confronting the researcher. Statistical analysis is based on hypotheses that are formulated and then tested. Often in published articles, these hypotheses or questions are described as an "objective" or "purpose" of the study.

## Hypothesis Testing

Sometimes referred to as **significance testing**, hypothesis testing is the process of inferring from a sample whether to accept a certain statement about the population from which the sample was taken.

| | |
|---|---|
| Hypothesis: | Fact A |
| Alternative: | Fact A is false |

Researchers must carefully define the population about which they plan to make inferences and then randomly select samples or subjects that should be representative of this population. For example, if 100 capsules were drawn at random from a particular batch of a medication and some analytical procedure was performed on the sample, this measurement could be considered indicative of the population. In this case, the population is only those capsules in that specific batch and cannot be generalized to other batches of the same medication. Similarly, pharmacokinetic results from a Phase I clinical trial performed only on healthy male volunteers between 18 and 55 years old, are not necessarily reflective of the responses expected in females, children, geriatric patients, or even individuals with the specific illness for which the drug is intended to treat.

In addition, with any inferential statistical test it is assumed that the individual measurements are independent of one another and any one measurement will not influence the outcome of any other member of the sample. Also, the stated hypotheses should be free from apparent prejudgment or bias. Lastly, the hypotheses should be well-defined and clearly stated. Thus, the results of the statistical test will determine which hypothesis is correct.

The hypothesis may be rejected, meaning the evidence from the sample casts enough doubt on the hypothesis for us to say with some degree of certainty that the hypothesis is false. If the null hypothesis is rejected we accept the **alternative hypothesis**, which is the statement the researcher is usually trying to prove. On the other hand, the hypothesis may not be rejected if we are unable to statistically contradict it. Using an inferential statistic there are two possible outcomes:

$H_0$: Hypothesis under test (null hypothesis)
$H_1$: Alternative hypothesis (research hypothesis)

By convention, the **null hypothesis** is stated as no real differences in the outcomes or a relationship of zero (a null relationship). For example, if we are comparing three levels of a discrete independent variable ($\mu_1$, $\mu_2$, $\mu_3$), the null hypothesis would be stated $\mu_1 = \mu_2 = \mu_3$. The evaluation then attempts to nullify the hypothesis of no significant difference in favor of an alternative research hypothesis. The type of null hypothesis will depend upon the type of variables and the outcomes the researcher is interested in measuring. These two hypotheses are mutually exclusive and exhaustive:

$H_0$: Hypothesis A
$H_1$: Hypothesis A is false

They cannot both occur and they include all possible outcomes. The sample values, if they are randomly sampled and measured independently, are the best estimate of the population values, therefore, in the case of two levels of a discrete independent variable:

$$\bar{X}_1 \approx \mu_1 \quad \text{and} \quad \bar{X}_2 \approx \mu_2$$

With the null hypothesis as a hypothesis of no difference, we are stating that the two populations under the hypothesis are the same:

$$H_0:\ \mu_1 = \mu_2$$

We are really testing our sample data $\bar{X}_1 = \bar{X}_2$ and inferring that these data are representative of the population $\mu_1 = \mu_2$, allowing for a certain amount of error in our decision. The alternative hypothesis is either accepted or rejected based upon the decision about the hypothesis under test. Thus, an **inference** can be defined as any conclusion that is drawn from a statistical evaluation.

Statistics from our sample provide us with a basis for estimating the probability that some observed difference between samples should be expected due to sampling error. Two approaches could be used: 1) creation of a confidence interval or 2) a comparison of a test value with a critical value. The former has already been employed in the previous chapter, with the establishment of a confidence interval for a population parameter based on sample results.

$$\begin{matrix} \textit{Population} \\ \textit{Mean} \end{matrix} = \begin{matrix} \textit{Estimate} \\ \textit{Sample Mean} \end{matrix} \pm \begin{matrix} \textit{Reliability} \\ \textit{Coefficient} \end{matrix} \; x \; \begin{matrix} \textit{Standard} \\ \textit{Error} \end{matrix}$$

In the second method we would calculate a “test statistic” (a value based on the manipulation of sample data). This value is compared to a preset “critical” value (usually found in a special table) based on a specific acceptable error rate (i.e., 5%). If the test statistic is extremely rare it will be to the extreme of our critical value and we will reject the hypothesis under test in favor of the research hypothesis, which is the only possible alternative. For example, assume that we are interested in the hypothesis $H_0$: $\mu_1 = \mu_2$. If we calculate a number (result of the statistical test) to test this hypothesis we would expect our calculated statistic to equal zero if the two populations are identical. As this number becomes larger, or to an extreme of zero (either in the positive or negative direction), it becomes more likely that the two populations are not equal. In other words, as the absolute value of the calculated statistic becomes large, there is a smaller probability that $H_0$ is true and that this difference is not due to chance error alone. The critical values for most statistical tests indicate an extreme at which we reject $H_0$ and conclude that $H_1$ is the true situation (in this case that $\mu_1 \neq \mu_2$).

The statistical test results have only two possible outcomes, either we cannot reject $H_0$ or we reject $H_0$ in favor of $H_1$. At the same time, if all the facts were known (the real world) or we had data for the entire population, the hypothesis ($H_0$) is either true or false for the population that the sample represents. This may be represented as follows, where we want our results to fall into either of the two clear areas. If the results fall into either of the shaded areas, these are considered mistakes or errors.

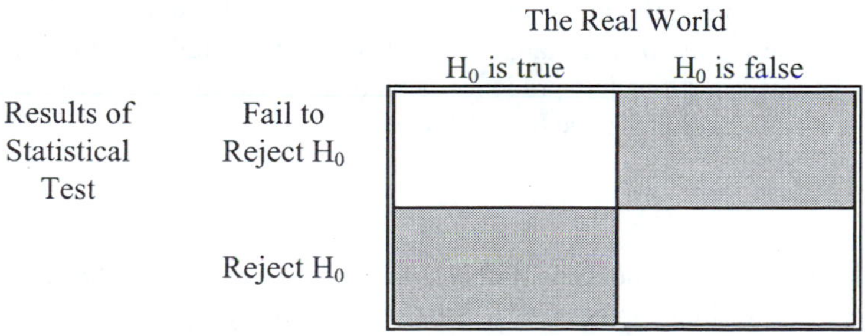

| | | The Real World | |
|---|---|---|---|
| | | $H_0$ is true | $H_0$ is false |
| Results of Statistical Test | Fail to Reject $H_0$ | (clear) | (shaded) |
| | Reject $H_0$ | (shaded) | (clear) |

An analogy to hypothesis testing can be seen in American jurisprudence (Kachigan, 1991). Illustrated below are the possible results from a jury trial.

$H_0$: Person is innocent of crime
$H_1$: Person is guilty of crime

| | | All the Facts are Known | |
|---|---|---|---|
| | | Person is Innocent | Person is Guilty |
| Jury's Verdict | Not Guilty | | ERROR II |
| | Guilty | ERROR I | |

During the trial, the jury will be presented with data (information, exhibits, testimonies, evidence) that will help, or hinder, their decision-making process. The original hypothesis is that the person is innocent until proven guilty. Evidence will conflict and the jury will never know the true situation, but will be required to render a decision. They will find the defendant either guilty or not guilty, when in fact if all the data were known, the person is either guilty or innocent of the crime. Two errors are possible: 1) sending an innocent person to prison (error I) or 2) freeing a guilty person (error II). For most, the former error would be the more grievous of the two mistakes.

Note that in this analogy, if the jury fails to find the person guilty their decision is not that the person is "innocent." Instead they present a verdict of "not guilty" (they failed to have enough evidence to prove guilt). In a similar vein, the decision is not to accept a null hypothesis, but to fail to reject it. If we cannot reject the null hypothesis, it does not prove that the statement is actually true. It only indicates that there is insufficient evidence to justify rejection. One cannot prove a null hypothesis, only fail to reject it.

It is hoped that outcomes from our court system will end in the clear areas of the previous illustration and the innocent are freed and the guilty sent to jail. Similarly, it is hoped that the results of our statistical analysis will not fall into the shaded error regions. Like our system of jurisprudence, a statistical test can only disprove the null hypothesis, it can never prove the hypothesis is true.

## Types of Errors

Similar to our jurisprudence example, there are two possible errors associated with hypothesis testing. Type I error is the probability of rejecting a true null hypothesis ($H_0$) and Type II error is the probability of accepting a false $H_0$. Type I error is also called the **level of significance** and uses the symbol $\alpha$ or $p$. Like sending an innocent person to jail, this is the most important error to minimize or control. Fortunately, the researcher has more control over the amount of acceptable Type I error. Alternatively, our level of confidence in our decision, or **confidence level**, is $1 - \alpha$ (the probability of all outcomes less Type I error).

Type II error is symbolized using the Greek letter beta ($\beta$). The probability of rejecting a false $H_0$ is called **power** $(1 - \beta)$. In hypothesis testing we always want to minimize the α and maximize $1 - \beta$. Continuing with our previous example of two populations being equal or not equal, the hypotheses are

$$H_0:\ \mu_1 = \mu_2$$
$$H_1:\ \mu_1 \neq \mu_2$$

with the four potential outcomes being:

$1 - \alpha$: Do not reject $H_0$ when in fact $\mu_1 = \mu_2$ is true
$\alpha$: Reject $H_0$ when in fact $\mu_1 = \mu_2$ is true
$1 - \beta$: Reject $H_0$ when in fact $\mu_1 = \mu_2$ is false
$\beta$: Do not reject $H_0$ when in fact $\mu_1 = \mu_2$ is false

| Results of Statistical Test | | The Real World | |
|---|---|---|---|
| | | $H_0$ is true | $H_0$ is false |
| | Fail to Reject $H_0$ | $1 - \alpha$ | $\beta$ |
| | Reject $H_0$ | $\alpha, p$ | $1 - \beta$ |

In Chapter 3 we discussed the different types of error in research (random and systematic). Statistics allow us to estimate the extent of our random errors or establish acceptable levels of random error. Systematic error is controlled through the experimental design used in the study (including random sampling and independence). In many cases systematic errors are predictable and often unidirectional. Random errors are unpredictable and relate to sample deviations that were discussed in the previous chapter.

### Type I Error

The Type I error rate should be established before making statistical computations. By convention, a probability of less than five percent ($p < 0.05$ or a 1/20 chance) is usually considered an unlikely event. However, we may wish to establish more stringent criteria (i.e., 0.01, 0.001) or a less demanding level (i.e., 0.10, 0.20) depending on the type of experiment and impact of erroneous decisions. For the purposes of this book, the error rates will usually be established at either 0.05 or 0.01. The term "statistically significant" is used to indicate that the sample data is incompatible with the null hypothesis for the proposed population and that it is rejected in favor of the alternate hypothesis.

If Type I error must be chosen before the data is gathered, it prevents the researcher from choosing a significance level to fit the $p$ values resulting from statistical testing of the data. A **decision rule** is established, which is a statement in hypothesis testing that determines whether the hypothesis under test should be rejected; for example, "with $\alpha = .05$, reject $H_0$ if … ."

In the previous illustration of pharmacokinetic data (Table 4.3), we found that there were over 234 million possible samples ($n$ = 5), which produced a normally distributed array of possible outcomes. Using any one of these samples it is possible to estimate the population mean (Eq. 7.5):

$$\mu = \overline{X} \pm Z_{(1-\alpha/2)} \times \frac{\sigma}{\sqrt{n}}$$

Using this equation we can predict a range of possible values within which the true population would fall. If we set the reliability coefficient to $\alpha = .05$, then 95% of the possible samples would create intervals that correctly include the population mean ($\mu$) based on the sample mean ($\overline{X}$). Unfortunately, 5% of the potential samples produce estimated ranges that do not include the true population mean.

As will be shown in the next chapter, the reverse of this procedure is to use a statistical formula, calculate a "test statistic" and then compare it to a critical number from a specific table in Appendix B. If the "statistic" is to the extreme of the table value, $H_0$ is rejected. Again, if we allow for a 5% Type I error rate, 95% of the time our results should be correct. However, through sampling distribution and random error, we could still be wrong 5% ($\alpha$) of the time due to chance error in sampling.

The **acceptance region** is that area in a statistical distribution where the outcomes will not lead to a rejection of the hypothesis under test. In contrast, the **rejection region**, or **critical region**, represents outcomes in a statistical distribution, which lead to the rejection of the hypothesis under test and acceptance of the alternative hypothesis. In other words, outcomes in the acceptance region could occur as a result of random or chance error. However, the likelihood of an occurrence falling in the critical region is so rare that this result cannot be attributed to chance alone.

The critical value is that value in a statistical test that divides the range of all possible values into an acceptance and a rejection region for the purposes of hypothesis testing. For example:

$$\text{With } \alpha = .05, \text{ reject } H_0 \text{ if } F > F_{3,120}(.95) = 2.68$$

In this particular case, if "F" (which is calculated through a mathematical procedure) is greater than "$F_{3,120}(.95)$" (which is found in a statistical table), then the null hypothesis is rejected in favor of the alternative.

To illustrate the above discussion, assume we are testing the fact that two samples come from different populations ($\mu_A \neq \mu_B$). Our null hypothesis would be that the two populations are equal and, if mutually exclusive and exhaustive, the only

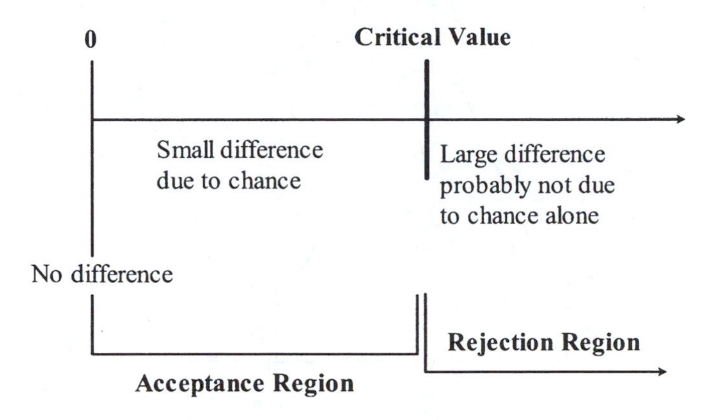


**Figure 8.1** The critical value.

alternate hypothesis would be that they are not the same.

$$H_0: \quad \mu_A = \mu_B$$
$$H_1: \quad \mu_A \neq \mu_B$$

The best, and only, estimate of the population(s) are the two sample means ($\overline{X}_A$, $\overline{X}_B$). Based on the discussion in the previous chapter on sampling distributions, we know that sample means can vary and this variability is the standard error of the mean. Obviously, if the two sample means are the same we cannot reject the null hypothesis. But what if one is 10% larger than the other? Or 20%? Or even 100%? Where do we "draw the line" and establish a point at which we must reject the null hypothesis of equality? At what point can the difference no longer be attributed to random error alone? As illustrated in Figure 8.1, this point is our critical value. If we exceed this point there is a significant difference. If the sample difference is zero or less than the critical value, then this difference could be attributed to chance error due to the potential distribution associated with samples.

Statistics provides us with tools for making statements about our certainty that there are real differences, as opposed to only chance differences between populations based on sample observations. The decision rule, with assistance from tables in Appendix B, establishes the **critical value**. The numerical manipulations presented in the following chapters will produce the **test statistic**. If we fail to reject the null hypothesis, then there is insufficient evidence available to conclude that $H_0$ is false.

Our hypothesis can be bidirectional or unidirectional. For example, assume we are not making a prediction that one outcome is better or worse than the other. Using the previous example:

$$H_0: \; \mu_A = \mu_B$$
$$H_1: \; \mu_A \neq \mu_B$$

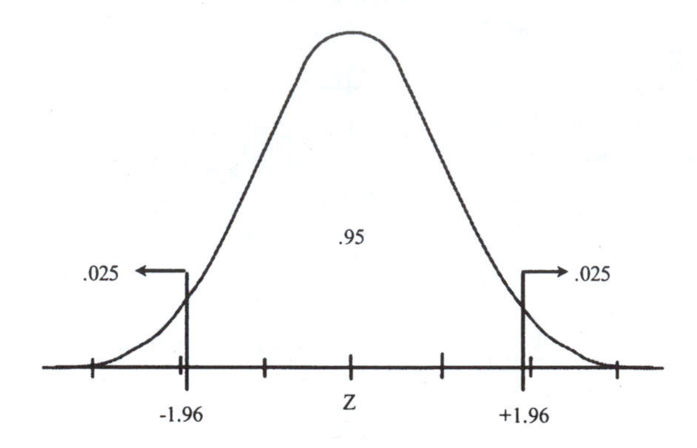


**Figure 8.2** Two-tailed 95% confidence interval.

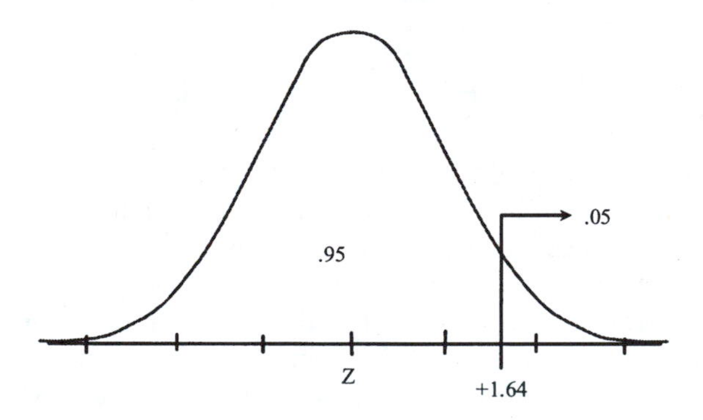


**Figure 8.3** One-tailed 95% confidence interval.

In this case the alternate hypothesis only measures that there is a difference, $\mu_A$ could be significantly larger or smaller than $\mu_B$. If $\alpha = .05$, then we need to divide it equally between the two extremes of our sampling distribution of outcomes and create two rejection regions (Figure 8.2). We then demarcate finite regions of their distribution. The range of these demarcations define the limits beyond which the null hypothesis will be rejected.

An alternative would be to create a **directional hypothesis** where we predict that one population is larger or smaller than the other:

$$H_0: \quad \mu_A \leq \mu_B$$
$$H_1: \quad \mu_A > \mu_B$$

In this case, if we reject $H_0$ we would conclude that population A is significantly larger than population B (Figure 8.3). Also referred to as **truncated**, **curtailed**, or

**one-sided hypotheses** we must be absolutely certain, usually on logical grounds, that the third omitted outcome ($\mu_A < \mu_B$) has a zero probability of occurring. The one-tailed test should never be used unless there is a specific reason for being directional.

### Type II Error and Power

Type II error and power are closely associated with sample size and the amount of difference the researcher wishes to detect. We are primarily interested in power, which is the complement of Type II error ($\beta$). Symbolized as $1 - \beta$, **power** is the ability of a statistical test to show if a significant difference truly exists. It is the probability that a statistical test will reveal a true difference when one exists. It is dependent on several factors including the size of the groups as well as the size of the difference in outcomes. In hypothesis testing, it is important to have a sizable sample to allow statistical tests to show significant differences where they exist.

Power is more difficult to understand than Type I error, where we simply select from a statistical table the amount of error we will tolerate in rejecting a true null hypotheses. We are concerned with the ability to reject a false $H_0$. In the simplest example ($H_0$: $\mu_1 = \mu_2$), we need the ability to reject this hypothesis if it is false and accept the alternative hypothesis ($H_1$: $\mu_1 \neq \mu_2$).

Let us assume for the moment that we know, or can approximate the population variance as a measure of dispersion. We could estimate our Type II error using the following equation:

$$z_\beta = \frac{\delta}{\sqrt{\frac{2\sigma^2}{n}}} - z_{\alpha/2} \qquad \text{Eq. 8.1}$$

In this equation, $\sigma^2$ represents the variance of the population (assuming the two samples are the same $\{\mu_1 = \mu_2\}$, then the dispersion will be the same for $\sigma_1$ and $\sigma_2$); $\delta$ is the detectable difference we want to be able to identify if $\mu_1 \neq \mu_2$; $n$ is the sample size for each level of the independent variable (assuming equal $n$); and $z_{\alpha/2}$ is the amount of Type I error preselected for our analysis. $z_{\alpha/2}$ is expressed as a $z$-value from the normal standardized distribution (Table B2 in Appendix B). Obviously, $z_\beta$ represents the amount of Type II error, again expressed as a value in the normalized standard distribution and reporting the probability ($\beta$) of being greater than $z_\beta$. The complement of our calculated $\beta$ would be the power associated with our statistical test $(1 - \beta)$.

As seen in Eq. 8.1, Type II error is a one-tailed distribution ($z_\beta$); whereas the Type I error rate may be set either unidirectional ($z_\alpha$) or bidirectional ($z_{\alpha/2}$). This can be explained through using the simplest hypothesis ($H_0$: $\mu_1 - \mu_2 = 0$), where we want to be able to reject this hypothesis if there is a true difference and accept the alternative hypothesis ($H_0$: $\mu_1 - \mu_2 \neq 0$). The question that needs to be asked is how large should the difference be in order to accept this alternative hypothesis? Figure 8.4 illustrates the relationship between Type I and II errors. In this figure, Type I

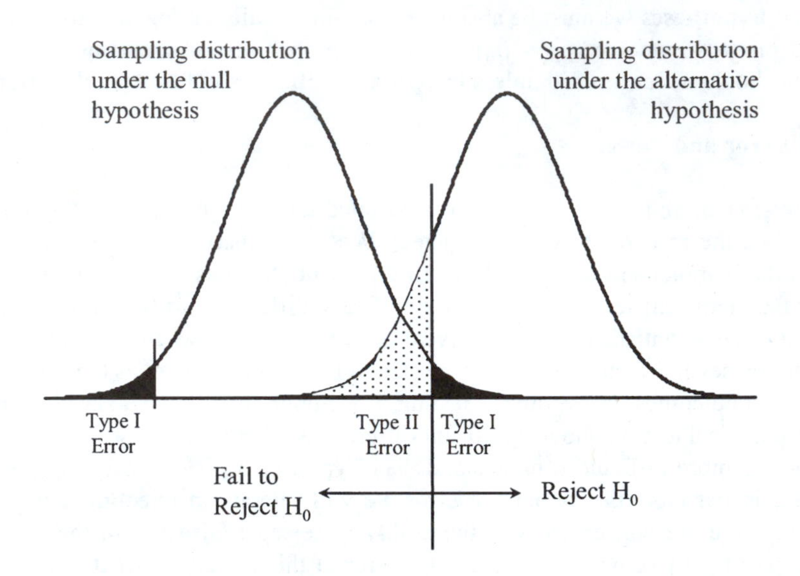


**Figure 8.4** Comparisons of sampling distributions under $H_0$ and $H_1$.

error is divided equally between the two tails of our null hypothesis and the Type II errors to the left side of the distribution for the alternative hypothesis (if it is true). Notice the common point where both types of errors end, which becomes our decision point to accept or reject the null hypothesis.

To illustrate this point, assume we are comparing samples from two tablet production runs (batches) and are concerned that there might be a difference in the average weights of the tablets. Based on historical data for the production of this dosage form, we expect a standard deviation of approximately 8 mg ($\sigma^2 = 64$) . If the two runs are not the same with respect to tablet weight ($\mu_1 \neq \mu_2$), we want to be able to identify true population differences as small as 10 mg ($\delta$). At the same time, we would like to be 95% confident in our decision ($z_{\alpha/2} = 1.96$). We sample 6 tablets from each batch. The Type II error calculation is as follows:

$$z_\beta = \frac{\delta}{\sqrt{\frac{2\sigma^2}{n}}} - z_{\alpha/2}$$

$$z_\beta = \frac{10}{\sqrt{\frac{2(8)^2}{6}}} - 1.96$$

$$z_\beta = 2.17 - 1.96 = 0.21$$

The value $z_\beta$ represents the point on a normal distribution, below which the β proportion of the curve falls. In other words the probability of being below this point is the Type II error. Looking at the normal standardized distribution table we see that the proportion of the curve between 0 and $z = 0.21$ is .0832. The area below the curve (Table B2, Appendix B), representing the Type II error, is .4168 (.5000 – .0832). Thus, for this particular problem we have power less than 60% (1 – .4168) to detect a 10-mg difference, if such a difference exists.

As will be discussed later, if we can increase our sample size we will increase our power. Let us assume that we double our sample, collecting 12 tablets from each batch, then $z_\beta$ would be:

$$z_\beta = \frac{10}{\sqrt{\frac{2(8)^2}{12}}} - 1.96 = 3.06 - 1.96 = 1.10$$

Once again referring to the normal standardized distribution table, we see that the proportion of the curve between 0 and $z = 1.10$ is .3643. In this case the area below the curve, representing the Type II error, is .1357 (.5000 – .3643). In this second case, by doubling the sample size we produce power greater than 86% (1 – .1357) to detect a 10-mg difference, if such a difference exists.

We can modify Eq. 8.1 slightly to identify the sample size required to produce a given power.

$$n \geq \frac{2\sigma^2}{\delta^2}(z_{\alpha/2} + z_\beta)^2 \qquad \text{Eq. 8.2}$$

Using the same example, assume that we still wish to be able to detect a 10-mg difference between the two batches with 95% confidence ($z_{\alpha/2} = 1.96$). In this case, we also wish to have at least 80% power (the ability to reject $H_0$ when $H_0$ is false). Therefore $\beta$ (1 – power) is the point on our normal standardized distribution below which 20% (or 0.20 proportion of the area of the curve) falls. At the same time 0.30 will fall between that point and 0 (.50 – .20). Once again looking at Table B2 in Appendix B we find that proportion (.2995) to be located at a $z$-value of 0.84. Note in Figure 8.4 that the critical values are based on α/2 (two-tailed) and $1 - \beta$ (one-tailed).

$$n \geq \frac{2\sigma^2}{\delta^2}(z_{\alpha/2} + z_\beta)^2 = \frac{2(64)}{(10)^2}(1.96 + 0.84)^2$$

$$n \geq (1.28)(2.80)^2 = 10.04$$

Therefore, to insure a power of at least 80% we should have 11 samples (rounding up the 10.04 to the next whole number).

Four characteristics are considered regarding power: 1) sample size; 2) the dispersion of the data; 3) amount of Type I error; and 4) the amount of difference to be detected.

$$\text{Type II Error} = \frac{\text{Detectable Difference}}{\sqrt{\frac{\text{Dispersion}}{n}}} + \text{Type I Error} \qquad \text{Eq. 8.3}$$

Using Eq. 8.1, it is possible to modify one of the four factors affecting power to detect differences: 1) as the detectable difference increases the power will increase; 2) as sample size increases the denominator decreases and the power once again increases; 3) as the dispersion increases the denominator increases and the power decreases; and 4) as the amount of Type I error decreases it will result in a decreased power. These are graphically illustrated in the following series of figures (Figures 8.5 through 8.8).

The only way to reduce both types of error is to increase the sample size. Thus, for a given level of significance ($\alpha$), larger sample sizes will result in greater power. Using data from the previous example, Figure 8.5 illustrates the importance of sample size. With $\alpha$, $\delta$ and the dispersion remaining the same, as we increase the sample size, the Type II error decreases and the power increases. Therefore, small sample sizes generally lack statistical power and are more likely to fail to identify important differences because the test results will be statistically insignificant.

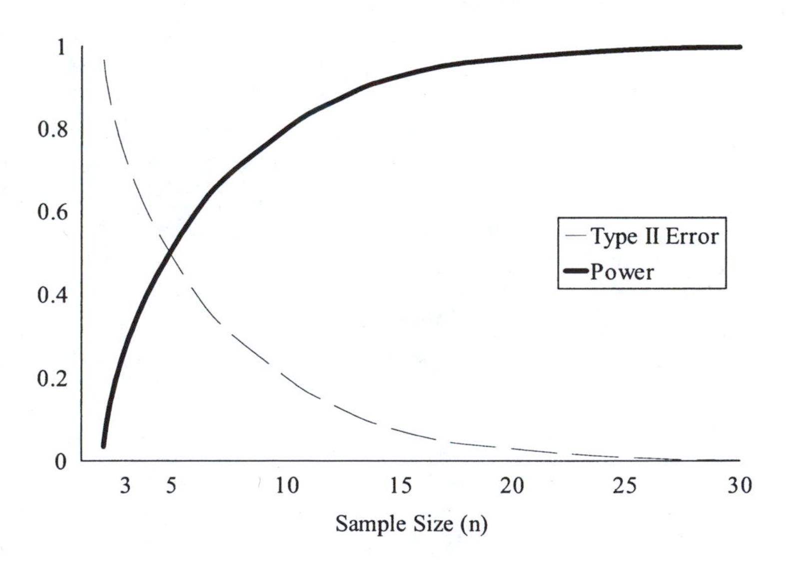


**Figure 8.5** Effect of changes in sample size on statistical power (constants $\delta = 10$, $\sigma^2 = 68$, $\alpha = 0.05$).

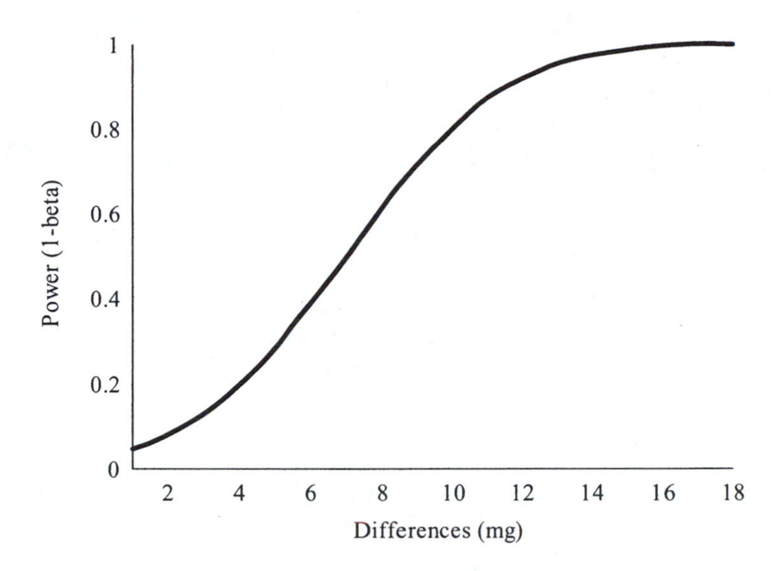


**Figure 8.6** Effect of changes in detectable differences on statistical power (constants n =10, σ2 = 64, α = 0.05).

Obviously, it is easier to detect large differences than very small ones. The importance of detectable differences is seen in Figure 8.6 where the sample size is constant ($n$ = 10), the estimated variance is 64 and α remains constant at 0.05. The only change is the amount of difference we wish to detect. As difference increases, power also increases. If we are interested in detecting a difference between two populations, obviously the larger the difference, the easier it is to detect. Again, the question we must ask ourselves is how small a difference do we want to be able to detect or how small should a difference be to be worth detecting?

As seen in Eq. 8.1, the amount of dispersion or variance can also influence power. Figure 8.7 displays the decrease in power that is associated with greater variance in the sample data. Conversely, as the variance within the population decreases, the power of the test to detect a fixed difference ($\delta$) will increase.

Generally Type II error is neither known nor specified in an experimental design. Both types of error are related inversely to each other. If we lower α without changing the sample size, we will increase the probability of having a Type II error and consequently decrease the power ($1 - \beta$). Figure 8.8 illustrates changes in power for two different levels of Type I error with increasing sample sizes. As we increase our confidence that there is a difference (making $\alpha$ smaller), we also increase the chance of missing a true difference, increasing $\beta$ or decreasing power.

In addition to the above four factors, the number of treatment levels must also be factored in when considering designs that are more complicated than comparing two levels of discrete independent variables.

The size of the sample, or number of observations, is extremely important to statistical research design. We can increase the power of a statistical test without sacrificing our confidence level ($1 - \alpha$) solely by increasing our sample size.

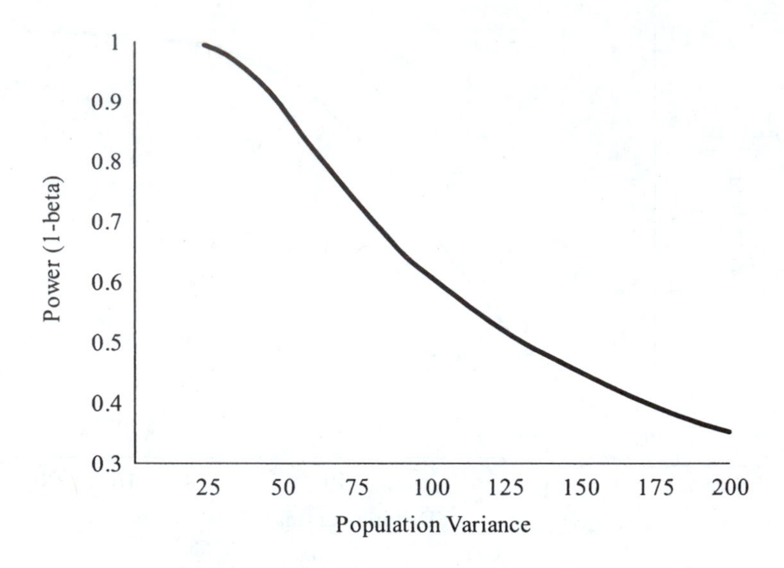


**Figure 8.7** Effect of changes in variance on statistical power (constants n = 10, $\delta = 10$, $\alpha = 0.05$).

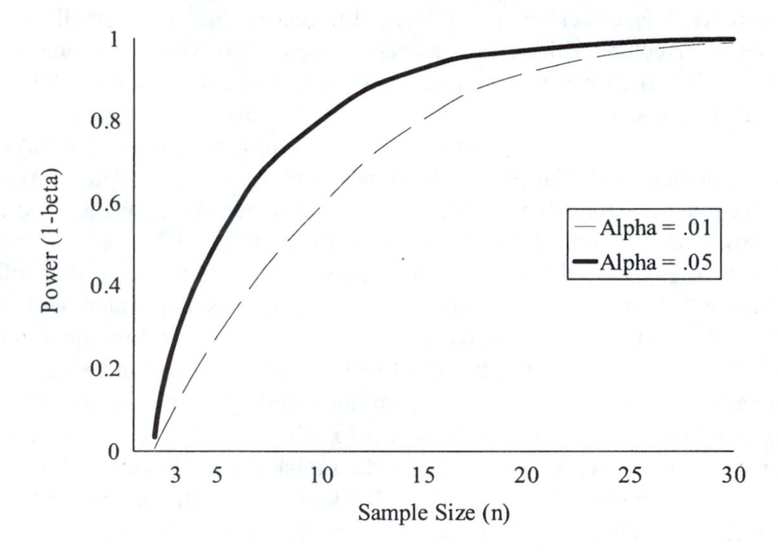


**Figure 8.8** Effect of changes in sample sizes on statistical power for two levels of Type I error (constants $\delta = 10$, $\sigma^2 = 68$).

Unfortunately, sometimes the sample sizes required to satisfy the desired power are extremely large with respect to time and cost considerations. The ways to reduce the required sample size are to increase the precision of the test, or instrument, or to increase the level of the minimal acceptable level of detectable differences. Even

**Table 8.1** Formulas for Determination of Statistical Power and Sample Size Selection

| Chapter | Statistical Test | Page(s) in Zar |
|---|---|---|
| 9 | One-sample t-test | 105-108 |
| 9 | Two-sample t-test | 132-136 |
| 9 | Paired t-test | 164 |
| 10 | One-way analysis of variance | 189-195 |
| 12 | Two-way analysis of variance | 261-263 |
| 13 | Correlation | 385-386 |
| 14 | Linear regression | 350-351 |
| 15 | Z-test of proportions | 539-542, 558-562 |

From: Zar, J.H. (1999). *Biostatistical Analysis*, Fourth edition, Prentice Hall, Englewood Cliffs, NJ.

though it is important to have a large enough sample size to be able to detect important differences; having too large a sample size may result in a significant finding even though for all practical purposes the difference is unimportant, thus producing results that are statistically significant, but have clinically insignificant differences.

The problem with the previous example is that the formula is limited to only two levels of discrete independent variables. Also, we must know the population variance. Therefore, Eq. 8.1 represents only one unique method of determining Type II error (specifically for the alternative hypothesis that two population means are not equal). Numerous formulas exist that can be used to calculate the appropriate sample size under different criteria. These include power curves presented by Kirk (1968), based on $\alpha$, $1 - \beta$, and the number of levels of the independent variable; and Young's nomograms (1983) for sample size determination (an excellent reference for many of these methods is presented by Zar). Listed in Table 8.1 are pages from Zar's book for power and sample size determination for many of the statistical tests presented in the remainder of this book. A discussion of power and sample size with the binomial tests was given by Bolton (1997).

Power is often calculated after the experiment has been completed. In these *post hoc* cases the sample standard deviation can be substituted for $\sigma$. In general, Type II error is neither known nor specified in an experimental design. For a given sample size, $\alpha$ and $\beta$ are inversely proportional. If we lower $\alpha$ without changing the sample size, we will increase the probability of a Type II error and consequently decrease the power ($1 - \beta$). The more "powerful" the test, the better the chances are that the null hypothesis will be rejected, when the null hypothesis is in fact false. The greater the power, the more sensitive the statistical test.

One of the advantages of statistical analysis and hypothesis testing is that its principles are general and applicable to data from any field of study (i.e., biological, physical, or behavioral). All of the tests presented apply to data regardless of the source of the information or the branch of science or academia from which it was derived. As mentioned in Chapter 1 and seen in Appendix A, the most important first step in selecting the most appropriate statistic is to identify the independent and dependent variables and define them as discrete or continuous.

In evaluating different tests for analyzing the same data set, we would like to use the most efficient test possible. **Efficiency** is a relative term, but provides a method for comparing the same size required with different tests that will provide the same amount of Type I and Type II errors. Obviously the test requiring the smallest sample size is the most efficient. Assume that TestA and TestB represent two statistical methods for testing the same $H_1$ against the same null $H_0$, with the same critical levels for $\alpha$ and $\beta$. The **relative efficiency** of TestA relative to TestB is the ratio of the sample size ($n_1/n_2$). The problem is finding power determination to estimate the sample size required for the desired levels of $\alpha$ and $\beta$. Finally, we can assess a potential bias nature of a test by evaluating $\alpha$ and $\beta$. An **unbiased test** is one in which the probability of rejecting $H_0$ when $H_0$ is false is always greater than or equal to the probability of rejecting $H_0$ when $H_0$ is true (i.e., $1 - \beta \geq \alpha$). It is possible to have a test result in an $\alpha = 0.60$ (obviously not significant and a failure to reject the null hypothesis. But at the same time we calculate the power (after the fact) to be 0.75. In this example we would have a biased test result.

## Experimental Errors and Propagation of Errors

In evaluating the results of data collected in a study, the value of the data will be dependent upon the accuracy of the experimental measurement. This accuracy will be reflected in the subsequent conclusions, and recommendations based on the study. The **experimental error** is then amount of uncertainty that is associated with any data set. The **true error** is the difference between the observed measurement and the true value of that quantity. For example the difference between a sample mean and the actual mean of the population from which the sample was taken. In the real world that true value is rarely known. This true error is composed of both systematic error and random error. As discussed previously, inaccuracy is a reflection of systematic error and can be reduced or eliminated using care in designing a study and measuring the results. Random error is our Type I and Type II errors and is the variability inherent in the variable being measured. One of the most effective ways to reduce random errors is through repeated measures or by replicating the experiment.

The process of error analysis is studying and evaluating experimental errors (both systematic and random). The primary goals are to: 1) estimate the magnitude of experimental errors and 2) reduce the amount of errors. The challenge is to minimize errors so that proper conclusion can be drawn from the experiment. Since "good" science is based on measurements and the interpretation of those measurements, it is important to keep uncertainties at a minimum. The topic of systematic error has already been discussed in Chapter 3. Control of random error has been focus of this chapter.

Random error exists in all measurement; if none exists, one needs a measurement instrument with greater precision. As seen in Chapter 5 the random error in a sample can be expressed by either the standard deviation (*S*) or the *RSD* (relative standard deviation). If we can directly measure our variable of interest, the *S* and *RSD* provide an assessment of the precision of the measurement. What if we cannot measure something directly, but need to calculate it based on several different variables? For example, consider the area of a flat rectangular surface. In this case we could measure the length and width of the rectangle and compute the area as A = L · W. However, several different measures of these same distances could have variable results (by different individuals, at different times, under different conditions, using different instruments, etc.). Both the length and width measurements could have an amount of associated uncertainty (measured as standard deviation):

$$L = \overline{X}_L \pm S_L \qquad W = \overline{X}_W \pm S_W$$

For calculation of the area our best estimate would involve the averages for the length and width.

$$A = \overline{X}_L \cdot \overline{X}_W$$

However, what about the measure of dispersion for this area? Could we simply sum the two standard deviations (for length and width), take the larger of the two, or create some average standard deviation? To handle this type of situation we need a method for dealing with the proliferation of error associated with the two dispersions that are related to each other, in the example the calculation of the area.

Often in experiments the final results may not be measurable, but are the result of some adding, subtracting, multiplying, or dividing of the results of the other original measurements. It becomes necessary to estimate the errors based on these types of mathematical manipulations. This combining of uncertainties from separate measures is referred to as **propagation of errors**. It is the resultant measure of dispersion where the results are dependent on a number of different independent variables, each of which is measured. Each of the independent variable will be associated with total measure of uncertainty (error). Similar to the previous example of surface areas, error components are estimated from repeating the measurement several times (or taking numerous samples) to calculate a measure of dispersion for the results (sample standard deviations or the relative standard deviations). The questions is how the handle the variability of these independent variables.

What if there is a serial progression and the first step involves a certain amount of error. The error would be compounded with the error associated with the second step in the procedure. Then further compounded with the third step, and so forth until the last step in a procedure.

There are two methods for dealing with the propagation of error and the choice depends on the mathematical process that takes place. For addition or subtraction (i.e., the previous serial example) the error term is based on the uncertainty measured by the variances of the independent measurements:

$$S_{Total} = \sqrt{S_1^2 + S_2^2 + S_3^2 + ...S_K^2} \quad \text{Eq. 8.4}$$

For multiplication or division (i.e., surface area example) the error term is based on the relative uncertainty (RSD) of the independent measurements:

$$RSD_{Total} = \sqrt{RSD_1^2 + RSD_2^2 + RSD_3^2 + ...RSD_K^2} \quad \text{Eq. 8.5}$$

This relative term is then converted to the standard deviation:

$$S_{Total} = \frac{RSD_{Total}(Final\ Mean)}{100} \quad \text{Eq. 8.6}$$

To illustrate these methods consider the following example. To calculate the molarity for mercuric nitrate it is necessary to calculate both a mass and volume measurement:

$$Molarity = \frac{Mass\ NaCl\,(mg)}{(58.44)(2)(ml_{titrant} - ml_{blank})}$$

Taking six samples, the mass (weight) will have a variance term and the volume will also have some variability. At the same time the blank used to measure the volume will vary. Listed in Table 8.2 are the results of the experiment. Without compensating for propagation of error the results for the six samples would be a mean of 0.02195 ± a standard deviation of 0.00003. However, the molarity is based on a division of the mass by the volume, but first there is the issue of variability in the volume term. The ml blank was based on the following triplicate measure:

| ml titrant | ml blank | ml used |
|---|---|---|
| 0.2003 | 0 | 0.2003 |
| 0.1754 | 0 | 0.1754 |
| 0.1956 | 0 | 0.1956 |
| | mean = | 0.1904 |
| | SD = | 0.0132 |

Therefore the propagation of error for the ($ml_{titrant} - ml_{blank}$) is calculated as follows:

$$S_{Total} = \sqrt{S_1^2 + S_2^2 + S_3^2 + ...S_K^2} = \sqrt{(0.0116)^2 + (0.0132)^2} = 0.0176$$

**Table 8.2** Results of Experiment for Mercuric Nitrate

| Mass (NaCl) | ml titrant | ml blank | ml used | Molarity |
|---|---|---|---|---|
| 16.24 | 6.5045 | 0.1904 | 6.3141 | 0.02201 |
| 16.22 | 6.5143 | 0.1904 | 6.3239 | 0.02194 |
| 16.27 | 6.5287 | 0.1904 | 6.3383 | 0.02196 |
| 16.17 | 6.5017 | 0.1904 | 6.3113 | 0.02192 |
| 16.23 | 6.5157 | 0.1904 | 6.3253 | 0.02195 |
| 16.24 | 6.5293 | 0.1904 | 6.3389 | 0.02192 |
| 16.228 | = Mean = | | 6.3253 | 0.02195 |
| 0.033 | = SD = | | 0.0116 | 0.00003 |

The calculation of the propagation of error for the molarity is further based on division and thus the relative deviations of the mass (0.033/16.228 · 100 = 0.2034%) and already propagated volume (RSD = 0.0176/6.3253 · 100 = 0.2782%):

$$RSD_{Total} = \sqrt{RSD_1^2 + RSD_2^2 + RSD_3^2 + \ldots RSD_K^2}$$

$$RSD_{Total} = \sqrt{(0.2034)^2 + (0.2782)^2} = 0.3446$$

$$S_{Total} = \frac{RSD_{Total}(Final\ Mean)}{100} = \frac{(0.3446)(0.02195)}{100} = 0.00008$$

As a result a more accurate measure of uncertainty associated with molarity, correction for the propagation of error, would be 0.02195 ± 0.00008.

**References**

Bolton, S. (1997). *Pharmaceutical Statistics: Practical and Clinical Applications*, Third edition, Marcel Dekker, Inc., New York, 1984, pp. 199-207.

Kachigan, S.K. (1991). *Multivariate Statistical Analysis*, Radius Press, New York, pp. 112, 113.

Kirk, R.E. (1968). *Experimental Design: Procedures for the Behavioral Science*, Brooks/Cole Publishing Co., Belmont, CA, pp. 9-11, 540-546.

Young, M.J., et al. (1983). "Sample size nomograms for interpreting negative clinical studies," *Annals of Internal Medicine* 99:248-251.

## Suggested Supplemental Readings

Daniel, W.W. (1999). *Biostatistics: A Foundation for Analysis in the Health Sciences*, Seventh edition, John Wiley and Sons, New York, pp. 204-270.

Kachigan, S.K. (1991). *Multivariate Statistical Analysis*, Radius Press, New York, pp. 104-116.

Snedecor, G.W. and Cochran W.G. (1989). *Statistical Methods*, Iowa State University Press, Ames, IA, pp. 64-82.

Taylor, J.R. (1982). *An Introduction to Error Analysis: The Study of Uncertainty in Physical Measurements*, University Science Books, Mill Valley, CA, 1982.

## Example Problems

1. Write the alternate hypothesis for each of the following null hypotheses:

   a. $\mu_A = \mu_B$

   b. $\mu_H \geq \mu_L$

   c. $\mu_1 = \mu_2 = \mu_3 = \mu_4 = \mu_5 = \mu_6$

   d. $\mu_A \leq \mu_B$

   e. $\mu = 125$

   f. populations C, D, E, F, and G are the same

   g. both samples come from the same population

2. If power is calculated to be 85%, with Type I error rate of 5%, what are the percentages associated with the four possible outcomes associated with hypothesis testing? What if the power was only 72%?

3. In order to calculate the average density of objects it is necessary to calculate the weight and volume of each object and calculated density using the formula: Density = mass/volume. Initial data based on 10 objects provide the following information (means and standard deviations):

   $$\text{Weight} = 10.6 \pm 0.6 \text{ gm}$$
   $$\text{Volume} = 4.9 \pm 0.3 \text{ ml}$$

   Report the mean and standard deviation for the density of these objects.

**Answers to Problems**

1. The null hypothesis and alternative hypothesis must create mutually exclusive and exhaustive statements.

   a. $H_0$: $\mu_A = \mu_B$
      $H_1$: $\mu_A \neq \mu_B$

   b. $H_0$: $\mu_H \geq \mu_L$
      $H_1$: $\mu_H < \mu_L$

   c. $H_0$: $\mu_1 = \mu_2 = \mu_3 = \mu_4 = \mu_5 = \mu_6$
      $H_1$: $H_0$ is false
      (As will be discussed in Chapter 10, traditional tests do not allow us to immediately identify which population means are different, only that at least two of the six means are significantly different. Further testing is required to determine the exact source of the difference(s).)

   d. $H_0$: $\mu_A \leq \mu_B$
      $H_1$: $\mu_A > \mu_B$

   e. $H_0$: $\mu = 125$
      $H_1$: $\mu \neq 125$

   f. $H_0$: Populations C, D, E, F, and G are the same
      $H_1$: Populations C, D, E, F, and G are not the same
      (Similar to c above, we do not identify the specific difference(s).)

   g. $H_0$: Both samples come from the same population
      $H_1$: Both samples do not come from the same population

2. In the first part of the question: $\alpha$ (Type I error) = 0.05; confidence level ($1 - \alpha$) = 0.95; power ($1 - \beta$) = 85%; therefore, $\beta$ (Type II error) = 0.15. If the power happens to be only 72% or 0.72, then the other outcomes in our test of null hypotheses are: $\beta$ (Type II error) = 1 – 0.72 = 0.28; $\alpha$ (Type I error) = 0.05; confidence level ($1 - \alpha$) = 0.95. Note that $\alpha$ and $1 - \alpha$ did not change because the researcher would have set these parameters prior to the statistical test.

3. This is an example of a propagation of error involving division, therefore the appropriate approach involved combining the relative standard deviations. Where the average density is:

$$\overline{X}_D = \frac{10.6}{4.9} = 2.16\ g/ml$$

Calculation of RSDs:

$$Weight\ RSD = \frac{0.6}{10.6} \cdot 100\% = 5.66\%$$

$$Volume\ RSD = \frac{0.3}{4.9} \cdot 100\% = 6.12\%$$

Calculation of measure of dispersion:

$$RSD_{Total} = \sqrt{(5.66)^2 + (6.12)^2} = 8.34\%$$

$$S_D = \frac{(8.34)(2.16)}{100} = 0.18$$

Result for the density: 2.16 ± 0.18 g/ml

# 9

# t-Tests

The initial eight chapters of this book focused on the "threads" associated with the statistical tests that will be discussed in the following 15 chapters. The order of presentation of these statistical tests are based on the types of variables (continuous or discrete) that researchers may encounter in the their design of experiments. As noted in Chapter 1, in this book independent variables are defined as those which the researcher can control (i.e., assignment to a control or experimental group); whereas, dependent variables fall outside the control of the researcher and are measured as outcomes or responses (i.e., pharmacokinetic responses). It should be noted that other authors may use the terms **factors** or **predictor variables** to describe what we have defined as an independent variables or **response variables** to describe dependent variables. We will continue to use the terms used in the preceding chapters.

Chapters 9 through 12 (t-tests, one-way analysis of variance, *post hoc* procedures and factorial designs) are concerned with independent variables that are discrete and outcomes measured on some continuum (dependent variable). Chapters 13, 14, and 20 present tests where both the dependent and independent variables are presented on continuous scales (i.e., correlation, regression, survival analyses). Chapters 15 through 19 (z-test of proportions, chi square tests, and measures of association) continue the presentation of tests concerned with discrete independent variables, but in these chapters the dependent variable is measured as a discrete outcome (i.e., pass or fail, live or die). Chapter 21 provides nonparametric or distribution-free statistics for evaluating data that does not meet the criteria required for many of the tests presented in Chapters 9 through 14.

### Parametric Procedures

The parametric procedures include such tests as the t-tests, analysis of variance (ANOVAs or F-tests), correlation and linear regression; Chapters 9, 10, 13, and 14 respectively. In addition to the requirements that the samples must be randomly selected from their population and independently measured, two additional "parameters" must be met. First, it must be assumed that the sample is drawn from a population whose distribution approximates that of a normal distribution. Second, when two or more distributions are being compared, there must be **homogeneity of**

**variance** or **homoscedasticity** (sample variances must be approximately equal). A rule of thumb is that if the largest variance divided by the smallest variance is less than two, then homogeneity may be assumed. More specific tests for homoscedasticity will be discussed in the next chapter. With both the t-tests and F-tests there is an independent discrete variable containing one or more levels and a dependent variable that is measured on a continuous scale. Three types of parametric tests are presented in this chapter: 1) one-sample t-test; 2) two-sample t-test; and 3) paired t-test. In each case, the independent variable is discrete and the dependent variable represents continuously distributed data.

### The t-Distribution

In Chapters 6 and 7, discussion focused on the standardized normal distribution, the standard error of the mean and the use of the z-test to create a confidence interval. This interval is the researchers "best guess" of a range of scores within which the true population mean will fall (Eq. 7.5):

$$\mu = \overline{X} \pm (1.96)\frac{\sigma}{\sqrt{n}}$$

The disadvantage with this formula is the requirement that the population standard deviation ($\sigma$) must be known. In most research, the population standard deviation is unknown or at best a rough estimate can be made based on previous research (i.e., initial clinical trials or previous production runs). As seen in Figure 7.1, the larger the sample size the more constant the value of the standard error of the mean; therefore, the z-test is accurate only for large samples. From this it would seem logical that the researcher should produce a more conservative statistic as sample sizes become smaller and less information is known about the true population variance. This was noted and rationalized by William S. Gossett in an excellent 1908 article (Student, 1908). He published this work under the pseudonym "student" because he worked for Guinness Brewing Company. At that time writing and publishing scientific papers was against company policy (Salsburg, 2002). The distribution became known as the Student t-distribution and subsequent tests are called Student t-tests or t-tests.

The t-tests, and their associated frequency distributions, are used 1) to compare one sample to a known population or value or 2) to compare two samples to each other and make inferences to their populations. These are the most commonly used tests to compare two samples because in most cases the population variances are unknown. To correct for this, the t-tables are used, which adjust the *z*-values of a normal distribution to account for sample sizes. Note in the abbreviated t-table below (Table 9.1), that any *t*-value at infinity degrees of freedom is equal to the corresponding *z*-value for a given Type I error ($\alpha$). In other words, the t-table is nothing more than a normal standardized distribution (z-table), which corrects for the number of observations per sample.

**Table 9.1** Selected Values for the t-distribution for (1-α/2)

| d.f. | $t_{.95}$ | $t_{.975}$ | $t_{.995}$ |
|---|---|---|---|
| 5 | 2.015 | 2.570 | 4.032 |
| 10 | 1.812 | 2.228 | 3.169 |
| 20 | 1.724 | 2.086 | 2.845 |
| 30 | 1.697 | 2.042 | 2.750 |
| 60 | 1.670 | 2.000 | 2.660 |
| 120 | 1.657 | 1.979 | 2.617 |
| ∞ | 1.645 | 1.960 | 2.576 |

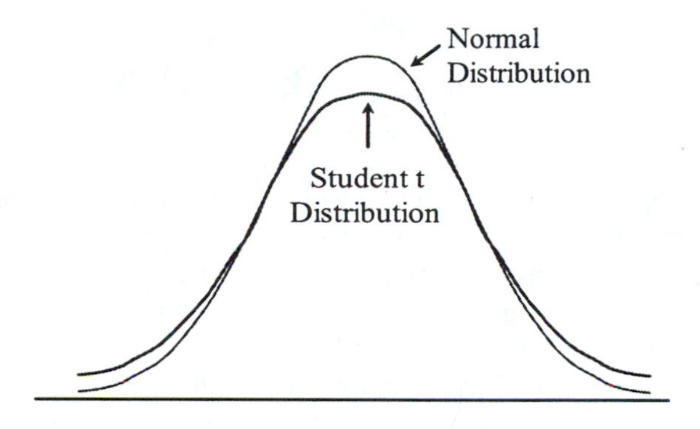


**Figure 9.1** Comparison of curves for a t-distribution and a z-distribution.

Like the normal distribution, the shape of the Student t-distribution is symmetrical and the mean value is zero. The exact shape of the curve depends on the degrees of freedom. As the sample sizes get smaller, the amplitude of the curve becomes shorter and the range becomes wider (Figure 9.1). A more complete table of *t*-values is presented in Table B5 in Appendix B. Note in Table 9.1 that this is a table designed for two-tailed bidirectional tests. The Type I error rate is divided in half ($\alpha/2$). In the case of 95% confidence, there is a 2.5% chance of being wrong to the high side of the distribution and a 2.5% chance of error to the lower tail of the distribution. Therefore, allowing for a 5% error divided in half and subtracted from all possible outcomes ($1 - \alpha/2$) the symbol of $t_{.975}$ presented in the second column of Table 9.1 represents the column for 95% confidence.

$$\alpha = 0.05$$
$$\alpha/2 = 0.025$$
$$1 - \alpha/2 = 0.975$$

Reviewing the table, the first column is degrees of freedom ($n - 1$), the third column represents critical values for 90% confidence levels, the fourth for 95%, and the last for 99.99% confidence intervals. As the number of observations decreases, the Student $t$-value increases and the spread of the distribution increases to give a more conservative estimate, because less information is known about the population variance.

**One-Tailed vs. Two-Tailed Tests**

There are two ways in which the Type I error ($\alpha$) can be distributed. In a **two-tailed test** the rejection region is equally divided between the two ends of the sampling distribution ($\alpha/2$) as described above. For example, assume we are comparing a new drug to a traditional therapeutic approach. With a two-tailed test we are not predicting that one drug is superior to the other. The alternative hypothesis is that they are different.

$$H_0: \quad \mu_{new\ drug} = \mu_{old\ drug}$$
$$H_1: \quad \mu_{new\ drug} \neq \mu_{old\ drug}$$

Assuming we would like to be 95% confident in our decision, the sampling error could result in a sample that is too high (2.5%) or too low (2.5%) based on chance sampling error. This would represent a total error rate of 5%. The rejection region for a two-tailed test where $p < .05$ and $df = \infty$ is illustrated as Figure 9.2.

In contrast, a **one-tailed test** is a test of hypothesis in which the rejection region is placed entirely at one end of the sampling distribution. In our current example, assume we want to prove that the new drug is superior to traditional therapy:

$$H_0: \quad \mu_{new\ drug} \leq \mu_{old\ drug}$$
$$H_1: \quad \mu_{new\ drug} > \mu_{old\ drug}$$

If a one-tailed test is used, all the $\alpha$ is loaded on one side of the equation and the decision rule with $\alpha = 0.05$, would be to reject $H_0$ if $t > t_{df}(1 - \alpha)$. Once again we would like to be 95% confident in our decision. The rejection region for a one-tailed test where $p < .05$ and $df = \infty$ is seen in Figure 9.3. In our example, what if our drug was truly inferior to the older drug? Using a one-tailed test we would not be able to prove this result. For that reason, the one-tailed test should never be used unless there is a specific justification for being directional. Table B6 in Appendix B provides critical $t$-values for both one-tailed and two-tailed tests.

Failure to reject the null hypothesis does not mean that this hypothesis is accepted as truth. Much like the jurisprudence example in the previous chapter, the defendant is acquitted as "not guilty," as contrasted to "innocent." Thus, we fail to reject the null hypothesis, we do not prove that the null hypothesis is true. Insufficient evidence is available to conclude that $H_0$ is false.

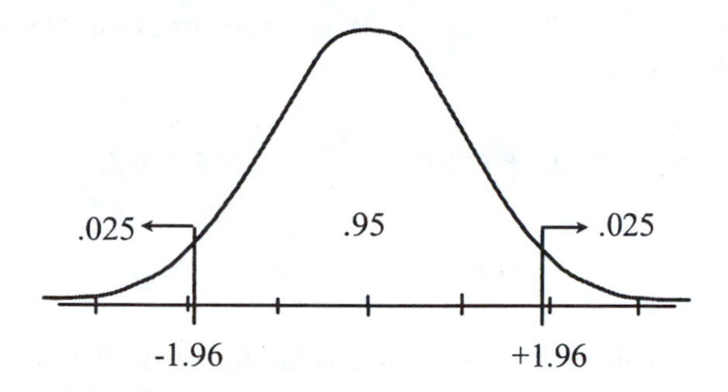


**Figure 9.2** Graphic representation of a two-tailed test.

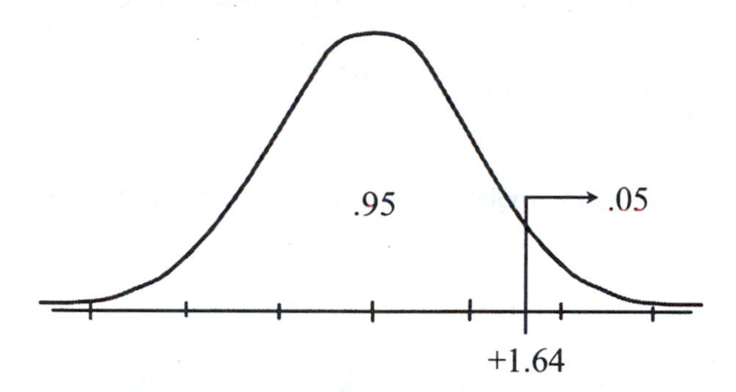


**Figure 9.3** Graphic representation of a one-tailed test.

## One-Sample t-Tests

The one-sample case can be used to either estimate the population mean or compare the sample mean to an expected population mean. In the first method, a sample is taken on some measurable continuous data and the researcher wishes to "guess" at the true population mean. In a previous chapter, 30 bottles of a cough syrup are randomly sampled from a production line (Table 5.1). From this information, it was found that the sample mean equaled 120.05 ml with a standard deviation of 0.84 ml. This data could be used to predict the mean for the entire population of cough syrup in this production lot. With 95% certainty, the confidence interval would be:

$$\mu = \overline{X} \pm t_{n-1}(1-\alpha/2) \cdot \frac{S}{\sqrt{n}} \qquad \text{Eq. 9.1}$$

Notice that the population standard deviation in the error term portion of the z-test (Eq. 7.5) has been replaced with the sample standard deviation. The expression

$t_{n-1}(1-\alpha/2)$ is the *t*-value in Tables B5 or B6 in Appendix B for 29 observations or $n-1$ degrees of freedom[1].

$$\mu = 120.05 \pm (2.045) \cdot \frac{0.84}{\sqrt{30}} = 120.05 \pm 0.31$$

$$119.74 < \mu < 120.36$$

The value 2.045 is an interpolation of the *t*-value between 30 and 25 degrees of freedom in Table B5. Therefore, based on our sample of 30 bottles, it is estimated with 95% confidence that the average volume per bottle for the true population (all bottles in the production lot) is between 119.74 and 120.34 ml.

With 99% confidence the values would be calculated as follows:

$$\mu = 120.05 \pm (2.757)\ \frac{0.84}{\sqrt{30}} = 120.05 \pm 0.42$$

where 2.757 represents an interpolated value off Tables B5 or B6 for 29 degrees of freedom at $\alpha = 0.01$.

$$119.63 < \mu < 120.47$$

Note that in order to express greater confidence in our decision regarding the population mean, the range of our estimate increases. If it were acceptable to be less confident (90% or 80% certain that the population mean was within the estimated range) the width of the interval would decrease.

One method for decreasing the size of the confidence interval is to increase the sample size. As seen in Equation 9.1, an increase in sample size will not only result in a smaller value for $t_{n-1}(1-\alpha/2)$, but the denominator (square root of *n*) will increase causing a decrease in the standard error portion of the equation. To illustrate this, assume the sample standard deviation remains constant for Sample B in the example of $C_{max}$ presented in Chapter 7 (Table 7.1), where the $\bar{X} = 752.8$, $S = 21.5$, and $n = 5$. With $t_4(.975) = 2.78$, our best guess of the population mean would be:

$$\mu = \bar{X} \pm t_{n-1}(1-\alpha/2)\ \frac{S}{\sqrt{n}}$$

---

[1] Note that exactly 29 degrees of freedom are not listed in Tables B5 or B6, but the value can be interpolated from a comparison of values for 25 and 30 df. The difference between 25 and 30 df is equivalent to 0.017 (2.059-2.042).

$$1/5 = x/0.017 \qquad x = 0.003$$

Therefore, $t_{29}(.975) = 2.042 + 0.003 = 2.045$

$$\mu = 752.8 \pm (2.78)\frac{21.5}{\sqrt{5}} = 752.8 \pm 26.73$$

$$726.07 < \mu < 779.53$$

If the sample size were increased to 25, where $t_{24}(.975) \approx 2.06$, the new confidence interval would be:

$$\mu = 752.8 \pm (2.06)\frac{21.5}{\sqrt{25}} = 752.8 \pm 8.86$$

$$743.94 < \mu < 761.66$$

If we had the ability, funds and time to have another five-fold increase to 125 samples, where $t_{124}(.975) \approx 1.98$, the confidence interval would shrink to the following size:

$$\mu = 752.8 \pm (1.98)\frac{21.5}{\sqrt{125}} = 752.8 \pm 3.81$$

$$748.99 < \mu < 756.61$$

This "shrinking" in the size of the confidence interval can be graphically seen in Figure 9.4. Obviously, the more we know about the population, as reflected by a large sample size, the more precisely we can estimate the population mean.

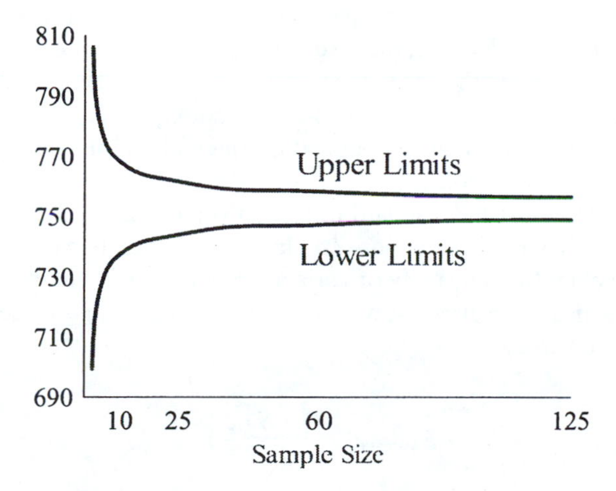


**Figure 9.4** Effect of sample size on width of confidence intervals.

## Two-Sample t-Tests

A two-sample t-test compares two levels of a discrete independent variable to determine, based on the sample statistics, if their respective populations are the same or different. Two approaches can be taken in performing a two-sample t-test: 1) establish a confidence interval for the population differences or 2) compare test results to a critical value. Either method will produce the same results and the same decision will be made with respect to the null hypothesis. The same example for the two-sample t-test will be used to illustrate these two methods of hypothesis testing. The hypotheses can be written as two identical statements.

| | Confidence Interval | Critical Value |
|---|---|---|
| The population means are the same: | $H_0$: $\mu_1 - \mu_2 = 0$ | $H_0$: $\mu_1 = \mu_2$ |
| The population means are different: | $H_1$: $\mu_1 - \mu_2 \neq 0$ | $H_1$: $\mu_1 \neq \mu_2$ |

Note that the hypotheses are saying the same thing. For the null hypothesis $\mu_1$ and $\mu_2$ are the same and the alternative (mutually exclusive and exhaustive) statement is that they are different.

The first method for calculating a two-sample t-test is an extension of the methodology used in performing a one-sample t-test. An interval is established based upon the estimated centers of the distributions (sample means), their respective standard error of the means and a selected reliability coefficient to reflect how confident we wish to be in our final decision (Eq. 7.4).

$$\begin{matrix} \textit{Population} \\ \textit{Difference} \end{matrix} = \begin{matrix} \textit{Sample} \\ \textit{Difference} \end{matrix} \pm \begin{matrix} \textit{Reliability} \\ \textit{Coefficient} \end{matrix} \; x \; \begin{matrix} \textit{Standard} \\ \textit{Error} \end{matrix}$$

The statistical formula compares the central tendencies of two different samples and based on the results determines whether their respective populations are equal or not. For the resulting confidence interval, the researcher looks for the presence or absence of zero within the interval. If they are equal, $H_0$: $\mu_1 - \mu_2 = 0$, then a zero difference must fall within the confidence interval. If they are not equal, $H_1$: $\mu_1 - \mu_2 \neq 0$, then zero does not fall within the estimated population interval and the difference cannot be attributed only to random error.

In the one-sample t-test the standard deviation (or variance) was critical to the calculation of the error term in Equation 7.4. In the two-sample case, the variances should be close together (homogeneity of variance requirement), but more than likely they will not be identical. The simplest way to calculate a central variance term would be to average the two variances:

$$S^2_{average} = \frac{S_1^2 + S_2^2}{2} \qquad \text{Eq. 9.2}$$

Unfortunately the number of observations per level may not be the same; therefore, it is necessary to "pool" these two variances and weigh them by the number of observations per discrete level of the independent variable.

$$S_p^2 = \frac{(n_1-1)S_1^2+(n_2-1)S_2^2}{n_1+n_2-2} \qquad \text{Eq. 9.3}$$

Using this latter equation, differences in sample sizes are accounted for by producing a **pooled variance** ($S_p^2$).

The confidence interval for the difference between the population means, based on the sample means, is calculated using the following equation:

$$\mu_1 - \mu_2 = (\bar{X}_1 - \bar{X}_2) \pm t_{n_1+n_2-2}(1-\alpha/2)\sqrt{\frac{S_p^2}{n_1}+\frac{S_p^2}{n_2}} \qquad \text{Eq. 9.4}$$

Obviously, $\bar{X}_1$ and $\bar{X}_2$ represent the two sample means and $n_1$ and $n_2$ are the respective sample sizes. The expression ($\bar{X}_1 - \bar{X}_2$) serves as our best estimate of the true population difference ($\mu_1 - \mu_2$).

The second, alternative method for testing the hypothesis is to create a statistical ratio and compare this to the critical value for a particular level of confidence. We can think of this t-test as a ratio:

$$t = \frac{\text{difference between the means}}{\text{distribution of the means}} \qquad \text{Eq. 9.5}$$

Obviously, if the difference between the samples is zero, the numerator would be zero, the resultant *t*-value would also be zero and the researcher would conclude no significant difference. As the difference between the sample mean becomes larger, the numerator increases, the *t*-value increases and there is a greater likelihood that the difference is not due to chance error alone. Looking at the illustrations in Figure 9.5, it is more likely that the groups to the left are significantly different because the numerator will be large; whereas the pair to the right will have a larger denominator because of the large overlap of the spreads of the distributions. But how far to the extreme does the calculated *t*-value in Equation 9.5 need to be in order to be significant? Greater than 1? Or 2? Or 50? The critical value is selected off the Student t-table (Table B5, Appendix B) based on the number of degrees of freedom. This is the same value we previously referred to as the reliability coefficient. In the case of a two-sample t-test the degrees of freedom are $n_1 - 1$ plus $n_2 - 1$, or more commonly written $n_1 + n_2 - 2$.

$$df = n_1 + n_2 - 2 = (n_1 - 1) + (n_2 - 1)$$

Notice this was the denominator in our calculation of the pooled variance (Eq. 9.3).

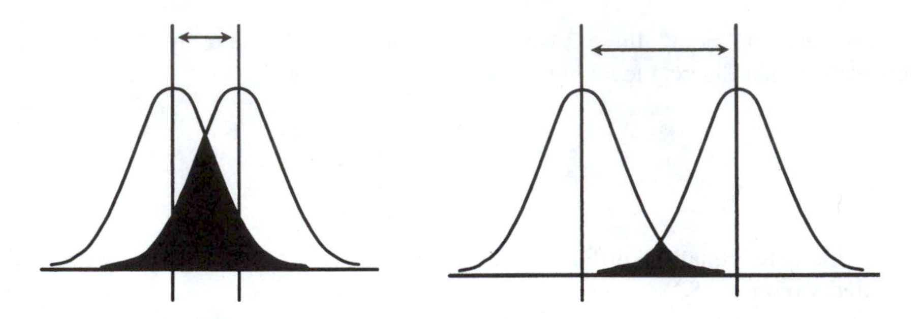

**Figure 9.5** Comparison of two different means with similar dispersions.

The variance also influences the calculated *t*-value. As observations cluster closer together, it is likely that smaller differences between means may be significant. With respect to Equation 9.5, as the variance becomes smaller the denominator in the ratio becomes smaller and the *t*-value will increase. If the *t*-value is to the extreme of the critical value then the null hypothesis will be rejected in favor of the alternative hypothesis. Once again the pooled variance (Eq. 9.3) is used to calculate this *t*-value:

$$t = \frac{\overline{X}_1 - \overline{X}_2}{\sqrt{\frac{S_P^2}{n_1} + \frac{S_P^2}{n_2}}} \qquad \text{Eq. 9.6}$$

As discussed in the next section, the t-test can be either one-tailed or two tailed. For the moment we shall focus only on two-tailed tests:

$$H_0: \mu_1 = \mu_2$$
$$H_1: \mu_1 \neq \mu_2$$

and no prediction is made whether $\mu_1$ or $\mu_2$ is larger. In this case the decision rule is, with $\alpha$ equal to a set value (usually 0.05), reject $H_0$ if $t > t_{df}(1 - \alpha/2)$ or if $t < -t_{df}(1 - \alpha/2)$. Note that the calculated *t*-value can be either positive or negative depending on which sample mean is considered first. Thus, the resultant *t*-value can be either positive or negative. Again, if the value resulting from Equation 9.6. is to the extreme (farther from zero to the positive or negative direction) than the critical value there is sufficient reason to reject the null hypothesis and conclude that this difference cannot be explained by chance error alone.

The use of these two different approaches for using the t-test in hypothesis testing is presented in the following example. An investigator used a study to compare two formulations of a drug to determine the time to maximum concentration ($C_{max}$). Is there a significant difference between the two formulations (Table 9.2)? The first approach is to establish a confidence interval where the hypotheses are:

**Table 9.2** $C_{max}$ Values for Two Formulations of the Same Drug

| Formulation A | | | | | | Formulation B | | | | | |
|---|---|---|---|---|---|---|---|---|---|---|---|
| 125 | 130 | 135 | 126 | 140 | 135 | 130 | 128 | 127 | 149 | 151 | 130 |
| 128 | 121 | 123 | 126 | 121 | 133 | 141 | 145 | 132 | 132 | 141 | 129 |
| 131 | 129 | 120 | 117 | 126 | 127 | 133 | 136 | 138 | 142 | 130 | 122 |
| 119 | 133 | 125 | 120 | 136 | 122 | 129 | 150 | 148 | 136 | 138 | 140 |
| Mean (ng/ml) | | | 127.00 | | | Mean (ng/ml) | | | 136.54 | | |
| Standard deviation | | | 6.14 | | | Standard deviation | | | 8.09 | | |
| Subjects | | | 24 | | | Subjects | | | 24 | | |

$$H_0: \mu_A - \mu_B = 0$$
$$H_1: \mu_A - \mu_B \neq 0$$

The test statistic is Equation 9.4 and the decision rule is, with $\alpha = .05$, reject $H_0$ if zero does not fall within the confidence interval. The computations involve first calculating the pooled variance and then the confidence interval with 95% confidence:

$$S_p^2 = \frac{23(6.14)^2 + 23(8.09)^2}{24+24-2} = \frac{2372.40}{46} = 51.57$$

$$\mu_A - \mu_B = (127.00 - 136.54) \pm 2.01\sqrt{\frac{51.57}{24} + \frac{51.57}{24}}$$

$$\mu_A - \mu_B = -9.54 \pm 2.01(2.07) = -9.54 \pm 4.16$$

$$-13.70 < \mu_A - \mu_B < -5.38$$

Thus, since zero is not within the confidence interval, reject $H_0$ and conclude that there is a significant difference, with formulation A reaching a significantly lower $C_{max}$. A zero outcome ($H_0$) is not a possible outcome with 95% confidence.

The second approach is to compare a calculated *t*-value to its corresponding critical value on the t-table (Table B5), where the hypotheses are the same:

$$H_0: \mu_A = \mu_B$$
$$H_1: \mu_A \neq \mu_B$$

The test statistic is Equation 9.6 and the decision rule is, with $\alpha = .05$, reject $H_0$ if $t > t_{46}(.025)$ or $t < -t_{46}(.025)$. In this case with 46 degrees of freedom reject $H_0$ if $t > 2.01$ or $t < -2.01$. The computations are as follows:

$$S_p^2 = \frac{23(6.14)^2 + 23(8.09)^2}{24 + 24 - 2} = 51.57$$

$$t = \frac{127.0 - 136.54}{\sqrt{\frac{51.57}{24} + \frac{51.57}{24}}} = \frac{-9.54}{2.07} = -4.61$$

The results show that the calculated $t$-value is smaller than (to the extreme negative side of) the critical-t of −2.01. Therefore; we would reject $H_0$, conclude that there is a significant difference, with formulation B reaching a significantly higher $C_{max}$. In both cases, the results of the statistical test were identical, the rejection of the null hypothesis. With only two formulas being compared, the initial data can be looked at and the results can state that there was a significant difference between the two formulations, and that with 95% confidence ($\alpha = .05$) Formula B has a significantly higher $C_{max}$.

**Corrected Degrees of Freedom for Unequal Variances**

As a parametric procedure, the two-sample t-test assumes that the population(s) from which the samples are taken are normally distributed and that they are approximately equal in their dispersion (homogeneity of variance). Tests for normality were discussed in Chapter 6 and tests for homogeneity of variance will be discussed in Chapter 10. As seen previously, the degrees of freedom involved with the two-sample case is $n_1 + n_2 - 2$. However in certain computer software packages the number of degrees of freedom reported on the output may be value less than $n_1 + n_2 - 2$. This is due to a correction factor based on deviations from the ideal situation where the variances are identical and both sample sizes are equal. This correction factor (Satterthwaite, 1946) is referred to as **Welch-Satterthwaite solution** or simply the **Satterthwaite solution**:

$$df = \frac{\left(\frac{S_1^2}{n_1} + \frac{S_2^2}{n_2}\right)^2}{\frac{\left(\frac{S_1^2}{n_1}\right)^2}{n_1 - 1} + \frac{\left(\frac{S_2^2}{n_2}\right)^2}{n_2 - 1}} \qquad \text{Eq. 9.7}$$

This corrected, producing a reduced number of degrees of freedom, is used as the reliability coefficients in our confidence interval or the new critical value in the ratio method for determining significance. For example, if the data presented in Table 9.2 were run on Minitab®, Version 13, the resultant output would be as follows:

### Two Sample T-Test and Confidence Interval

```
Two sample T for Cmax

Formulation        N      Mean      StDev   SE Mean
A                 24    127.00       6.14       1.3
B                 24    136.54       8.09       1.7

95% CI for mu (A) - mu (B): ( -13.7,   -5.4)
T-Test mu (A) = mu (B) (vs not =): T = -4.60  P = 0.0000  DF = 42
```

Equation 9.7 can be used as a check to determine if the degrees of feedom are the same as those calculated using the Satterthwaite solution.

$$S_1^2 = (6.14)^2 = 37.70 \quad and \quad S_2^2 = (8.09)^2 = 65.45$$

$$df = \frac{\left(\frac{37.70}{24} + \frac{65.45}{24}\right)^2}{\frac{\left(\frac{37.70}{24}\right)^2}{23} + \frac{\left(\frac{65.45}{24}\right)^2}{23}}$$

$$df = \frac{(1.571 + 2.727)^2}{\frac{(1.571)^2}{23} + \frac{(2.727)^2}{23}}$$

$$df = \frac{18.472}{0.107 + 0.323} = \frac{18.472}{0.430} = 42.9 \approx 42$$

Therefore the adjusted degrees of freedom are the same as those on the computer program and the reliability coefficient would be adjusted for 42 rather than the original 46 degrees of freedom. For this example, the reliability coefficient or critical value for rejection would still be 2.01. However, when sample sizes get small this correction factor and can result in a much larger reliability coefficient.

Basically three factors influence the t-test (and other parametric procedures): 1) normality; 2) similar variances; and 3) sample size. Parametric statistics are robust and moderate violations of these parametric assumptions have little effect in most cases (Cohen, pp. 266,267). But what if there are violations in normality, homogeneity, and sample size at the same size? This may invalidate the use of parametric statistics. The one factor that the researcher can control is sample size. Thus every effort should be made to keep the sample sizes the same, allowing for minor deviations from normality and slightly different variances.

### One-Sample t-Test Revisited for Critical Values

The one-sample t-test can also use an established critical value as a method for testing the null hypothesis that a sample is taken from a certain population. Using the previous sample of 30 bottles of cough syrup (Table 5.1), assume that we expect this particular syrup to have a fill volume of 120.0 ml. In this case our expected population center ($\mu_0$) is 120 ml. Is this sample taken from that population?

$$H_0: \mu = \mu_0 = 120.0$$
$$H_1: \mu \neq \mu_0$$

The null hypothesis is that the samples come from a given population and that any difference has arisen simply by chance. The one-sample t-test enables us to determine the likelihood of this hypothesis. The test statistic is:

$$t = \frac{\overline{X} - \mu_0}{\frac{S}{\sqrt{n}}} \qquad \text{Eq. 9.8}$$

The decision rule can be established based on the researcher's desired confidence (acceptable amount of Type I error) in the outcome of the hypothesis testing. With $1 - \alpha$ equal to 0.95 (95% confidence) the decision rule is, reject $H_0$ if $t > t_{29}(1 - \alpha/2)$ or if $t < -t_{29}(1 - \alpha/2)$, where $t_{29}(1 - \alpha/2)$ is 2.045. For 99% confidence, the decision rule would be, with $\alpha = .01$, reject $H_0$ if $t > +2.756$ or if $t < -2.756$. Therefore if the *t*-value we calculate is to the extreme of 2.045 (positive or negative) $H_0$ can be rejected with 95% confidence in the decision. If the result is to the extreme of 2.756, $H_0$ is rejected with 99% confidence. The calculation of the *t*-value or *t*-statistic is:

$$t = \frac{120.05 - 120.00}{\frac{0.84}{\sqrt{30}}} = \frac{0.05}{0.15} = 0.33$$

Similar to both the 95% and 99% confidence interval created in a previous section, where 120.0 fell within the interval, we cannot reject the hypothesis that the sample is equal to the expected population mean of 120 ml. Stated differently, we cannot reject the hypothesis that our sample is taken from a population with a mean of 120 ml.

### Matched Pair t-Test (Difference t-Test)

The matched pair, or **paired t-test**, is used when complete independence does not exist between the two samples, two time periods or **repeated measures**. For example, in a pretest-posttest design, where the same individual takes both tests, it is assumed that his/her results on the posttest will be affected (not independently) by the pretest. The individual actually serves as his/her own control. Therefore the test statistic is not concerned with differences between groups, but actual individual subject differences. The hypotheses are associated with the mean difference in the population based on sample data:

$$H_0: \mu_d = 0$$
$$H_1: \mu_d \neq 0$$

To perform the test a table showing the differences must be created and used to calculate the mean difference and the standard deviation of the difference between the two sample measurements.

| Before | After | d (After – Before) | $d^2$ |
|---|---|---|---|
| $x_1$ | $x'_1$ | $d_1 = (x'_1 - x_1)$ | $d_1^2$ |
| $x_2$ | $x'_2$ | $d_2 = (x'_2 - x_2)$ | $d_2^2$ |
| $x_3$ | $x'_3$ | $d_3 = (x'_3 - x_3)$ | $d_3^2$ |
| ... | ... | ... | ... |
| $x_n$ | $x'_n$ | $d_n = (x'_n - x_n)$ | $d_n^2$ |
| | | $\Sigma d$ | $\Sigma d^2$ |

Each row represents an individual's score or response. The first two columns are the actual outcomes. The third column is the difference between the first two columns per individual. Traditionally the first measure (before) is subtracted from the second measurement (after). Therefore a positive difference represents a larger outcome on the second measure. The mean difference is calculated:

$$\overline{X_d} = \frac{\Sigma d}{n} \qquad \text{Eq. 9.9}$$

and the standard deviation of the difference is the square root of the variance difference:

$$S_d^2 = \frac{n(\Sigma d^2) - (\Sigma d)^2}{n(n-1)} \qquad \text{Eq. 9.10}$$

$$S_d = \sqrt{S_d^2} \qquad \text{Eq. 9.11}$$

The *t*-value calculations are as follows, depending on use of the confidence interval or ratio approach for evaluating the results. Very similar to the one-sample t-test, the confidence interval would be:

$$\mu_d = \overline{X}_d \pm t_{n-1}(\alpha/2) \cdot \frac{S_d}{\sqrt{n}} \qquad \text{Eq. 9.12}$$

Interpreted the same as the two-sample t-test, if zero falls within the confidence interval, a zero outcome is possible and we fail to reject the $H_0$. Alternatively, if all the possible values in the confidence interval are positive or all are negative, we reject the null hypothesis and conclude that there is a significant difference.

The second method for hypothesis testing would be to: 1) establish a decision rule based on a critical *t*-value from Tables B5 or B6; 2) calculate a *t*-value based on the ratio of the difference divided by the distribution; and 3) reject the hypothesis under test if the *t*-value that is calculated is greater than the critical value off the table. Similar to previous tests, our estimator is in the numerator and an error term in the denominator:

$$t = \frac{\overline{X}_d}{\frac{S_d}{\sqrt{n}}} \qquad \text{Eq. 9.13}$$

Like the decision rules for hypothesis testing with the two-sample case, the test can be either one-tailed or two-tailed. In the one-tailed paired t-test the hypotheses would be either:

$$H_0: \mu_d \leq 0 \qquad \text{or} \qquad H_0: \mu_d \geq 0$$
$$H_1: \mu_d > 0 \qquad\qquad\quad H_1: \mu_d < 0$$

and the decision rule would be, with $\alpha = 0.05$, reject $H_0$ if $t > t_{df}(1 - \alpha)$. In the two-tailed test we again split the Type I error between the two tails with our hypotheses being:

$$H_0: \mu_d = 0$$
$$H_1: \mu_d \neq 0$$

the decision rule with $\alpha = 0.05$, is to reject $H_0$ if $t > t_{df}(1 - \alpha/2)$ or if $t < -t_{df}(1 - \alpha/2)$.

Because we are interested in differences in each individual, with the matched-paired t-test the degrees of freedom (*df*) is concerned with the number of pairs of individual differences rather than the total number of data points collected.

$$df = n - 1 \text{ (number of pairs)}$$

The following illustrates the use of a one-tailed matched paired t-test. A preliminary study was conducted to determine if a new antihypertensive agent could lower the diastolic blood pressure in normal individuals. Initial clinical results are presented in the second and third columns of Table 9.3. Because this is a one-tailed test (did the new drug <u>lower</u> the blood pressure, indicating a desired direction for the

**Table 9.3** Diastolic Blood Pressure before and after Administration of a New Antihypertensive

| Subject | Before | After | d(after – before) | $d^2$ |
|---|---|---|---|---|
| 1 | 68 | 66 | –2 | 4 |
| 2 | 83 | 80 | –3 | 9 |
| 3 | 72 | 67 | –5 | 25 |
| 4 | 75 | 74 | –1 | 1 |
| 5 | 79 | 70 | –9 | 81 |
| 6 | 71 | 77 | +6 | 36 |
| 7 | 65 | 64 | –1 | 1 |
| 8 | 76 | 70 | –6 | 36 |
| 9 | 78 | 76 | –2 | 4 |
| 10 | 68 | 66 | –2 | 4 |
| 11 | 85 | 81 | –4 | 16 |
| 12 | 74 | 68 | –6 | 36 |
| | | Σ = | –35 | 253 |

alternate hypothesis) the hypotheses are as follows:

$$H_0: \mu_d \geq 0$$
$$H_1: \mu_d < 0$$

In this case a rise in blood pressure or no change in blood pressure would result in a failure to reject $H_0$. Only if there was a significant decrease in the blood pressure would we reject $H_0$ in favor of the alternative hypothesis.

In this first example we will first establish a critical *t*-value and use the ratio method (Eq. 9.13) for testing the null hypothesis. The decision rule would be, with $\alpha$ = .05, reject $H_0$ if $t < -t_{11}(.95)$, which is 1.795 in Table B5 (note that this is a one-tailed test; therefore, the critical value comes from the third column, $t_{95}$ the same value is listed in the second column in Table B6). In this case we have set up our experiment to determine if there is a significant decrease in blood pressure and the difference we record is based on the second measure (after) minus the original results (before). Therefore a "good" or "desirable" response would be a negative number. If the ratio we calculate using the t-test is a negative value to the extreme of the critical value we can reject the $H_0$. Because we are performing a one-tailed test we need to be extremely careful about the signs (positive or negative).

The calculations for the mean difference and standard deviation of the difference are as follows:

$$\overline{X_d} = \frac{\Sigma d}{n} = \frac{-35}{12} = -2.92$$

$$S_d^2 = \frac{n(\sum d^2) - (\sum d)^2}{n(n-1)} = \frac{12(253) - (-35)^2}{12(11)} = 13.72$$

$$S_d = \sqrt{S_d^2} = \sqrt{13.72} = 3.70$$

The calculation of the *t*-value would be:

$$t = \frac{-2.92}{\frac{3.70}{\sqrt{12}}} = \frac{-2.92}{1.07} = -2.73$$

Therefore, based on a computed *t*-value less than the critical t-value of −1.795, the decision is to reject $H_0$ and conclude that there was a significant decrease in the diastolic blood pressure.

Using this same example, it is possible to calculate a confidence interval with $\alpha$ = 0.05. If zero falls within the confidence interval, then zero difference between the two measures is a possible outcome and the null hypothesis cannot be rejected. From the previous example we know that $\overline{X}_d$ = −2.92, $S_d$ = 3.70 and $n$ = 12. From Table B6 in Appendix B the reliability coefficient for 11 degrees of freedom ($n$ − 1) is $t_{11}(1 - \alpha) = 1.795$ at 95% confidence. Calculation of the confidence interval is

$$\mu_d = \overline{X}_d \pm t_{n-1}(\alpha - 1/2) \frac{S_d}{\sqrt{n}}$$

$$\mu_d = -2.92 \pm (1.795) \frac{3.70}{\sqrt{12}} = -2.92 \pm 1.92$$

$$-4.84 < \mu_d < -1.00$$

Since zero does not fall within the interval and in fact all possible outcomes are in the negative direction, it could be concluded with 95% certainty that there was a significant decrease in blood pressure. The results are exactly the same as found when the *t*-ratio was calculated the first time.

**References**

Cohen, J. (1969). *Statistical Power Analysis for the Behavioral Sciences*. Academic Press, New York.

Salsburg, D. (2002). *The Lady Tasting Tea: How Statistics Revolutionized Science in the Twentieth Century*, Henry Holt and Company, New York, p. 26.

Satterthwaite, F.E. (1946). "An approximate distribution of estimates of variance components," *Biometrics Bulletin* 2:110-114.

Student (1908). "The probable error of a mean," *Biometrika* 6(1):1-25.

**Suggested Supplemental Readings**

Bolton, S. (1997). *Pharmaceutical Statistics: Practical and Clinical Applications*, Third edition, Marcel Dekker, New York, pp. 141-148, 151-158.

Daniel, W.W. (1999). *Biostatistics: A Foundation for Analysis in the Health Sciences*, Seventh edition, John Wiley and Sons, New York, pp. 230-234, 241-247.

Snedecor, G.W. and Cochran W.G. (1989). *Statistical Methods*, Iowa State University Press, Ames, IA, pp. 83-105.

**Example Problems**

1. Two groups of physical therapy patients are subjected to two different treatment regimens. At the end of the study period, patients are evaluated on specific criteria to measure the percent of desired range of motion. Do the results listed below indicate a significant difference between the two therapies at the 95% confidence level?

| Group 1 | | Group 2 | |
|---|---|---|---|
| 78 | 82 | 75 | 91 |
| 87 | 87 | 88 | 79 |
| 75 | 65 | 93 | 81 |
| 88 | 80 | 86 | 86 |
| 91 | | 84 | 89 |
| | | 71 | |

2. Twelve subjects in a clinical trial to evaluate the effectiveness of a new bronchodilator were assessed for changes in their pulmonary function. Forced expiratory volume in one second ($FEV_1$) measurements were taken before and three hours after drug administration (Table 9.4).

   a. What is $t_{(1-\alpha/2)}$ for $\alpha = 0.05$?

   b. Construct a 95% confidence interval for the difference between population means.

   c. Use a t-test to compare the two groups.

**Table 9.4** $FEV_1$ Data

| Subject number | Before administration | $FEV_1$ three hours past administration |
|---|---|---|
| 1 | 3.0 | 3.1 |
| 2 | 3.6 | 3.9 |
| 3 | 3.5 | 3.7 |
| 4 | 3.8 | 3.8 |
| 5 | 3.3 | 3.2 |
| 6 | 3.9 | 3.8 |
| 7 | 3.1 | 3.4 |
| 8 | 3.2 | 3.3 |
| 9 | 3.5 | 3.6 |
| 10 | 3.4 | 3.4 |
| 11 | 3.5 | 3.7 |
| 12 | 3.6 | 3.5 |

3. Calculate the mean, standard deviation, relative standard deviation, and 95% confidence interval for each of the time periods presented in the following dissolution profile (percentage of label claim):

| | Time (minutes) | | | | |
|---|---|---|---|---|---|
| Sample | 10 | 20 | 30 | 45 | 60 |
| 1 | 60.3 | 95.7 | 97.6 | 98.6 | 98.7 |
| 2 | 53.9 | 95.6 | 97.5 | 98.6 | 98.7 |
| 3 | 70.4 | 95.1 | 96.8 | 97.9 | 98.0 |
| 4 | 61.7 | 95.3 | 97.2 | 98.0 | 98.2 |
| 5 | 64.4 | 92.8 | 95.0 | 95.8 | 96.0 |
| 6 | 59.3 | 96.3 | 98.3 | 99.1 | 99.2 |

4. Samples are taken from a specific batch of drug and randomly divided into two groups of tablets. One group is assayed by the manufacturer's own quality control laboratories. The second group of tablets is sent to a contract laboratory for identical analysis.

| Manufacturer | Contract Lab |
|---|---|
| 101.1 | 97.5 |
| 100.6 | 101.1 |
| 98.8 | 99.1 |
| 99.0 | 98.7 |
| 100.8 | 97.8 |
| 98.7 | 99.5 |

Is there a significant difference between the results generated by the two labs?

a. What is $t_{(1-\alpha/2)}$ for $\alpha = 0.05$?

b. Construct a 95% confidence interval for the difference between population means.

c. Use a t-test to compare the two groups.

5. A first-time-in-man clinical trial was conducted to determine the pharmacokinetic parameters for a new calcium channel blocker. The study involved 20 healthy adult males and yielded the following $C_{max}$ data (maximum serum concentration in ng/ml):

715, 728, 735, 716, 706, 715, 712, 717, 731, 709,
722, 701, 698, 741, 723, 718, 726, 716, 720, 721

Compute a 95% confidence interval for the population mean for this pharmacokinetic parameter.

6. Following training on content uniformity testing, comparisons are made between the analytical result of the newly trained chemist with those of a senior chemist. Samples of four different drugs (compressed tablets) are selected from different batches and assayed by both individuals. These results are listed below:

| Sample Drug, Batch | New Chemist | Senior Chemist |
|---|---|---|
| A,42 | 99.8 | 99.9 |
| A,43 | 99.6 | 99.8 |
| A,44 | 101.5 | 100.7 |
| B,96 | 99.5 | 100.1 |
| B,97 | 99.2 | 98.9 |
| C,112 | 100.8 | 101.0 |
| C,113 | 98.7 | 97.9 |
| D,21 | 100.1 | 99.9 |
| D,22 | 99.0 | 99.3 |
| D,23 | 99.1 | 99.2 |

**Answers to Problems**

1. Comparison of two groups of physical therapy patients.

| | |
|---|---|
| Independent variable: | group 1 vs. group 2 (discrete) |
| Dependent variable: | percent range of motion (continuous) |
| Statistical test: | two-sample t-test |

| | Group 1 | Group 2 |
|---|---|---|
| Mean = | 81.44 | 83.91 |
| S.D. = | 8.08 | 6.80 |
| n = | 9 | 11 |

Hypotheses: $H_0$: $\mu_1 = \mu_2$
$H_1$: $\mu_1 \neq \mu_2$

Decision rule: With $\alpha = .05$, reject $H_0$ if $t > t_{18}(.025)$ or $t < -t_{18}(.025)$.
With $\alpha = .05$, reject $H_0$ if $t > 2.12$ or $t < -2.12$.

$$S_p^2 = \frac{(n_1-1)S_1^2 + (n_2-1)S_2^2}{n_1+n_2-2} = \frac{8(8.08)^2 + 10(6.80)^2}{9+11-2} = 54.70$$

$$t = \frac{\overline{X}_1 - \overline{X}_2}{\sqrt{\frac{S_p^2}{n_1} + \frac{S_p^2}{n_2}}} = \frac{81.44 - 83.91}{\sqrt{\frac{54.7}{9} + \frac{54.7}{11}}} = \frac{-2.47}{3.32} = -0.74$$

Decision: With $t > -2.12$ cannot reject $H_0$, conclude that there is no significant difference between the two types of treatment regimens.

2. Clinical trial to evaluate the effectiveness of a new bronchodilator
Independent variable: two time periods (patient serves as own control)
Dependent variable: forced expiratory volume (continuous)
Test statistic: paired t-test

| Subject number | $FEV_1$ before administration | Three hours past administration | d | $d^2$ |
|---|---|---|---|---|
| 1 | 3.0 | 3.1 | +0.1 | 0.01 |
| 2 | 3.6 | 3.9 | +0.3 | 0.09 |
| 3 | 3.5 | 3.7 | +0.2 | 0.04 |
| 4 | 3.8 | 3.8 | 0 | 0 |
| 5 | 3.3 | 3.2 | −0.1 | 0.01 |
| 6 | 3.9 | 3.8 | −0.1 | 0.01 |
| 7 | 3.1 | 3.4 | +0.3 | 0.09 |
| 8 | 3.2 | 3.3 | +0.1 | 0.01 |
| 9 | 3.5 | 3.6 | +0.1 | 0.01 |
| 10 | 3.4 | 3.4 | 0 | 0 |
| 11 | 3.5 | 3.7 | +0.2 | 0.04 |
| 12 | 3.6 | 3.5 | −0.1 | 0.01 |
| | | $\Sigma =$ | +1.0 | 0.32 |

Mean difference and standard deviation difference:

$$\overline{X_d} = \frac{\Sigma d}{n} = \frac{+1.0}{12} = 0.083$$

$$S_d^2 = \frac{n(\Sigma d^2) - (\Sigma d)^2}{n(n-1)} = \frac{12(0.32) - (1.0)^2}{12(11)} = 0.022$$

$$S_d = \sqrt{S_d^2} = \sqrt{0.022} = 0.148$$

a. What is $t_{(1-\alpha/2)}$ for $\alpha = 0.05$? $t_{11}(.975) = 2.201$

b. Construct a 95% confidence interval for the difference between population means.

$$\mu_d = \overline{X_d} \pm t_{n-1}(1-\alpha/2)\frac{S_d}{\sqrt{n}}$$

$$\mu_d = +0.083 \pm 2.201\frac{0.148}{\sqrt{12}} = +0.083 \pm 0.094$$

$$-0.011 < \mu_d < +0.177 \quad \underline{\textit{not significant}}$$

c. Use a t-test to compare the two groups.

$$t = \frac{\overline{X_d}}{\frac{S_d}{\sqrt{n}}}$$

$$t = \frac{0.083}{\frac{0.148}{\sqrt{12}}} = 1.94$$

Decision: With $t < 2.20$, fail to reject $H_0$, fail to show a significant difference between the two time periods.

3. Calculation of measures of central tendency and 95% confidence interval.
Independent variable: 5 time periods (discrete)
Dependent variable: percent active ingredient (continuous)
Test statistic: one-sample t-test

| | Time (minutes) | | | | |
|---|---|---|---|---|---|
| Sample | 10 | 20 | 30 | 45 | 60 |
| 1 | 60.3 | 95.7 | 97.6 | 98.6 | 98.7 |
| 2 | 53.9 | 95.6 | 97.5 | 98.6 | 98.7 |
| 3 | 70.4 | 95.1 | 96.8 | 97.9 | 98.0 |
| 4 | 61.7 | 95.3 | 97.2 | 98.0 | 98.2 |
| 5 | 64.4 | 92.8 | 95.0 | 95.8 | 96.0 |
| 6 | 59.3 | 96.3 | 98.3 | 99.1 | 99.2 |

Example of the first (10-minute) time period:

Sample mean

$$\overline{X} = \frac{\sum x}{n} = \frac{60.3 + 53.9 + 70.4 + 61.7 + 64.4 + 59.3}{6} = 61.67\%$$

Sample variance/standard deviation

$$S^2 = \frac{\sum (x_i - \overline{X})^2}{n - 1}$$

$$S^2 = \frac{(60.3 - 61.67)^2 + \ldots(59.3 - 61.67)^2}{5} = 30.305$$

$$S = \sqrt{S^2} = \sqrt{30.305} = 5.505\%$$

Relative standard deviation

$$C.V. = \frac{S}{\overline{X}} = \frac{5.505}{61.67} = 0.089267$$

$$RSD = C.V. \, x \, 100 = 0.08927 \, x \, 100 = 8.927\%$$

95% Confidence interval: $\overline{X} = 61.67$, $S = 5.505$, $n = 6$

$$\mu = \overline{X} \pm t_{1-\alpha/2} \, x \, \frac{S}{\sqrt{n}}$$

$$\mu = 61.67 \pm 2.57 \cdot \frac{5.505}{\sqrt{6}} = 61.67 \pm 5.78$$

$$55.89 < \mu < 67.45 \quad 95\%\ C.I.$$

Results for all five time periods:

| | Time (minutes) | | | | |
|---|---|---|---|---|---|
| Sample | 10 | 20 | 30 | 45 | 60 |
| 1 | 60.3 | 95.7 | 97.6 | 98.6 | 98.7 |
| 2 | 53.9 | 95.6 | 97.5 | 98.6 | 98.7 |
| 3 | 70.4 | 95.1 | 96.8 | 97.9 | 98.0 |
| 4 | 61.7 | 95.3 | 97.2 | 98.0 | 98.2 |
| 5 | 64.4 | 92.8 | 95.0 | 95.8 | 96.0 |
| 6 | 59.3 | 96.3 | 98.3 | 99.1 | 99.2 |
| Mean | 61.67 | 95.13 | 97.07 | 98.00 | 98.13 |
| SD | 5.505 | 1.214 | 1.127 | 1.164 | 1.127 |
| RSD | 8.927 | 1.276 | 1.161 | 1.188 | 1.148 |
| 95% confidence interval | | | | | |
| Upper limit | 67.45 | 96.40 | 98.25 | 99.22 | 99.31 |
| Lower limit | 55.89 | 93.86 | 95.89 | 96.78 | 96.95 |

4. Comparison of results from a contract laboratory and manufacturer's quality control laboratory.
   Independent variable: manufacturer vs. contract laboratory (discrete)
   Dependent variable: assay results (continuous)
   Statistical test: two-sample t-test

Percentage of labeled amount of drug:

| Manufacturer | | Contract Lab | |
|---|---|---|---|
| 101.1 | | 97.5 | |
| 100.6 | $\overline{X} = 99.83$ | 101.1 | $\overline{X} = 98.95$ |
| 98.8 | | 99.1 | |
| 99.0 | S = 1.11 | 98.7 | S = 1.30 |
| 100.8 | | 97.8 | |
| 98.7 | n = 6 | 99.5 | n = 6 |

a. What is $t_{(1-\alpha/2)}$ for $\alpha = 0.05$? Critical $t = t_{10}(.975) = 2.228$

b. Construct a 95% confidence interval for the difference between population means.

$$S_p^2 = \frac{(n_1-1)S_1^2+(n_2-1)S_2^2}{n_1+n_2-2} = \frac{5(1.11)^2+5(1.30)^2}{6+6-2} = 1.46$$

$$\mu_1 - \mu_2 = (\overline{X}_1 - \overline{X}_2) \pm t_{n_1+n_2-2}(1-\alpha/2)\sqrt{\frac{S_P^2}{n_1}+\frac{S_P^2}{n_2}}$$

$$\mu_1 - \mu_2 = (99.83-98.95) \pm 2.228\sqrt{\frac{1.46}{6}+\frac{1.46}{6}}$$

$$\mu_1 - \mu_2 = (0.88) \pm 2.228(0.698) = 0.88 \pm 1.55$$

$$-0.67 < \mu_1 - \mu_2 < +2.43$$

Zero falls within the confidence interval; therefore assume there is a significant difference between the results from the two laboratories.

c. Use a t-test to compare the two groups.

Hypotheses: $H_0: \mu_m = \mu_c$
$H_1: \mu_m \neq \mu_c$

Test statistic:

$$t = \frac{\overline{X}_h - \overline{X}_c}{\sqrt{\frac{S_P^2}{n_h}+\frac{S_P^2}{n_c}}}$$

Decision Rule: With $\alpha = .05$, reject $H_0$ if $t > t_{10}(.025)$ or $< -t_{10}(.025)$.
With $\alpha = .05$, reject $H_0$ if $t > 2.228$ or $t < -2.228$.

Computation:

$$t = \frac{\overline{X}_1 - \overline{X}_2}{\sqrt{\frac{S_P^2}{n_1}+\frac{S_P^2}{n_2}}} = \frac{0.88}{\sqrt{\frac{1.46}{6}+\frac{1.46}{6}}} = \frac{0.88}{0.698} = 1.26$$

Decision: With $t < 2.228$, fail to reject $H_0$, fail to show a significant difference between the results from the two laboratories.

5. First-time-in-humans clinical trial
   Independent variable: volunteer assignment
   Dependent variable: $C_{max}$ (continuous)
   Test statistic: one-sample t-test

   Results: $\overline{X} = 718.5$ $S^2 = 114.6$ $S = 10.7$ $n = 20$

   Calculation:

$$\mu = \overline{X} \pm t_{(1-\alpha/2)} \frac{S}{\sqrt{n}}$$

$$\mu = 718.5 \pm 2.09 \frac{10.7}{\sqrt{20}} = 718.5 \pm 5.00$$

$$713.5 < \mu_{C_{max}} < 723.5 \ ng/ml$$

   Conclusion, with 95% confidence, the true population $C_{max}$ is between 713.5 and 723.5 ng/ml.

6. Comparisons between the analytical result of the newly trained chemist and senior chemist.
   Independent variable: two time periods (each sample serves as own control)
   Dependent variable: assay results (continuous)
   Test statistic: paired t-test

| Sample Drug, Batch | New Chemist | Senior Chemist | d | $d^2$ |
|---|---|---|---|---|
| A,42 | 99.8 | 99.9 | 0.1 | 0.01 |
| A,43 | 99.6 | 99.8 | 0.2 | 0.04 |
| A,44 | 101.5 | 100.7 | –0.8 | 0.64 |
| B,96 | 99.5 | 100.1 | 0.6 | 0.36 |
| B,97 | 99.2 | 98.9 | –0.3 | 0.09 |
| C,112 | 100.8 | 101.0 | 0.2 | 0.04 |
| C,113 | 98.7 | 97.9 | –0.8 | 0.64 |
| D,21 | 100.1 | 99.9 | –0.2 | 0.04 |
| D,22 | 99.0 | 99.3 | 0.3 | 0.09 |
| D,23 | 99.1 | 99.2 | 0.1 | 0.01 |
| | | Σ = | –0.6 | 1.96 |

Confidence interval:

$$\overline{X_d} = \frac{-0.6}{10} = -0.06$$

$$S_d^2 = \frac{10(1.96) - (-0.6)^2}{10(9)} = 0.214$$

$$S_d = \sqrt{0.214} = 0.463$$

$$\mu_d = -0.06 \pm 2.262 \frac{0.463}{\sqrt{10}} = -0.06 \pm 0.33$$

$$-0.39 < \mu_d < +0.27$$

Use a t-test to compare the two measures.

$\overline{X}_d = -0.06$
$S_d = 0.466$

Hypotheses: $H_0: \mu_h = \mu_c$
$H_1: \mu_h \neq \mu_c$

Test statistic:

$$t = \frac{\overline{X_d}}{\frac{S_d}{\sqrt{n}}}$$

Decision rule: With $\alpha = .05$, reject $H_0$ if $t > t_9(.025)$ or $< -t_9(.025)$.
With $\alpha = .05$, reject $H_0$ if $t > 2.26$ or $t < -2.26$.

Calculations:

$$t = \frac{-0.06}{\frac{.463}{\sqrt{10}}} = \frac{-0.06}{.146} = -0.41$$

Decision: With $t > -2.26$, fail to reject $H_0$, fail to show a significant difference assay results for the two scientists.

# 10

# One-Way Analysis of Variance (ANOVA)

Where the t-test was appropriate for the one- or two-sample cases (one or two levels of the discrete independent variable), the F-test or one-way analysis of variance provides an extension to $k$ levels of the independent variable. The calculation involves an *analysis of variance* of the individual sample means around a central grand mean. Like the t-test, the dependent variable represents data from a continuous distribution. The analysis of variance is also referred to as the F-test, after R.A. Fisher, a British statistician who developed this test in during the 1920s (Salsburg, 2002). This chapter will focus on the one-way analysis of variance (abbreviated with the acronym ANOVA), which involves on independent discrete variable and one dependent continuous variable.

## Hypothesis Testing with the One-Way ANOVA

There are numerous synomyms for the one-way ANOVA including: **univariate ANOVA, simple ANOVA, single-classification ANOVA or one-factor ANOVA.** The hypotheses associated with the one-way analysis of variance can be expanded to any number ($k$) levels of the discrete independent variable.

$$H_0: \mu_1 = \mu_2 = \mu_3 \ldots = \mu_k$$
$$H_1: H_0 \text{ is false}$$

The null hypothesis states that there are no differences among the population means, and that any fluctuations in the sample means are due to chance error only.

The ANOVA represents a variety of techniques used to identify and measure sources of variation within a collection of observations, hence the name analysis of variance. The ANOVA has the same assumption as those seen with the t-test: 1) sample sizes are relatively equal; 2) the variances are similar (homogeneity of variance); and 3) the dependent variable is from a normally distributed population. In fact the t-test could be considered a special case of the one-way ANOVA where $k$ = 2. Factors that can affect whether differences are statistically significant include: 1) amount of the difference between the sample means; 2) the variances of the dependent variable (wide or narrow dispersion); and 3) the sample size (larger samples provide more reliable the information).

Note that the alternative hypothesis does not say that all samples are unequal, nor does it tell where any inequalities exist. The test results merely identify that a difference does occur somewhere among the population means. In order to find where these differences are, some form of multiple comparison procedure should be performed once the null hypothesis is rejected (Chapter 11).

### The F-Distribution

A full discussion of the derivation of the sampling distribution associated with the analysis of variance is beyond the scope of this text. A more complete description can be found in Daniel (1999) or Kachigan (1991). The simplest approach would be to consider the ratio of variances for two samples randomly selected from a normally distributed population. The ratio of the variances, based on sample sizes of $n_1$ and $n_2$, would be:

$$F = \frac{S_1^2}{S_2^2}$$

Assuming the sample was taken from the same population, the ratio of the variances would be:

$$E(F) = E(\frac{S_1^2}{S_2^2}) = \frac{\sigma^2}{\sigma^2} = 1$$

However, due to the variations in sampling distributions (Chapter 7), some variation from E(F) = 1 would be expected by chance alone due to expected difference between the two sample variances. Based on previous discussions in Chapter 7 it would be expected that the variation of the sampling distribution of $S^2$ should depend on the sample size *n* and the larger the sample size, the smaller that variation. Thus, sample size is important to calculating the various F-distributions.

As will be shown in the next section, the F-test will create such a ratio comparing the variation among the levels of the independent variable and the variation within the samples. Curves have been developed that provide values that can be exceeded only 5% or 1% of the time by chance alone (Figure 10.1). Obviously if the calculated *F*-value is much larger than one and exceeds the critical value indicated below, it is most likely not due to random error. Because of the mathematical manipulations discussed later in this chapter the calculated *F*-statistic must be positive. Therefore, unlike the t-test, we are only interested in positive values to the extreme of our critical value. Similar to the t-distribution, the F-distribution is a series of curves, whose shape differs based on the degrees of freedom. As will be seen later in the chapter, the decision to accept or reject the null hypothesis, based on the shape of the F-distribution, is dependent on both the total sample size and the number of levels

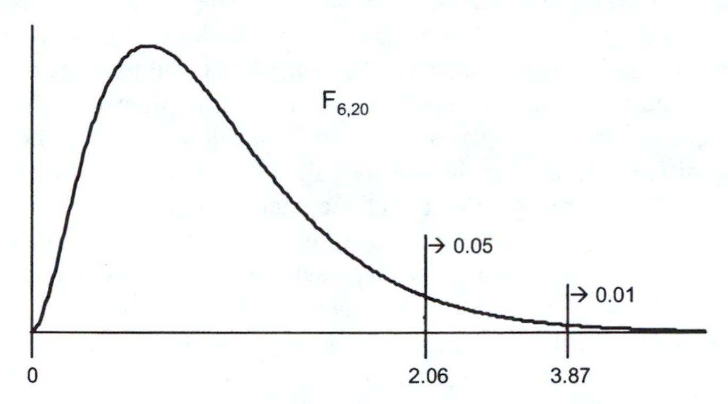


**Figure 10.1** Example of an F-distribution.

associated with the discrete independent variable. As the number of degrees of freedom get larger, the F-distribution will approach the shape of a normal distribution. A listing of the critical F-values ($F_c$) is given in Table B7 of Appendix B.

**Test Statistic**

The analysis of variance involves determining if the observed values belong to the same population, regardless of the level of the discrete variable (group), or whether the observations in at least one of these groups come from a different population.

$$H_0: \mu_1 = \mu_2 = \mu_3 \ldots = \mu_k = \mu$$

To obtain an *F*-value we need two estimates of the population variance. It is necessary to examine the variability (analysis of variance) of observations within groups as well as between groups. With the t-test, we computed a *t*-statistic by calculating the ratio of the difference between the two means over the distribution of the means (represented by the pooled variance). The *F*-statistic is computed using a simplified ratio similar to the t-test.

$$F = \frac{\text{difference between the means}}{\text{standard error of the difference of the means}} \qquad \text{Eq. 10.1}$$

The actual calculation of the *F*-statistic is as follows:

$$F = \frac{MS_B}{MS_W} \qquad \text{Eq. 10.2}$$

This formula shows the overall variability between the samples means (***$MS_B$*** or **mean squared between**) and at the same time it corrects for the dispersion of data points within each sample ($MS_W$ or **mean squared within**). The actual calculations for the $MS_B$ and $MS_W$ will be discussed in the following two sections. Obviously, the greater the differences among the sample means (the numerator), the less likely that all the samples were selected from the same population (all the samples represent population that are the same or are equal). If all the sample means are equal, the numerator measuring the differences among the means will be zero and the corresponding *F*-statistics also will be zero. As the *F*-statistic increases it becomes likely that a significant difference exists. Like the t-test, it is necessary to determine if the calculated *F*-value is large enough to represent a true difference between the populations sampled or if the difference is merely due to chance error or sampling variation. The decision rule to reject the null hypothesis of equality is stated as follows:

$$\text{with } \alpha = 0.05, \text{ reject } H_0 \text{ if } F > F_{v1,v2}(1-\alpha).$$

The critical F-value is associated with two separate degrees of freedom. The numerator degrees of freedom ($v_1$) equals $k - 1$ or the number of treatment levels minus one; and the denominator degrees of freedom ($v_2$) equals $N - k$ or the total number of observations minus the number of treatment levels ($k$).

An analogy can be made between the F-distribution and the t-distribution. As will be seen in the following sections, the process involves a squaring of the differences between sample means the total mean for all the sample observations. Values for the F-distribution for two levels of the discrete independent variable will be identical to the corresponding t-distribution value, squared. In other words, with only two levels of the independent variable $F_{1,N-2}$ equals $(t_{N-2})^2$, or $(t_{n1+n2-2})^2$, for the same level of confidence ($1 - \alpha$). This is illustrated in Table 10.1. As might be expected, the outcome for an F-test on data with only two levels of a discrete independent variable will be the same as a t-test if performed on the same information.

To calculate the *F*-statistic for the decision rule either a definitional or computational formulas may be used. With the exception of rounding errors, both methods will produce the same results. In the former case the sample means and standard deviations are used:

$\bar{X}_1, \bar{X}_2, \ldots \bar{X}_k$ = sample means
$S_1^2, S_2^2, \ldots S_k^2$ = sample variance
$n_1, n_2, \ldots n_k$ = sample sized
$N$ = total number of observations
$k$ = number of discrete levels (treatment levels) of the independent variable

Whereas, in the computational formula: 1) individual observations; 2) the sum of observations for each level of the discrete independent variable; and 3) the total sum of all observations, are squared and manipulated to produce the same outcome. The analysis of variance is a statistical procedure to analyze the overall dispersion for data in our sample outcomes.

**Table 10.1** Comparison of Critical Value between t- and F-Distributions

| | $\alpha = 0.05$ | | | $\alpha = 0.01$ | | |
|---|---|---|---|---|---|---|
| df | $t_{N-2}$ | $(t_{N-2})^2$ | $F_{1,N-2}$ | $t_{N-2}$ | $(t_{N-2})^2$ | $F_{1,N-2}$ |
| 15 | 2.131 | 4.54 | 4.54 | 2.946 | 8.68 | 8.68 |
| 30 | 2.042 | 4.17 | 4.17 | 2.750 | 7.56 | 7.56 |
| 60 | 2.000 | 4.00 | 4.00 | 2.660 | 7.08 | 7.08 |
| 120 | 1.979 | 3.92 | 3.92 | 2.617 | 6.85 | 6.85 |
| ∞ | 1.960 | 3.84 | 3.84 | 2.576 | 6.63 | 6.63 |

t- and F-Values taken from Tables B5 and B7 in Appendix B, respectively.

## ANOVA Definitional Formula

The denominator of the F-statistic (Eq. 10.2), the **mean square within** ($MS_W$), is calculated in the same way as the pooled variance is calculated for the t-test, except there are *k* levels instead of only two levels as found in the t-test.

$$MS_W = \frac{(n_1-1)S_1^2 + (n_2-1)S_2^2 + (n_3-1)S_3^2 + \ldots + (n_k-1)S_k^2}{N-K} \qquad \text{Eq. 10.3}$$

Note the similarity of this formula and the pooled variance for the t-test (Eq. 9.3). Since no single sample variance is a better measure of dispersion than the other sample variances, our best estimate is to pool the variances and create a single estimate for within variation. The mean square within is often referred to as the **mean-squared error** ($MS_E$) or **pooled-within-group variance** ($S_w^2$) and these terms are synonymous.

$$MS_W = MS_E = S_w^2$$

The mean squared within is a measure of random variability or random "error" among the measured objects and is not the same as the variability of the total set (*N*).

In the t-test, the numerator was the difference between two means (Eq. 9.6), which was easily calculated by subtracting one mean from the other. But how do we calculate a measure of difference when there are more than two means? In the ANOVA, there are *k* different means, therefore a measure is calculated to represent the variability among the different means. This measure of dispersion of the means is calculated similarly to a previous dispersion term, the variance (Eq. 5.3). First, the center (the grand mean) for all sample observations is calculated. Then the squared differences between each sample mean and the grand central mean are calculated. This measures an analysis of the variance between the individual sample means and the total center for all the sample observations. The **grand mean** or **pooled mean** is computed:

$$\overline{X}_G = \frac{(n_1\overline{X}_1)+(n_2\overline{X}_2)+(n_3\overline{X}_3)+...+(n_k\overline{X}_k)}{N} \qquad \text{Eq. 10.4}$$

This grand mean represents a weighted combination of all the sample means and an approximation of the center for all the individual sample observation. From it, the mean squared between ($MS_B$) is calculated similar to a sample variance (Eq. 5.3) by squaring the difference between each sample mean and the grand mean, and multiplying by the number of observations associated with each sample mean:

$$MS_B = \frac{n_1(\overline{X}_1-\overline{X}_G)^2+n_2(\overline{X}_2-\overline{X}_G)^2+...+n_k(\overline{X}_k-\overline{X}_G)^2}{K-1} \qquad \text{Eq. 10.5}$$

Finally the *F*-statistic is based on the ratio of the difference between the means over the distribution of their data points (Eq. 10.2):

$$F = \frac{MS_B}{MS_W}$$

In both the F-test and the t-test, the numerator of the final ratio considers differences between the means and the denominator takes into account how data are distributed around these means. The greater the spread of the sample observations, the larger the denominator, the smaller the calculated statistic; and thus a lesser the likelihood of rejecting $H_0$. The greater the differences between the means, the larger the numerator, the larger the calculated statistic, and the greater the likelihood of rejecting $H_0$ in favor of $H_1$. In other words, as the centers (means) get further apart the calculated *F*-value will increase and there is a greater likelihood that the difference will be significant. Conversely, as the dispersion becomes larger, the calculated *F*-value will decrease and the observed difference will more than likely be caused by random error.

To illustrate this method of determining the *F*-statistic, assume that during the manufacturing of a specific enteric coated tablet, samples were periodically selected from production lines at three different facilities. Weights were taken for fifteen tablets and their average weights are listed in Table 10.2. The research question would be: is there any significant difference in weights of the tablets among the three facilities? The hypotheses would be:

$H_0$: $\mu_{\text{facility A}} = \mu_{\text{facility B}} = \mu_{\text{facility C}}$
$H_1$: $H_0$ is false

The decision rule is with $\alpha = .05$, reject $H_0$ if $F > F_{2,42}(.95) = 3.23$. The value is approximated from Table B7 in Appendix B, where 2 is selected from the first column ($k - 1$) and 42 approximated from the second column ($N - k$) and the value is selected from the fourth column, ($1 - \alpha = .95$) is 3.24 (an interpolation between 3.23 for 40 *df* and 3.15 for 60 *df*). The computations are as follows:

**Table 10.2** Average Weights in Enteric Coated Tablets (in mg)

| Facility A | | Facility B | | Facility C | |
|---|---|---|---|---|---|
| 277.3 | 278.4 | 271.6 | 275.5 | 275.5 | 272.3 |
| 280.3 | 272.9 | 274.8 | 274.0 | 274.2 | 273.4 |
| 279.1 | 274.7 | 271.2 | 274.9 | 267.5 | 275.1 |
| 275.2 | 276.8 | 277.6 | 269.2 | 274.2 | 273.7 |
| 273.6 | 269.1 | 274.5 | 283.2 | 270.5 | 268.7 |
| 276.7 | 276.3 | 275.7 | 280.6 | 284.4 | 275.0 |
| 281.7 | 273.1 | 276.1 | 274.6 | 275.6 | 268.3 |
| 278.7 | | 275.9 | | 277.1 | |
| Mean = 276.26 | | Mean = 275.29 | | Mean = 273.70 | |
| S.D. = 3.27 | | S.D. = 3.46 | | S.D. = 4.16 | |

$$MS_W = \frac{(n_A - 1)S_A^2 + (n_B - 1)S_B^2 + (n_C - 1)S_C^2}{N - K}$$

$$MS_W = \frac{14(3.27)^2 + 14(3.46)^2 + 14(4.16)^2}{42} = 13.32$$

$$\overline{X}_G = \frac{(n_A\overline{X}_A) + (n_B\overline{X}_B) + (n_C\overline{X}_C)}{N}$$

$$\overline{X}_G = \frac{15(276.26) + 15(275.29) + 15(273.70)}{45} = 275.08$$

$$MS_B = \frac{n_A(\overline{X}_A - \overline{X}_G)^2 + n_B(\overline{X}_B - \overline{X}_G)^2 + n_C(\overline{X}_C - \overline{X}_G)^2}{K - 1}$$

$$MS_B = \frac{15(276.26 - 275.08)^2 + 15(275.29 - 275.08)^2 + 15(273.70 - 275.08)^2}{2}$$

$$MS_B = 25.06$$

$$F = \frac{MS_B}{MS_W} = \frac{25.06}{13.32} = 1.88$$

Thus based on the test results, the decision is with $F < 3.23$, do not reject $H_0$, and conclude that there is inadequate information to show a significant difference between the three facilities.

| | Treatments (levels) | | | | | |
|---|---|---|---|---|---|---|
| | A | B | C | ... | K | |
| | $x_{a1}$ | $x_{b1}$ | $x_{c1}$ | ... | $x_{k1}$ | |
| | $x_{a2}$ | $x_{b2}$ | $x_{c2}$ | ... | $x_{k2}$ | |
| | $x_{a3}$ | $x_{b3}$ | $x_{c3}$ | ... | $x_{k3}$ | |
| | ... | ... | ... | ... | ... | |
| | $x_{an}$ | $x_{bn}$ | $x_{cn}$ | ... | $x_{kn}$ | |
| | $\Sigma x_A$ | $\Sigma x_B$ | $\Sigma x_C$ | ... | $\Sigma x_K$ | |
| Observations per level = | $n_A$ | $n_B$ | $n_C$ | ... | $n_K$ | $\Sigma x_T$ = total sum of observations |

**Figure 10.2** Data format for the ANOVA computational formula.

### ANOVA Computational Formula

The computation technique is an alternative "short cut," which arrives at the same results as the computational method, except the formulas involve the raw data, and the means and standard deviations are neither calculated nor needed in the equations. Using this technique the $MS_W$ and $MS_B$ (also known as the **mean sum of squares**) are arrived at by two steps. First a sum of the squared deviations are obtained and then these sums are divided by their respective degrees of freedom (i.e., numerator or denominator degrees of freedom). Figure 10.2 illustrates the layout for data treated by the computational formula. This type of mathematical notation will be used with similar formulas in future chapters. In the notation scheme, $x_{jk}$ refers to the $j$th observation in the $k$th level of the discrete independent variable, where $k$ varies from 1 to $k$ (the number of groups in the analysis), and $j$ varies from 1 to $n_j$ (the number of observations in the $k$th group). In addition, the sums for each of the columns are added together ($\Sigma x_T$), represent the sum total for all the observations ($N_K$).

A series of intermediate equations are calculated. Intermediate $I$ is the sum of all the squared individual observations.

$$I = \sum_{k=1}^{K} \sum_{i=1}^{n} x_{jk}^2 = (x_{a1})^2 + (x_{a2})^2 + \ldots + (x_{kn})^2 \qquad \text{Eq. 10.6}$$

Intermediate $II$ is the square of the total sum of all observations, divided by the total number of observations.

$$II = \frac{\left[\sum_{k=1}^{K} \sum_{i=1}^{n} x_{jk}\right]^2}{N_K} = \frac{(\Sigma x_T)^2}{N_K} \qquad \text{Eq. 10.7}$$

Intermediate *III* involves summing each column (level of the discrete variable), squaring that sum, and dividing by the number of observations in the column. Then the results for each column are summed.

$$III = \sum_{k=1}^{K} \frac{\left[\sum_{i=1}^{n} x_{jk}\right]^2}{n_K} = \frac{(\Sigma x_A)^2}{n_A} + \frac{(\Sigma x_B)^2}{n_B} + \ldots + \frac{(\Sigma x_K)^2}{n_k} \qquad \text{Eq. 10.8}$$

These intermediate equations are used to determine the various sums of squares that appear in a traditional ANOVA table:

$$SS_B = III - II \qquad \text{Eq. 10.9}$$

$$SS_W = I - III \qquad \text{Eq. 10.10}$$

$$SS_T = I - II \qquad \text{Eq. 10.11}$$

Note that the sum of squared deviations for the within groups ($SS_W$) and between groups ($SS_B$) should add to the total sum of the squares ($SS_T$) and this relationship can serve as a quick check of our mathematical calculations.

$$SS_B + SS_W = SS_T$$

The ANOVA table is used to calculate the *F*-statistic. Each sum of squares is divided by their respective degrees of freedom and the resultant mean squares are used in the formula present for determining the *F*-statistic (Eq. 10.2):

| Source | Degrees of Freedom | Sum of Squares | Mean Square | F |
|---|---|---|---|---|
| Between Groups | k − 1 | III − II | $\frac{III - II}{k - 1}$ | $\frac{MS_B}{MS_W}$ |
| Within Groups | N − k | I − III | $\frac{I - III}{N - k}$ | |
| Total | N − 1 | I − II | | |

This method can be applied to the same problem that was used for the definitional formula. The hypotheses, test statistic, decision rule, and critical value ($F_{critical} = 3.23$) remain the same for the data presented in Table 10.2. In Table 10.3 the same data is presented, but includes the sums of the various columns. The mathematics for the computational formula are as follows:

**Table 10.3** Average Weights in Enteric Coated Tablets (in mg)

| Facility A | Facility B | Facility C |
|---|---|---|
| 277.3 | 271.6 | 275.5 |
| 280.3 | 274.8 | 274.2 |
| 279.1 | 271.2 | 267.5 |
| ... | ... | ... |
| 273.1 | 274.6 | 268.3 |
| $\Sigma x_A = 4143.9$ | $\Sigma x_B = 4129.4$ | $\Sigma x_C = 4105.5$ |
| | $\Sigma\Sigma x = 12378.8$ | |

$$I = \Sigma\Sigma x_{jk}^2 = (277.3)^2 + (280.3)^2 + ...(268.3)^2 = 3,405,824.58$$

$$II = \frac{\left[\Sigma\Sigma x_{jk}\right]^2}{N_k} = \frac{(12378.8)^2}{45} = 3,405,215.32$$

$$III = \Sigma\frac{\left[\Sigma x_{jk}\right]^2}{n_k} = \frac{(4143.9)^2}{15} + \frac{(4129.4)^2}{15} + \frac{(4105.5)^2}{15} = 3,405,265.45$$

$$SS_B = III - II = 3,405,265.45 - 3,405,215.32 = 50.13$$

$$SS_W = I - III = 3,405,824.58 - 3,405,265.45 = 559.13$$

$$SS_T = I - II = 3,405,824.58 - 3,405,215.32 = 609.26$$

$$SS_B + SS_W = SS_T \qquad 609.26 = 559.13 + 50.13$$

The ANOVA table for this example would be:

| Source | df | SS | MS | F |
|---|---|---|---|---|
| Between | 2 | 50.13 | 25.07 | 1.88 |
| Within | 42 | 559.13 | 13.31 | |
| Total | 44 | 609.26 | | |

The decision rule is the same, with $F < 3.23$, do not reject $H_0$. Note that the results are identical to those using the definitional formula, with minor rounding differences in the mean square column.

A second example of a one-way analysis of variance, seen below, is a case where $C_{max}$ measurements (maximum concentrations in mcg/ml) were found for four different formulations of a particular drug[1]. The researcher wished to determine if there was a significant difference in the time required to $C_{max}$.

| $C_{max}$ in mcg/ml: | Mean | S.D. | n |
|---|---|---|---|
| Formulation A | 123.2 | 12.8 | 20 |
| Formulation B | 105.6 | 11.6 | 20 |
| Formulation C | 116.4 | 14.6 | 19 |
| Formulation D | 113.5 | 10.0 | 18 |

In this case the hypotheses are:

$$H_0: \quad \mu_A = \mu_B = \mu_C = \mu_D$$
$$H_1: \quad H_0 \text{ is false}$$

The hypothesis under test is that the four formulas of the study drug produce the same $C_{max}$, on the average. If this is rejected then the alternate hypothesis is accepted, namely, that some difference exists between the four formulations. Using Eq. 10.2, our decision rule is, with $\alpha = .05$, reject $H_0$ if $F > F_{3,73}(.95) = 2.74$. This critical value comes from Table B7 in Appendix B, with $k - 1$ or 3 in the first column, $N - k$ or 73 approximated in the second column and 2.74 interpolated from the fourth column (between 60 and 120 *df*) at 95% confidence.

The computations using the definitional formula would be:

$$MS_W = \frac{(n_A - 1)S_A^2 + (n_B - 1)S_B^2 + (n_C - 1)S_C^2 + (n_D - 1)S_D^2}{N - K}$$

$$MS_W = \frac{19(12.8)^2 + 19(11.6)^2 + 18(14.6)^2 + 17(10.0)^2}{73} = 153.51$$

$$\overline{X}_G = \frac{(n_A\overline{X}_A) + (n_B\overline{X}_B) + (n_C\overline{X}_C) + (n_D\overline{X}_D)}{N}$$

$$\overline{X}_G = \frac{20(123.2) + 20(105.6) + 19(116.4) + 18(113.5)}{77} = 114.68$$

[1] It should be noted that in most cases distributions of $C_{max}$ data would be positively skewed and a lognormal transformation be required. However, for our purposes we will assume that the sample data approximates a normal distribution. Also note that the variances, squares of the standard deviations, are similar and we can assume homogeneity of variances. Specific tests for homogeneity are presented in the last section of this chapter.

$$MS_B = \frac{n_A(\overline{X}_A - \overline{X}_G)^2 + n_B(\overline{X}_B - \overline{X}_G)^2 + n_C(\overline{X}_C - \overline{X}_G)^2 + n_D(\overline{X}_D - \overline{X}_G)^2}{K-1}$$

$$MS_B = \frac{20(123.2 - 114.68)^2 + 20(105.6 - 114.68)^2 + \ldots 18(113.5 - 114.68)^2}{3}$$

$$MS_B = 1060.67$$

$$F = \frac{MS_B}{MS_W} = \frac{1060.67}{153.51} = 6.91$$

The decision based on the sample data is, with $F > 2.74$, reject $H_0$ and conclude there is a difference between the various formulations.

This last example shows an important feature of the analysis of variance. In this particular case, $H_0$ was rejected, therefore $\mu_A = \mu_B = \mu_C = \mu_D$ is not true. However, the results of the statistical test do *not* tell us where the difference or differences among the four population means occur. Looking at the data it appears that Formulation A has a $C_{max}$ that is significantly longer than the other formulations. Yet, at the same time Formulation B has a significantly shorter $C_{max}$. In fact, all four formulations could be significantly different from each other. The *F*-value that was calculated does not provide an answer to where the significant differences occur. In order to determine this, some type of *post hoc* or multiple comparisons procedure needs to be performed (Chapter 11).

**Randomized Block Design**

Whereas the one-way analysis of variance was presented as a logical extension of the t-test to more than two levels of the independent variable, the **randomized block design** can be thought of as an expansion of the paired t-test to three or more measures of the same subject or sample. Also known as the **randomized complete block design**, it represents a two-dimensional design for repeated measures with one observation per cell.

The randomized block design was developed in the 1920s by R. A. Fisher, to evaluate methods for improving agricultural experiments (Fisher, 1926). To eliminate variability between different locations of fields, his research design first divided the land into blocks. The area within each block was assumed to be relatively homogeneous. Then each of the blocks were further subdivided into plots and each plot within a given block received one of the treatments under consideration. Therefore, only one plot within each block received a specific treatment and each block contained plots that represented all the treatments.

Using this design, subjects are assigned to blocks in order to reduce variability within each treatment level. The randomized block design can be used for a variety of situations where there is a need for homogeneous blocks. The observations or

**Table 10.4** Randomized Block Design

| Age | Treatment 1 | Treatment 2 | Treatment 3 |
|---|---|---|---|
| 21-25 | 1 volunteer | 1 volunteer | 1 volunteer |
| 26-30 | 1 volunteer | 1 volunteer | 1 volunteer |
| 31-35 | 1 volunteer | 1 volunteer | 1 volunteer |
| ... | ... | ... | ... |
| 61-65 | 1 volunteer | 1 volunteer | 1 volunteer |

subjects within each block are more homogeneous than subjects within the different blocks. For example, assume that the age of volunteers may influence the study results and the researcher wants to include all possible age groups with each of the possible treatment levels. Volunteers are divided into groups based on age (i.e., 21-25, 26-30, 31-35, etc.), then one subject from each age group is randomly selected to receive each treatment (Table 10.4). In this randomized block design, each age group represents one block and there is only one observation per cell (called **experimental units**). Like Fisher's agricultural experiments, each treatment is administered to each block and each block receives every treatment. The rows represent the blocking effect and the columns show the treatment effect.

As a second example, with three treatment levels (three assay methods), assume that instead of twenty-four tablets randomly sampled from one production run, we sample from eight different runs and give one sample from each run to each of three analytical chemists to assay. In this case we assume that each of our individual production runs are more homogeneous than total mixing of all twenty-four samples across the eight runs. As seen in Figure 10.3, three samples in each row comprise a block from the same production run. Note there is still only one observation per cell. Differences between the means for the columns reflect treatment effects (in this case the difference between the three chemists) and differences between the mean for each row reflect the differences between the production runs.

As seen in Figure 10.3 the independent variables are 1) the treatment levels that appear in the columns (main effect) and 2) the blocks seen in the rows that are sub-levels of the data. The assumptions are that: 1) there has been random independent sampling; 2) at each treatment level, the outcomes are normally distributed and variances for groups at different treatment levels are similar (homogeniety of variance); and 3) block and treatment effects are additive (no interaction between the treatments and blocks). The hypotheses are as follows:

$H_0$: $\mu_A = \mu_B$ for two treatment levels
$H_1$: $\mu_A \neq \mu_B$

$H_0$: $\mu_A = \mu_B = ... \mu_K$ for three or more treatment levels
$H_1$: $H_0$ is false

As seen in the hypotheses, the main interest is in treatment effects and the blocking is used to eliminate any extraneous source of variation. The decision rule is, with $\alpha =$

| | $AC_1$ | $AC_2$ | | $AC_k$ | Sum by Block | Block Means |
|---|---|---|---|---|---|---|
| Block (batch) $b_1$ | $x_{11}$ | $x_{12}$ | ... | $x_{1k}$ | $\sum x_{b1}$ | $\bar{X}_{b1}$ |
| Block (batch) $b_2$ | $x_{21}$ | $x_{22}$ | ... | $x_{2k}$ | $\sum x_{b2}$ | $\bar{X}_{b2}$ |
| Block (batch) $b_3$ | $x_{31}$ | $x_{32}$ | ... | $x_{3k}$ | $\sum x_{b3}$ | $\bar{X}_{b3}$ |
| Block (batch) $b_4$ | $x_{41}$ | $x_{42}$ | ... | $x_{4k}$ | $\sum x_{b4}$ | $\bar{X}_{b4}$ |
| ... | ... | ... | ... | ... | ... | ... |
| Block (batch) $b_8$ | $x_{j1}$ | $x_{j2}$ | ... | $x_{jk}$ | $\sum x_{bj}$ | $\bar{X}_{b8}$ |
| Sum by column | $\sum x_{t1}$ | $\sum x_{t2}$ | ... | $\sum x_{tk}$ | $\sum\sum x_{jk}$ | |
| Treatment means | $\bar{X}_{t1}$ | $\bar{X}_{t2}$ | $\bar{X}_{t3}$ | | | |

**Figure 10.3** Data format for a randomized block design.

0.05, reject $H_0$ if $F > F_{k-1,j-1}(1 - \alpha)$. The critical $F$-value is based on $k - 1$ treatment levels as the numerator degrees of freedom, and $j - 1$ blocks as the denominator degrees of freedom. The data is presented as follows:

| | Treatment Levels | | | |
|---|---|---|---|---|
| Blocks | $K_1$ | $K_2$ | ... | $K_k$ |
| $B_1$ | $x_{11}$ | $x_{21}$ | ... | $x_{k1}$ |
| $B_2$ | $x_{12}$ | $x_{22}$ | ... | $x_{k2}$ |
| ... | ... | ... | ... | ... |
| $B_j$ | $x_{1j}$ | $x_{2j}$ | ... | $x_{kj}$ |

The formula and ANOVA table are similar to those involved in the computational formula for the one-way ANOVA. In this case there are four intermediate calculations, including one that measures the variability of blocks as well as the column treatment effect. The total sum of squares for the randomized block design is composed of the sums of squares attributed to the treatments, the blocks, and random error. Similar to the computational formula for the one-way ANOVA, Intermediate $I$ is the sum of all the squared individual observations.

$$I = \sum_{k=1}^{K} \sum_{j=1}^{J} x_{kj}^2 \qquad \text{Eq. 10.12}$$

Intermediate II is the square of the total sum of all observations, divided by the product of the number of treatments ($K$) times the number of blocks ($J$).

$$II = \frac{\left[\sum_{k=1}^{K}\sum_{j=1}^{J} x_{kj}\right]^2}{kj} \qquad \text{Eq. 10.13}$$

Intermediate III for the block effect is calculated by adding up all the sums (second to the last column in Figure 10.3) for each block and dividing by the number of treatment levels.

$$III_R = \frac{\sum_{k=1}^{K}\left[\sum_{j=1}^{J} x_{kj}\right]^2}{k} \qquad \text{Eq. 10.14}$$

Intermediate III for the treatment effect is calculated by adding up all the sums second to the last row in Figure 10.3) for each treatment and dividing by the number of blocks.

$$III_C = \frac{\sum_{j=1}^{J}\left[\sum_{k=1}^{K} x_{kj}\right]^2}{j} \qquad \text{Eq. 10.15}$$

The intermediate results are used to calculate each of these various sum of squares:

$$SS_{Total} = SS_T = I - II \qquad \text{Eq. 10.16}$$

$$SS_{Blocks} = SS_B = III_R - II \qquad \text{Eq. 10.17}$$

$$SS_{Treatment} = SS_{Rx} = III_C - II \qquad \text{Eq. 10.18}$$

$$SS_{Error} = SS_{Residual} = SS_T - SS_B - SS_{Rx} \qquad \text{Eq. 10.19}$$

An ANOVA table is constructed and each sum of squares is divided by its corresponding degrees of freedom to produce a mean square (Figure 10.4).

The $F$-value is calculated by dividing the mean square for the treatment effect by the mean square error (or **mean square residual**):

$$F = \frac{MS_{Rx}}{MS_R} \qquad \text{Eq. 10.20}$$

| Source | df | SS | MS | F |
|---|---|---|---|---|
| Treatment | k – 1 | $SS_{Rx}$ | $\frac{SS_{Rx}}{k-1}$ | $\frac{MS_{Rx}}{MS_R}$ |
| Blocks | j – 1 | $SS_B$ | $\frac{SS_B}{j-1}$ | |
| Residual | (k – 1)(j – 1) | $SS_R$ | $\frac{SS_R}{(k-1)(j-1)}$ | |
| Total | N – 1 | $SS_T$ | | |

**Figure 10.4** ANOVA Table for a randomized block design.

If the calculated *F*-value exceeds the critical value ($F_c$) for $k - 1$ and $j - 1$ degrees of freedom, $H_0$ is rejected and it is assumed that there is a significant difference between the treatment effects.

One of the most common uses for the randomized block design involves crossover clinical drug trials. **Crossover studies**, are experimental designs in which each patient receives two or more treatments that are being evaluated. The order in which patients receive the various treatments is decided through a random assignment process (for example, if only treatments A and B are being evaluated, half the patients would be randomly assigned to receive A first, the other half would receive A second). This design contrasts with two others designs already presented, parallel studies and self-controlled studies. In **parallel studies**, two or more treatments are evaluated concurrently in separate, randomly assigned, groups of patients. An example of a parallel study would be the first question in the problem set in Chapter 9, where physical therapy patients were assigned (presumably by a randomized process) to two different treatment regimens and evaluated (using a two-sample t-test) for outcomes as measured by range of motion. A **self-controlled study**, is one in which only one treatment is evaluated and the same patients are evaluated during treatment and at least one period when no treatment is present. The second question in the problem set for Chapter 9 offers an example of a self-controlled study in which the same patients were measured before and after treatment with a new brochodilator and their response evaluated using a paired t-test.

The major advantage of the crossover design is that each patients serves as his or her own control, which eliminates subject-to-subject variability in response to the treatments being evaluated. The term "randomized" in the title of this design refers to the order in which patients are assigned to the various treatments. With each patient serving as a block in the design there is increased precision, because of decreased random error and a more accurate estimate of true treatment differences. Major disadvantages with crossover experiments are that: 1) the patient may change over time (the disease state becomes worse, affecting later measurements); 2) with increased time there is a chance for subjects to withdraw or drop out of the study, which results in decreased sample size; 3) there may be a carryover effect of the first

**Table 10.5** Diastolic Blood Pressure before and after Administration of a New Antihypertensive

| Blocks (Subject) | Treatment 1 (Before) | Treatment 2 (After) | Σ | Mean |
|---|---|---|---|---|
| 1 | 68 | 66 | 134 | 67 |
| 2 | 83 | 80 | 163 | 81.5 |
| 3 | 72 | 67 | 139 | 69.5 |
| 4 | 75 | 74 | 149 | 74.5 |
| 5 | 79 | 70 | 149 | 74.5 |
| 6 | 71 | 77 | 148 | 74 |
| 7 | 65 | 64 | 129 | 64.5 |
| 8 | 76 | 70 | 146 | 73 |
| 9 | 78 | 76 | 154 | 77 |
| 10 | 68 | 66 | 134 | 67 |
| 11 | 85 | 81 | 166 | 83 |
| 12 | 74 | 68 | 142 | 71 |
| Σ = | 894 | 859 | 1753 | |
| Mean = | 74.50 | 71.58 | | |

treatment affecting subsequent treatments; and 4) the first treatment may introduce permanent physiological changes affecting later measurements. These latter two problems can be evaluated using a two-way analysis of variance design, discussed in Chapter 12, where two independent variables (treatment and order of treatment) can be assessed concurrently. Additional information about these types of experimental designs are presented by Bolton (1997) and Freidman and colleagues (1985).

As mentioned previously, a paired t-test could be considered a special case of the randomized block design with only two treatment levels. For example, the data appearing in the first three columns of Table 9.3 could be considered a randomized design (Table 10.5). Each subject represents one of twelve blocks, with two treatment measures (before and after). In this particular case the null hypothesis states that there is no difference between the two treatment periods (before vs. after):

$$H_0:\ \mu_B = \mu_A$$
$$H_1:\ \mu_B \neq \mu_A$$

The decision rule is with $\alpha$ = 0.05, reject $H_0$ if $F > F_{1,11}(.95)$, which is 4.90 (interpolated from Table B7). The calculations are as follows:

$$I = \sum_{k=1}^{K} \sum_{j=1}^{J} x_{kj}^2$$

$$I = (68)^2 + (83)^2 + (72)^2 + \ldots (68)^2 = 128{,}877$$

$$II = \frac{\left[\sum_{k=1}^{K}\sum_{j=1}^{J} x_{kj}\right]^2}{KJ}$$

$$II = \frac{(1753)^2}{24} = 128{,}042.0417$$

$$III_R = \frac{\sum_{k=1}^{K}\left[\sum_{j=1}^{J} x_{kj}\right]^2}{K}$$

$$III_R = \frac{(134)^2 + (163)^2 + \ldots(142)^2}{2} = 128{,}750.5$$

$$III_C = \frac{\sum_{j=1}^{J}\left[\sum_{k=1}^{K} x_{kj}\right]^2}{J}$$

$$III_C = \frac{(894)^2 + (859)^2}{12} = 128{,}093.0833$$

$$SS_{Total} = SS_T = I - II$$

$$SS_T = 128{,}877 - 128{,}042.0417 = 834.9583$$

$$SS_{Blocks} = SS_B = III_R - II$$

$$SS_B = 128{,}750.5 - 128{,}042.0417 = 708.4583$$

$$SS_{Treatment} = SS_{Rx} = III_C - II$$

$$SS_{Rx} = 128{,}093.0833 - 128{,}042.0417 = 51.0416$$

$$SS_{Error} = SS_{Residual} = SS_T - SS_B - SS_{Rx}$$

$$SS_{Residual} = 834.9583 - 708.4583 - 51.0416 = 75.4584$$

The ANOVA table is:

| Source | df | SS | MS | F |
|---|---|---|---|---|
| Treatment | 1 | 51.0416 | 51.0416 | 7.44 |
| Blocks | 11 | 708.4583 | 64.4053 | |
| Residual | 11 | 75.4584 | 6.8599 | |
| Total | 23 | 834.9583 | | |

With the calculated $F$-value greater than the critical value of 4.90, the decision is to reject $H_0$ and conclude that there is a significant difference between the before and after measurements with the after measure of diastolic blood pressure significantly lower than that before therapy. These results are exactly the same as observed in the paired t-test example in the previous chapter (both test results with a $p < 0.02$)[2].

### Homogeneity of Variance

It is important that we address the issue of homoscedasticity. One of the criteria required to perform any parametric procedure is that the dispersion within the different levels of the independent discrete variable be approximately equal. The reason that homogeneity of variance is important is that the error term denominator of the $F$-ratio ($MS_W$) is an average for variances as the different levels of the independent variable weighted by the size of each group. When these individual variances differ greatly this average becomes a useless summary for these measures of dispersions. As mentioned in Chapter 9 a simple rule of thumb is that the ratio of largest to smallest group variances should be 2.0 or less. Because of the robustness of the F-distribution, differences with variances can be tolerated if sample sizes are equal (Cochran, 1947; Box, 1954). However, for samples that are unequal in size, a marked difference in variances can affect the statistical outcomes.

Several tests are also available to determine if there is a lack of homogeneity. The simplest is **Hartley's F-max test**. Using this test the following hypotheses of equal variances are tested:

$$H_0: \sigma_1^2 = \sigma_2^2 = \sigma_3^2 \ldots = \sigma_k^2$$
$$H_1: H_0 \text{ is false}$$

The test statistic is a simple ratio between the largest and smallest variances:

$$F_{\max} = \frac{S^2_{largest}}{S^2_{smallest}} \qquad \text{Eq. 10.21}$$

---

[2] Using Excel® 2002 the p-value can be calculated for t = 2.73 using the TDIST function (p = 0.01958) as well as the p-value for F = 7.44 using the FDIST function (p = 0.01966). The minor difference is due to rounding before the final t- and F-values were reported.

The resultant $F_{max}$ value is compared to a critical value from Table B8 (Appendix B) for $k$ levels of the discrete independent variable and $n - 1$ degrees of freedom, based on $n$ observations per level of the independent variable (equal cell size). If $F_{max}$ exceeds the critical value, $H_0$ is rejected and the researcher cannot assume that there is homogeneity. For example, consider the previous example comparing the weights of tablets from three different facilities (Table 10.2). The largest variance is from facility C at 17.31 ($4.16^2$) and the smallest from Facility A is 10.69 ($3.27^2$). Can the investigator assume that there is homogeneity of variance?

$$H_0: \quad \sigma_A^2 = \sigma_B^2 = \sigma_C^2$$
$$H_1: \quad H_0 \text{ is false}$$

With $\alpha = 0.05$, $H_0$ would be rejected if $F_{max}$ exceeds the critical $F_{3,14}$, which is approximately 3.75. Calculation of the test statistic is:

$$F_{\max} = \frac{S_{largest}^2}{S_{smallest}^2} = \frac{17.31}{10.69} = 1.62$$

With $F_{max}$ less than 3.75 the researcher would fail to reject the null hypothesis with 95% confidence and would assume that the sample variances are all equal.

A second procedure that can be used for unequal cell sizes (differing numbers of observations per level of the independent variable) would be **Cochran's C test,** which compares the ratio of the largest sample variance with the sum of all variances:

$$C = \frac{S_{largest}^2}{\Sigma S_k^2} \qquad \text{Eq. 10.22}$$

Once again a table of critical values is required (Table B9, Appendix B). The calculated $C$ ratio is compared to a critical value from Table B7 for $k$ levels of the independent variable in the samples and $n - 1$ observations per sample. If $C$ exceeds the critical value, $H_0$ is rejected and the researcher cannot assume that there is homogeneity. Using the same example as above, with $\alpha = 0.05$, $H_0$ would be rejected if $C$ exceeds the critical C-value, which is approximately 0.5666. Calculation of the test statistic is:

$$C = \frac{S_{largest}^2}{\Sigma S_k^2} = \frac{(4.16)^2}{(3.27)^2 + (3.46)^2 + (4.16)^2} = \frac{17.31}{39.97} = 0.4331$$

With $C$ less than 0.5666 the exact same result occurs as was found with the $F_{max}$ results.

If the cell size differs slightly, the largest of the $n$'s can be used to determine the degrees of freedom. Consider the second ANOVA example with four different formulations (A, B, C, and D) and cell sizes of 20, 20, 19, and 18, respectively. In this case $n = 20$, $n - 1 = 19$ and the critical values for C by interpolation would be 0.4355. The test statistic would be:

$$C = \frac{(14.6)^2}{(12.8)^2 + (11.6)^2 + (14.6)^2 + (10.0)^2} = 0.3486$$

In both cases, the statistics are less than the critical values, the researcher fails to reject $H_0$ and assume that there is homogeneity of variance.

Another alternative procedure that involves more complex calculations is **Bartlett's test**, which is an older test based on a chi-square test (Chapter 16) with $(k - 1)$ degrees of freedom (Barlett, 1937). This test is described in Kirk's book (1968). **Levene's test** and **Brown and Forsythe's test** are two other tests for homogeneity that might be found on computer software packages. The Brown and Forsythe's test is based on Levene's test is more robust when groups are unequal in size. However, because the F-test is so robust regarding violations of the assumption of homogeneity of variance, in most cases these tests of homogeneity are usually not required if equal sample sizes are maintained.

**References**

Bartlett, M.S. (1937). "Properties of sufficient and statistical tests," *Proceedings Royal Society of London, Series A* 160:280-282.

Bolton, S. (1997). *Pharmaceutical Statistics: Practical and Clinical Applications*, Third edition, Marcel Dekker, Inc., New York, pp. 397-425.

Box, G.E.P. (1954). "Some theorems on quadratic forms applied in the study of analysis of variance problems," *Annals of Statistics* 25:290-302.

Cochran, W.G. (1947). "Some consequences when the assumptions of analysis of variance are not satisfied," *Biometrics* 3:22-38.

Daniel, W.W. (1999). *Biostatistics: A Foundation for Analysis in the Health Sciences*, Seventh edition, John Wiley and Sons, New York, pp. 295-298.

Fisher, R.A. (1926). "The arrangement of field experiments," *Journal of Ministry of Agriculture* 33:503-513.

Friedman, L.M., Furberg, C.D., and DeMets, D.L. (1985). *Fundamentals of Clinical Trials*, PSG Publishing Company, Inc., Littleton, MA, pp. 33-47.

Kachigan, S.K. (1991). *Multivariate Statistical Analysis*, Second edition, Radius Press, New York, pp. 195-197.

Kirk, R.E. (1968). *Experimental Design: Procedures for the Behavioral Sciences*, Brooks/Cole, Belmont, CA, pp. 61,62.

Salsburg, D. (2002). *The Lady Tasting Tea: How Statistics Revolutionized Science in the Twentieth Century*. Henry Holt and Company, New York, pp. 48-50.

## Suggested Supplemental Readings

Bolton, S. (1997). *Pharmaceutical Statistics: Practical and Clinical Applications*, Third edition, Marcel Dekker, Inc., New York, pp. 265-273.

Daniel, W.W. (1999). *Biostatistics: A Foundation for Analysis in the Health Sciences*, Seventh edition, John Wiley and Sons, New York, pp. 295-341.

Kirk, R.E. (1968). *Experimental Design: Procedures for the Behavioral Sciences*, Brooks/Cole, Belmont, CA, pp. 104-109, 131-134.

## Example Problems

1. In a collaborative trial, four laboratories were sent samples from a reservoir and requested to perform ten assays and report the results based on percentage of a labeled amount of the drug (Table 10.6). Were there any significant differences based on the laboratory performing the analysis?

2. Acme Chemical and Dye received from the same raw material supplier three batches of oil from three different production sites. Samples were drawn from drums at each location and compared to determine if the viscosity was the same for each batch (Table 10.7). Are the viscosities the same regardless of the batch?

**Table 10.6** Data from Four Different Laboratories

| | Lab(A) | Lab(B) | Lab(C) | Lab(D) |
|---|---|---|---|---|
| | 100.0 | 99.5 | 99.6 | 99.8 |
| | 99.8 | 100.0 | 99.3 | 100.5 |
| | 99.5 | 99.3 | 99.5 | 100.0 |
| | 100.1 | 99.9 | 99.1 | 100.1 |
| | 99.7 | 100.3 | 99.7 | 99.4 |
| | 99.9 | 99.5 | 99.6 | 99.6 |
| | 100.4 | 99.6 | 99.4 | 100.2 |
| | 100.0 | 98.9 | 99.5 | 99.9 |
| | 99.7 | 99.8 | 99.5 | 100.4 |
| | 99.9 | 100.1 | 99.9 | 100.1 |
| Σ = | 999.0 | 996.9 | 995.1 | 1000.0 |

**Table 10.7** Viscosity of Different Batches of a Product

| | Viscosity Batch A | Viscosity Batch B | Viscosity Batch C | |
|---|---|---|---|---|
| | 10.23 | 10.24 | 10.25 | |
| | 10.33 | 10.28 | 10.20 | |
| | 10.28 | 10.20 | 10.21 | |
| | 10.27 | 10.21 | 10.18 | |
| | 10.30 | 10.26 | 10.22 | |
| $\Sigma =$ | 51.41 | 51.19 | 51.06 | $\Sigma\Sigma = 153.66$ |

3. During a clinical trial, Acme Chemical wants to compare two possible generic formulations to the currently available brand product (reference standard). Based on the following results (Table 10.8), is there a significant difference between the two Acme formulations and the reference standard?

**Answers to Problems**

1. Collaborative trial with assays from four laboratories (Table 10.6)
   Independent variable: laboratories (discrete, 4 levels)
   Dependent variable: assay results (continuous)
   Statistical test: ANOVA (example of the computational formula)

   Hypotheses: $H_0$: $\mu_A = \mu_B = \mu_C = \mu_D$
   $H_1$: $H_0$ is false

   Decision rule: With $\alpha = .05$, reject $H_0$ if $F > F_{3,36}(.95) \approx 2.87$.

**Table 10.8** Original Data for Two Different Formulations

| | Plasma Elimination Half-Life (in minutes) | | |
|---|---|---|---|
| | Formulation A | Formulation B | Reference Standard |
| Subject 001 | 206 | 207 | 208 |
| Subject 002 | 212 | 218 | 217 |
| Subject 003 | 203 | 199 | 204 |
| Subject 004 | 211 | 210 | 213 |
| Subject 005 | 205 | 209 | 209 |
| Subject 006 | 209 | 205 | 209 |
| Subject 007 | 217 | 213 | 225 |
| Subject 008 | 197 | 203 | 196 |
| Subject 009 | 208 | 207 | 212 |
| Subject 010 | 199 | 195 | 202 |
| Subject 011 | 208 | 208 | 210 |
| Subject 012 | 214 | 222 | 219 |

Calculations:

$$I = \sum_{k=1}^{K}\sum_{i=1}^{n} x_{jk}^2 = (100)^2 + (99.8)^2 + ...(100.1)^2 = 398,207.04$$

$$II = \frac{\left[\sum_{k=1}^{K}\sum_{i=1}^{n} x_{jk}\right]^2}{N_K} = \frac{(3991)^2}{40} = 398,202.025$$

$$III = \sum_{k=1}^{K} \frac{\left[\sum_{i=1}^{n} x_{jk}\right]^2}{n_K} = \frac{(999.0)^2}{10} + ... \frac{(1000)^2}{10} = 398,203.462$$

$$SSB = III - II = 398,203.462 - 398,202.025 = 1.437$$

$$SSW = I - III = 398,207.04 - 398,203.462 = 3.578$$

$$SST = I - II = 398,207.04 - 398,202.025 = 5.015$$

ANOVA Table

| Source | DF | SS | MS | F |
|---|---|---|---|---|
| Between | 3 | 1.437 | 0.479 | 4.84 |
| Within | 36 | 3.578 | 0.099 | |
| Total | 39 | 5.015 | | |

Decision: With $F > 2.87$, reject $H_0$, conclude that $\mu_A = \mu_B = \mu_C = \mu_D$ is not true.

2. Comparison of a raw material at three different production sites (Table 10.7)
   Independent variable: production site (discrete, 3 levels)
   Dependent variable: oil viscosity (continuous)
   Statistical test: ANOVA (example of the computational formula)

   Hypotheses: $H_0$: $\mu_A = \mu_B = \mu_C$
   $H_1$: $H_0$ is false

   Decision rule: With $\alpha = .05$, reject $H_0$ if $F > F_{2,12}(.95) \approx 3.70$.

Calculations:

$$I = \sum_{k=1}^{K} \sum_{i=1}^{n} x_{jk}^2 = (10.23)^2 + (10.33)^2 + \ldots (10.22)^2 = 1574.1182$$

$$II = \frac{\left[ \sum_{k=1}^{K} \sum_{i=1}^{n} x_{jk} \right]^2}{N_k} = \frac{(153.66)^2}{15} = 1574.0930$$

$$III = \sum_{k=1}^{K} \frac{\left[ \sum_{i=1}^{n} x_{jk} \right]^2}{n_K} = \frac{(51.41)^2}{5} + \frac{(51.19)^2}{5} + \frac{(51.06)^2}{5} = 1574.1056$$

$$SS_B = III - II = 1574.1056 - 1574.0930 = 0.0126$$

$$SS_W = I - III = 1574.1182 - 1574.1056 = 0.0126$$

$$SS_T = I - II = 1574.1182 - 1574.0930 = 0.0252$$

ANOVA table:

| Source | DF | SS | MS | F |
|---|---|---|---|---|
| Between | 2 | 0.0126 | 0.0063 | 6.3 |
| Within | 12 | 0.0126 | 0.0010 | |
| Total | 14 | 0.0252 | | |

Decision: With $F > 2.83$, reject $H_0$, conclude that $\mu_A = \mu_B = \mu_C$ is not true

3. Evaluation of two formulations compared to the reference standard (Table 10.9).
   Independent variable: formulations (discrete, 3 levels)
   subjects (blocks)
   Dependent variable: plasma elimination half-life (continuous)
   Statistical design: randomized block design

   Hypotheses: $H_0$: $\mu_A = \mu_B = \mu_{RS}$
   $H_1$: $H_0$ is false

   Decision rule: With $\alpha = 0.05$, reject $H_0$ if $F > F_{2,11} \approx 3.98$

**Table 10.9** Plasma Elimination Half-Life (in minutes)

| Blocks (Subjects) | Form. A | Form. B | Reference Standard | Σ | Mean |
|---|---|---|---|---|---|
| 001 | 206 | 207 | 208 | 621 | 207.0 |
| 002 | 212 | 218 | 217 | 647 | 215.7 |
| 003 | 203 | 199 | 204 | 606 | 202.0 |
| 004 | 211 | 210 | 213 | 634 | 211.3 |
| 005 | 205 | 209 | 209 | 623 | 207.7 |
| 006 | 209 | 205 | 209 | 623 | 207.7 |
| 007 | 217 | 213 | 225 | 655 | 218.3 |
| 008 | 197 | 203 | 196 | 596 | 198.7 |
| 009 | 208 | 207 | 212 | 627 | 209.0 |
| 010 | 199 | 195 | 202 | 596 | 198.7 |
| 011 | 208 | 208 | 210 | 626 | 208.7 |
| 012 | 214 | 222 | 219 | 655 | 218.3 |
| Σ | 2489 | 2496 | 2524 | 7509 | |
| Mean | 207.4 | 208.0 | 210.3 | | |

Calculations:

$$I = \sum_{k=1}^{K} \sum_{j=1}^{J} x_{kj}^2$$

$$I = (206)^2 + (212)^2 + (203)^2 + \ldots (219)^2 = 1567969$$

$$II = \frac{\left[ \sum_{k=1}^{K} \sum_{j=1}^{J} x_{kj} \right]^2}{KJ}$$

$$II = \frac{(7509)^2}{36} = 1566252.25$$

$$III_R = \frac{\sum_{k=1}^{K} \left[ \sum_{j=1}^{J} x_{kj} \right]^2}{K}$$

$$III_R = \frac{(621)^2 + (647)^2 + \ldots (655)^2}{3} = 1567729$$

$$III_C = \frac{\sum_{j=1}^{J}\left[\sum_{k=1}^{K} x_{kj}\right]^2}{J}$$

$$III_C = \frac{(2489)^2 + (2496)^2 + (2524)^2}{12} = 1566309.417$$

$$SS_{Total} = SS_T = I - II$$

$$SS_{Total} = 1567969 - 1566252.25 = 1716.75$$

$$SS_{Blocks} = SS_B = III_R - II$$

$$SS_{Blocks} = 1567729 - 1566252.25 = 1476.75$$

$$SS_{Treatment} = SS_{Rx} = III_C - II$$

$$SS_{Treatment} = 1566309.417 - 1566252.25 = 57.167$$

$$SS_{Error} = SS_{Residual} = SS_T - SS_B - SS_{Rx}$$

$$SS_{Residual} = 1716.75 - 1476.75 - 57.167 = 182.833$$

ANOVA Table

| Source | df | SS | MS | F |
|---|---|---|---|---|
| Treatment | 2 | 57.167 | 28.58 | 3.44 |
| Blocks | 11 | 1476.75 | 134.25 | |
| Residual | 22 | 182.833 | 8.31 | |
| Total | 35 | 1716.75 | | |

Decision: With $F < 3.98$, fail to reject $H_0$ and conclude that there is no significant difference among the three products.

# 11

# Multiple Comparison Tests

As discussed in the previous chapter, rejection of the null hypothesis in the one-way analysis of variance simply proves that some significant difference exists between at least two levels of the discrete independent variable. Unfortunately the ANOVA does not identify the exact location of the difference(s). Multiple comparison tests can be used to reevaluate the data for a *significant* ANOVA and identify where the difference(s) exist while maintaining an overall Type I error rate ($\alpha$) at a level similar to that used to test the original null hypothesis for the one-way ANOVA. Assuming an analysis of variance was conducted with $\alpha = .05$ and the $H_0$ was rejected, then the multiple comparison tests should keep the error rate constant at .05.

**Error Associated with Multiple t-Tests**

Sometimes researchers err in performing multiple t-tests between the various two levels of the independent variable (called pair-wise combinations). It should be noted that the use of the term "pair-wise" refers to comparisons involving two levels of the discrete independent variable and should not be confused with "paired" tests, which involve repeated measures (i.e. paired t-test). By using **multiple t-tests** the researcher actually compounds the Type I error rate. This compounding of the error is referred to as **the experimentwise error rate**. For example, if there are three levels to the independent variable, there are three possible comparisons:

$$\binom{3}{2} = \frac{3!}{2!1!} = 3$$

which are A vs. B, B vs. C, and A vs. C. Alternative formula for number pair-wise comparisons is simply using the *k* number of levels of the independent variable:

$${}_kC_2 = \frac{k(k-1)(k-2)!}{2!(k-2)!} = \frac{k(k-1)}{2} \qquad \text{Eq. 11.1}$$

**Table 11.1** Experimentwise Error Rates for Multiple Paired t-Tests after a Significant ANOVA

| Number of Groups (Discrete levels) | Number of Possible Paired Comparisons | Level of Significance Used in Each t-Test 0.05 | 0.01 |
|---|---|---|---|
| 2 | 1 | 0.05 | 0.01 |
| 3 | 3 | 0.143 | 0.030 |
| 4 | 6 | 0.265 | 0.059 |
| 5 | 10 | 0.401 | 0.096 |
| 6 | 15 | 0.536 | 0.140 |
| 7 | 21 | 0.659 | 0.190 |
| 8 | 28 | 0.762 | 0.245 |

In the previous example with $k = 3$, the results would be identical:

$$_3C_2 = \frac{3(2)}{2} = 3$$

A simple way of thinking about this compounding error rate would be that if each t-test were conducted with $\alpha = .05$, then the error rate would be three comparisons times .05, or a .15 error rate. As can be seen in Table 11.1, as the number of levels of the independent variable increases, the number of intersample comparisons (i.e., pair-wise comparisons) increases at a rapid rate, thus greatly increasing the level of $\alpha$. The actual calculation for compounding the error or experimentwise error rate is:

$$\alpha_{ew} = 1 - (1 - \alpha)^C \qquad \text{Eq. 11.2}$$

where $C$ is the total possible independent t-tests comparing only two levels of the discrete independent variable. Table 11.1 lists the experimental error rate for various pair-wise combinations. The third column is for the 95% confidence level and the fourth for the 99% confidence level. One could also think of these comparison as a "family" of possible pair-wise comparisons. These tests are used to ensure that the probability is held constant for the family's multiple comparisons. Thus, a synonym for experimentalwise error rate is **familywise error rate** (FWE = $\alpha_{ew}$).

**Overview of Multiple Comparison Tests**

As will be seen, there are many multiple comparison tests. Multiple comparison procedures can be divided into *a priori* and *post hoc* tests (planned and unplanned tests). This chapter will present most of the multiple comparison tests in that order: 1) planned pair-wise comparisons; 2) *post hoc* pair-wise tests; and 3) complex comparisons using Scheffé's procedures.

**Table 11.2.** Multiple Comparison Tests

| Single Step Methods | Stepwise (Step-Down) Methods |
|---|---|
| Bonferroni | Student-Newman-Keul |
| Sidák | REGWQ |
| Dunnett | REGWF |
| Fisher LSD | Duncan |
| Tukey HSD | Tukey's-b |
| Tukey-Kramer | Bonferroni-Holm |
| Scheffé | Sidák-Holm |
| Hochbeg's GF2 | |
| Gabriel | |

A second way to divide these tests is into: 1) single-step methods and 2) stepwise, sequential methods (Table 11.2). In the former case, there are simultaneous confidence intervals that allow directional decisions. Tests in the latter group are limited to hypotheses testing, but are usually more powerful. Thus, if the primary goal is not hypothesis testing or confidence intervals are not needed, the stepwise methods are preferable. Stepwise tests usually involve a range test. Most of these multiple comparison tests listed in Table 11.2 will be discussed in this chapter.

Certain multiple comparison tests are defined as "exact tests." These exact tests are procedures where the experimentwise error rate is exactly equal to α for balanced as well as unbalanced one-way designs (balanced designs involve an equal number of observations per level of the independent variable). Other tests, such as the REGWQ, REGWF, SNK, and Duncan tests are recommend for balanced designs only.

The standard error term used for most multiple comparison tests is based on modifications of the following:

$$SE = \sqrt{MS_E}\sqrt{\frac{1}{n_1}+\frac{1}{n_2}} \qquad \text{Eq. 11.3}$$

where the $MS_E$ (which is the same as the $MS_W$) is taken from the original ANOVA table.

The one-way ANOVA is a robust test and can tolerate some deviation from the parameter of equal variances. However, most of the commonly used *post hoc* procedures require equal variances (Tukey HSD, Fisher LSD, Student-Newman-Keul, Duncan); other more obscure tests do not require this assumption (Games-Howell, Dunnett's T3, Dunnett's C, and Tamhane's T2. tests)

Because there are a variety of multiple comparison tests to choose from, it is important to understand these tests and choose the most appropriate one. The test should not be picked at random, and more importantly, it should not be chosen based on the results of the various tests (for example, looking at the results for many different multiple comparison tests and picking the one that gives researcher's desired outcome). Just like any other statistical test it should be chosen before the initial ANOVA is computed. Different situations require the use of different multiple comparison tests and there does not appear to be agreement on a "best" procedure to use routinely. Figure 11.1 provide a rough algorithm for selecting a multiple comparison test.

### The *q*-Statistic

The *q*-statistic (also known as the *q* range statistic or **Studentized range statistic**) is commonly used in coefficients for multiple comparison tests (planned and *post hoc*). As the number of comparisons between group increases, there is an expected increase in variability and the researcher should compensate for this by using a more conservative test; if not, the likelihood of Type I errors increases considerably. The *q*-statistic provides this more conservative approach. Both the *q*- and *t*-statistics use the difference between means in the numerator. However, the *q*-statistic uses the standard error of the mean in the denominator, whereas the *t*-statistic

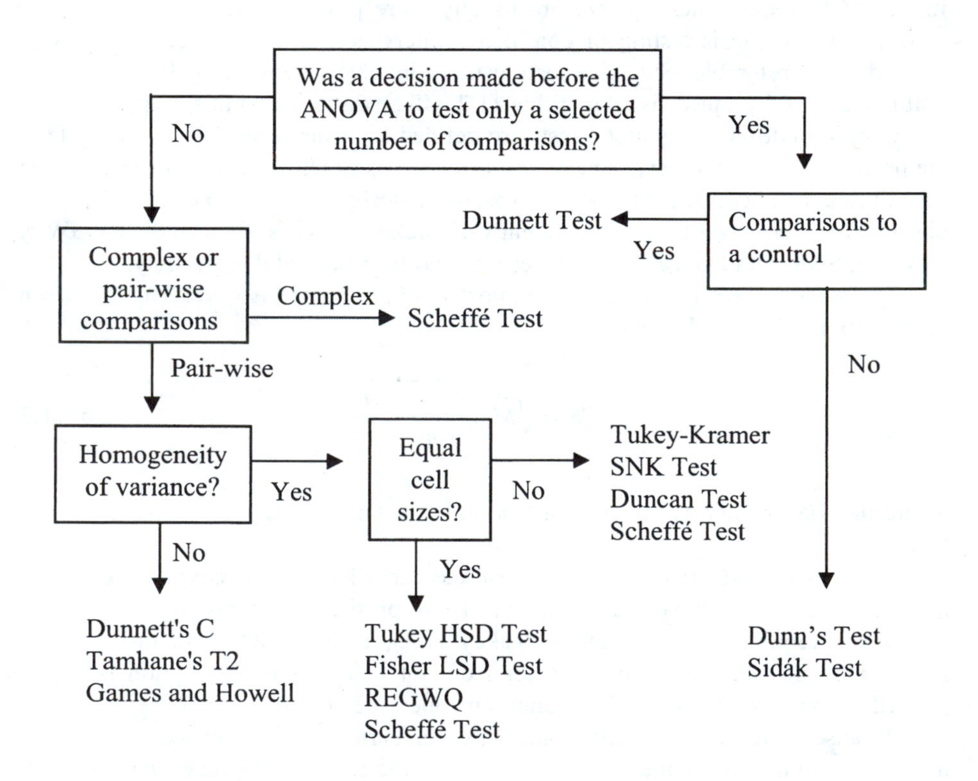


**Figure 11.1** Algorithm for choosing multiple comparison procedures.

uses the standard error of the difference between the means. Thus, instead of measuring the difference between two means in *t*-statistic, the *q*-statistic tests the probability that the largest and smallest sample means were sampled from the same population. Similar to using the *t*-statistic, if the computed *q*-statistic is not as large as the critical q-value from a table, then the researcher cannot reject the null hypothesis that the groups do not differ at the given alpha significance level. It follows that if the null hypothesis is not rejected comparing the largest and smallest sample means, then all intermediate means representing the other levels of the discrete independent variable are also drawn from the same population. The general formula for the q-statistic is:

$$q = \frac{\overline{X}_A - \overline{X}_B}{SE} \qquad \text{Eq. 11.4}$$

The SE term is defined differently for various multiple comparison procedures, the more popular of these will be discussed below. Also, the *q*-value can be used as a reliability coefficient to build a confidence interval:

$$\mu_A - \mu_B = (\overline{X}_A - \overline{X}_B) \pm (q_{critical})(SE) \qquad \text{Eq. 11.5}$$

The q-critical can be found in the Studentized range distribution in Table B10 in Appendix B and is usually defined as $q_{1-\alpha,k-1,N-k}$ where $k - 1$ and $N - k$ are the degrees of freedom from the ANOVA table for the within and between effects. Certain multiple comparison statistics define these numerator and denominator degrees of freedom differently and these will be noted below.

One can think of the Studentized range test as a traditional t-test, where the critical values have been adjusted base on the number of sample means being compared. It replaces the traditional one-way analysis of variance with a test that compares only the largest and the smallest mean in the experiment. The *q*-statistic is basically an adjusted t-test between the largest and smallest means. The formula is similar, except for a missing square root of two in the denominator.

$$t = \frac{\overline{X}_1 - \overline{X}_2}{\sqrt{\frac{S_p^2}{n_1} + \frac{S_p^2}{n_2}}} = \frac{\overline{X}_1 - \overline{X}_2}{\sqrt{\frac{2S_p^2}{n}}} = \frac{\overline{X}_1 - \overline{X}_2}{\sqrt{\frac{2MS_E}{n}}} \qquad \text{Eq. 11.6}$$

Above is an expansion of the t-statistic: 1) for equal sample sizes and 2) replacing the pooled variance for the $MS_{error}$, which are the same. The *q*-statistics is the same with the removal of the square root of two in the denominator:

$$q = \frac{\bar{X}_1 - \bar{X}_2}{\sqrt{\frac{MS_E}{n}}} \qquad \text{Eq. 11.7}$$

**Planned Multiple Comparisons**

The student t-test can be used to compare only two levels of the independent variable and is only recommended when the researcher has a single **planned comparison,** based on *a priori* theory, established before running the initial analysis of variance. Bonferroni, Sidák, Dunn, and Dunnett's tests are really planned multiple comparison tests, not *post hoc* procedures since decisions are made prior to calculating the original analysis of variance. Following the rejection of the global null hypothesis for the one-way ANOVA, a *post hoc* procedure should be used to identify specific significant differences. These *post hoc* methods are described following the *a priori* methods described below. Most results will be expressed as confidence intervals similar to the previous example (Eq. 11.5).

**Bonferroni Adjustment**

The Bonferroni adjustment (or **Bonferroni test**) is the simplest multiple comparison test and involves multiple t-tests. In this procedure the experimentwise error rate is kept constant (usually .05) by dividing the Type I error by the total number of possible or planned pair-wise comparisons ($C$).

$$\alpha' = \frac{\alpha}{C} \qquad \text{Eq. 11.8}$$

Experimentalwise error rate is not exactly equal to α, but is less than α in most situations. Unfortunately, the Bonferroni test may be too conservative and not have enough power to detect significant differences. Plus, tables of critical *t*-values may be hard to find for the required $\alpha'$. For example, with three levels of an independent variable, $C = 3$ and $\alpha' = .0167$ (if the original ANOVA was tested at .05). Table 11.3 lists various adjustments for an infinite number of observations. These were calculated under the assumption that the *t*-value is at infinity and uses the standardized normal distribution and *z*-values for the various adjusted *p*-values ($\alpha$). Notice how the critical value increases as the number of levels of the discrete independent variable increases, thus controlling increased experimentwise error rate.

What if there are less than an infinite number of observations? Other tables are available in various textbooks for smaller sample sizes and smaller α values than those in the third column of Table 11.3. As seen in Table B5 (Appendix B), for larger sample sizes the reliability coefficient is very close to the *t*-value at infinity (1.96). For example, at 80 degrees of freedom the critical *t*-value = 2.00. Therefore,

**Table 11.3** Bonferroni Adjustment for Maintaining an Experimental Error Rate of 0.05

| Number of Discrete Levels | Number of Possible Paired Comparisons | Bonferroni Adjustment | Estimate Critical Value for Infinite Degrees of Freedom |
|---|---|---|---|
| 2 | 1 | 0.0500 | 1.960 |
| 3 | 3 | 0.0167 | 2.394 |
| 4 | 6 | 0.0083 | 2.638 |
| 5 | 10 | 0.0050 | 2.807 |
| 6 | 15 | 0.0037 | 2.935 |
| 7 | 21 | 0.0024 | 3.038 |
| 8 | 28 | 0.0018 | 3.124 |
| 9 | 36 | 0.0014 | 3.197 |
| 10 | 45 | 0.0011 | 3.261 |

Table 11.3 can be used as a rough approximation for the required critical value[1].

To illustrate both multiple t-tests and Bonferroni's adjustment, consider the first example in the problem set in Chapter 10 where a significant difference was found with a Type I error rate of .05, leading to the rejection of the following "global" null hypothesis associated with the original one-way analysis of variance:

$$H_0: \mu_A = \mu_B = \mu_C = \mu_D$$

The data used for this example were:

| Concentration in mcg/ml: | Mean | S.D. | n |
|---|---|---|---|
| Formulation A | 123.2 | 12.8 | 20 |
| Formulation B | 105.6 | 11.6 | 20 |
| Formulation C | 116.4 | 14.6 | 19 |
| Formulation D | 113.5 | 10.0 | 18 |

Since there are four levels of the discrete independent variable, there are six possible pair-wise comparisons, the Bonferroni's adjustment of the α would be 0.008 and a *very rough approximation* for the reliability coefficient would be 2.65 from Table 11.3. Confidence intervals can be created using the following formula (Eq. 9.4):

$$\mu_1 - \mu_2 = (\overline{X}_1 - \overline{X}_2) \pm 2.65\sqrt{\frac{S_P^2}{n_1} + \frac{S_P^2}{n_2}}$$

[1] The t-values can be obtained using Microsoft Excel by determining $\alpha'$ ($\alpha/C$) and using the function TINV ($\alpha'$, df).

**Table 11.4** Comparison of Results with Multiple t-Tests and the Bonferroni Adjustment

| | Multiple t-Tests | Bonferroni Adjustments |
|---|---|---|
| Pairing | Confidence Interval | Confidence Interval |
| $\overline{X}_A - \overline{X}_B$ | $+9.79 < \mu_A - \mu_B < +25.41$ * | $+7.38 < \mu_A - \mu_B < +27.82$ * |
| $\overline{X}_A - \overline{X}_C$ | $-2.07 < \mu_A - \mu_C < +15.674$ | $-0.24 < \mu_A - \mu_C < +13.84$ |
| $\overline{X}_A - \overline{X}_D$ | $+2.11 < \mu_A - \mu_D < +17.29$ * | $+3.29 < \mu_A - \mu_D < +16.11$ * |
| $\overline{X}_B - \overline{X}_C$ | $-19.31 < \mu_B - \mu_C < -2.29$ * | $-21.95 < \mu_B - \mu_C < +0.35$ |
| $\overline{X}_B - \overline{X}_D$ | $-15.04 < \mu_B - \mu_D < -0.76$ * | $-17.26 < \mu_B - \mu_D < +1.46$ |
| $\overline{X}_C - \overline{X}_D$ | $-5.46 < \mu_C - \mu_D < +11.26$ | $-8.06 < \mu_C - \mu_D < +13.86$ |

* Significant at $p < 0.05$.

If we compare the results for all six pair-wise t-tests and six tests with Bonferroni's adjustment, there are more significant findings with the multiple t-test due to the experimentwise error (Table 11.4).

Performing unadjusted multiple t-tests is one of the major errors found in the literature (Glantz, 1980). When the independent variable has more than two discrete levels, an ANOVA followed by an appropriate multiple comparison procedure is the correct test, not multiple t-tests. As seen in Table 11.4, when multiple independent t-tests are applied to one set of data, it becomes increasingly likely that a significant outcome will result by chance alone.

## Sidák Test

The Sidák test (or **Dunn-Sidák test**) is a variation of the Bonferroni test using a t-test for pair-wise multiple comparisons. For this test, the Type I error rate is modified to slightly smaller adjusted *p*-values than for the Bonferroni test (a slightly smaller adjusted *p*-value). The Sidák procedure is slightly more powerful than the Bonferroni procedure and guarantees to control for experimentwise error when there are independent comparisons (orthogonal contrasts).

$$\alpha' = 1 - (1 - \alpha)^{1/C} \qquad \text{Eq. 11.9}$$

Once again the problems of identifying appropriate tables, limits the usefulness of this procedure (in the precious example C = 3 and $\alpha' = .01695$).

## Dunn's Multiple Comparisons

Dunn's procedure (also called a **Bonferroni t statistic, Bonferroni corrected test,** or **Fisher protected LSD test**) calculates mean differences for all pair-wise comparisons and compares these differences to a critical value extracted from a table. As an extension of the Bonferroni adjustment it is recommended for multiple planned comparisons, if the number of pair-wise comparisons is not large. As seen in Table 11.1, as larger numbers of comparisons are made, one is increasing the likelihood of a Type I error. Thus, as the number of comparisons increase, the more stringent the $\alpha$ level must be used to maintain an overall experimentwise Type I error rate consistent with the Type I error rate in the original analysis of variance. For most of the multiple comparison tests we will continue using the same example from Chapter 10, where it was found that a significant difference existed somewhere between the following means:

| Concentration in mcg/ml: | Mean | n | |
|---|---|---|---|
| Formulation A | 123.2 | 20 | $MS_W = MS_E = 153.51$ |
| Formulation B | 105.6 | 20 | |
| Formulation C | 116.4 | 19 | $\nu_2 = N - K = 73$ |
| Formulation D | 113.5 | 18 | |

The total number of possible pair-wise comparisons is:

$$C = \binom{4}{2} = \frac{4!}{2!2!} = 6$$

The absolute difference for each pair-wise comparison is computed:

$$|\bar{X}_A - \bar{X}_B| = 17.6 \qquad |\bar{X}_B - \bar{X}_C| = 10.8$$
$$|\bar{X}_A - \bar{X}_C| = 6.8 \qquad |\bar{X}_B - \bar{X}_D| = 7.9$$
$$|\bar{X}_A - \bar{X}_D| = 9.7 \qquad |\bar{X}_C - \bar{X}_D| = 2.9$$

A value is extracted from the table of Dunn's percentage points (Table B11, Appendix B). This value takes into consideration: 1) the total number of possible pair-wise comparisons ($C$); 2) the original denominator degrees of freedom ($N - k$) for the ANOVA; and 3) the Type I error rate used in the original ANOVA (i.e., $\alpha$ = .05). As seen in Table B11, the first column is the number of possible combinations, the Type I error rate is in the second column, and the remaining columns relate to the $N - k$ degrees of freedom. In this particular example the table value is

$$t'D_{\alpha;C;N\text{-}K} = t'D_{.05;6;73} \approx 2.72$$

This number is then inserted into the calculation of a critical Dunn's value:

$$d = t'D_{\alpha/2;C;N-K}\sqrt{MS_E \cdot (\frac{1}{n_1} + \frac{1}{n_2})} \qquad \text{Eq. 11.10}$$

If the mean difference is greater than the calculated *d*-value there is a significant difference between the two means. The calculation of the *d*-value for the first pair-wise comparison is:

$$d = (2.72)\sqrt{153.51 \cdot (\frac{1}{20} + \frac{1}{20})} = (2.72)(3.92) = 10.66$$

Our decision, with $|\bar{X}_A - \bar{X}_B|$ greater than the calculated *d*-value of 10.66, is to reject $\mu_A = \mu_B$ and conclude that there is a significant difference between these two population means.

An alternative method would be to create a confidence interval similar to the t-test:

$$\mu_1 - \mu_2 = (\bar{X}_1 - \bar{X}_2) \pm t'D_{\alpha/2;C;N-K}\sqrt{MS_E \cdot (\frac{1}{n_1} + \frac{1}{n_2})} \qquad \text{Eq. 11.11}$$

Notice how this equation is exactly the same in layout as all previous confidence intervals (estimate ± reliability coefficient x error term). For the first pair-wise comparison:

$$\mu_A - \mu_B = (123.2 - 105.6) \pm 2.72\sqrt{153.51\ (\frac{1}{20} + \frac{1}{20})}$$

$$\mu_A - \mu_B = (17.6) \pm 10.66$$

$$6.94 < \mu_A - \mu_B < 28.26$$

Since zero does not fall within the interval, there is a significant difference between Formulations A and B. Note the same results occurred with the Bonferroni adjustment. However, two important features appear with Dunn's procedure: 1) the table of critical values allows for better corrections for smaller sample sizes and 2) by using the $MS_E$ the entire variance from the original ANOVA is considered rather than only the pooled variance for the pair-wise comparison.

Using the original method for the calculation of the *d*-value, the *d*-value for this second pair-wise comparison is:

$$d = (2.72)\sqrt{153.51\ (\frac{1}{20} + \frac{1}{19})} = (2.72)(3.97) = 10.80$$

**Table 11.5** Results of Dunn's Multiple Comparisons

| Pairing | Confidence Interval | Results |
|---|---|---|
| $\overline{X}_A - \overline{X}_B$ | $+6.94 < \mu_A - \mu_B < +28.26$ | Significant |
| $\overline{X}_A - \overline{X}_C$ | $-4.00 < \mu_A - \mu_C < +17.60$ | |
| $\overline{X}_A - \overline{X}_D$ | $-1.25 < \mu_A - \mu_D < +20.65$ | |
| $\overline{X}_B - \overline{X}_C$ | $-21.64 < \mu_B - \mu_C < +0.04$ | |
| $\overline{X}_B - \overline{X}_D$ | $-18.85 < \mu_B - \mu_D < +3.05$ | |
| $\overline{X}_C - \overline{X}_D$ | $-8.18 < \mu_C - \mu_D < +13.98$ | |

Here the decision, with $|\overline{X}_A - \overline{X}_C| < 10.80$, is that we fail to reject $\mu_A - \mu_C$, thus we fail to find that there is a significant difference between these two levels. Similarly the confidence interval is:

$$\mu_A - \mu_C = (123.2 - 116.4) \pm 2.72\sqrt{153.51 \cdot (\frac{1}{20} + \frac{1}{19})}$$

$$-4.00 < \mu_A - \mu_B < 17.60$$

With zero within the confidence interval, the same results are obtained and we cannot conclude that there is a difference. The Dunn's test is not recommended when the investigator plans to perform all possible pair-wise comparisons, but for this example all possible pair-wise comparisons will be tesets.

Table 11.5 presents a summary of all pair-wise comparisons. Thus, we can conclude that Formulation B has a significantly lower maximum concentration than Formulation A, and that there appears to be no other significant pair-wise comparisons.

### Dunnett's Test

The last planned multiple comparison test is used when various treatment groups are compared to a single control group. This test was developed by C.W. Dunnett and is based on a modification of the $q$-statistic. It is an exact test (the experimentwise error rated exactly equal to $\alpha$) for both balanced and unbalanced one-way designs. It generally has better power than alternative tests. Significance can be tested using the following ratio based on the $q$-statistic:

$$q = \frac{\overline{X}_C - \overline{X}_i}{\sqrt{MS_E\left(\frac{1}{n_C} + \frac{1}{n_i}\right)}} \qquad \text{Eq. 11.12}$$

where $\overline{X}_i$ is the sample mean for one experimental groups, the $\overline{X}_C$ is the mean for the control group and $n$'s are the sample sizes for the experimental and control groups. For this test the null hypothesis would be that each experimental group equals the control group.

$$H_0: \mu_I = \mu_C$$
$$H_1: \mu_I \neq \mu_C$$

All the experimental groups and the control group are placed in order based on the magnitude of their means. Then a range ($p$) is determined for the number of inclusive means between the experimental group being considered and the control group. For example, consider the following means ranked from smallest to largest:

$$\overline{X}_5 \qquad \overline{X}_1 \qquad \overline{X}_C \qquad \overline{X}_3 \qquad \overline{X}_4 \qquad \overline{X}_2$$

In this example, if group 5 were to be compared to the control, the $p$-range would be three (three mean are included in the range between $\overline{X}_5$ and $\overline{X}_C$). Similarly, if the second group ($\overline{X}_2$) were compared to the control, the $p$-range would be four. This $p$-value is used in the decision rule:

$$\text{Reject } H_0 \text{ if } q > q_{\alpha,p,N-k}$$

The critical $q$-values are found in Table B12 (Appendix B). This table represents values for a two-tailed tests only; tables are available in other texts for one-tailed Dunnett tests (Zar, 1999).

An alternative approach would be to create a confidence interval:

$$\mu_C - \mu_i = \left(\overline{X}_C - \overline{X}_i\right) \pm q_{\alpha,p,N-k}\sqrt{MS_E\left(\frac{1}{n_C} + \frac{1}{n_i}\right)} \qquad \text{Eq.11.13}$$

The interpretation of this test would be similar to the two-sample t-test confidence interval. If zero falls with in the confidence interval, the null hypothesis cannot be rejected. If all the values in the interval are positive or negative values, the null hypothesis is rejected.

For these comparisons, the control group should have more observations than the other comparison groups. It is recommended that the ideal size for the control groups should be approximately $\sqrt{k-1}$ times larger than the sample sizes for the

**Table 11.6** Approximate Sample Sizes for the Control Group in a Dunnett's Test Based on Number of Samples in the Other Treatment Levels

| Sample size in Other Treatment Groups | k-Levels of Independent including Control Group | | | | | | |
|---|---|---|---|---|---|---|---|
| | 3 | 4 | 5 | 6 | 7 | 8 | 10 |
| 10 | 14 | 17 | 20 | 22 | 24 | 26 | 30 |
| 15 | 21 | 25 | 30 | 33 | 36 | 39 | 45 |
| 20 | 28 | 34 | 40 | 44 | 48 | 52 | 60 |
| 25 | 35 | 43 | 50 | 55 | 60 | 65 | 75 |
| 30 | 42 | 51 | 60 | 66 | 72 | 78 | 90 |
| 50 | 70 | 85 | 100 | 110 | 120 | 130 | 150 |
| 100 | 140 | 170 | 200 | 220 | 240 | 260 | 300 |

experimental groups. Table 11.6 lists a comparison of the number of observations required in the control group for various numbers of observations in each treatment group.

As an example of Dunnett's test, consider a study to evaluate the responsiveness of individuals receiving various commercially available benzodiazepines, volunteers were administered these drugs and subjected to a computer-simulated driving test. Volunteers are randomly assigned to three treatment groups receiving different benzodiazepines ($n_i = 12$) and a control group receiving a placebo ($n = 24$). For the results: the higher the score, the greater the number of driving errors. The results of the study are presented in Table 11.7. Performing an ANOVA on this data, it was determined that there was a significant difference and the null hypotheses of $\mu_A = \mu_B = \mu_D = \mu_{Placebo}$ was rejected (decision rule: with $\alpha = .05$, reject $H_0$ if $F > F_{.05,3,56}(.95) \approx 2.77$):

$$F = \frac{MS_B}{MS_W} = \frac{190.6}{28.93} = 6.59$$

The order of the different sample means is:

$$\bar{X}_B \; < \; \bar{X}_A \; < \; \bar{X}_D \; < \; \bar{X}_C$$

With the $MS_E = MS_W = 28.93$ and $q_{\alpha/2,p,N-k} = q_{.05,3,56} = 2.27$, the comparison for benzodiazepine A to the control group using Dunnett's test and subsequent confidence interval is as follows:

$$\mu_C - \mu_A = (50.33 - 54.42) \pm 2.27\sqrt{28.93\left(\frac{1}{24} + \frac{1}{12}\right)}$$

**Table 11.7** Data for a Dunnett Example

| | Drug A | Drug B | Drug D | Placebo (Control) | |
|---|---|---|---|---|---|
| | 57 | 60 | 53 | 50 | 57 |
| | 53 | 56 | 45 | 51 | 58 |
| | 51 | 56 | 48 | 53 | 49 |
| | 61 | 54 | 46 | 52 | 50 |
| | 50 | 58 | 58 | 61 | 55 |
| | 54 | 50 | 61 | 49 | 40 |
| | 46 | 69 | 52 | 50 | 47 |
| | 62 | 55 | 51 | 60 | 46 |
| | 55 | 62 | 55 | 45 | 43 |
| | 56 | 53 | 48 | 47 | 50 |
| | 49 | 66 | 62 | 48 | 51 |
| | 59 | 64 | 49 | 43 | 53 |
| Mean = | 54.42 | 58.58 | 52.33 | 50.33 | |

$$\mu_C - \mu_A = -4.09 \pm 4.32$$

$$-8.41 < \mu_C - \mu_A < +0.23$$

With zero within the interval, there is no significant difference between benzodiazepine A and the control. Similar results are seen with benzodiazepine D where $p = 2$:

$$\mu_C - \mu_D = (50.33 - 52.33) \pm 2.00\sqrt{28.93\left(\frac{1}{24} + \frac{1}{12}\right)}$$

$$-5.80 < \mu_C - \mu_A < +1.80$$

But there is a significant difference between benzodiazepine B and the control group ($p = 4$):

$$\mu_C - \mu_B = (50.33 - 58.58) \pm 2.41\sqrt{28.93\left(\frac{1}{24} + \frac{1}{12}\right)}$$

$$-12.83 < \mu_C - \mu_A < -3.67$$

### *Post hoc* Procedures

*Post hoc* procedures or ***a posteriori* tests** are used when the researcher is interested in evaluating differences, but not limited to those specified in advance (in contrast to Bonferroni, Dunn, or Dunnett's tests). Many of these types of tests are based on a q-statistic. As seen in Chapter 10 there are two underlying assumptions associated with the one-way analysis of variance, namely, population normality and homogeneity of variance. Homogeneity of variance is the more serious assumption. However, the ANOVA is a robust statistic and can tolerate minor deviations from the ideal. Also, equal sample sizes should be the goal to maximum power and robustness of the ANOVA. These same rule applies to *post hoc* procedures.

### Tukey HSD Test

The Tukey HSD test (honestly significant difference test) is a *post hoc* procedure that can be used for all pair-wise comparisons between level of the discrete independent variable. The Tukey HSD test is also referred to as **HDS test** or the **Tukey test**. It is based on the Studentized range distribution ($q$-statistic) and is preferred when the number of groups is large since it is a conservative pair-wise comparison test. Large numbers of groups threaten to inflate the Type I error rate. It is recommended to use the Tukey HSD test if it is required to test all pair-wise comparisons of the means and present confidence intervals. When all pair-wise comparisons are being tested, the Tukey HSD test is more powerful than the Dunn test. Therefore, the Dunn test would be recommended for a small partial set of pair-wise comparisons and the Tukey test would be employed when all pair-wise comparisons are considered *a posteriori*. The Tukey HSD test is limited to only pair-wise comparisons and preferably equal sample sizes (balanced design).

For each pair-wise comparison the following hypotheses are tested.

$$H_0:\ \mu_A = \mu_B$$
$$H_1:\ \mu_A \neq \mu_B$$

Using the following statistic

$$q = \frac{\bar{X}_A - \bar{X}_B}{\sqrt{\frac{MS_E}{n}}} \qquad \text{Eq. 11.14}$$

the decision rule is

With $\alpha = .05$, reject $H_0$ if $q > q_{\alpha,k,N\text{-}k}$ or $q < -q_{\alpha,k,N\text{-}k}$

Where $\alpha$ is usually consistent with the value used for the original one-way analysis of variance, $k$ is the number of levels of the independent variable and $N - k$ represent the denominator degrees of freedom from the ANOVA . The $q$-value is obtained from Table B10 (Appendix B).

The **Tukey-Kramer test** is a modification of the formula to accommodate for unequal cell sizes:

$$q = \frac{\bar{X}_A - \bar{X}_B}{\sqrt{\frac{MS_E}{2}\left(\frac{1}{n_A} + \frac{1}{n_B}\right)}} \quad \text{Eq. 11.15}$$

Both these formulas (Eqs. 11.14 and 11.15) can be modified to create confidence intervals:

$$\mu_A - \mu_B = (\bar{X}_A - \bar{X}_B) \pm (q_{\alpha,k,N-k})\sqrt{\frac{MS_E}{n}} \quad \text{Eq. 11.16}$$

$$\mu_A - \mu_B = (\bar{X}_A - \bar{X}_B) \pm (q_{\alpha,k,N-k})\sqrt{\frac{MS_E}{2}\left(\frac{1}{n_A} + \frac{1}{n_B}\right)} \quad \text{Eq. 11.17}$$

Interpretation of the results would be similar to those used for confidence intervals involving two-sample t-tests; if zero is within the interval there is no significant difference, if zero is outside the interval there is a significant difference between the two sample means being tested.

Using the previous example with the four formulations, the critical value from Table B10 is 3.73 for $q$ with $k$ = 4 number of means and $N - k$ = 73 degrees of freedom with 95% confidence $(1 - \alpha)$. A comparison between Formulas A and D would be computed as follows:

$$q = \frac{123.2 - 113.5}{\sqrt{\frac{153.51}{2}\left(\frac{1}{20} + \frac{1}{18}\right)}} = \frac{9.7}{2.85} = 3.40$$

Since 3.40 is less than the critical value of 3.73 we would fail to reject the hypothesis that $\mu_A - \mu_D$ and conclude that no difference could be found between these two formulas. Similar results would obtained creating a confidence interval:

$$\mu_A - \mu_D = (123.2 - 113.5) \pm 3.73 \cdot \sqrt{\frac{153.51}{2}\left(\frac{1}{20} + \frac{1}{18}\right)}$$

$$\mu_A - \mu_D = (9.7) \pm 10.62$$

$$-0.92 < \mu_A - \mu_D < 20.32$$

Again, since zero falls within the interval, the decision is that there is no significant difference between Formulations A and D. A summary of all possible pair-wise comparisons using the Tukey-Kramer test is presented in Table 11.8.

**Table 11.8** Results of the Tukey-Kramer Test Comparisons

| Pairing | Confidence Interval | Results |
|---|---|---|
| $\bar{X}_A - \bar{X}_B$ | $+7.27 < \mu_A - \mu_B < +27.93$ | Significant |
| $\bar{X}_A - \bar{X}_C$ | $-3.68 < \mu_A - \mu_C < +17.28$ | |
| $\bar{X}_A - \bar{X}_D$ | $-0.92 < \mu_A - \mu_D < +20,32$ | |
| $\bar{X}_B - \bar{X}_C$ | $-21.28 < \mu_B - \mu_C < -0.32$ | Significant |
| $\bar{X}_B - \bar{X}_D$ | $-18.53 < \mu_B - \mu_D < +2.73$ | |
| $\bar{X}_C - \bar{X}_D$ | $-7.84 < \mu_C - \mu_D < +13.64$ | |

It is possible to reject $H_0$ with the original ANOVA and the Tukey tests fail to detect a pair-wise difference. This is due to the fact that the ANOVA is a more powerful test than multiple comparison tests. In this case repeating the study with a larger sample size would tend to result in a greater likelihood of identifying a significant difference using one of the multiple comparison tests. Alternatively, tests like Scheffé could be used to make more complex comparisons.

Two other *post hoc* procedures are modifications of the Tukey HSD test based on the $q$-statistic. The first is the **Tukey's wholly significant difference (WSD) test** (also called the **Tukey WDS** or **Tukey-b** test**).** It is a less conservative stepwise procedure. The critical value of Tukey WSD is the average of the corresponding values for the Tukey's HSD test and the Newman-Keuls test. The second procedure is **Games-Howell test** (also know as the Games and Howell's modification of Tukey's HSD or **GH test**). This pair-wise test is designed for unequal variances and/or unequal sample sizes. The GH test is a relatively liberal *post hoc* procedure and can be too liberal when sample size is small and it is recommended that individual levels of the independent variable have sample sizes greater than five. Discussions of these tests can be found in Toothaker's book on multiple comparisons (Toothaker, 1991).

### Student Newman-Keuls Test

The Student Newman-Keul test (also referred to as the **Newman-Keuls test** or **SNK test**) is a stepwise, multiple range *post hoc* procedure, based on the $q$-statistic, which compares every mean with every other mean in a pair-wise fashion. Notice the formula is identical to that used for the Tukey and Tukey-Kramer tests. For balanced designs the formula is:

$$q = \frac{\bar{X}_A - \bar{X}_B}{\sqrt{\frac{MS_E}{n}}} \qquad \text{Eq. 11.18}$$

For unbalanced designs use:

$$q = \frac{\overline{X}_A - \overline{X}_B}{\sqrt{\frac{MS_E}{2}\left(\frac{1}{n_A} + \frac{1}{n_B}\right)}} \qquad \text{Eq. 11.19}$$

The Tukey HSD and Student Newman-Keuls tests are run exactly the same except the Tukey test maintains a constant *k*-value for the number of levels of the independent variable and with the SNK test the value is based on the number of steps inclusive of the means being compared. The Tukey test is more conservative, but it is an exact test and will keep alpha at .05 for all pair-wise comparisons, regardless of the number of means in the study.

Sample means are first rank-ordered in ascending or descending order. The number of means between two means being compared (including those two means) become the range. In these cases, the critical values is $q_{\alpha,p,N-k}$, where *p* is the range. The *p*-range is some times referred to as "steps." The difference in the process compared to the HSD test is that the critical values for the Tukey test remains constant for all comparisons but the critical values for the SNK differ based on the size of the stepwise differences. SNK tends to be less conservative than the Tukey test and will result in the identification of more significantly different pair-wise comparisons than Tukey. Also, it should be used cautiously for unbalanced cases.

The calculated *q*-statistic is compared to the critical values listed in Table B10 of Appendix B. The denominator degrees of freedom used, similar to previous procedures, is the same as the original denominator degrees of freedom for the F-test ($N - k$). One additional piece of information is required to read the critical value, namely the distance in "steps." For example, listed below are means used previously, but reordered from the highest to the lowest mean:

| | |
|---|---|
| Formulation A | 123.2 |
| Formulation C | 116.4 |
| Formulation D | 113.5 |
| Formulation B | 105.6 |

The step difference between Formulation A and Formulation C is two ($p = 2$) and the number of steps between Formulation A and Formulation B is four ($p = 4$). This difference is used to select the appropriate column from Table B10. As seen in Table B10, the first column is the denominator degrees of freedom ($N - k$), the Type I error rate is in the second column, and the remaining columns relate to the number of mean steps. In the above example if we were to select the critical value for a comparison between Formulations A and D the step difference would be three and the $N - k$ degrees of freedom is 73, giving a critical value for $\alpha = .05$ of approximately 3.39. The decision rule is with $\alpha = .05$, reject the $H_0$: $\mu_A = \mu_D$ if $q > q_{.05,3,73} \approx 3.39$ and the computation is:

$$q = \frac{123.2 - 113.5}{\sqrt{\dfrac{153.51}{2}\left(\dfrac{1}{20} + \dfrac{1}{18}\right)}} = \frac{9.7}{2.85} = 3.40$$

In this case, $q$ is greater than the critical q-value; therefore, we would reject the $H_0$ that they are equal. Step-down procedures (such as the SNK test) do not provide confidence intervals, but just divide pair-wise differences into possible overlapping groups.

Similarly, the comparison between Formulations B and D would involve only two means in the "step difference"; therefore, the decision rule for this comparison is, with $\alpha = .05$, reject $H_0$: $\mu_B = \mu_D$ if $q > q_{.05,2,73} \approx 2.82$ and the computation is:

$$q = \frac{113.5 - 105.6}{\sqrt{\dfrac{153.51}{2}\left(\dfrac{1}{20} + \dfrac{1}{18}\right)}} = \frac{7.9}{2.85} = 2.77$$

Here the calculated q-value is less than the critical $q$-value, therefore we cannot reject the hypothesis that the formulations are equal. A summary of all possible pair-wise comparisons using the Newman-Keuls test is presented in Table 11.9.

A modification of the SNK test is the **Ryan-Einot-Gabriel-Welch range test**, which is abbreviated as the **REGWQ test** or **Ryan test**. In this adjustment the critical values decrease as stretch size deceases (the range from highest to lowest mean in the set being considered). It is based on the q-distribution. Like the Newman-Keuls test, the Ryan test is a step-down procedure and is not recommended for unbalanced design, but is a more conservative test for balanced designs. In this case the family-wise error rate does not exceed alpha and the REGWQ is generally considered more powerful than the Tukey test. The **Ryan test F** (or **REGWF**) is a further modification of the SNK test, but based on the F-distribition and it is more computationally intense and more powerful than the REGWQ. More information about these tests can be found in Toothaker's book (Toothaker, 1991).

**Fisher LSD test:**

The Fisher LSD (least significant difference) test is a *post hoc* procedure based on the $t$-statistic and not a range test ($q$-statistic). Developed by R.A. Fisher, this test is also referred to as the **LSD test** or **protected t-test**. The process compares all possible pair-wise means after a significant F-test rejects the null hypothesis that all levels of the independent variable are equal. The Fisher LSD can handle all pair-wise comparisons and equal sample sizes are not required.

$$\mu_1 - \mu_2 = \left(\bar{X}_1 - \bar{X}_2\right) \pm t_{1-\alpha/2,N-k}\sqrt{\frac{MS_E}{n_1} + \frac{MS_E}{n_2}} \qquad \text{Eq. 11.20}$$

**Table 11.9** Results of Newman-Keuls' Comparisons

| Pairing | q-Statistic | Critical Value | Results |
|---|---|---|---|
| $\overline{X}_A - \overline{X}_B$ | 6.35 | 3.73 | Significant |
| $\overline{X}_A - \overline{X}_C$ | 2.24 | 2.82 | |
| $\overline{X}_A - \overline{X}_D$ | 3.41 | 3.39 | Significant |
| $\overline{X}_B - \overline{X}_C$ | 3.85 | 3.39 | Significant |
| $\overline{X}_B - \overline{X}_D$ | 2.78 | 2.82 | |
| $\overline{X}_C - \overline{X}_D$ | 1.01 | 2.82 | |

This method is quick, though a less rigorous *post hoc* procedure and has some control over the experimental-wise error rate. The problem with this approach is that it can lead to a high experimental-wise error rate if most population means are equal but only one or two are different. Homogeneity of variance is typically assumed for Fisher's LSD. Even though the LSD test can handle unpaired contrasts, it is not to be recommended for multiple comparisons. The Scheffé test is suited for multiple contrasts (complex comparisons).

Similar to previous examples, using this test, let us compare Formulations A and D once again:

$$\mu_A - \mu_D = (123.2 - 113.5) \pm 1.99\sqrt{\frac{153.51}{20} + \frac{153.51}{18}}$$

$$\mu_A - \mu_D = 9.7 \pm 8.01$$

$$+1.69 < \mu_A - \mu_D < +17.71$$

Similar to previous methods, there is a significant difference because zero is not within the confidence interval, and cannot be a possible outcome. Results for all pair-wise *post hoc* comparisons using Fisher LSD are presented in Table 11.10.

As seen in the above example and Table 11.10, the LSD test is the most liberal of the *post hoc* tests and controls the experimentwise Type I error rate at a selected level (typically 5%). In contrast to the HSD test, the LSD intervals are narrower than the HSD intervals, making it easier to find a significant difference. Thus the LSD test is a less conservative *post hoc* procedure than the HSD test. The **Fisher-Hayter test** is a modification of the LSD test designed to control for the liberal $\alpha$ significance level seen with the LSD test. It can be used when all pair-wise comparisons are done *post hoc*, unfortunately the power may be low for fewer comparisons.

**Table 11.10** Results of Fisher LSD Pair-wise Comparisons

| Pairing | Confidence Interval | Results |
|---|---|---|
| $\overline{X}_A - \overline{X}_B$ | $+9.80 < \mu_A - \mu_B < +25.40$ | Significant |
| $\overline{X}_A - \overline{X}_C$ | $-1.10 < \mu_A - \mu_C < +14.70$ | |
| $\overline{X}_A - \overline{X}_D$ | $+1.69 < \mu_A - \mu_D < +17.71$ | Significant |
| $\overline{X}_B - \overline{X}_C$ | $-2.90 < \mu_B - \mu_C < +18.70$ | |
| $\overline{X}_B - \overline{X}_D$ | $-0.11 < \mu_B - \mu_D < +15.91$ | |
| $\overline{X}_C - \overline{X}_D$ | $-5.20 < \mu_C - \mu_D < +11.00$ | |

### Scheffé Procedure

Scheffé's procedure for multiple comparisons offers several advantages over the previous methods: 1) this procedure allows not only pair-wise, but also complex comparisons; 2) Scheffé's procedure guarantees finding a significant comparison if there was a significant F-value in the original ANOVA, this significant *post hoc* comparison; however, may not be expressible in logical terms; and 3) the Type I error rate remains constant with the error rate used in the original ANOVA for both pair-wise and complex comparisons. Regarding the second point, results that might not be logical or interpretable, a hypothetical example may be useful for illustrative purposes. Assume that pharmacists are administered a cognitive test to assess their knowledge of some therapeutic class of medication. The findings below result in a significant one-way ANOVA for the four levels of a discrete independent variable (note that the levels are mutually exclusive and exhaustive).

| Level | Years of Experience | Mean Score |
|---|---|---|
| A | 10 or less | 94.8 |
| B | 11-20 | 85.1 |
| C | 21-30 | 91.3 |
| D | More than 30 | 87.9 |

However, no significant pair-wise comparisons could be found and when each experience level was compared to all the other three levels there were no significant differences. The only statistically significant difference was between levels A and C combined and levels B and D combined. With levels B and D significantly lower. How can these results be logically explained? Do pharmacists have a mental dormancy during their second decade of practice, but awaken during the third decade? What about the old adage, that parents appear to become smarter as a child passes into adulthood? Could it be that during the second decade that many of the pharmacists had teenage sons or daughters and really were not very bright, but the pharmacists become smarter as their children enter adulthood and the real world? Whatever the reason, a logical assessment of the finding is difficult, if not impossible, and makes interpretation difficult.

The first step is to establish a Scheffé value, which is expressed as follows:

$$(Scheffe\ value)^2 = S^2 = (K-1)(F_{K-1,N-K}(1-\alpha))$$

This procedure does not require any additional tables. The Scheffé value is nothing more than the $F_c$ value used in the original ANOVA multiplied by the numerator degrees of freedom ($k - 1$). The Scheffé value is used in the following to create a confidence interval:

$$\psi_i = \hat{\psi}_i \pm \sqrt{S^2 \cdot Var(\hat{\psi}_i)} \qquad \text{Eq. 11.21}$$

where $\psi_i$ (psi) is the estimated population difference and $\hat{\psi}_i$ (psi hat) is the sample difference. This $\hat{\psi}_i$ can represent either a pair-wise or complex comparison:

$$\hat{\psi}_i = \overline{X}_1 - \overline{X}_2 \ \ (pair\text{-}wise\ comparison)$$

$$\hat{\psi}_i = \overline{X}_1 - 1/2(\overline{X}_2 + \overline{X}_3) \ \ (complex\ comparison)$$

The measure of the standard error term for this equation is slightly more complex than the previous two methods:

$$Var(\hat{\psi}_i) = MS_E \cdot \Sigma \frac{a_k^2}{n_k} \qquad \text{Eq. 11.22}$$

In this formula, $a_k$ represents the prefix to each of the mean values.

$$\hat{\psi}_i = (a_1)\overline{X}_1 + (a_2)\overline{X}_2 + \ldots (a_n)\overline{X}_n$$

For example, consider the following simple pair-wise example:

$$\hat{\psi}_i = \overline{X}_1 - \overline{X}_2$$

This also can be written as:

$$\hat{\psi}_i = (+1)\overline{X}_1 + (-1)\overline{X}_2$$

where the two $a_k$s equal +1 and −1. A second example, involving a complex comparison is:

$$\hat{\psi}_i = \overline{X}_1 - 1/2(\overline{X}_2 + \overline{X}_3)$$

Once again the formula can be rewritten as:

$$\hat{\psi}_i = (+1)\overline{X}_1 + (-1/2)\overline{X}_2 + (-1/2)\overline{X}_3$$

where the three $a_k$s equal +1, −1/2, and −1/2. As a quick check, for all comparisons the sum of the absolute $a_k$s ($\Sigma|a_k|$) must equal 2. In each example the $a_k$ is squared and divided by the number of observations associated with the sample mean and the sum of these ratios is multiplied by $MS_E$, or $MS_W$, taken from the ANOVA table in the original analysis of variance (Eq. 11.22).

$$Var(\hat{\psi}_i) = MS_E \cdot \Sigma \frac{a_k^2}{n_k}$$

If zero does not fall within the confidence interval produced by the formula (Eq. 11.21), then it is assumed that there is a significant difference in the comparison being made. Conversely, if zero falls in the interval no significant difference is found.

Using the same example for the previous *post hoc* procedures, where do the significant pair-wise differences exist between the various formulations?

$$(Scheffe\ \ value\ )^2 = S^2 = (3)(F_{3,73}(.95)) = 3(2.74) = 8.22$$

The first pair-wise comparison is between Formulations A and B, where:

$$\psi_1 = Formulation\ A\ vs.\ B \qquad \hat{\psi}_1 = 17.6$$

The computation is as follows:

$$var(\hat{\psi}_1) = 153.51\left[\frac{(+1)^2}{20} + \frac{(-1)^2}{20}\right] = 15.35$$

$$\psi_1 = +17.6 \pm \sqrt{(8.22)(15.35)}$$

$$+6.37 < \psi_1 < +28.83$$

Because zero does not fall in the confidence interval, the decision is to reject $H_0$, that Formulation A and Formulation B have the same $C_{max}$, and conclude that a difference exists. The second pair-wise comparison is between Formulation A and C, with:

$$\psi_2 = Formulation\ A\ vs.\ C \qquad \hat{\psi}_2 = 6.8$$

**Table 11.11** Results of Scheffé's Pair-wise Comparisons

| Pairing | Confidence Interval | Results |
|---|---|---|
| $\overline{X}_A - \overline{X}_B$ | $+6.37 < \mu_A - \mu_B < +28.83$ | Significant |
| $\overline{X}_A - \overline{X}_C$ | $-4.58 < \mu_A - \mu_C < +18.18$ | |
| $\overline{X}_A - \overline{X}_D$ | $-1.84 < \mu_A - \mu_D < +21.24$ | |
| $\overline{X}_B - \overline{X}_C$ | $-22.18 < \mu_B - \mu_C < +0.58$ | |
| $\overline{X}_B - \overline{X}_D$ | $-19.44 < \mu_B - \mu_D < +3.64$ | |
| $\overline{X}_C - \overline{X}_D$ | $-8.78 < \mu_C - \mu_D < +14.58$ | |

The calculation of the confidence interval is:

$$var(\hat{\psi}_2) = 153.51\left[\frac{(+1)^2}{20} + \frac{(-1)^2}{19}\right] = 15.75$$

$$\psi_2 = +6.8 \pm \sqrt{(8.22)(15.75)}$$

$$-4.58 < \psi_2 < +18.18$$

In this case, with zero inside the confidence interval, the decision is that the null hypothesis that Formulation A has the same $C_{max}$ as Formulation C cannot be rejected.

A summary of all possible pair-wise comparisons using Scheffé's procedure appears in Table 11.11.

The Scheffé test is not appropriate for planned comparisons. It should be restricted to *post hoc* comparisons where there are a large number of pair-wise comparisons and mainly for complex comparisons. Interestingly each of the three

**Table 11.12** Comparison of Results for Various *Post hoc* Procedures

| Pairing | Mean Δ | Bonferroni Adjustment | Dunn's | Newman-Keuls | Scheffé |
|---|---|---|---|---|---|
| A vs. B | 17.6 | Significant | Significant | Significant | Significant |
| B vs. C | 10.8 | Significant | | Significant | |
| A vs. D | 9.5 | | | Significant | |
| B vs. D | 7.9 | | | | |
| A vs. C | 6.8 | | | | |
| C vs. D | 2.9 | | | | |

methods give slightly different results. From this one example, the Scheffé and Dunn procedures appear to be the most conservative tests and the Newman-Keuls test more liberal (Table 11.12). All three procedures found a significant difference between the two extreme means (Formulations A and B); however, results varied for the other pair-wise comparisons.

### Scheffé Procedure for Complex Comparisons

In the above example it was possible, by all four methods used, to identify significant pair-wise differences comparing the means of sample groups and extrapolating those differences to the populations which they represent. But what if all possible pair-wise comparisons were made and no significant differences were found? For example, suppose we actually found slightly different data among the four formulations:

| Concentration in mcg/ml: | Mean | S.D. | n |
|---|---|---|---|
| Formulation A | 119.7 | 11.2 | 20 |
| Formulation B | 110.9 | 9.9 | 20 |
| Formulation C | 117.7 | 9.5 | 19 |
| Formulation D | 112.6 | 8.9 | 18 |

In this case the calculated *F*-value (3.48) exceeds the critical F-value of (2.74). Therefore, the null hypothesis that all formulations are equal is rejected. Unfortunately, none of the Scheffé pair-wise comparisons are significant.

As mentioned previously, the Scheffé test also can be used for complex comparisons. This process begins by comparing individual levels (one formulation), to the average of the other combined levels (average of remaining three formulations) and determining if one is significantly larger or smaller than the rest. For example, the formulation with the smallest $C_{max}$ can be compared to the remaining three groups:

$$\hat{\psi}_7 = 110.9 - 1/3(119.7 + 117.7 + 112.6)$$

with the appropriate $a_k$ being:

$$\hat{\psi}_7 = (+1)\,110.9 + (-1/3)\,119.7 + (-1/3)\,117.7 + (-1/3)\,112.6 = -5.77$$

The computations for the confidence interval, with the calculated $MS_E$ of 98.86 from the original ANOVA, are:

$$var(\hat{\psi}_7) = 98.86\left[\frac{(+1)^2}{20} + \frac{(-.33)^2}{20} + \frac{(-.33)^2}{19} + \frac{(-.33)^2}{18}\right] = 6.65$$

$$\psi_7 = -5.77 \pm \sqrt{(8.22)(6.65)} = -5.77 \pm 7.39$$

$$-13.16 < \psi_7 < +1.62$$

Unfortunately, in this particular example all of the single group comparisons were found to be not significant.

| Compared to All Others | Confidence Interval |
|---|---|
| Formulation A | $-1.45 < \psi_8 < +13.39$ |
| Formulation B | $-13.16 < \psi_8 < +1.62$ |
| Formulation C | $-4.25 < \psi_8 < +10.85$ |
| Formulation D | $-11.19 < \psi_8 < +4.19$ |

With such results, the next logical step is to compare the two larger results with the two smallest. In this case the complex comparison would appear as follows:

$$\frac{\mu_A + \mu_C}{2} - \frac{\mu_D + \mu_B}{2} = 0$$

and also could be written as follows:

$$+\frac{1}{2}(\mu_A) + \frac{1}{2}(\mu_C) - \frac{1}{2}(\mu_D) - \frac{1}{2}(\mu_B) = 0$$

The +1/2s and –1/2s before each population mean become the $a_k$ in the equation for calculating the variance term:

$$Var(\hat{\psi}_i) = MS_E \cdot \Sigma \frac{a_k^2}{n_k}$$

Notice that in both this and the previous example, the $\Sigma / a_k /$ equals 2.

The calculations for the confidence interval are as follows:

$$\psi_{11} = \textit{Formulations A and C vs. Formulations D and B}$$

$$\hat{\psi}_{11} = 1/2(119.7 + 117.7) - 1/2(110.9 + 112.6) = 6.95$$

$$var(\hat{\psi}_{11}) = 98.86 \left[ \frac{(+.5)^2}{20} + \frac{(+.5)^2}{19} + \frac{(-.5)^2}{20} + \frac{(-.5)^2}{18} \right] = 5.15$$

$$\psi_{11} = 6.95 \pm \sqrt{(8.22)(5.15)} = 6.95 \pm 6.51$$

$$+0.44 < \psi_7 < +13.46$$

Here we find a significant difference if we compare the two formulations with the highest means to those with the smallest means.

If a significant pair-wise comparison is found, then more complex comparisons do not need to be computed unless the researcher wishes to analyze specific combinations. Once again it is assumed that the original analysis of variance was found to be significant, and rejection of the hypothesis that all the means are equal. In all the tests performed in this section the Type I error (α) remained constant with the original error rate used to test the analysis of variance for *k* levels of the independent variable. While the Scheffé test can evaluate more complex comparisons it does so at the expense of statistical power. Event though the Scheffé test is low in power it can be used when one wishes to do all or a large number of comparisons.

### Unbalanced Designs

Many multiple comparison procedure assume that there are equal sample sizes in the groups being compared. Since multiple comparison tests are robust and can contend with minor violations in this assumption, tests specifically designed for unequal sample sizes (unbalanced) are rare. The Tukey-Kramer test has been discussed previously and represents a modified Tukey HSD test for unbalanced designs. It assumes that there is homogeneity comparing the various sample variances. For unbalanced designs with equal variances, it is recommended to use the Tukey-Kramer test if all pair-wise comparisons of the means are tested. This test is not an exact test, but it is conservative for unbalanced one-way ANOVAs and the experimentwise error rate will not exceed alpha. It is less conservative when the designs are only slightly unbalanced, but more conservative when there are large differences in samples sizes. Also, the Scheffé and Student-Neuman-Kuels tests can be adjusted for unbalanced designs. Other procedures specifically designed to handle unequal sample sizes include the **Miller-Winer test**, **Hochberg GT2 test**, and **Gabriel test**.

### Lack of Homogeneity

Ideally, the one-way ANOVA would be preformed only when the assumption of homogeneity of variances is met. However, because it is a robust statistic it can be employed when there is a deviation from this assumption. When the design involves unequal variances, there are several lesser used *post hoc* procedures including Games-Howell, Dunnett's C, Dunnett's T3, and Tamhane's T2 tests, which have been mentioned previously. None of these tests are exact tests, but the T2, T3 and C are conservative procedures and the experimental-wise error rate will not exceed $\alpha$. For larger samples that are approximately equal in size (balanced), the T2 is more conservative than T3. Where as, the T3 is more conservative than C for large samples, while C is more conservative for smaller.

The **Games-Howell test** (GH test) is designed for both unequal variances and unequal sample sizes. It is pair-wise procedure based on the *q*-distribution. The Games-Howell test may be too liberal when sample sizes are small and is therefore recommended for sample sizes greater than five. The Games-Howell is an extension of the Tukey-Kramer test, more powerful (narrower confidence intervals) than C, T2 or T3, and is recommended over these tests. It is most liberal (experimentalwise error rate is likely to exceed alpha) when the sample variances are approximately equal.

Both the **Dunnett's T3 and Dunnett's C** are similar post hoc procedures for use then the assumption of homogeneity of variance is not met or questionable. The T3 and C should be used for pair-wise comparisons. The **Tamhane's T2** is a pair-wise procedure based on the Student t-distribution. It uses Sidak test to define the alpha level. Tamhane's T2 is a more conservative post hoc comparison for data with unequal variances and is appropriate when variances are unequal and/or when the sample sizes are different. Toothaker's textbook discussed most of the *post hoc* procedures discussed in these last two sections (Toothaker, 1991).

**Other *Post hoc* Tests**

The **Hsu's MCB** (multiple comparison with the best) test creates confidence intervals for the difference between the mean for each level of the independent variable and the best of the remaining level means (Hsu, 1981). In other words each sample mean is compared to the "best" of the other means. Best is a default or the largest mean for the remaining levels. The test calculates q values associated with each sample. Hsu's MCB test is an exact test for a one-way analysis of variance with levels that have equal sample sizes (balanced). If unbalanced group sizes the experimentalwise error rate will be smaller than stated and results will be slightly more conservative confidence intervals. Results are comparable to Tukey LDS and Dunnett's tests when confidence intervals are larger. For comparing all pair-wise comparisons, the Tukey confidence intervals will be wider and the hypothesis tests less powerful for the experimentalwise error rate.

The **Bonferroni-Holm** test is a step down test that does not require any assumptions regarding the population distribution. It can be applied to any pair-wise comparison and is a conservative test (the exeprimentalwise error rate does not exceed alpha). The **Sidák-Holm** procedure is similar to the Bonferroni-Holms method except the difference are not compared to alpha, but to the Sidák adjust alpha. The Sidák-Holm test is slightly less conservative than Bonferroni-Holm test.

The **Duncan test**, also referred to as the Duncan new multiple range test, is a multiple range test based on the q-statistic. It is a stepwise test for ordered means. The test is not recommended for unbalanced cases (Duncan, 1955).

### References

Daniel, W.W. (1999). *Biostatistics: A Foundation for Analysis in the Health Sciences*, Seventh edition, John Wiley and Sons, New York, pp. 314-317.

Duncan, D.B. (1955). "Multiple range and multiple F tests," *Biometrics* 11:1-42

Glantz, S.A. (1980). "Biostatistics: How to detect correct and prevent errors in the medical literature," *Circulation* 61(1):1-7.

Hsu, J.C. (1981). "Simultaneous confidence intervals for all distances from the 'best'," *Annals of Statistics* 9:1026-1034.

Toothaker, L.E. (1991). *Multiple Comparisons for Researchers*, Sage Publications, Newbury Park, CA.

Zar, J.H. (1999). *Biostatistical Analysis*, Fourth edition, Prentice-Hall, Englewood Cliffs, NJ, Table B.6, p. App.74.

### Suggested Supplemental Readings

Fisher, L.D. and van Belle, G. (1993). *Biostatistics: A Methodology for the Health Sciences*, John Wiley and Sons, New York, pp. 596-661.

Hochberg Y. and Tamhane, A.C. (1987). *Multiple Comparison Procedures*, John Wiley and Sons, New York, 1987.

Kirk, R.E. (1968). *Experimental Design: Procedures for the Behavioral Sciences*, Brooks/Cole, Belmont, CA, pp. 69-98.

Toothaker, L.E. (1991). *Multiple Comparisons for Researchers*, Sage Publications, Newbury Park, CA.

Zar, J.H. (1999). *Biostatistical Analysis*, Fourth edition, Prentice-Hall, Englewood Cliffs, NJ, pp. 208-230.

### Example Problems

Based on the information presented, identify where the significant differences exist using the various *post hoc* procedures for the following problems.

1. A prospective study was conducted on 105 patient randomly assigned to one of three HMG-CoA reductase inhibitors for lowering cholesterol levels. After twelve months 94 of the patients were still being followed. Table 11.13 represents the change in total cholesterol reported for the patients (different

**Table 11.13** Change in Total Cholesterol Levels (mg/dl) for Patients Treated with Three Different HMG-CoA Reductase Inhibitors

| | Drug A | | Drug B | | Drug C | |
|---|---|---|---|---|---|---|
| | 1 | −3 | −20 | −3 | −54 | −33 |
| | −42 | −14 | 16 | −35 | −7 | −24 |
| | −7 | 2 | 3 | 9 | −30 | 2 |
| | −33 | −23 | −32 | −37 | −48 | −36 |
| | −2 | −45 | 10 | 10 | 9 | −14 |
| | 8 | 6 | −33 | 13 | 12 | −23 |
| | 15 | −36 | −24 | 0 | −39 | −18 |
| | 7 | 20 | −29 | −37 | −39 | 1 |
| | −16 | 21 | −35 | 3 | −32 | −26 |
| | 20 | 33 | −21 | −45 | −48 | −46 |
| | −21 | −23 | −22 | −12 | −55 | −35 |
| | 8 | −21 | 34 | −4 | −68 | −5 |
| | −38 | −19 | −9 | 14 | 7 | −12 |
| | −3 | −39 | 13 | 15 | −10 | −3 |
| | 7 | 11 | −9 | 7 | 13 | −10 |
| | 1 | | | | 12 | −8 |
| | | | | | −39 | |
| Mean = | −7.26 | | −8.67 | | −21.39 | |
| Standard Deviation = | 21.03 | | 20.90 | | 22.13 | |
| n = | 31 | | 30 | | 33 | |

between pretreatment level and most recent cholesterol level). There was a significant ANOVA ($p < .05$) comparing the three agents and rejection of the null hypothesis that $\mu_A = \mu_B = \mu_C$. The ANOVA table shows that the *F*-statistic exceeded the critical F-value of 3.111:

| Source | DF | SS | MS | F |
|---|---|---|---|---|
| Between | 2 | 3900.30 | 1950.15 | 4.27 |
| Within | 91 | 41604.48 | 457.19 | |
| Total | 93 | 45505 | | |

Use the most appropriate multiple comparison test(s), to identify significant difference(s) among these different agents, given the following scenarios.

a. Scenario 1: The researcher decided before the study to compare the newest agent (Drug C) to each of the other drugs (currently on the hospital formulary) if there was a significant ANOVA.

b. Scenario 2: The researcher decided before the study to consider Drug C and the "control" agent and compare each of the other drugs to this product.

c. Scenario 3: After identifying a significant ANOVA the researcher decided to compare the three agents "after the fact" to determine where the difference(s) exist.

2. Problem 3 in Chapter 10, which compares the viscosity of a raw material delivered to three different sites.

Hypotheses: $H_0$: $\mu_A = \mu_B = \mu_C$
$H_1$: $H_0$ is false

Decision rule: With $\alpha = .05$, reject $H_0$ if $F > F_{2,12}(.95) \approx 3.70$.

| Data: | Batch A | Batch B | Batch C |
|---|---|---|---|
| Mean = | 10.28 | 10.24 | 10.21 |
| S.D. = | 0.037 | 0.033 | 0.026 |
| n = | 5 | 5 | 5 |

Results:

$$F = \frac{MS_B}{MS_W} = \frac{0.0063}{0.0010} = 6.3$$

Decision: With $F > 3.70$, reject $H_0$, conclude that $\mu_A = \mu_B = \mu_C$ is not true.

Use the appropriate post hoc test(s) for results with equal sample sizes.

**Answers to Problems**

Possible examples for multiple comparison tests

1. Several different possible multiple comparisons.

a. Scenario 1: Prior to the ANOVA the researcher has decided on only two possible pair-wise comparisons. There are three possible tests, multiple t-tests with adjusted $\alpha$, or Dunn's test.

Multiple t-tests with adjusted $\alpha$:

Keeping $\alpha$ constant at .05 and doing two separate t-test the $\alpha = .05/2 = .025$ and a reliability coefficient = 2.297 for $t_{0.9875,62}$ for A vs. C and 2.298 for $t_{0.9875,61}$ for B vs. C (using Microsoft® Excel, TINV(0.025,*df*)).

$$\mu_A - \mu_C = (\overline{X}_A - \overline{X}_C) \pm t_{n_1+n_2-2}(1-\alpha/2)\sqrt{\frac{s_p^2}{n_A} + \frac{s_p^2}{n_C}}$$

$$S_p^2 = \frac{(n_A - 1)S_A^2 + (n_C - 1)S_C^2}{n_A + n_C - 2}$$

$$S_p^2 = \frac{(30)(21.03)^2 + (32)(22.13)^2}{62} = 466.765$$

$$\mu_A - \mu_C = (14.13) \pm 2.298\sqrt{\frac{466.765}{31} + \frac{466.765}{33}}$$

$$+1.712 < \mu_A - \mu_C < +26.548$$

$$\mu_B - \mu_C = (12.72) \pm 2.298\sqrt{\frac{464.575}{30} + \frac{464.575}{33}}$$

$$+0.225 < \mu_B - \mu_C < +25.215$$

Results: Since zero was not within the interval in both cases, Drug C showed a significantly larger decrease in total cholesterol than either Drug A or Drug B.

Dunn Test:

The Dunn reliability coefficient for is $t'D_{.05;3;91} \approx 2.45$ (Table B11).

Computation for $\overline{X}_A - \overline{X}_B$:

$$\mu_A - \mu_B = (\overline{X}_A - \overline{X}_B) \pm t'D_{\alpha/2;C;N-K}\sqrt{MS_E \cdot (\frac{1}{n_A} + \frac{1}{n_B})}$$

$$\mu_A - \mu_B = (1.41) \pm 2.45\sqrt{457.19 \cdot (\frac{1}{31} + \frac{1}{30})}$$

$$\mu_A - \mu_B = (1.41) \pm 13.416$$

$$-12.006 < \mu_A - \mu_B < +14.826$$

Results:

| Pairing | Confidence Interval | Results |
|---|---|---|
| $\bar{X}_A - \bar{X}_B$ | $-12.006 < \mu_A - \mu_B < +14.826$ | |
| $\bar{X}_A - \bar{X}_C$ | $+1.027 < \mu_A - \mu_C < +27.233$ | Significant |
| $\bar{X}_B - \bar{X}_C$ | $-0.495 < \mu_B - \mu_C < +25.935$ | |

b. Scenario 2: Prior to the ANOVA the researcher has decided on a control group and wishes to compare each alternative therapy to the control group. Only one possibility, the Dunnett test.

In this case the means of the sample are ranked from smallest to largest:

| $\bar{X}_C$ | $\bar{X}_B$ | $\bar{X}_A$ |
|---|---|---|
| −21.39 | −8.67 | −7.26 |

Thus, the *p* and subsequent q-value for A vs. C is 3 and 1.99, respectively, and for B vs. C it is 2 and 2.26 (Table B12).

$$\mu_C - \mu_A = (\bar{X}_C - \bar{X}_A) \pm q_{\alpha,p,N-k}\sqrt{MS_E\left(\frac{1}{n_C} + \frac{1}{n_A}\right)}$$

$$\mu_C - \mu_A = (14.13) \pm 1.99\sqrt{457.19\left(\frac{1}{33} + \frac{1}{31}\right)}$$

$$+3.487 < \mu_C - \mu_A < +24.773$$

$$\mu_C - \mu_B = (12.72) \pm 2.26\sqrt{457.19\left(\frac{1}{33} + \frac{1}{30}\right)}$$

$$+0.530 < \mu_C - \mu_B < +24.910$$

Results: In both cases zero did not fall within the interval. Thus, when Drug C is designated the "control" *a priori*, both pair-wise comparisons were significant and Drug C showed a significantly larger decrease in total cholesterol than either Drug A or Drug B.

c. Scenario 3: *Post hoc* comparison is required. With unequal cell sizes and equal variances the possible tests are Tukey-Kramer, SNK, and Scheffé tests.

Tukey-Kramer Test:

With slightly difference sample sizes the Tukey-Kramer test would be used over the Tukey test. In this case the $q$-value for the reliability coefficient would be the same for all three pair-wise comparisons, $q_{.05,3,91} = 3.38$ (Table B10).

Computation for $\overline{X}_A - \overline{X}_B$:

$$\mu_A - \mu_B = (\overline{X}_A - \overline{X}_B) \pm (q_{\alpha,k,N-k})\sqrt{\frac{MS_E}{2}\left(\frac{1}{n_A}+\frac{1}{n_B}\right)}$$

$$\mu_A - \mu_B = (1.41) \pm (3.38)\sqrt{\frac{457.19}{2}\left(\frac{1}{31}+\frac{1}{30}\right)}$$

$$\mu_A - \mu_B = (1.41) \pm (13.088)$$

$$-11.678 < \mu_A - \mu_B < +14.498$$

Results:

| Pairing | Confidence Interval | Results |
|---|---|---|
| $\overline{X}_A - \overline{X}_B$ | $-11.678 < \mu_A - \mu_B < +14.498$ | |
| $\overline{X}_A - \overline{X}_C$ | $+1.348 < \mu_A - \mu_C < +26.912$ | Significant |
| $\overline{X}_B - \overline{X}_C$ | $-0.171 < \mu_B - \mu_C < +25.611$ | |

Student Newman-Keul:

For unbalanced designs the Student Newman-Keul equation is exactly the same as the Tukey-Kramer and would give the exact same results, except that the $q$-statistic calculated as:

$$q = \frac{\overline{X}_1 - \overline{X}_2}{\sqrt{\frac{MS_E}{2}\left(\frac{1}{n_1}+\frac{1}{n_2}\right)}}$$

would be compared to the critical value of 3.38. In these cases for:

$$\mu_A - \mu_B \qquad q = 0.364 \qquad \textit{not significant}$$

$$\mu_A - \mu_C \qquad q = 3.736 \qquad \textit{significant}$$

$$\mu_B - \mu_C \qquad q = 3.335 \qquad \textit{not significant}$$

Results: The only significant difference was that Drug C showed a significantly larger decrease in total cholesterol than either Drug A.

Scheffé Procedure:

For all three possible pair-wise comparisons, the Scheffe value ($S^2$) would equal $(k-1)(F_{k-1,N-k(1-\alpha)}) = (2)(3.111) = 6.222$. The error term is slightly different based on the pairing.

Computation for $\overline{X}_A - \overline{X}_B$:

$$var(\hat{\psi}_{AB}) = 457.19\left[\frac{(+1)^2}{31} + \frac{(-1)^2}{30}\right] = 29.988$$

$$\psi_{AB} = \hat{\psi}_{AB} \pm \sqrt{S^2 \cdot Var(\hat{\psi}_{AB})}$$

$$\psi_{AB} = 1.41 \pm \sqrt{(6.222)(29.988)}$$

$$\psi_{AB} = 1.41 \pm 13.659$$

$$-12.249 < \psi_{AB} < +15.069$$

Results:

| Pairing | Confidence Interval | Results |
|---|---|---|
| $\overline{X}_A - \overline{X}_B$ | $-12.249 < \mu_A - \mu_B < +15.069$ | |
| $\overline{X}_A - \overline{X}_C$ | $+0.790 < \mu_A - \mu_C < +27.470$ | Significant |
| $\overline{X}_B - \overline{X}_C$ | $-0.734 < \mu_B - \mu_C < +26.174$ | |

2. Three *post hoc* tests, discussed in this chapter, would be appropriate for results with equal sample sizes: 1) Tukey HSD; 2) Fisher LSD; and 3) Scheffe tests. Data comparing the site of raw materials and viscosity.

Sample Differences: $\overline{X}_A - \overline{X}_B = +0.04$
$\overline{X}_A - \overline{X}_C = +0.07$ $MS_W = MS_E = 0.001$
$\overline{X}_B - \overline{X}_C = +0.03$

Tukey HSD Test:

For the Tukey HSD test the reliability coefficient for is $q_{.05;3;12} = 3.77$ (Table B10).

Computation for $\overline{X}_A - \overline{X}_B$:

$$\mu_A - \mu_B = (\overline{X}_A - \overline{X}_B) \pm (q_{\alpha,k,N-k})\sqrt{\frac{MS_E}{n}}$$

$$\mu_A - \mu_B = (+0.04) \pm (3.77)\sqrt{\frac{0.001}{5}}$$

$$\mu_A - \mu_B = +0.04 \pm 0.053$$

$$-0.013 < \mu_A - \mu_B < +0.093$$

Results:

| Pairing | Confidence Interval | Results |
|---|---|---|
| $\overline{X}_A - \overline{X}_B$ | $-0.013 < \mu_A - \mu_B < +0.093$ | |
| $\overline{X}_A - \overline{X}_C$ | $+0.017 < \mu_A - \mu_C < +0.123$ | Significant |
| $\overline{X}_B - \overline{X}_C$ | $-0.023 < \mu_B - \mu_C < +0.083$ | |

Fisher LSD Test:

For the Fisher LSD test the reliability coefficient for is $t_{.025;12} = 2.1788$ (Table B5).

Computation for $\overline{X}_A - \overline{X}_C$:

$$\mu_A - \mu_C = \left(\overline{X}_A - \overline{X}_C\right) \pm t_{1-\alpha/2,N-k}\sqrt{\frac{MS_E}{n_A} + \frac{MS_E}{n_C}}$$

$$\mu_A - \mu_C = (+0.07) \pm (2.1788)\sqrt{\frac{0.001}{5} + \frac{0.001}{5}}$$

$$\mu_A - \mu_c = (0.07) \pm 0.044$$

$$+0.026 < \mu_A - \mu_C < +0.114$$

Results:

| Pairing | Confidence Interval | Results |
|---|---|---|
| $\overline{X}_A - \overline{X}_B$ | $-0.004 < \mu_A - \mu_B < +0.084$ | |
| $\overline{X}_A - \overline{X}_C$ | $+0.026 < \mu_A - \mu_C < +0.114$ | Significant |
| $\overline{X}_B - \overline{X}_C$ | $-0.014 < \mu_B - \mu_C < +0.074$ | |

Scheffé procedure

Scheffé value is:

$$(Scheffe\ \ value)^2 = S^2 = (K-1)(F_{K-1,N-K}(1-\alpha)) = 2(3.70) = 7.40$$

Computation for $\overline{X}_B - \overline{X}_C$:

$$var(\hat{\psi}_3) = 0.001\left[\frac{(+1)^2}{5} + \frac{(-1)^2}{5}\right] = 0.0004$$

$$\psi_3 = +0.03 \pm \sqrt{(7.40)(0.0004)} = 0.03 \pm 0.054$$

$$-0.024 < \psi_3 < +0.084$$

Results:

| Pairing | Confidence Interval | Results |
|---|---|---|
| $\overline{X}_A - \overline{X}_B$ | $-0.014 < \mu_A - \mu_B < +0.094$ | |
| $\overline{X}_A - \overline{X}_C$ | $+0.016 < \mu_A - \mu_C < +0.124$ | Significant |
| $\overline{X}_B - \overline{X}_C$ | $-0.024 < \mu_B - \mu_C < +0.084$ | |

# 12

# Factorial Designs: An Introduction

As presented in Chapter 10, the simple, one-way analysis of variance is used to test the effect of one independent discrete variable. When using factorial designs it is possible to control for multiple independent variables and determine their effect on a single dependent continuous variable.

Through random sampling and an appropriate definition of the population, in an ideal world, the researcher should be able to control all variables not of interest to the particular research design. For example in a laboratory, the researcher should be able to control the temperature of the experiment, the quality of the ingredients used (the same batch, the same bottle), the accuracy of the measurements, and numerous other factors that might produce bias in the statistical analyses performed. However, in many research situations, several different factors must be considered at the same time as well as the relationship of these variables to each other. Therefore, the study must be designed to consider two or more independent variables at one time and their influence on the outcome of the dependent variable.

## Factorial Designs

The ANOVA model discussed in Chapter 10 is referred to as a "simple" or "one-way" analysis of variance because only a single independent variable or **factor** is being assessed. The term factor is synonymous with the terms **independent variable, treatment variable**, **predictor variable**, or **experimental variable**. Throughout this chapter the terms factor and independent variable will be used interchangeably.

Instead of repeating our experiment for each independent variable or factor, we can design a more efficient experiment that evaluates the effects of two or more factors at the same time. These types of designs are referred to as **factorial designs** because each level of one factor is combined with each level of the other factor, or independent variable. The primary advantage of a factorial design is that it allows us to evaluate the effects of more than one independent variable, both separately and in combination with each other. As will be seen, these factorial designs can be used to increase the control we have over our experiment by reducing the within-group variance. The factorial designs also offer economical advantages by reducing the total number of subjects or observations, which would be needed if the two main effects were evaluated separately.

To illustrate this situation, consider the following example. A school of pharmacy is working on developing a new method of delivering their recently developed Pharm.D. curriculum to B.S. pharmacists desiring to obtain this new degree, but unable to take a one- or two-year sabbatical to return to school. Therefore, the school is working with different delivery systems to provide distance learning for the didactic portion of the course work. The primary investigator has developed a satisfaction index on a linear scale for the pharmacist, to evaluate the convenience, flexibility, and usefulness of the course materials, as well as the user friendliness of the course work. It is assumed that the better the response (maximum score of 10), the more likely that pharmacists beginning the course work will continue to the end of the didactic portion of the program. A pilot study was conducted on a random sample of pharmacists. Two different delivery methods were considered: written monographs ($M_1$) and computer-based training using CD-ROMs ($M_2$). However, early in the development of course work there was concern that institutional (primarily hospital) and ambulatory (mostly retail) pharmacists may possess different learning signs and may react differently with respect to their evaluation of the course materials. Therefore, the pilot study was designed to evaluate two independent variables, the delivery system used, and the pharmacist's practice setting, either institutional ($S_1$) or ambulatory ($S_2$). This can be illustrated in the simplest possible experimental design, a 2 x 2 factorial design:

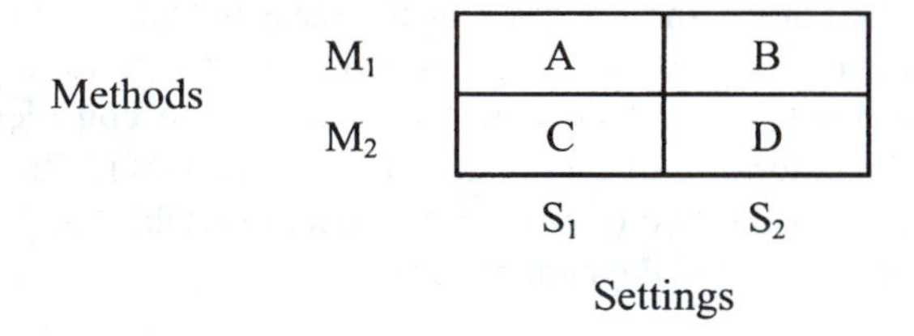

| Methods | | $S_1$ | $S_2$ |
|---|---|---|---|
| | $M_1$ | A | B |
| | $M_2$ | C | D |

Settings

where A,B,C, and D represent the mean results for the continuous dependent variable (satisfaction index), and rows and columns represent the main factors tested. For example, A represents the responses for pharmacist practicing in institutional settings who receive the written monongraphs; whereas D represents ambulatory pharmacists exposed to computer-based training.

In this design we are interested in evaluating the main effects of both the factors used and the interaction of these two factors. In this case we are dealing with three different hypotheses:

$H_{01}$: $\mu_{M1} = \mu_{M2}$ (Main effect of the delivery method)

$H_{02}$: $\mu_{S1} = \mu_{S2}$ (Main effect of the practice setting)

$H_{03}$: $(\mu_{M1,S1} - \mu_{M1,S2}) = (\mu_{M2,S1} - \mu_{M2,S2})$ (Interaction of method and setting)

The first hypotheses ($H_{01}$) evaluates the main factor for the two methods used for distance learning ($M_1$, $M_2$). Are they approximately the same or are they statistically different? The second hypothesis ($H_{02}$) assesses the influence of the pharmacists' practice setting ($S_1$, $S_2$) and what influence they might have on evaluations of the course materials. These first two hypotheses are called **tests of main effects** and are similar to separate tests using a one-way analysis of variance. The third hypothesis ($H_{03}$) evaluates the possibility of relationships between the row and column variables. As discussed below, two independent variables are considered to interact if differences in an outcome for specific levels of one factor are different at two or more levels of the second factor.

Whenever we evaluate the effect of two or more independent variables on a dependent variable, we must be cautious of a possible interaction between these independent variables. The **interaction effect** measures the joint effects of two or more factors on the dependent variable. If the factors are independent of each other, or have no relationship, there will be no interaction. We are interested in detecting interactions because the overall tests of main effects, without considering interactions, may cause us to make statements about our data that are incorrect or misleading. The validity of most multifactorial designs is contingent on an assumption of no interaction effects among the independent variables. One might argue that a more appropriate procedure is to test for any interaction first and if no interaction is detected (i.e., the test is not significant), then perform separate tests for the main effects. However, if interaction exists, it is meaningless to test the main effects or to try to interpret the main effects. The approach used in this book is to evaluate the main effect and interactions in concert as a more efficient and time-saving method. Granted, if the interaction is found to be significant, the results of the evaluation of main effects are without value, because the factors are not independent of each other.

To illustrate the various outcomes, consider the possible outcomes in Figure 12.1 for our experiment with the factors of delivery system and practice setting. Here results are plotted for one main factor (setting) on the x-axis and the second main factor (delivery system) on the y-axis. In Outcome I the results are the same for all four observations, therefore the investigator would fail to reject any of the three hypotheses and conclude that there was no significant effect for either of the main effects and there was no interaction between the two factors. For Outcome II, there is a significant difference between the two delivery methods used ($M_1 > M_2$) and the investigator could reject $H_{01}$, but would fail to reject the other two hypotheses. The opposite results are seen in Outcome III, where the investigator would find there is a significant difference between the two practice settings ($S_2 > S_1$) and reject $H_{02}$, but would fail to reject the other two hypotheses. Outcome IV represents a rejection of both $H_{01}$ and $H_{02}$ where $M_1 > M_2$ and $S_2 > S_1$, but there is no significant interaction and $H_{03}$ cannot be rejected.

Outcomes V and VI illustrate two possible interactions. In Outcome V there are significant differences in the main effects and a significant interaction between the two main factors. We can see that the two lines cross and there is a significant interaction between methods and settings. In this example, it appears that

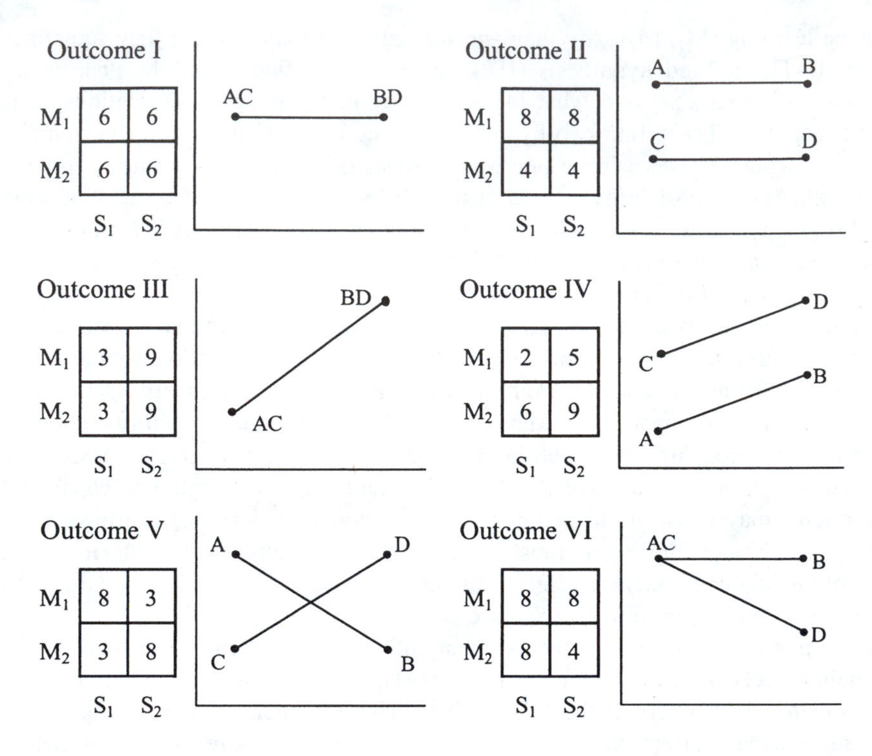


**Figure 12.1** Examples of possible outcomes with a 2 x 2 factorial design.

institutional pharmacists prefer monographs and ambulatory pharmacists favor the computer-based training. Because of the interaction, it becomes meaningless to evaluate the results of the main effects, because if there was a significant difference between methods of delivery, it may be influenced by the practice setting of the pharmacists. In Outcome VI there is no difference in $M_1$ based on the practice setting, but there is a difference for $M_2$. Is this significant? Is there an interaction between the two main effects (factors)? A two-way analysis of variance can determine, with a certain degree of confidence, which hypotheses should be rejected as false.

**Two-Way Analysis of Variance**

In the one-way ANOVA, we were only concerned with one major treatment effect or factor:

$$H_0: \mu_1 = \mu_2 = \mu_3 = \ldots \mu_k$$
$$H_1: H_0 \text{ is false}$$

However, in a two-way ANOVA, we are concerned about the major effects of two variables and their potential interaction.

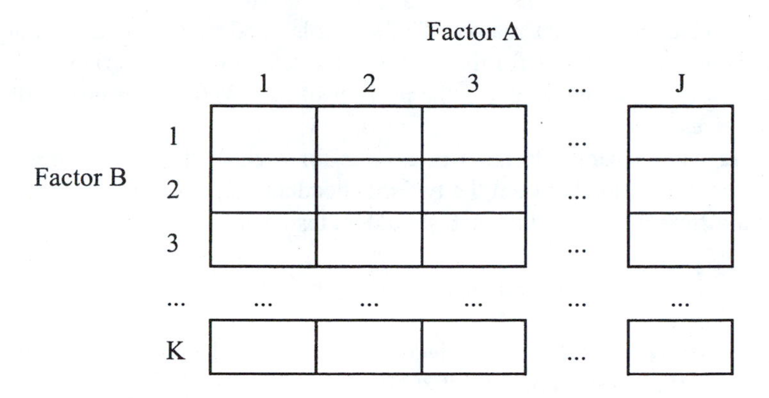


**Figure 12.2** Layout for a two-way analysis of variance.

The number of factors and levels within each factor determine the dimensions of a factorial design. For example, if Factor A consists of three levels and Factor B only two, it would be presented as a 3 x 2 (read three by two) factorial design. Areas within the factorial design, where dependent variable outcomes are reported, are called **cells**. In the case of a 4 x 5 factorial design, there are 20 cells (4 x 5 = 20). In factorial designs there must be more than one observation per cell. If there were only one observation per cell, there would be no variance within the cells and therefore a sum-of-squares error term would not be available. Each of the two major factors is a discrete independent variable and the significance of each factor is measured based on a single continuous dependent variable. The design for a two-way analysis of variance is presented in Figure 12.2. The column factor is represented by *J*-levels and the row factor by *K*-levels for each discrete independent variable. As seen in the previous illustration there are three hypotheses that are being tested simultaneously: two testing for the main effects and one for the interaction:

$H_{01}: \mu_{A1} = \mu_{A2} = \mu_{A3} = \ldots \mu_{AJ}$ (Main effect of Factor A)
$H_{02}: \mu_{B1} = \mu_{B2} = \mu_{B3} = \ldots \mu_{BK}$ (Main effect of Factor B)
$H_{03}: (\mu_{A1,B1} - \mu_{A1,B2}) = (\mu_{A2,B1} - \mu_{A2,B2}) = \text{etc.}$ (Interaction of A and B)

Similarly, there are three alternative hypotheses to complement each of the null hypotheses:

$H_{11}$: $H_{01}$ is false
$H_{12}$: $H_{02}$ is false
$H_{13}$: $H_{03}$ is false

With the one-way analysis of variance, the degrees of freedom for the critical F-value were associated with the number of levels of the independent variable $(k - 1)$ and the total number of observations $(N - k)$. Because the two-way analysis of variance deals with two independent variables, we have a different $F_c$ associated with each null hypotheses tested and these are directly associated with the number of rows and columns presented in the data matrix. The symbols used are: $j$ for the number of levels of the column variable; $k$ for the number of levels of the row variable; $N_k$ is the total number of observations; and $n$ is the number of observations per cell in the case of equal cell sizes.

There are three separate decision rules, one for each of the two main variables and one for the interaction between the two independent variables. Each hypothesis is tested with a different F-value, but each should be tested at the same $\alpha$.

$$\text{Reject } H_0 \text{ if } F > F_{\nu 1 \nu 2}(1-\alpha).$$

Where the $\nu_2$ degrees of freedom is always $j \cdot k \cdot (n-1)$ and $\nu_1$ will vary depending upon which null hypothesis is being tested, then:

$$H_{01}: \quad \nu_1 = j-1$$
$$H_{02}: \quad \nu_1 = k-1$$
$$H_{03}: \quad \nu_1 = (j-1)(k-1)$$

For equal cell sizes (the numbers of observations in each cell of the matrix are equal), the formulas are similar to those of the one-way ANOVA computational formulas. For intermediate value I, each observation ($x_i$) is squared, and then summed.

$$I = \sum_{k=1}^{K} \sum_{j=1}^{J} \sum_{i=1}^{I} x_i^2 \qquad \text{Eq. 12.1}$$

In the case of equal cell sizes the number observations in each cell for $i = 1$ to $I$ for be equal to n then Eq. 12.1 could be written as follows:

$$I = \sum_{k=1}^{K} \sum_{j=1}^{J} \sum_{i=1}^{n} x_i^2$$

However, in a later section of this chapter, equations will be presented for unequal cell sizes and the "$i$" summation notation will be used for continuity.

In intermediate value II the total sum of all observations is squared and divided by the total number of observations in the data set.

$$II = \frac{\left[ \sum_{k=1}^{K} \sum_{j=1}^{J} \sum_{i=1}^{I} x_i \right]^2}{N} \qquad \text{Eq. 12.2}$$

To compute the intermediate value IV, the sum of values for each cell of the matrix is squared and then all these values are summed and finally divided by the number of observations in each cell:

$$IV = \frac{\sum_{k=1}^{K} \sum_{j=1}^{J} \left[ \sum_{i=1}^{I} x_i \right]^2}{n} \qquad \text{Eq. 12.3}$$

There are two intermediate III values, one for the main effect of Factor A (columns) and one for the main effect of Factor B (rows). In the former case the sum of all values for each column is totaled and squared. These squared values are then summed and divided by the product of the number columns multiplied by the number of observations per cell:

$$III_C = \frac{\sum_{j=1}^{J} \left[ \sum_{k=1}^{K} \sum_{i=1}^{I} x_i \right]^2}{k \cdot n} \qquad \text{Eq. 12.4}$$

A similar procedure is used for the intermediate III rows, where the sum of all values for each row is totaled and squared. These squared values are then summed and divided by the product of the number of rows multiplied by the number of observations per cell:

$$III_R = \frac{\sum_{k=1}^{K} \left[ \sum_{j=1}^{J} \sum_{i=1}^{I} x_i \right]^2}{j \cdot n} \qquad \text{Eq. 12.5}$$

The $SS_{total}$ and $SS_{error}$ are calculated in a similar way to the one-way ANOVA. Note that the former error term $SS_W$ is now referred to as $SS_E$ or $SS_{error}$.

$$SS_{Error} = SS_E = I - IV \qquad \text{Eq. 12.6}$$

$$SS_{Total} = SS_T = I - II \qquad \text{Eq. 12.7}$$

In the two-way ANOVA, $SS_{rows}$, $SS_{columns}$ and $SS_{interactions}$ are calculated from the sum of squares formulas $III_R$ and $III_C$.

$$SS_{(Rows)} = SS_R = III_R - II \qquad \text{Eq. 12.8}$$

$$SS_{Columns} = SS_C = III_C - II \qquad \text{Eq. 12.9}$$

$$SS_{Interaction} = SS_{RC} = IV - III_R - III_C + II \qquad \text{Eq. 12.10}$$

The key difference with this design is that the between-group variance is further divided into the different sources of variation (row variable, column variable, and interaction). A certain amount of variation can be attributed to the row variable and

| Source | Degrees of Freedom | Sum of Squares | Mean Squares (MS) | F |
|---|---|---|---|---|
| Between: | | | | |
| Rows | $k-1$ | $SS_R$ | $\frac{SS_R}{k-1}$ | $\frac{MS_R}{MS_E}$ |
| Columns | $j-1$ | $SS_C$ | $\frac{SS_C}{j-1}$ | $\frac{MS_C}{MS_E}$ |
| Interaction | $(k-1)(j-1)$ | $SS_{RC}$ | $\frac{SS_{RC}}{(k-1)(j-1)}$ | $\frac{MS_{RC}}{MS_E}$ |
| Within: | | | | |
| Error | $k \cdot j \cdot (n-1)$ | $SS_E$ | $\frac{SS_E}{k \cdot j \cdot (n-1)}$ | |
| Total | $N-1$ | $SS_T$ | | |

**Figure 12.3** Computations for the ANOVA table for a two-way design.

some to the column variable. The remaining left over or **residual variation** is attributable to the "interaction" between these two factors.

The sum-of-squares information is inserted into an ANOVA table (Figure 12.3) where there are three levels for the between mean variability, the main effect of the rows variable, the main effect of the columns variable, and the effect of their interactions. The first column indicates the source of the variance. The second column is the degrees of freedom associated with each source. Note that the total number of degrees of freedom is one less than the total number of observations, again to correct for bias ($N-1$). The third column is the sum of squares calculated by Equations 12.6 through 12.10. The fourth column contains the mean-square terms that are calculated by dividing the sum of squares by the corresponding degrees of freedom for each row. Finally, the *F*-values are calculated by dividing each of the mean square between values by the mean-square error. Figure 12.4 represents other symbols that can be used to represent an analysis of variance table. Computer programs, such as SPSS or SAS, present results of factorial design calculations in formats similar to those in Tables 12.1 or 12.2.

The within or error line in the ANOVA table represents the error factor or **residual variance,** which cannot be accounted for by the variability among the row means, column means, or cell means. As will be discussed later, the mean-square error serves as the error term in the fixed-effects ANOVA. As seen in Figure 12.3, the denominator of each ratio in the last column, is the variance estimate based on the pooled within-groups sum of squared deviations. Once again this within groups variance ($MS_E$) is a measure of random "error" or chance differences among the variables.

| Source | df | SS | MS | F |
|---|---|---|---|---|
| Between: | | | | |
| Rows | k – 1 | $SS_R$ | $MS_R$ | $F_R$ |
| Columns | j – 1 | $SS_C$ | $MS_C$ | $F_C$ |
| Interaction | (k – 1)(j – 1) | $SS_{RC}$ | $MS_{RC}$ | $F_{RC}$ |
| Within: | | | | |
| Error | k·j·(n – 1) | $SS_E$ | $MS_E$ | |
| Total | N – 1 | $SS_T$ | | |

**Figure 12.4** ANOVA table for a two-way design.

If one or more of the *F* values calculated in the ANOVA table exceed their parallel critical $F_c$ value defined in the decision rule, the hypothesis or hypotheses will be rejected in favor of the alternative hypothesis. It could be possible for all three null hypotheses rejected, meaning that both column and row variables were significantly different and that there was a significant interaction between the two variables. If a significant outcome is not identified for the interaction portion of the ANOVA table then the outcome of the *F* tests for the two main effects can be interpreted the same way as the *F*-ratio in the one-way ANOVA. This measure of interaction is based upon the variability of the cell means. Therefore, when significant interaction occurs, caution must be used in interpreting the significance of the main effects. As mentioned previously, the validity of most factorial designs assume that there is no significant interaction between the independent variables. When interpreting the outcome of the two-way ANOVA, especially if there is a significant interaction, a plotting of the means (similar to Figure 12.1) can be extremely helpful to visualize the outcomes and identify the interaction.

As an example of a two-way ANOVA we will use a previous example associated with a two-sample t-test, where the investigator compared two formulations of the same drug and was interested in determining the maximum concentration (Table 9.2). However, in this case the study involved a two-period crossover study and the researcher wanted to make certain that the order in which the subjects received the formulation did not influence the $C_{max}$ for the formulation received during the second period. The three hypotheses under test were:

$$H_{01}: \mu_{\text{Formula A}} = \mu_{\text{Formula B}}$$
$$H_{02}: \mu_{\text{Order 1}} = \mu_{\text{Order 2}}$$
$$H_{03}: (\mu_{\text{Formula A,First}} - \mu_{\text{Formula B,First}}) = (\mu_{\text{Formula A,Second}} - \mu_{\text{Formula B,Second}})$$

and the decision rules were: 1) with $\alpha = .05$ and $n = 12$, reject $H_{01}$ if $F > F_{1,44}(.95) \approx 4.06$; 2) with $\alpha = .05$ and $n = 12$, reject $H_{02}$ if $F > F_{1,44}(.95) \approx 4.06$; and 3) with $\alpha = .05$ and $n = 12$, reject $H_{03}$ if $F > F_{1,44}(.95) \approx 4.06$.

**Table 12.1** Sample Data for a Two-way Crossover Clinical Trial ($C_{max}$)

| | Formulation A | | | Formulation B | | | $\sum_{j=1}^{J}\sum_{i=1}^{I}$ | $\sum_{k=1}^{K}\sum_{j=1}^{J}\sum_{i=1}^{I}$ |
|---|---|---|---|---|---|---|---|---|
| Formula A | 125 | 130 | 135 | 14 | 15 | 13 | | |
| Received | 128 | 121 | 123 | 9 | 1 | 0 | | |
| First | 131 | 129 | 120 | 13 | 14 | 12 | | |
| | 119 | 133 | 125 | 2 | 1 | 9 | | |
| | | | | 14 | 13 | 12 | | |
| | | | | 2 | 0 | 2 | | |
| | | | | 13 | 13 | 14 | | |
| | | | | 6 | 8 | 0 | | |
| $\sum_{i=1}^{I}$ = | 1,519 | | | 1,640 | | | 3,159 | |
| Formula B | 126 | 140 | 135 | 13 | 12 | 12 | | |
| Received | 126 | 121 | 133 | 0 | 8 | 7 | | |
| First | 117 | 126 | 127 | 14 | 14 | 13 | | |
| | 120 | 136 | 122 | 1 | 5 | 2 | | |
| | | | | 13 | 13 | 13 | | |
| | | | | 3 | 6 | 8 | | |
| | | | | 12 | 15 | 14 | | |
| | | | | 9 | 0 | 8 | | |
| $\sum_{i=1}^{I}$= = | 1,529 | | | 1,637 | | | 3,166 | |
| $\sum_{k=1}^{K}\sum_{i=1}^{I}$ = | 3,048 | | | 3,277 | | | | 6,325 |

The data observed by the investigator is presented in Table 12.1. Also included are: 1) the sum of observations for each cell (2 x 2 design); 2) the sum for each column (formulations A and B); 3) the sum for each row (order in which formulations were received); and 4) the total sum of all the observations. The initial computations of the intermediate values are:

$$I=\sum_{k=1}^{K}\sum_{j=1}^{J}\sum_{i=1}^{I}x_i^2=(125)^2+(130)^2+...(148)^2=836{,}917$$

$$III_R = \frac{\sum_{k=1}^{K}\left[\sum_{j=1}^{J}\sum_{i=1}^{I} x_i\right]^2}{j \cdot n} = \frac{(3,159)^2 + (3,166)^2}{24} = 833,451.54$$

$$III_C = \frac{\sum_{j=1}^{J}\left[\sum_{k=1}^{K}\sum_{i=1}^{I} x_i\right]^2}{k \cdot n} = \frac{(3,048)^2 + (3,277)^2}{24} = 834,543.04$$

$$IV = \frac{\sum_{k=1}^{K}\sum_{j=1}^{J}\left[\sum_{i=1}^{I} x_i\right]^2}{n} = \frac{(1,519)^2 + \ldots (1,637)^2}{12} = 834,547.58$$

The sum of squares required for the ANOVA table are:

$$SS_R = III_R - II = 833,451.54 - 833,450.52 = 1.02$$

$$SS_C = III_C - II = 834,543.04 - 833,450.52 = 1,092.52$$

$$SS_{RC} = IV - III_R - III_C + II$$

$$SS_{RC} = 834,547.58 - 833,451.54 - 834,543.04 + 833,450.52 = 3.52$$

$$SS_E = I - IV = 836,917 - 834,547.58 = 2,369.42$$

$$SS_T = I - II = 836,917 - 833,450.52 = 3,466.48$$

The resultant ANOVA table is as follows:

| Source | df | SS | MS | F |
|---|---|---|---|---|
| Between | | | | |
| Rows (order) | 1 | 1.02 | 1.02 | 0.02 |
| Column (formula) | 1 | 1,092.52 | 1,092.52 | 20.29* |
| Interaction | 1 | 3.52 | 3.52 | 0.07 |
| Within (error): | 44 | 2,369.42 | 53.85 | |
| Total | 47 | 3,466.48 | | |

In this example, with $\alpha = .05$, the decision is to reject $H_{02}$ and conclude that there is a significant difference between the two formulations. Note that this is a valid decision since there is not a significant interaction between the two factors. Also, there is no

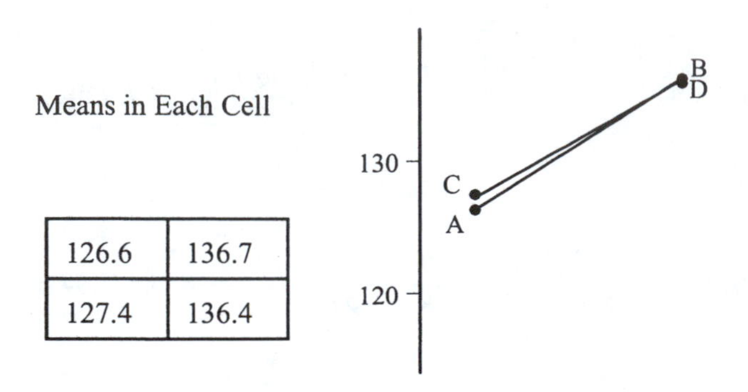


**Figure 12.5** Visual representation of clinical trial data.

significant difference based on the order in which the drugs were administered. If the data is visually represented similar to the examples in Figure 12.5, it is possible to see the significance in formulation, the closeness and insignificance of the order in which the drugs were administered, and the lack of any interaction (Figure 12.5).

A second example involving more levels of the independent variable involves a pharmaceutical manufacturer wishing to evaluate two automated systems for dissolution testing. Four separate batches of a particular agent were tested using each of the two automated systems and a technician-operated traditional dissolution system. Presented in Table 12.2 are the results of the experiment. Is there a significant difference between the batches or procedure used, or is there a significant interaction between the two factors?

Once again three hypotheses are being tested simultaneously ($H_{01}$ for differences in the method used, $H_{02}$ for differences in the batches tested, and $H_{03}$ for possible interaction between the two factors):

$$H_{01}: \mu_{Traditional} = \mu_{Automated\ I} = \mu_{Automated\ II}$$
$$H_{02}: \mu_{Batch\ A} = \mu_{Batch\ B} = \mu_{Batch\ C} = \mu_{Batch\ D}$$
$$H_{03}: (\mu_{Traditional,Batch\ A} - \mu_{Traditional,Batch\ B}) \ldots = (\mu_{Automated\ II,Batch\ C} - \mu_{Automated\ II,Batch\ D})$$

and the decision rules are, with $\alpha = .05$ and $n = 6$: 1) reject $H_{01}$ if $F > F_{2,60}(.95) = 3.15$; 2) reject $H_{02}$ if $F > F_{3,60}(.95) = 2.76$; and 3) reject $H_{03}$ if $F > F_{6,60}(.95) = 2.25$. The computations are:

$$I = \sum_{k=1}^{K} \sum_{j=1}^{J} \sum_{i=1}^{I} x_i^2$$

$$I = (57)^2 + (62)^2 + (65)^2 + \ldots (44)^2 = 271{,}245$$

**Table 12.2** Comparison of Methods of Dissolution Testing

| | | Dissolution Results at 10 Minutes (%) n = 6 | | | |
|---|---|---|---|---|---|
| Batch | Statistic | Traditional Method | Automated System I | Automated System II | ∑∑x |
| A | ∑x = | 391 | 378 | 310 | 1079 |
| | ∑x² = | 25,627 | 23,968 | 16,189 | |
| | Mean = | 65.17 | 63.00 | 51.67 | |
| | SD = | 5.41 | 5.55 | 5.72 | |
| B | ∑x = | 369 | 360 | 358 | 1087 |
| | ∑x² = | 22,831 | 21,734 | 21,510 | |
| | Mean = | 61.50 | 60.00 | 59.67 | |
| | SD = | 5.24 | 5.18 | 5.46 | |
| C | ∑x = | 406 | 362 | 330 | 1098 |
| | ∑x² = | 27,612 | 21,982 | 18,284 | |
| | Mean = | 67.67 | 60.33 | 55.00 | |
| | SD = | 5.27 | 5.32 | 5.18 | |
| D | ∑x = | 401 | 383 | 345 | 1129 |
| | ∑x² = | 26,945 | 24,579 | 19,993 | |
| | Mean = | 66.83 | 63.83 | 57.50 | |
| | SD = | 5.38 | 5.11 | 5.09 | |
| | ∑∑x = | 1567 | 1483 | 1343 | 4393 |

$$II = \frac{\left[\sum_{k=1}^{K}\sum_{j=1}^{J}\sum_{i=1}^{I} x_i\right]^2}{N}$$

$$II = \frac{(4393)^2}{72} = 268{,}034.0139$$

$$III_R = \frac{\sum_{k=1}^{K}\left[\sum_{j=1}^{J}\sum_{i=1}^{I} x_i\right]^2}{j \cdot n}$$

$$III_R = \frac{(1079)^2 + (1087) + \ldots (1129)^2}{18} = 268{,}114.1667$$

$$III_C = \frac{\sum_{j=1}^{J}\left[\sum_{k=1}^{K}\sum_{i=1}^{I} x_i\right]^2}{k \cdot n}$$

$$III_C = \frac{(1567)^2 + (1483)^2 + (1343)^2}{24} = 269{,}101.1250$$

$$IV = \frac{\sum_{k=1}^{K}\sum_{j=1}^{J}\left[\sum_{i=1}^{I} x_i\right]^2}{n}$$

$$IV = \frac{(391)^2 + (378)^2 + (345)^2 + \ldots (310)^2}{6} = 269{,}514.1667$$

$$SS_R = III_R - II = 268{,}114.1667 - 268{,}034.0139 = 80.1528$$

$$SS_C = III_C - II = 269{,}101.1250 - 268{,}034.0139 = 1067.1111$$

$$SS_{RC} = IV - III_R - III_C + II$$

$$SS_{RC} = 269{,}514.1667 - 268{,}114.1667 - 269{,}101.1250 + 268{,}034.0139$$

$$SS_{RC} = 332.8889$$

$$SS_E = I - IV = 271{,}245 - 269{,}514.1667 = 1730.8333$$

$$SS_T = I - II = 271{,}245 - 268{,}034.0139 = 3210.9861$$

The results of the statistical analysis are presented in an ANOVA table:

| Source | df | SS | MS | F |
|---|---|---|---|---|
| Between | | | | |
| Rows (batch) | 3 | 80.1528 | 26.72 | 0.93 |
| Column (method) | 2 | 1067.1111 | 533.56 | 18.49* |
| Interaction | 6 | 332.8889 | 55.48 | 1.92 |
| Within (error): | 60 | 1730.8333 | 28.85 | |
| Total | 71 | 3210.9861 | | |

There was no significant interaction between the two factors; therefore, our decision is to reject the null hypothesis $H_{02}$ for the main effect of methods used and assume that all three methods of dissolution testing are not all equal. There was no significant difference based on the batches tested.

### Computational Formula with Unequal Cell Size

Every attempt should be made to have an equal number of observations in each cell. Unfortunately, sometimes data are lost despite the best intentions of the researcher. When data are available that do not contain equal cell sizes, the exact same procedure is used except that slightly modified formulas are substituted for Eqs. 12.3 through 12.5. For intermediate value IV, each cell is summed, that value is squared and divided by the number of observations within the cell, and these values for all individual cells are summed:

$$IV = \sum_{k=1}^{K} \sum_{j=1}^{J} \frac{\left[ \sum_{i=1}^{I} x_i \right]^2}{n_i} \qquad \text{Eq. 12.11}$$

For the intermediate step involving the rows factor, all values within a row are summed, squared, and then divided by the number of observations within that row ($N_R$). Finally, all the calculated squared sums for each row are added together:

$$III_R = \sum_{k=1}^{K} \frac{\left[ \sum_{j=1}^{J} \sum_{i=1}^{I} x_i \right]^2}{N_R} \qquad \text{Eq. 12.12}$$

The intermediate step for the column is calculated in a similar manner as the $III_R$ except the values in each column and the total number of observations per column ($N_C$) are used:

$$III_C = \sum_{j=1}^{J} \frac{\left[ \sum_{k=1}^{K} \sum_{i=1}^{I} x_i \right]^2}{N_C} \qquad \text{Eq. 12.13}$$

These modified intermediate steps, along with values I and II are then used to calculate the sum of squares value using the same formulas (Eqs. 12.6 through 12.10) used for data with equal cell sizes.

As an example of this application, consider the previous clinical trials example. However in this case, due to dropouts in the study, there were three fewer subjects on the second leg of the clinical trial (Table 12.3). In this case the decision rules remain the same, except the denominator degrees of freedom decreases. With $\alpha = .05$ and $n = 12$: 1) reject $H_{01}$ if $F > F_{1,41}(.95) \approx 4.08$; 2) reject $H_{02}$ if $F > F_{1,41}(.95) \approx 4.08$; and 3)

**Table 12.3** Sample Data of a Clinical Trial with Unequal Cells ($C_{max}$)

| | Formulation A | | | Formulation B | | | ΣΣ | ΣΣΣ |
|---|---|---|---|---|---|---|---|---|
| Formula A Received First | 125 | 130 | 135 | 149 | 151 | ... | | |
| | 128 | 121 | 123 | 132 | 141 | 129 | | |
| | 131 | 129 | 120 | 142 | 130 | 122 | | |
| | 119 | 133 | 125 | ... | 138 | 140 | | |
| | Σ = | 1,519 | | | 1,374 | | 2,893 | |
| Formula B Received First | 126 | 140 | 135 | 130 | 128 | 127 | | |
| | 126 | 121 | 133 | 141 | 145 | 132 | | |
| | 117 | 126 | ... | 133 | 136 | 138 | | |
| | 120 | 136 | 122 | 129 | 150 | 148 | | |
| | Σ = | 1,402 | | | 1,637 | | 3,039 | |
| ΣΣ = | | 2,921 | | | 3,011 | | | 5,932 |

reject $H_{03}$ if $F > F_{1,41}(.95) \approx 4.08$.

The initial computational steps are:

$$I = \sum_{k=1}^{K}\sum_{j=1}^{J}\sum_{i=1}^{I} x_i^2$$

$$I = (125)^2 + (130)^2 + (135)^2 + \ldots (150)^2 + (148)^2 = 785{,}392$$

$$II = \frac{\left[\sum_{k=1}^{K}\sum_{j=1}^{J}\sum_{i=1}^{I} x_i\right]^2}{N}$$

$$II = \frac{(5{,}932)^2}{45} = 781{,}969.42$$

$$III_R = \sum_{k=1}^{K} \frac{\left[\sum_{j=1}^{J}\sum_{i=1}^{I} x_i\right]^2}{N_R}$$

$$III_R = \frac{(2{,}893)^2}{22} + \frac{(3{,}039)^2}{23} = 781{,}973.89$$

$$III_C = \sum_{j=1}^{J} \frac{\left[\sum_{k=1}^{K}\sum_{i=1}^{I} x_i\right]^2}{N_C}$$

$$III_C = \frac{(2,921)^2}{23} + \frac{(3,011)^2}{22} = 783,063.41$$

$$IV = \frac{\sum_{k=1}^{K}\sum_{j=1}^{J}\left[\sum_{i=1}^{I} x_i\right]^2}{n}$$

$$IV = \frac{(1,519)^2}{12} + \frac{(1.374)^2}{10} + \frac{(1,402)^2}{11} + \frac{(1,637)^2}{12} = 783,073.03$$

Calculation of the sum of squares:

$$SS_R = 781,973.89 - 781,969.42 = 4.47$$

$$SS_C = 783,063.41 - 781,969.42 = 1,093.99$$

$$SS_{RC} = 783,073.03 - 781,973.89 - 783,063.41 + 781,969.42 = 5.15$$

$$SS_E = 785,392 - 783,073.03 = 2,318.97$$

$$SS_T = 785,392 - 781,969.42 = 3,422.58$$

The ANOVA table from the sum of squares data and appropriate degrees of freedom appears as follows:

| Source | df | SS | MS | F |
|---|---|---|---|---|
| Between | | | | |
| Rows (order) | 1 | 4.47 | 4.47 | 0.08 |
| Column (formula) | 1 | 1,093.99 | 1,093.99 | 19.34* |
| Interaction | 1 | 5.15 | 5.15 | 0.09 |
| Within (error): | 41 | 2,318.97 | 56.56 | |
| Total | 44 | 3,422.58 | | |

There is no significant interaction and the results, with $\alpha = .05$, is to reject $H_{02}$ and conclude that there is a significant difference between the two formulations, but there is no significant difference based on the order that the drugs were administered. These results are identical to the ones found when all of the cell sizes were equal.

## *Post Hoc* Procedures

Similar to the one-way ANOVA, if there are significant findings for the tests of main effect in the two-way analysis, *post hoc* procedures must be used to determine where those differences occur. If there are no significant interactions, then the *post hoc* procedures described in Chapter 11 can be performed on significant main effect factors. For example, consider the results of the analysis of the three methods for dissolution testing presented above. The findings were as follows, with the method providing the only significant difference:

| Source | df | SS | MS | F |
|---|---|---|---|---|
| Between | | | | |
| Column (method) | 2 | 1067.1111 | 533.56 | 18.49* |

Since there were no effects from the batch factor or a significant interaction, the data can be combined for each method tested.

Dissolution Results at 10 Minutes (%) $n = 6$

| | Traditional Method | Automated System I | Automated System II |
|---|---|---|---|
| $\sum x =$ | 1567 | 1483 | 1343 |
| $\sum x^2 =$ | 103,015 | 92,263 | 75,976 |
| Mean = | 65.29 | 61.79 | 55.96 |
| SD = | 5.52 | 5.21 | 5.99 |

One-way analysis of this data would produce an $F = 17.11$ with an $MS_E = 31.165$. Using Scheffé's procedure, the following results were observed:

| Pairing | Confidence Interval | Results |
|---|---|---|
| $\overline{X}_T - \overline{X}_I$ | $-0.54 < \mu_T - \mu_I < +7.54$ | |
| $\overline{X}_T - \overline{X}_{II}$ | $+5.28 < \mu_T - \mu_{II} < +13.37$ | Significant |
| $\overline{X}_I - \overline{X}_{II}$ | $+5.28 < \mu_I - \mu_{II} < +9.87$ | Significant |

Thus, based on the *post hoc* analysis there was no significant difference between the traditional dissolution testing method and the first automated process. However, both of these methods were significantly different than the second automated process.

When there is a significant interaction, *post hoc* analyses are required for each independent variable separately to determine significant differences between or among the levels of each variable. In other words we must perform a one-way

**Table 12.4** Different Comparison of Methods of Dissolution Testing Involving New Data

| | | Dissolution Results at 10 Minutes (%) n = 6 | | | |
|---|---|---|---|---|---|
| Batch | Statistic | Traditional | System I | System II | ∑∑x |
| A | ∑x = | 391 | 378 | 345 | 1114 |
| | Mean = | 65.17 | 63.00 | 57.50 | |
| B | ∑x = | 369 | 360 | 358 | 1087 |
| | Mean = | 61.50 | 60.00 | 59.67 | |
| C | ∑x = | 406 | 362 | 330 | 1098 |
| | Mean = | 67.67 | 60.33 | 55.00 | |
| D | ∑x = | 401 | 383 | 310 | 1094 |
| | Mean = | 66.83 | 63.83 | 51.67 | |
| ∑∑x = | | 1567 | 1483 | 1343 | 4393 |

ANOVA on each level of the main effect variable(s), which are found to be significant with a two-way ANOVA. For illustrative purposes assume the data previously shown in Table 12.2 was instead found to be the data in Table 12.4. A resultant ANOVA table shows there is also a significant interaction between the batch and method used.

| Source | df | SS | MS | F |
|---|---|---|---|---|
| Column (method) | 2 | 1067.1111 | 533.56 | 18.49* |
| Interaction | 6 | 391.2223 | 65.20 | 2.26* |

The method for evaluating this data is to divide up the total variance for both the significant main effect and the interaction. This is accomplished by creating a sum of squares comparison ($SS_{comparison}$) for each level of the significant main effect. For illustrative purposes we will assume that the column factor is significant:

$$\sum SS_{comparison} = SS_C + SS_{RC} \qquad \text{Eq. 12.14}$$

Estimating this $SS_{comparison}$ for each row involves the following equation:

$$SS_{comparison} = \frac{\sum_{j=1}^{J}\left[\sum_{i=1}^{I} x_i\right]^2}{n} - \frac{\left[\sum_{k=1}^{K} x_i\right]^2}{j \cdot n} \qquad \text{Eq. 12.15}$$

where the first part of the equation involves summing each squared cell ∑x and the second portion is the square for the sum for the row divided by the number of levels multiplied by the number of observations per cell. For example with the first row in Table 11.6:

$$SS_{comparison}\ for\ Row\ 1 = \frac{(391)^2 + (378)^2 + (345)^2}{6} - \frac{(1114)^2}{3(6)} = 187.45$$

The results for the second row would be:

$$SS_{comparison}\ for\ Row\ 2 = \frac{(369)^2 + (360)^2 + (358)^2}{6} - \frac{(1087)^2}{3(6)} = 11.45$$

The information from these comparisons is placed in an ANOVA table along with the error measurement ($SS_E$) from the original two-way ANOVA table. The results from Table 12.5 are presented below (* indicating significant outcomes):

| Source | df | SS | MS | F |
|---|---|---|---|---|
| Row 1 | 2 | 187.45 | 93.73 | 3.24* |
| Row 2 | 2 | 11.45 | 5.73 | 0.20 |
| Row 3 | 2 | 485.33 | 242.67 | 8.41* |
| Row 4 | 2 | 774.11 | 387.06 | 13.41* |
| Error | 60 | 1730.83 | 28.85 | |

As usual, the sum of squares term is divided by the appropriate degrees of freedom and each of the row mean squares is divided by the $MS_E$. Each F-value would be compared to a critical $F_{(j-1),(J \cdot K \cdot (n-1))}$ $F(1 - \alpha)$. In this case the critical value is $F_{2,60}$ = 3.15, and all but the second row showed significant differences. Note that the sum of SS terms fulfills Equation 12.15:

$$187.45 + 11.45 + 485.33 + 774.11 = 1067.11 + 391.22$$

This same process can be modified if a significant main effect is identified for the column independent variable.

## Repeated Measures Design

A **repeated measures design** is an experimental design in which a variable is measured for each subject at two or more points in time or different conditions. The design is to control for the variability among subjects, where each subject will serve as his/her own control. When only one independent factor is used in the design it is called a single-factor repeated measure. This design is exactly the same as a randomized complete block design (Chapter 10) where the subjects make up the blocking variable and the *k* points in time or different conditions make up the factor associated with the repeated measures. The *k* treatments are a fixed effect model. The same calculations and interpretations presented in the randomized complete block design are used for the repeated measures design.

**Repeatability and Reproducibility**

A special application of a two-way analysis of variance is to estimate the repeatability and reproducibility of intra- and interlaboratory studies on test data. The simplest study design is to send samples to each of several different laboratories. Each laboratory follows specific instructions for measuring specific traits of the samples with at least two repeated measures. The **repeatability**, the with-run or within-laboratory precision, is an assessment of the variability of replicate runs for the same sample preparation within a short period of time. It can also be the evaluation of data obtained by one person while repeatedly measuring the same item or sample. A synonymous term for repeatability is **inherent precision**. In contrast the **reproducibility** of a method, the between-laboratory or between-run precision, involves replicated runs at different times, at different locations or by different operators. It could also be considered a measure of variability of the data caused by differences in analyst behavior. Both measures are associated with random error in the system.

To complicate the situation, International Conference on Harmonization guidelines (ICH, 1995) define repeatability as the precision under the same operating conditions over a short time interval (**intra-assay precision**) and reproducibility is the precision between laboratories (collaborative studies that are usually applied to standardizing a method). ICH also includes a third term, **intermediate precision**, as an assessment of within laboratory variability due to different days, different analysts, or different equipment. Thus, internal precision and reproducibility are calculated the same way, but defined differently depending on what is being assessed. For example, if we have three different technicians in the same laboratory it is intermediate precision; if the three technicians work at three different laboratories (example below) it is reproducibility.

The two-way ANOVA is the most accurate method for quantifying repeatability and reproducibility. In addition, the analysis of variance method can quantify the interaction between repeatability and reproducibility (the variability of the interaction between the analyst/laboratory and the samples). The two-way fixed effects model with replications is calculated in the traditional manner using the analyst/laboratory as the column variable and the samples tested as the row variable. Each sample is tested multiple times by the same observer and these results appear within a given cell (replicate measurements). All samples should be tested an equal number of times by each analyst/laboratory, thus creating equal cell sizes. Repeatability and reproducibility are calculated using values that are found in the two-way ANOVA table (Figure 12.3) where the columns are the analyst (or laboratory) variable and the rows variable represents the samples run by each analyst (or laboratory).

Calculations are based on the degree of certainty the investigator requires. Most calculations are dependent on a reliability coefficient ($Z_0$) that is based in the normal distribution and include the range of area under the standardized curve. Thus, if one wants to be 95% confident, $Z_0 = 3.92$ (1.96 times 2 or a range from $-1.96$ to $+.196$). Listed in Table 12.5 are various commonly used $Z_0$-values. In the case of

**Table 12.5** Common $Z_0$-values

| % Confidence | $Z_0$ |
|---|---|
| 90 | 3.29 |
| 95 | 3.92 |
| 99 | 5.15 |
| 99.5 | 5.62 |
| 99.9 | 6.60 |

repeatability and reproducibility, 99% confidence is usually desired and will be used in the following example.

When performing a two-way ANOVA there are four sources of variability and since sample data is the best estimate of population variances ($\sigma^2$), we will use our sample measures of variance ($S^2$):

| Sources of variability | Variance Component |
|---|---|
| Analyst (or laboratory) | $S_j^2$ |
| Sample | $S_k^2$ |
| Analyst/Sample interaction | $S_{jk}^2$ |
| Error (repeatability) | $S_{error}^2$ |

The total variability in the data is:

$$Total\ variation = Z_0 \cdot S_{Total}$$

The $S_{Total}$ is calculated by taking into consideration the variability attributed to the samples ($k$) as well as the repeatability and reproducibility:

$$S_{Total} = \sqrt{S_k^2 + S_{repeatibility}^2 + S_{reproducility}^2}$$

The specific calculation for repeatability is as follows:

$$Repeatability = Z_0 \cdot \sqrt{MS_E} \qquad \text{Eq. 12.16}$$

The $MS_E$ is the error term taken from the two-way ANOVA table. Similar values are extracted from the ANOVA table for reproducibility:

$$Reproducibility = Z_0 \cdot \sqrt{\frac{MS_C - MS_{RC}}{k \cdot n}} \qquad \text{Eq. 12.17}$$

where $k$ is the number of samples evaluated by each analyst (or laboratory) and $n$ is the number of repeated trials on each sample. The interaction between variability for the samples and analysts/laboratories is:

$$Interaction = Z_0 \cdot \sqrt{\frac{MS_{RC} - MS_E}{n}} \qquad \text{Eq. 12.18}$$

Note that it is possible to have such small interaction (small $MS_{RC}$) that the equation may attempt to take the square root of a negative number. Since this is impossible to calculate (square roots of negatives are imaginary numbers), the interactive effect in this case equals zero. The measurement systems repeatability and repeatability is:

$$R \,\&\, R = \sqrt{Repeatability^2 + Reproducibility^2 + Interaction^2} \qquad \text{Eq. 12.19}$$

The sample variation is:

$$V_P = Z_0 \cdot \sqrt{\frac{MS_R - MS_{RC}}{j \cdot n}} \qquad \text{Eq. 12.20}$$

where j is the number of analysts/laboratories. The total system variation is:

$$V_T = \sqrt{R \,\&\, R^2 + V_P^2} \qquad \text{Eq. 12.21}$$

As an example, consider three different laboratories, analyzing 10 different samples and each laboratory performs two assays on each sample (it is assumed that the same analyst performs the tests on the same equipment for each laboratory to remove possible additional variability). The data for this assessment is present in Table 12.6 along with the results of the two-way ANOVA calculations. With 99% confidence in our results ($Z_0 = 5.15$), the various calculations are as follows:

$$Repeatability = 5.15\sqrt{0.92} = 4.94$$

$$Reproducibility = 5.15\sqrt{\frac{191.19 - 3.25}{10(2)}} = 15.79$$

$$Interaction = 5.15\sqrt{\frac{3.25 - 0.92}{2}} = 5.56$$

$$R \,\&\, R = \sqrt{(4.94)^2 + (15.79)^2 + (5.56)^2} = 17.45$$

**Table 12.6** Sample Data for Measures of Repeatability and Reproducibility

| | Laboratory A | | Laboratory B | | Laboratory C | |
|---|---|---|---|---|---|---|
| Sample | Trial 1 | Trial 2 | Trial 1 | Trial 2 | Trial 1 | Trial 2 |
| 1 | 101.5 | 101.3 | 96.7 | 97.1 | 102.3 | 103 |
| 2 | 92 | 92.2 | 90.3 | 91 | 92.5 | 92.2 |
| 3 | 104.6 | 105.4 | 99.5 | 99.7 | 105.3 | 105 |
| 4 | 114.3 | 114 | 108.9 | 103.6 | 113.6 | 115.5 |
| 5 | 101.4 | 101.6 | 96.5 | 96.1 | 104 | 103.7 |
| 6 | 99.7 | 99.4 | 91.8 | 92.4 | 99.9 | 99.5 |
| 7 | 101.1 | 101.4 | 96.8 | 97.5 | 103.3 | 102.9 |
| 8 | 100.3 | 101.1 | 97.4 | 97 | 102.6 | 100.9 |
| 9 | 102 | 101.3 | 101.3 | 99.1 | 103.4 | 104.8 |
| 10 | 105.5 | 102.9 | 98.8 | 97.5 | 105.3 | 105.9 |

Two-way ANOVA for data

| Source | df | SS | MS | F | p |
|---|---|---|---|---|---|
| Laboratory (column) | 2 | 382.37 | 191.19 | 207.44 | <0.0005 |
| Sample (row) | 9 | 1355.37 | 150.60 | 163.40 | <0.0005 |
| Interaction | 18 | 58.49 | 3.25 | 3.53 | <0.01 |
| Error | 30 | 27.65 | 0.92 | | |
| Total | 59 | 1823.88 | | | |

$$V_P = 5.15\sqrt{\frac{150.60 - 3.25}{(3)(2)}} = 25.52$$

$$V_T = \sqrt{(17.45)^2 + (25.52)^2} = 30.92$$

How can the above results be interpreted? As noted previously, each type of random variability contributes a certain proportion to the total variability of the system. Therefore, the calculation of the percentage each contributes to the total variability is:

$$\%\,Contribution = \left(\frac{Source}{V_T}\right)^2 x\,100 \qquad \text{Eq. 12.22}$$

For this particular example the contributions of the repeatability, reproducibility, and samples are:

$$\% \, repeatibility = \left( \frac{Repeatibility}{V_T} \right)^2 x \, 100 = \left( \frac{4.94}{30.92} \right)^2 x \, 100 = 2.55\%$$

$$\% \, reproducibility = \left( \frac{reproducibility}{V_T} \right)^2 x \, 100 = \left( \frac{15.79}{30.92} \right)^2 x \, 100 = 26.08\%$$

$$\% \, R \,\&\, R = \left( \frac{R \,\&\, R}{V_T} \right)^2 x \, 100 = \left( \frac{17.45}{30.92} \right)^2 x \, 100 = 31.85\%$$

$$\% \, sample = \left( \frac{V_P}{V_T} \right)^2 x \, 100 = \left( \frac{25.52}{30.92} \right)^2 x \, 100 = 68.12\%$$

Potential guidelines for interpreting the results are as follows: 1) the percent contributed by the repeatability should be 5% or less (if greater than 5%, the measurement system may not be adequate for its intended application); 2) the percent contribution for the R&R term should be less than 30% (if greater than 30% effort should be made to reduce the variability before further analyses are performed). In this particular example, the repeatability was acceptable, but the R&R was unacceptably large and improvements are required before interlaboratory testing can be performed with confidence.

## Latin Square Designs

As discussed in Chapter 10, the one-way ANOVA (referred to as a **completely randomized block design**) allows the researcher to minimize experimental error by creating relatively homogeneous subgroups, by blocking the data. Similarly, the two-way ANOVA described earlier in this chapter is also an complete randomized block design. We could think of the levels of dependent variable can be deemed as "blocks." It is assumed that the only variability within the blocks is due to difference in the levels of the independent variable. Also in Chapter 10 we discussed the **randomized block design** where treatments are repeated once per block in only one direction, where we expanded the paired t-test to more than two levels and each subject or unit served as its own control.

An extension of the randomized block design to include two extraneous factors in the same study is called the **Latin square design**. In the Latin square design one possible source of extraneous variation is assigned to the columns of the two-way matrix and the second source of extraneous variation is assigned to the rows. Like the randomized block design the outcome is measured once and only once in each row and each column. Therefore, the number of columns, rows, and treatments are all equal. This design is sometime referred to as **Youden square plan.** The purpose of the design is to control the variation in the experiment. Because of its design, the Latin square is more powerful than either the randomized block design or completely randomized block design.

This design was originally used in agricultural experiments, where fields were divided into units or plots to account for variations in soil quality and other environmental factors. Treatments are assigned at random within the rows and columns (each treatment once per row and once per column). Number of rows and columns must be the same and it is assumed that there is no interaction between the row and column variables. An example of four treatments administered in four rows (I-IV) and four columns (1-4) as illustrated below.

| | | Column Factor | | | |
|---|---|---|---|---|---|
| | | 1 | 2 | 3 | 4 |
| | I | A | B | C | D |
| Row | II | C | D | A | B |
| Factor | III | D | C | B | A |
| | IV | B | A | D | C |

In this example (1, 2, 3, and 4) represent different patients and (I, II, III, and IV) represent the order in which the four patients will receive the treatments. For example patient 1 will receive A first, C second, D third, and B fourth. Whereas, patient 4 will receive D first, B second, A third, and C last. In the Latin Square design there are $t$ treatments and $t^2$ experimental units ($R$ x $C$). In the above example, $t$ = 4 with 16 experimental units. Examples of other possible Latin square designs would include the following permutations:

| 3 x 3 | 4 x 4 | 5 x 5 |
|---|---|---|
| ABC | ABCD | ABCDE |
| BCA | BADC | BAECD |
| CAB | CDBA | CDAEB |
| | DCAB | DEBAC |
| | | ECDBA |

In all cases, each treatment appears only once in each column and once in each row. An advantage of the Latin square design is that it allows the researcher to control for two sources of variation by blocking the variables. One disadvantage is that the number of levels of each blocking variable must equal the number of treatment levels (requiring $t^2$ number of experimental units). Another disadvantage is that the researcher must assume there is no interaction between the treatment and blocking variables. Also, the smallest possible Latin square is a 3 x 3 design (Mason, 1989, p. 149).

In the Latin-square design the hypothesis being tested concerns equality among the levels of the discrete independent variable and in this experimental design we have a three-factor ANOVA, with one fixed and two random factors. In this design there are no replicate measures. Similar to the two-way ANOVA, the Latin square design tests three null hypotheses simultaneously. That there is no significant difference among

**Table 12.7** Critical Values for Latin Square Designs

| Design | $\upsilon_1,\upsilon_2$ | $(1 - \alpha) = 0.95$ | $(1 - \alpha) = 0.99$ |
|---|---|---|---|
| 3 x 3 | 3,2 | 19.1642 | 99.1640 |
| 4 x 4 | 4,6 | 4.5337 | 9.1484 |
| 5 x 5 | 5,12 | 3.1059 | 5.0644 |
| 6 x 6 | 6,20 | 2.5990 | 3.8714 |
| 7 x 7 | 7,30 | 2.3343 | 3.3045 |
| 8 x 8 | 8,42 | 2.1681 | 2.9681 |
| 9 x 9 | 9,56 | 2.0519 | 2.7420 |
| 10 x 10 | 10,72 | 1.9649 | 2.5775 |

This table was created using Microsoft® Excel 2002 using function command FINV(alpha,df1,df2).

the level of the treatment and no difference for the two extraneous factors in the design:

$$H_{01}: \mu_{C1} = \mu_{C2} \ldots = \mu_{Cj} \quad \text{(extraneous factor in the column)}$$
$$H_{02}: \mu_{R1} = \mu_{R2} \ldots = \mu_{Rk} \quad \text{(extraneous factor in the row)}$$
$$H_{03}: \mu_{T1} = \mu_{T2} \ldots = \mu_{Tn} \quad \text{(treatment variable)}$$

In this design we are primarily concerned with the significance of the third hypothesis (treatment effect) and at the same time that the extraneous variable is not significantly different. The critical value for rejecting each of the null hypotheses is the same since $j = k = t$. In this case the numerator degrees of freedom would be the $t$ and the denominator (or error) degrees of freedom is $(t - 1)(t - 2)$. Thus for Latin square the critical value would be:

$$F_{t,(t-1)(t-2)}(1 - \alpha)$$

For example, in the case of a 4 x 4 Latin square design shown above the denominator degrees of freedom is (4 – 1)(3 – 1) = 6. With a decided 95% level of confidence, the critical value would be $F_{4,6}(.95) = 4.5337$ (from Table B7). The difficulty of fewer errors degrees of freedom can be corrected by using replicates or repeated measures. Listed in Table 12.7 are critical values for various Latin square designs.

The Latin square design involves a $t$ x $t$ matrix design with an equal number or rows and columns and $t$ is the number of treatments. Each cell will contain only one observation and the formulas used are similar to those already used in the two-way ANOVA computational formulas. Intermediates *I* and *II* are similar, except for the fact that there is only one observation per cell (even though it is a $t$ x $t$ design we will continue to use the previous $j$ and $k$ notations to refer to column and row functions, respectively) .

$$I = \sum_{k=1}^{K} \sum_{j=1}^{J} x_i^2 \qquad \text{Eq. 12.23}$$

$$II = \frac{\left[ \sum_{k=1}^{K} \sum_{j=1}^{J} x_i \right]^2}{k \cdot j} \qquad \text{Eq. 12.24}$$

where $k{\cdot}j$ is the total number of cells within the Latin square design. For intermediate value $I$ each value is squared and summed. For intermediate II the values are all summed and then squared before dividing by $N$.

The two intermediates associated with the variability due to the rows and columns are calculated by squaring the sum of each column and summing these results (for $III_C$) or squaring the sum of each row and summing these results (for $III_R$). Each of these sums are divided by the number of columns or rows.

$$III_C = \frac{\sum_{j=1}^{J} \left[ \sum_{k=1}^{K} x_i \right]^2}{j} \qquad \text{Eq. 12.25}$$

$$III_R = \frac{\sum_{k=1}^{K} \left[ \sum_{j=1}^{J} x_i \right]^2}{k} \qquad \text{Eq. 12.26}$$

Where $j$ and $k$ are the number of columns and rows, these are always the same in a Latin square design. The last measure takes into account the variability of the treatment effects. In this case the sum for all the results for each individual level of treatment is calculated regardless of the column or row location.

$$III_T = \frac{(\sum x_1)^2 + (\sum x_2)^2 + (\sum x_3)^2 + ...(\sum x_T)^2}{T} \qquad \text{Eq. 12.27}$$

Where $T$ is the number of levels of the treatment or independent variable. Again, in a Latin square design, $j = k = T$.

The sum of squares terms are calculated similar to those for the one-way and two-way ANOVAs:

$$SS_{Total} = SS_T = I - II \qquad \text{Eq. 12.28}$$

$$SS_{(Rows)} = SS_R = III_R - II \qquad \text{Eq. 12.29}$$

$$SS_{Columns} = SS_C = III_C - II \qquad \text{Eq. 12.30}$$

$$SS_{Treatment} = III_T - II \qquad \text{Eq. 12.31}$$

$$SS_{Error} = I - III_R - III_C - III_T + 2II \qquad \text{Eq. 12.32}$$

The sum of squares information is inserted into an ANOVA table (Figure 12.6) where the effect of the treatment is evaluated in contrast to the other variables. Results from the ANOVA table are compared to the critical value defined above.

As an example, assume we are conducting a small study on the responses of pharmacy students to a series of case studies and we are considering two possible sources of extraneous variation: 1) the individual students and 2) the order in which the case studies are presented. Based on several questions the student's responses could range from 0 to 100 points. In this example the hypotheses are:

$H_{01}$: $\mu_{C1} = \mu_{C2} \ldots = \mu_{Cj}$ (no difference based on the student)
$H_{02}$: $\mu_{R1} = \mu_{R2} \ldots = \mu_{Rk}$ (no difference based on the order of case)
$H_{03}$: $\mu_{T1} = \mu_{T2} \ldots = \mu_{Tn}$ (no significant difference in case studies)

Here we are primarily concerned with the significance of the case studies themselves (treatment effect) and want to determine if the extraneous factors (students or order) have any effect. The five case studies (A, B, C, D, and E) are presented in the following Latin square design:

| | | Student | | | | |
|---|---|---|---|---|---|---|
| | | 1 | 2 | 3 | 4 | 5 |
| Order | 1st | B | E | A | C | D |
| | 2nd | D | A | E | B | C |
| | 3rd | E | B | C | D | A |
| | 4th | A | C | D | E | B |
| | 5th | C | D | B | A | E |

For a five-treatment model the Latin square design, the denominator degrees of freedom are (5 – 1)(5 – 2) = 12, the 95% confidence, the critical value would be $F_{5,12(.95)} = 3.106$ (from Table B7). In this example the first student would receive case study B first, followed by D, E, A, and conclude with case study C. The results are as follows (with the column and row sums included):

| | | Student | | | | | |
|---|---|---|---|---|---|---|---|
| | | 1 | 2 | 3 | 4 | 5 | |
| Order | 1st | 88 | 80 | 80 | 84 | 86 | 418 |
| | 2nd | 81 | 81 | 82 | 91 | 86 | 421 |
| | 3rd | 86 | 85 | 82 | 77 | 77 | 407 |
| | 4th | 80 | 81 | 83 | 84 | 87 | 415 |
| | 5th | 87 | 84 | 83 | 78 | 78 | 410 |
| | | 422 | 411 | 410 | 414 | 414 | 2071 |

| Source | df | SS | MS | F |
|---|---|---|---|---|
| Between: | | | | |
| Rows | k − 1 | $SS_R$ | $MS_R$ | $F_R$ |
| Columns | j − 1 | $SS_C$ | $MS_C$ | $F_C$ |
| Treatment | t − 1 | $SS_T$ | $MS_T$ | $F_T$ |
| Within: | | | | |
| Error | (j − 1)(k − 2) | $SS_E$ | $MS_E$ | |
| Total | N − 1 | $SS_T$ | | |

**Figure 12.6** ANOVA table for a Latin square design.

The results for the individual case studies are as follows:

| Case Study: | A | B | C | D | E |
|---|---|---|---|---|---|
| Σx: | 396 | 434 | 420 | 411 | 410 |
| Mean: | 79.2 | 86.8 | 84 | 82.2 | 82 |

The calculations for the Latin square design are as follows:

$$I = \sum_{k=1}^{K} \sum_{j=1}^{J} x_i^2 = 88^2 + 80^2 + 80^2 ... + 78^2 = 171,879$$

$$II = \frac{\left[ \sum_{k=1}^{K} \sum_{j=1}^{J} x_i \right]^2}{k \cdot j} = \frac{2071^2}{25} = 171,561.64$$

$$III_C = \frac{\sum_{j=1}^{J} \left[ \sum_{k=1}^{K} x_i \right]^2}{j} = \frac{418^2 + 421^2 + 407^2 + 415^2 + 410^2}{5} = 171,587.80$$

$$III_R = \frac{\sum_{k=1}^{K} \left[ \sum_{j=1}^{J} x_i \right]^2}{k} = \frac{422^2 + 411^2 + 410^2 + 414^2 + 414^2}{5} = 171,579.40$$

$$III_T = \frac{(\sum x_1)^2 + ...(\sum x_5)^2}{T} = \frac{396^2 + 434^2 + 420^2 + 411^2 + 410^2}{5} = 171,718.60$$

$$SS_T = I - II = 171,879 - 171,561.64 = 317.36$$

$$SS_R = III_R - II = 171,579.40 - 171,561.64 = 26.16$$

$$SS_C = III_C - II = 171{,}587.80 - 171{,}561.64 = 17.76$$

$$SS_{Treatment} = III_T - II = 171{,}718.60 - 171{,}561.64 = 156.96$$

$$SS_{Error} = I - III_R - III_C - III_T + 2II$$

$$SS_{Error} = 171{,}879 - 171{,}579.40 - 171{,}587.80 - 171{,}718.60 + 2(171{,}561.64)$$

$$SS_{Error} = 116.48$$

| Source | df | SS | MS | F |
|---|---|---|---|---|
| Between: | | | | |
| Rows | 4 | 26.16 | 6.54 | 0.67 |
| Columns | 4 | 17.76 | 4.44 | 0.46 |
| Treatment | 4 | 156.96 | 39.24 | 4.44* |
| Within: | | | | |
| Error | 12 | 116.48 | 9.71 | |
| Total | 24 | 317.36 | | |

Neither of the two nuisance variables (student or order) was significant, but the case studies (treatment) were significant. Thus, one should be concerned that the responses to the cases studies vary, but the order in which they are administered or the students reacting to the case studies did not have an impact.

## Other Designs

The **Graeco-Latin square design** is an extension of the Latin square design and allows for the identification and isolation of three extraneous sources of variation. Greek letters are superimposed on the Latin letters in such a way that each Greek letter occurs once in each column, once in each row, and once with each Latin letter. Another way to think of these designs, is that we are concerned with main factor outcome (or treatment factor) and several nuisance independent or predictor factors. For the previous Latin square design there were two nuisance (predictor) factors. For Graeco-Latin square designs there are three nuisance factors and for **hyper-Graeco-Latin square designs** there are four nuisance predictor factors. The predictor or nuisance variables are the blocking variables. The advantage with the Graeco-Latin design is a reduction in the number of experimental units, as illustrated in Table 12.8. Notice that with the Graeco-Latin square design you are testing four factors concurrently and with the hyper-Graeco-Latin square design there are five variables tested concurrently.

**Table 12.8** Number of Runs Associated with Various Latin Square Designs

| Design | Factors | Runs (experimental units) |
|---|---|---|
| 3 x 3 Latin Square | 3 | 9 |
| 4 x 4 Latin Square | 3 | 16 |
| 5 x 5 Latin Square | 3 | 25 |
| 6 x 6 Latin Square | 3 | 36 |
| 3 x 3 Graeco-Latin Square | 4 | 9 |
| 4 x 4 Graeco-Latin Square | 4 | 16 |
| 5 x 5 Graeco-Latin Square | 4 | 25 |
| 6 x 6 Graeco-Latin Square | 4 | 36 |
| 4 x 4 Hyper-Graeco-Latin Square | 5 | 16 |
| 5 x 5 Hyper-Graeco-Latin Square | 5 | 25 |
| 6 x 6 Hyper-Graeco-Latin Square | 5 | 36 |

In many cases a complete randomized block design will require a large number of treatments that may not be economically or practically feasible. The **balanced incomplete block design** includes only a part of the treatments in a block. There will be missing pieces of information but the design must be balanced; balanced by the fact that each level of each factor has the same number of observations. Because some of the information is missing at other levels for each factor, the method involves incomplete blocks.

Other types of designs include **fractional factorial designs**, **split plot designs**, and **orthogonal array designs**. Each of these types of designs require stringent assumptions about the absence of interaction effects. We will not discuss formulas and calculations involved in these multifactor designs because they are tedious and best run on a computer. Details can be found in advanced texts (Kirk, 1968; Mason, 1989).

## Fixed, Random, and Mixed Effect Models

As seen with the previous examples of the two-way analysis of variance, the levels of the independent variable were purposefully set by the investigator as part of the research design. Such a design is termed a **fixed effects model** because the levels of the independent variables have been “fixed” by the researcher. The result of a fixed effect model cannot be generalized to values of the independent variables beyond those selected for the study. Any factor can be considered fixed if the researcher uses the same levels of the independent variable on replications of a study. The fixed-effects design is normally used for cost considerations and because studies usually involve only a specific number of levels for the independent variables of interest.

If the levels under investigation are chosen at random from a population then the model used would be called a **random effects model** and results can be generalized to the population from which the samples were selected. Usually, the researcher will randomly select the number of levels that he/she feels represents that independent variable. It is assumed that the selected levels represent all possible levels of that variable.

Lastly, there can be **mixed effects models** that contain both fixed effect variable(s) and random effects variable(s). An illustration of a mixed random effects model is a general linear regression model where the effects of multiple predictor variables, both continuous and discrete, are evaluated on a single outcome. As will be discussed in Chapter 14 the ANOVA can be used to evaluate an interaction effect, but regression models cannot evaluate interactions.

The computational formulas for all three models are identical except for the numerator used to calculate the *F*-value in the ANOVA table. In certain situations the mean square interaction is substituted for the traditional mean squares error ($MS_E$) term. The fixed-effect model would be calculated as presented in Figure 12.3. Using the symbols presented in Figure 12.3 the following modifications are required. For the random effects model modifications, where both the row and column variables are random, both the row and column F-statistics are modified as follows:

$$F_R = \frac{MS_R}{MS_{RC}} \qquad \text{Eq. 12.33}$$

$$F_C = \frac{MS_C}{MS_{RC}} \qquad \text{Eq. 12.34}$$

With the mixed effect, either the row or column variable could be fixed. If the columns are fixed and the rows are random, then equation Eq. 12.34 would be used for the column statistic and the traditional F-statistic would be calculated for the row.

$$F_R = \frac{MS_R}{MS_E} \qquad \text{Eq. 12.35}$$

Similarly, with the mixed effect model where the row variable is fixed and the column variable is random, Eq. 12.33 would be used for the row effect and the traditional F-statistic would be used for the column:

$$F_C = \frac{MS_C}{MS_E} \qquad \text{Eq. 12.36}$$

**Beyond a Two-Way Factorial Design**

There are numerous other ANOVA designs, but they all employ the same logic as the one-way and two-way ANOVAs. One can increase the number of independent variables to create more complex **N-way ANOVA** designs. As we have seen the two-

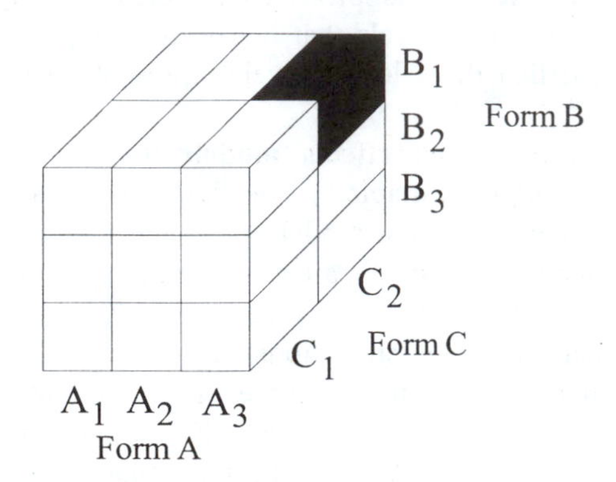


**Figure 12.7** Example of a three-way ANOVA.

way ANOVA we can evaluate both main and interaction effects. However, the two-way ANOVA is less sensitive than one-way ANOVA to moderate violations of the assumption of homogeneity and one needs approximately equal variances.

Figure 12.7 represents a three-dimensional schematic comparing three independent variables (a three-way ANOVA). Each of the three independent variables (A, B, and C) are represented by a dimension of the drawing. The shaded cube represents the combined effect of the third level of Factor A (columns), the first level of Factor B (rows), and the second level of Factor C (plains).

The advantage of these multifactor designs is the increased efficiency for comparing different levels of several independent variables or factors at one time instead of conducting several separate single-factor experiments. However, as the number of independent variables increases the number of possible outcomes increases and designs get extremely complicated to interpret, especially the interactions between two or possibly more variables. For example, with a two-way ANOVA there are two tests of the main effect and one interaction to interpret. With the three-way ANOVA these are increased to three tests of the main effect, three two-way interactions, and one three-way interaction. With the three-way ANOVA we would have the following numerator and denominator degrees of freedom and resultant F-statistic:

| Source of Variation | $\nu_1$ | $\nu_2$ | F-statistic |
|---|---|---|---|
| Column factor (A) | $j - 1$ | $j \cdot k \cdot m \cdot (n - 1)$ | $MS_C/MS_E$ |
| Row factor (B) | $k - 1$ | $j \cdot k \cdot m \cdot (n - 1)$ | $MS_R/MS_E$ |
| Plain Factor (C) | $m - 1$ | $j \cdot k \cdot m \cdot (n - 1)$ | $MS_P/MS_E$ |
| Interaction (AB) | $(j - 1)(k - 1)$ | $j \cdot k \cdot m \cdot (n - 1)$ | $MS_{RC}/MS_E$ |
| Interaction (AC) | $(j - 1)(m - 1)$ | $j \cdot k \cdot m \cdot (n - 1)$ | $MS_{CP}/MS_E$ |
| Interaction (CB) | $(k - 1)(m - 1)$ | $j \cdot k \cdot m \cdot (n - 1)$ | $MS_{RP}/MS_E$ |
| Interaction (ABC) | $(j - 1)(k - 1)(m - 1)$ | $j \cdot k \cdot m \cdot (n - 1)$ | $MS_{RCP}/MS_E$ |

**Table 12.9** Possible Significant Outcomes in Factorial Designs

| | Main Effects | Interactions | |
|---|---|---|---|
| One Factor | A | | |
| Two Factors | A | A x B | |
| | B | | |
| Three Factors | A | A x B | A x B x C |
| | B | A x C | |
| | C | B x C | |
| Four Factors | A | A x B | A x B x C |
| | B | A x C | B x C x D |
| | C | A x D | A x C x D |
| | D | B x C | |
| | | B x D | A x B x C x D |
| | | C x D | |
| Five Factors | A | A x B | A x B x C |
| | B | A x C | A x C x D |
| | C | A x D | A x D x E |
| | D | A x E | B x C x D |
| | E | B x C | B x D x E |
| | | B x D | C x D x E |
| | | B x E | |
| | | C x D | A x B x C x D |
| | | C x E | A x B x C x E |
| | | D x E | B x C x D x E |
| | | | A x B x C x D x E |

where *m* denotes the number of levels on the fixed plain variable. Similar to the two-way ANOVA, the denominator degrees of freedom remain constant. Random and mixed effect models can also be used in the three-way ANOVA design.

This same reasoning can be expanded to a four-way ANOVA where the complexity of the outcomes includes four tests of main effects, six two-way interactions, four three-way interactions, and one four-way interaction (Table 12.9). N-way ANOVAs are also referred to as **MANOVA** or multiple analysis of variance. MANOVAs are intended for large research studies where there are a number of different variables being assessed. Multiple one-way ANOVAs can result in a compounding of the error rate when the same data is used repeatedly. MANOVAs can detect mean differences for a number of different groups and their potential interactions where the Type I error rate remains constant.

Another type of related statistical procedure is the **analysis of covariance** or

**ANCOVA**. This procedure is useful for detecting mean differences among three or more groups when the researcher wishes to hold one variable constant. For example, evaluating the patients' knowledge of their particular disease state, controlling the level of education (i.e., less than high school education to graduate degrees). ANCOVA is useful in pharmacoeconomic studies where variables such as age, gender, educational background, or income could bias the study results. The measures are typical covariates and could also include a measure of people's aptitude, prior experience, or pretest scores.

In addition to MANOVAs and ANCOVAs there are **MANCOVA** (**multivariate analysis of covariance**), which is, combination of ANCOVA and MANOVA designs. Multivariate Analysis of Covariance (MANCOVA) is used when the researcher wishes to detect mean differences among a number of different levels of the independent variable, while holding one or more other variables constant. The MANCOVA is useful for when there are a variety of levels being evaluated on a number of different measures.

Finally, there are **fractional factorial designs** or **incomplete block designs.** These are experimental design in which only a part of the treatment blocks are included in the statistical analysis. Because of this increased complexity, factorial designs involving more than three factors pose difficulties in the interpretation of the interaction effects. Therefore, most factorial designs are usually limited to three factors. Factorial designs are well beyond the scope of this book. Excellent references for any of the methods described in this last section of the chapter would be Petersen (1985) or Box et al. (1978).

**References**

Box, G.E., Hunter, W.G. and Hunter, J.S. (1978). *Statistics for Experimenters*, John Wiley and Sons, New York, NY.

"ICH Topic Q2A Validation of Analytical Methods: Definitions and Terminology," *International Conference on Harmonization*, London, England, 1995.

Kirk, R.E. (1968). *Experimental Design: Procedures for the Behavioral Sciences*, Brooks/Cole Publishing, Belmont, CA.

Mason, R.L., Gunst, R.F., and Hess, J.L (1989). *Statistical Design and Analysis of Experiments*, John Wiley and Sons, New York.

Petersen, R.G. (1985). *Design and Analysis of Experiments*, Marcel Dekker, New York, NY.

**Suggested Supplemental Readings**

Havilcek, L.L. and Crain, R.D. (1988). *Practical Statistics for the Physical Sciences*, American Chemical Society, Washington, pp. 255-333.

Kachigan, S.K. (1991). *Multivariate Statistical Analysis*, Radius Press, New York, pp. 203-215.

Kirk, R.E. (1968). *Experimental Design: Procedures for the Behavioral Sciences*, Brooks/Cole Publishing, Belmont, CA, pp. 164-169, 403-420.

Zar, J.H. (1999). *Biostatistical Analysis*, Fourth edition, Prentice-Hall, Englewood Cliffs, NJ, pp. 286,287.

**Example Problems**

1. A preformulation department is experimenting with different fillers and various speeds on a tableting machine (Table 12.10). Are there any significant differences in hardness based on the following samples?

2. An investigator compares three different indexes for measuring the quality of life of patients with a specific disease state. She randomly selects four hospitals and identifies twelve individuals with approximately the same state of disease. These patients are randomly assigned to each of the indexes and evaluated (note one patient's information was lost due to incomplete information). The results are presented in Table 12.11. Are there any differences based on indexes or hospital used?

**Table 12.10** Results of an Experiment Involving Tablet Hardness

| | Hardness (kP) | | | | | | | |
|---|---|---|---|---|---|---|---|---|
| | Speed of Tableting Machine (1000 units/hour) | | | | | | | |
| Filler | 80 | | 100 | | 120 | | 180 | |
| | 7 | 8 | 6 | 7 | 5 | 7 | 6 | 7 |
| Lactose | 5 | 7 | 8 | 8 | 8 | 9 | 8 | 9 |
| | 8 | 9 | 6 | 7 | 7 | 7 | 7 | 7 |
| | 7 | 7 | 8 | 10 | 9 | 10 | 8 | 9 |
| | 7 | 7 | 8 | 9 | 5 | 7 | 7 | 6 |
| Microcrystalline | 7 | 9 | 6 | 7 | 8 | 8 | 6 | 6 |
| Cellulose | 5 | 7 | 8 | 7 | 5 | 7 | 8 | 7 |
| | 8 | 9 | 6 | 7 | 8 | 8 | 9 | 9 |
| | 7 | 5 | 4 | 6 | 6 | 7 | 4 | 6 |
| Dicalcium | 5 | 7 | 6 | 7 | 4 | 5 | 9 | 7 |
| Phosphate | 7 | 7 | 5 | 6 | 7 | 7 | 5 | 6 |
| | 5 | 8 | 7 | 8 | 5 | 6 | 7 | 6 |

**Table 12.11** Results of a Study on Patients' Quality of Life

| | Quality of Life Index (Scores 0-100) | | | | | |
|---|---|---|---|---|---|---|
| | Index 1 | | Index 2 | | Index 3 | |
| Hospital A | 67 | 73 | 85 | 91 | 94 | 95 |
| | 61 | 69 | 81 | 87 | 99 | 92 |
| Hospital B | 81 | 83 | 83 | ... | 86 | 85 |
| | 85 | 80 | 81 | 84 | 89 | 80 |
| Hospital C | 82 | 77 | 79 | 74 | 81 | 85 |
| | 80 | 86 | 80 | 84 | 82 | 77 |

**Table 12.12** Comparison of Sample Results in Various Laboratories

| | Laboratory | | | | | | |
|---|---|---|---|---|---|---|---|
| | 1 | 2 | 3 | 4 | 5 | 6 | 7 |
| | 80.22 | 80.49 | 80.23 | 80.93 | 80.20 | 80.80 | 80.00 |
| Sample 1 | 80.80 | 80.19 | 80.58 | 79.14 | 80.14 | 80.35 | 80.87 |
| | 80.38 | 80.35 | 80.44 | 80.46 | 80.79 | 80.65 | 80.99 |
| | 80.99 | 80.12 | 79.21 | 80.38 | 80.45 | 80.55 | 80.35 |
| | 75.94 | 76.24 | 76.72 | 77.99 | 76.84 | 76.52 | 75.95 |
| Sample 2 | 75.85 | 75.22 | 76.34 | 76.45 | 76.10 | 76.69 | 76.15 |
| | 75.74 | 76.49 | 76.08 | 75.85 | 76.82 | 76.8 | 76.45 |
| | 76.45 | 76.36 | 76.71 | 76.21 | 76.03 | 75.77 | 75.87 |
| | 74.83 | 75.00 | 75.77 | 76.32 | 76.17 | 75.30 | 75.28 |
| Sample 3 | 74.98 | 75.81 | 75.09 | 75.96 | 75.88 | 75.38 | 75.79 |
| | 75.40 | 74.21 | 75.54 | 75.17 | 77.36 | 75.14 | 75.45 |
| | 75.06 | 74.39 | 75.33 | 75.08 | 75.06 | 74.39 | 75.65 |

3. In a multicenter study, individuals at seven laboratories trained to perform a specific analyses using identical equipment from an instrument manufacturer. Following training, three samples were sent to each laboratory and four assays were performed on each sample (Table 12.12). Was there good repeatability and reproducibility in the results from the seven laboratories?

## Answers to Problems

1. Experiment with different fillers and various speeds on a tableting machine.

Hypotheses: $H_{01}$: $\mu_{Speed\ 1} = \mu_{Speed\ 2} = \mu_{Speed\ 3} = \mu_{Speed\ 4}$
$H_{02}$: $\mu_{Filler\ 1} = \mu_{Filler\ 2} = \mu_{Filler\ 3}$
$H_{03}$: No interaction between speed and filler

Hardness (kP)

Speed of Tableting Machine

| Filler | | 80 | 100 | 120 | 180 | |
|---|---|---|---|---|---|---|
| Lactose | $\Sigma =$ | 56 | 60 | 62 | 61 | $\Sigma\Sigma = 239$ |
| Microcrystalline Cellulose | $\Sigma =$ | 59 | 58 | 56 | 58 | $\Sigma\Sigma = 231$ |
| Dicalcium Phosphate | $\Sigma =$ | 51 | 49 | 47 | 50 | $\Sigma\Sigma = 197$ |
| $\Sigma\Sigma =$ | | 166 | 167 | 165 | 169 | $\Sigma\Sigma\Sigma = 667$ |

Decision Rules: With $\alpha = .05$ and n = 8: reject $H_{01}$ if $F > F_{3,84}(.95) \approx 2.72$; reject $H_{02}$ if $F > F_{2,84}(.95) \approx 3.11$; and reject $H_{03}$ if $F > F_{6,84}(.95) \approx 2.21$.

Calculations:

$$I = \sum_{k=1}^{K} \sum_{j=1}^{J} \sum_{i=1}^{I} x_i^2$$

$$I = (7)^2 + (5)^2 + (8)^2 \ldots + (6)^2 + (6)^2 = 4809$$

$$II = \frac{\left[ \sum_{k=1}^{K} \sum_{j=1}^{J} \sum_{i=1}^{I} x_i \right]^2}{N}$$

$$II = \frac{(667)^2}{96} = 4634.26$$

$$III_R = \frac{\sum_{k=1}^{K} \left[ \sum_{j=1}^{J} \sum_{i=1}^{I} x_i \right]^2}{j \cdot n}$$

$$III_R = \frac{(239)^2 + (231)^2 + (197)^2}{(4)(8)} = \frac{149291}{32} = 4665.344$$

$$III_C = \frac{\sum_{j=1}^{J}\left[\sum_{k=1}^{K}\sum_{i=1}^{I} x_i\right]^2}{k \cdot n}$$

$$III_C = \frac{(166)^2 + (167)^2 + (165)^2 + (169)^2}{(3)(8)} = \frac{111231}{24} = 4634.625$$

$$IV = \frac{\sum_{k=1}^{K}\sum_{j=1}^{J}\left[\sum_{i=1}^{I} x_i\right]^2}{n}$$

$$IV = \frac{(56)^2 + (60)^2 ... + (47)^2 + (50)^{(2)}}{8} = \frac{37357}{8} = 4669.625$$

$$SS_R = III_R - II = 4{,}665.344 - 4{,}634.26 = 31.084$$

$$SS_C = III_C - II = 4{,}634.625 - 4{,}634.26 = 0.365$$

$$SS_{RC} = IV - III_R - III_C + II$$

$$SS_{RC} = 4{,}669.625 - 4{,}665.344 - 4{,}634.625 = 3.916$$

$$SS_E = I - IV = 4{,}809 - 4{,}669.625 = 139.375$$

$$SS_T = I - II = 4{,}809 - 4{,}634.26 = 174.74$$

ANOVA Table:

| Source | df | SS | MS | F |
|---|---|---|---|---|
| Between | | | | |
| Rows (filler) | 2 | 31.084 | 15.542 | 9.368* |
| Column (speed) | 3 | 0.365 | 0.122 | 0.074 |
| Interaction | 6 | 3.916 | 0.653 | 0.394 |
| Within (error): | 84 | 139.375 | 1.659 | |
| Total | 95 | 174.740 | | |

Decision: With $\alpha$ = .05, reject $H_{01}$ and conclude that there is a significant difference between the three fillers used in the experiment, but there is no significant difference based on the speed of the tableting machine and no significant interaction between these two factors.

2. Experiment with quality of life indexes and various hospitals.

Hypotheses: $H_{01}$: $\mu_{Index\ 1} = \mu_{Index\ 2} = \mu_{Index\ 3}$
$H_{02}$: $\mu_{Hospital\ A} = \mu_{Hospital\ B} = \mu_{Hospital\ C}$
$H_{03}$: No interaction between index and hospital

Decision Rules: With $\alpha = .05$: reject $H_{01}$ if $F > F_{2,26}(.95) \approx 3.39$; reject $H_{02}$ if $F > F_{2,26}(.95) \approx 3.39$; and reject $H_{03}$ if $F > F_{4,26}(.95) \approx 3.00$.

| | | Index 1 | Index 2 | Index 3 | |
|---|---|---|---|---|---|
| Hospital A | $\Sigma =$ | 270 | 344 | 380 | $\Sigma\Sigma = 994$ |
| Hospital B | $\Sigma =$ | 329 | 248 | 340 | $\Sigma\Sigma = 917$ |
| Hospital C | $\Sigma =$ | 325 | 317 | 325 | $\Sigma\Sigma = 967$ |
| | $\Sigma\Sigma =$ | 924 | 909 | 1045 | $\Sigma\Sigma\Sigma = 2878$ |

Calculations:

$$I = \sum_{k=1}^{K} \sum_{j=1}^{J} \sum_{i=1}^{I} x_i^2$$

$$I = (67)^2 + (73)^2 + (61)^2 \ldots + (82)^2 + (77)^2 = 238{,}646$$

$$II = \frac{\left[\sum_{k=1}^{K} \sum_{j=1}^{J} \sum_{i=1}^{I} x_i\right]^2}{N}$$

$$II = \frac{(2{,}878)^2}{35} = 236{,}653.83$$

$$III_R = \sum_{k=1}^{K} \frac{\left[\sum_{j=1}^{J} \sum_{i=1}^{I} x_i\right]^2}{N_R}$$

$$III_R = \frac{(994)^2}{12} + \frac{(917)^2}{11} + \frac{(967)^2}{12} = 236{,}704.87$$

$$III_C = \sum_{j=1}^{J} \frac{\left[\sum_{k=1}^{K}\sum_{i=1}^{I} x_i\right]^2}{N_C}$$

$$III_C = \frac{(924)^2}{12} + \frac{(909)^2}{11} + \frac{(1045)^2}{12} = 237{,}266.54$$

$$IV = \sum_{k=1}^{K}\sum_{j=1}^{J} \frac{\left[\sum_{i=1}^{I} x_i\right]^2}{N_i}$$

$$IV = \frac{(270)^2}{4} + \frac{(344)^2}{4} + \frac{(380)^2}{4} + \ldots \frac{(325)^2}{4} = 238{,}305.33$$

$$SS_R = III_R - II = 236{,}704.87 - 236{,}653.83 = 51.04$$

$$SS_C = III_C - II = 237{,}266.54 - 236{,}653.83 = 612.71$$

$$SS_{RC} = IV - III_R - III_C + II$$

$$SS_{RC} = 238{,}305.33 - 236{,}704.87 - 237{,}266.54 + 236{,}653.83 = 987.75$$

$$SS_E = I - IV = 238{,}646 - 238{,}305.33 = 340.67$$

$$SS_T = I - II = 238{,}646 - 236{,}653.83 = 1992.17$$

ANOVA Table:

| Source | df | SS | MS | F |
|---|---|---|---|---|
| Between | | | | |
| Rows (hospital) | 2 | 51.04 | 25.52 | 1.95 |
| Column (index) | 2 | 612.71 | 306.36 | 23.39* |
| Interaction | 4 | 987.75 | 246.94 | 18.85* |
| Within (error): | 26 | 340.67 | 13.10 | |
| Total | 34 | 1992.17 | | |

Decision: With $\alpha = .05$, reject $H_{02}$, conclude that there is a significant difference between the indexes used in this study. Reject $H_{03}$, conclude that a significant interaction exists between the two main factors, but there is no significant difference based on the hospital.

3. Repeatability and reproducibility between seven laboratories.

$H_{01}$: $\mu_{L1} = \mu_{L2} = \mu_{L3} = \mu_{L4} = \mu_{L5} = \mu_{L6} = \mu_{L7}$ (Main effect of laboratories)

$H_{02}$: $\mu_{S1} = \mu_{S2} = \mu_{S3}$ (Main effect of samples)

$H_{03}$: $(\mu_{L1,S1} - \mu_{L1,S2}) = (\mu_{L2,S1} - \mu_{L2,S2}) =$ etc. (Interaction)

Results of Two-Way ANOVA for Data

| Source | df | SS | MS | F | p |
|---|---|---|---|---|---|
| Sample (row) | 2 | 398.01 | 199.00 | 752.53 | <0.0005 |
| Laboratory (column) | 6 | 2.50 | 0.42 | 1.58 | |
| Interaction | 12 | 4.28 | 0.36 | 1.35 | |
| Error | 63 | 16.66 | 0.26 | | |
| Total | 83 | 421.45 | | | |

Application to repeatability and reproducibility where with 99% confidence, $Z_0 =$ 5.15.

$$Repeatability = 5.15\sqrt{0.26} = 2.63$$

$$Reproducibility = 5.15\sqrt{\frac{0.42 - 0.36}{3(4)}} = 0.36$$

$$Interaction = 5.15\sqrt{\frac{0.36 - 0.26}{4}} = 0.81$$

$$R \& R = \sqrt{(2.63)^2 + (0.36)^2 + (0.81)^2} = 2.88$$

$$V_P = 5.15\sqrt{\frac{199.00 - 0.36}{(7)(4)}} = 13.72$$

$$V_T = \sqrt{(2.88)^2 + (13.72)^2} = 14.02$$

$$\%\ repeatibility = \left(\frac{2.63}{14.02}\right)^2 x100 = 3.52\%$$

$$\%\ reproducibility = \left(\frac{0.36}{14.02}\right)^2 x100 = 0.07\%$$

$$\% \, R \,\&\, R = \left( \frac{2.88}{14.02} \right)^2 x100 = 4.23\%$$

$$\% \, Sample = \left( \frac{13.72}{14.02} \right)^2 x100 = 95.77\%$$

Result: Good repeatability (<5%) and good reproducibility (<30%).

# 13

# Correlation

Both correlation and regression analysis are concerned with continuous variables. Correlation does not require an independent (or predictor) variable, which as we will see in the next chapter, is a requirement for the regression model. With correlation, two or more variables may be compared to determine if there is a relationship and to measure the strength of that relationship. Correlation describes the degree to which two or more variables show interrelationships within a given population. The correlation may be either positive or negative. Correlation results do not explain why the relation occurs, only that such a relationship exists. Although a correlation line will be defined and can be drawn on a scatter plot, this line of best fit should be reserved for linear regression (Chapter 14) where at least one independent variable exists.

## Graphic Representation of Two Continuous Variables

Graphs offer an excellent way of showing relationships between continuous variables based on either an interval or ratio scales. The easiest way to visualize this relationship graphically is by using a **bivariate scatter plot**. Correlation usually involves only dependent or response variables. If one or more variables are under the researcher's control (for example, varying concentrations of a solution or specific speeds for a particular instrument) then the linear regression model would be more appropriate. Traditionally, with either correlation or regression, if an independent variable exists it is plotted on the horizontal $x$-axis of the graph or the **abscissa**. The second, dependent variable is plotted on the vertical $y$-axis or the **ordinate** (Figure 13.1). In the correlation model, both variables are evaluated with equal import, vary at random (both referred to as dependent variables), and may be assigned to either axis.

The first role of correlation is to determine the strength of the relationship between the two variables represented on the $x$-axis and the $y$-axis. The measure of this magnitude is called the correlation coefficient (discussed in the next section). The data required to compute this coefficient are two continuous measurements $(x,y)$ obtained on the same entity (a person, object, or data point) and is referred to as the **unit of association**. As will be seen, the **correlation coefficient** is a well-defined mathematical index that measures the strength of relationships. This index measures both the magnitude and the direction of the relationships.

| | |
|---|---|
| +1.0 | perfect positive correlation |
| 0.0 | no correlation |
| −1.0 | perfect negative correlation |

If there is a perfect relationship (a correlation coefficient of +1.00 or −1.00), a straight line can be drawn through all of the data points. The greater the change in *Y* for a constant change in *X*, the steeper the slope of the line. In a less than perfect relationship between two variables, the closer the data points are located on a straight line, the stronger the relationship and greater the correlation coefficient. In contrast, a zero correlation would indicate absolutely no linear relationship between the two variables.

Graph A in Figure 13.1 represents a **positive correlation** where data points with larger *x*-values tend to have corresponding large *y*-values. As seen later, an example of a positive correlation is the height and weight of individuals. As the heights of people increase their weights also tend to increase. Graph B is a **negative correlation**, where *Y* appears to decrease as values for *X* increase (approaching a perfect negative correlation of −1.00). An example of a negative or **inverse correlation** might be speed versus accuracy. The faster an individual completes a given task, the lower the accuracy; whereas, the slower the person's speed, the greater the accuracy of the task. Graph C in Figure 13.1 shows a scattering of points with no correlation or discernible pattern.

More visual information can be presented by drawing a circle or an ellipse to surround the points in the scatter plot (D in Figure 13.1). If the points fall within a circle there is no correlation. If the points fall within an ellipse, the flatter the ellipse the stronger the correlation until the ellipse produces a straight line or a perfect correlation. The orientation of the ellipse indicates the direction of the correlation. An orientation from the lower left to the upper right is positive and from the upper left to the lower right is a negative correlation. Dashed lines can be drawn on the *x*- and *y*-axis to represent the centers of each distribution. These lines divide the scatter plot into **quadrants**. In an absolute 0.00 correlation, each quadrant would have an equal number of data points. As the correlation increases (in the positive or negative direction) the data point will increasingly be found in only two diagonal quadrants. An additional assumption involved with the correlation coefficient is that the two continuous variables possess a **joint normal distribution**. In other words, for any given value on the *x*-axis variable, the *y*-variable is sampled from a population that is normally distributed around some central point. If the populations, from which the samples are selected are not normal, inferential procedures are invalid (Daniel, 1999). In such cases the strength of the relationship can be calculated using an alternative nonparameteric procedure such as Spearman rank correlation (Chapter 21) or transformation procedure can be used to create an approximate normal distribution

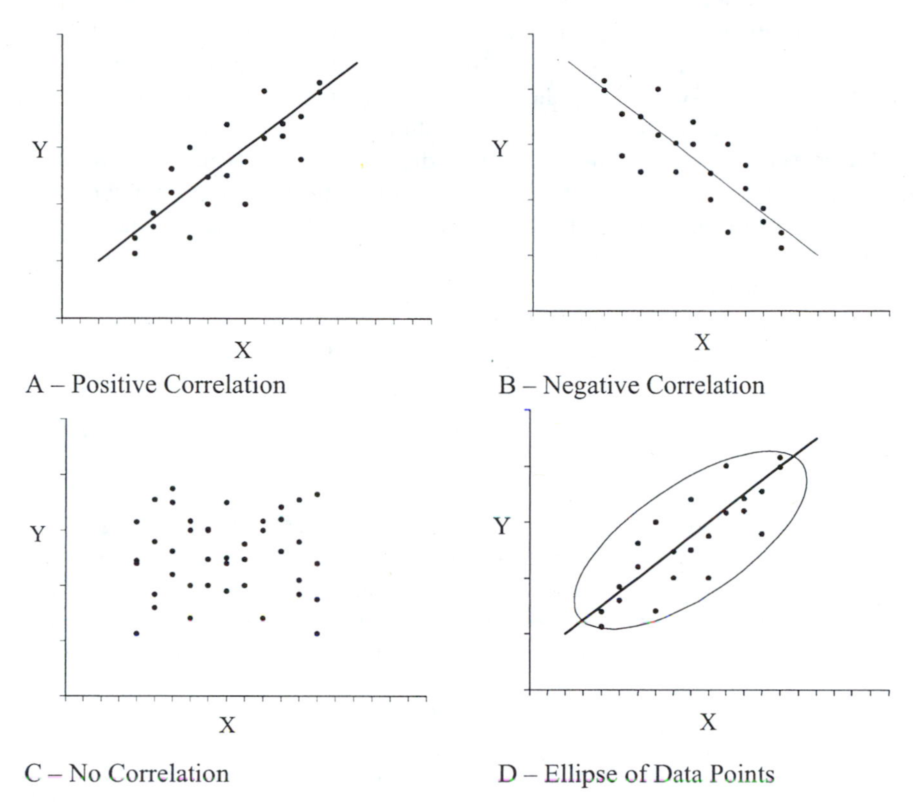


**Figure 13.1** Examples of graphic representations of correlation data.

(Chapter 6).

There are several different methods for calculating measures of correlation; the most widely used is the Pearson Product-Moment Correlation Coefficient ($r$).

## Pearson Product-Moment Correlation Coefficient

The simplest approach to discussing correlation is to focus first on only two continuous variables. The **correlational relationship** can be thought of as an association that exists between the values representing two random variables. In this relationship we, as the investigators, have no control over the observed values for either variable.

**Covariance** is a measure of how the deviations (differences between individual data points and the respective means) for the two variables compare. It is calculated as follows:

$$Cov(x,y) = \sum (x_i - \overline{X}_x)(y - \overline{X}_y) \qquad \text{Eq. 13.1}$$

When there is a strong comparison, large positive deviations for $x$-values will match with large positive deviations for $y$-values. At the same time large negatives will match with large negatives. However, it is difficult to compare the covariance between the x- and y-variables if they differ in magnitude (i.e., comparing patients' weights in kilograms to heights in centimeters), therefore some type of **standardization** is required and this will be discussed below. This is accomplished by creating standardized values (subtracting the mean from each value and dividing by the standard deviation. This will result in a mean of 0 and standard deviation of 1.

The correlation coefficient assumes that the continuous variables are randomly selected from normally distributed populations. This coefficient is the average of the products for each $x$- and $y$-variable result measured as units in standardized normal distribution. Therefore $r$ is the sum of the products divided by $n - 1$, or

$$r_{xy} = \frac{\sum z_x z_y}{n-1} \qquad \text{Eq. 13.2}$$

where $z_x$ and $z_y$ are standard scores for the variables at each data point and $n$ is the number of data points (each point representing an $x$- and $y$-value), or the sample size. Ideally, we would know the population mean ($\mu$) and standard deviation ($\sigma$) for each variable. This can be a very laborious process and involves computing the mean of each distribution, and then determining the deviation from the mean for each value in terms of a standard score.

$$z_x = \frac{x_i - \mu_x}{\sigma_x} \quad \text{and} \quad z_y = \frac{y_i - \mu_y}{\sigma_y} \qquad \text{Eq. 13.3}$$

Unfortunately, we usually do not know the parameters for the population and we must approximate the means and standard deviations using sample information.

A slightly more convenient formula for calculating the association of two variables is the **Pearson r** or the **Pearson product-moment correlation**. This coefficient is the product of the **moments** ($x_i - \mu$) of the two variable observation. Where the moment deviation ($x_i - \overline{X}$) is the difference between the individual observations and the sample mean for that variable. Using the covariance term (Eq. 13.1) in the numerator, the formula for this correlation coefficient is as follows:

$$r = \frac{\Sigma(x - \overline{X}_x)(y - \overline{X}_y)}{\sqrt{\Sigma(x - \overline{X}_x)^2 (y - \overline{X}_y)^2}} \qquad \text{Eq. 13.4}$$

These calculations involve a determination of how values deviate from their respective sample means: how each $x$-value deviates from the mean for the $x$-variable ($\overline{X}_x$) and how each $y$-value varies from the mean for the $y$-variable ($\overline{X}_y$). The convenience comes from not having to compute the individual $z$-values for each data point. Normally a table is set up for the terms required in the equation (Table

**Table 13.1** Data Layout for Computation of the Pearson Product-Moment Correlation Coefficient – Definitional Formula

| x | y | $x-\overline{X}_x$ | $Y-\overline{X}_y$ | $(x-\overline{X}_x)(y-\overline{X}_y)$ | $(x-\overline{X}_x)^2$ | $(y-\overline{X}_y)^2$ |
|---|---|---|---|---|---|---|
| $x_1$ | $y_1$ | ... | ... | ... | ... | ... |
| $x_2$ | $y_2$ | ... | ... | ... | ... | ... |
| $x_3$ | $y_3$ | ... | ... | ... | ... | ... |
| ... | ... | ... | ... | ... | ... | ... |
| $x_n$ | $y_n$ | ... | ... | ... | ... | ... |
| | | | | $\Sigma(x-\overline{X}_x)(y-\overline{X}_y)$ | $\Sigma(x-\overline{X}_x)^2$ | $\Sigma(y-\overline{X}_y)^2$ |

13.1). Using this method, the researcher must first calculate the sample mean for both the *x*- and *y*-variable. As seen in Table 13.1, values for the observed data are represented in the first two columns, where *x* is the value for each measurement associated with the *x*-axis and *y* is the corresponding measure on the *y*-axis for that same data point. The third and fourth columns reflect the deviations of the *x*- and *y*-scores about their respective sample means. The fifth column is the product of these deviations, the sum of which becomes the numerator in the Pearson product-moment equation. The last two columns are the deviations squared for both the *x*- and *y*-variables and are used in the denominator.

As an example, consider the data collected on six volunteer subjects during a Phase I clinical trial (Table 13.2). For whatever reason, the investigator is interested in determining if there is a correlation between the subjects' weight and height. First, both the volunteers' mean weight and mean height are calculated:

$$\overline{X}_x = \frac{\Sigma x}{n} = \frac{511.1}{6} = 85.18$$

$$\overline{X}_y = \frac{\Sigma y}{n} = \frac{10.86}{6} = 1.81$$

Table 13.3 shows the required information for: 1) the deviations from the respective means; 2) the squares of those deviations; and 3) the products of deviations. Finally, each of the last three columns are summed and entered into the equation:

$$r = \frac{\Sigma(x-\overline{X}_x)(y-\overline{X}_y)}{\sqrt{\Sigma(x-\overline{X}_x)^2(y-\overline{X}_y)^2}}$$

$$r = \frac{2.6690}{\sqrt{(607.15)(0.015)}} = \frac{2.6690}{3.0178} = +0.884$$

**Table 13.2** Clinical Trial Data for Six Volunteers

| Subject | Weight (kg) | Height (m) |
|---|---|---|
| 1 | 96.0 | 1.88 |
| 2 | 77.7 | 1.80 |
| 3 | 100.9 | 1.85 |
| 4 | 79.0 | 1.77 |
| 5 | 73.0 | 1.73 |
| 6 | 84.5 | 1.83 |
| $\Sigma =$ | 511.1 | 10.86 |

**Table 13.3** Sample Data for Pearson's $r$ Calculation – Definitional Formula

| x | y | $X-\overline{X}_x$ | $Y-\overline{X}_y$ | $(x-\overline{X}_x)(y-\overline{X}_y)$ | $(x-\overline{X}_x)^2$ | $(y-\overline{X}_y)^2$ |
|---|---|---|---|---|---|---|
| 96.0 | 1.88 | 10.52 | 0.07 | 0.7574 | 117.07 | 0.0049 |
| 77.7 | 1.80 | −7.48 | −0.01 | 0.0748 | 55.96 | 0.0001 |
| 100.9 | 1.85 | 15.72 | 0.04 | 0.6288 | 247.12 | 0.0016 |
| 79.0 | 1.77 | −6.18 | −0.04 | 0.2472 | 38.19 | 0.0016 |
| 73.0 | 1.73 | −12.18 | −0.08 | 0.9744 | 148.35 | 0.0064 |
| 84.5 | 1.83 | −0.68 | 0.02 | −0.0136 | 0.46 | 0.0004 |
| | | | $\Sigma =$ | 2.6690 | 607.15 | 0.0150 |

The resulting $r$-value is the **product-moment correlation coefficient**, or simply the correlation coefficient, shows a positive relationship and can be noted as a very strong relationship considering a perfect correlation is +1.00.

A third formula is available that further simplifies the mathematical process and is easier to compute, especially for hand-held calculators or computers. This computational formula is:

$$r = \frac{n\sum xy - \sum x \sum y}{\sqrt{n\sum x^2 - (\sum x)^2}\sqrt{n\sum y^2 - (\sum y)^2}} \qquad \text{Eq. 13.5}$$

Once again a table is developed based on the sample data (Table 13.4). In this case there are only five columns and the calculation of the sample means ($\overline{X}_x, \overline{X}_y$) are not required. Similar to Table 13.3, these first two columns represent the observed data, paired for both the $x$ and $y$ measurement scale. The third and fourth columns represent the individual $x$- and $y$-values squared and the last column is the product of $x$ and $y$ for each data point. Using this method to compute the correlation coefficient for the previous example of height and weight would produce the results seen in Table 13.5. The calculation of the correlation coefficient would be:

**Table 13.4** Data Layout for Computation of the Pearson Product Moment Correlation Coefficient – Computational Formula

| x | y | $x^2$ | $y^2$ | xy |
|---|---|---|---|---|
| $x_1$ | $y_1$ | $x_1^2$ | $y_1^2$ | $x_1y_1$ |
| $x_2$ | $y_2$ | $x_2^2$ | $y_2^2$ | $x_2y_2$ |
| $x_3$ | $y_3$ | $x_3^2$ | $y_3^2$ | $x_3y_3$ |
| ... | ... | ... | ... | ... |
| $x_n$ | $y_n$ | $x_n^2$ | $y_n^2$ | $x_ny_n$ |
| $\Sigma x$ | $\Sigma y$ | $\Sigma x^2$ | $\Sigma y^2$ | $\Sigma xy$ |

**Table 13.5** Sample Data for Pearson's *r* Calculation – Computational Formula

| x | y | $x^2$ | $y^2$ | xy |
|---|---|---|---|---|
| 96.0 | 1.88 | 9216.00 | 3.5344 | 180.480 |
| 77.7 | 1.80 | 6037.29 | 3.2400 | 139.860 |
| 100.9 | 1.85 | 10180.81 | 3.4225 | 186.665 |
| 79.0 | 1.77 | 6241.00 | 3.1329 | 139.830 |
| 73.0 | 1.73 | 5329.00 | 2.9929 | 126.290 |
| 84.5 | 1.83 | 7140.25 | 3.3489 | 154.635 |
| 511.1 | 10.86 | 44144.35 | 19.6716 | 927.760 |

$$r = \frac{n\sum xy - \sum x \sum y}{\sqrt{n\sum x^2 - (\sum x)^2}\sqrt{n\sum y^2 - (\sum y)^2}}$$

$$r = \frac{6(927.76) - (511.1)(10.86)}{\sqrt{6(44144.35) - (511.1)^2}\sqrt{6(19.6716) - (10.86)^2}}$$

$$r = \frac{5566.56 - 5550.546}{(60.356)(0.3)} = \frac{16.014}{18.107} = +0.884$$

The results from using either formula (Eq. 13.4 or 13.5) produce the identical answers since algebraically these formulas are equivalent.

Correlations can be measured on variables that have completely different scales with completely different units (i.e., a correlation between weight in kilograms and height in meters). Thus, the value of the correlation coefficient is completely independent of the values for the means and standard deviations of the two variables being compared. Thus, even though the correlation coefficient is a parametric procedure, we do not need be concerned about the homogeneity of variance because each axis may involve a different measurement scale. However, it is critical that the underlying population distributions are assumed to be normally distributed.

**Correlation Line**

The correlation coefficient is an index that can be used to describe the linear relationship between two continuous variables and deals with paired relationships (each data point represents a value on the $x$-axis as well as a value on the $y$-axis). As will be seen in the next chapter, the best line to be fitted between the points on the bivariate scatter plot is very important for the linear regression model where prediction is required for $y$ at any given value on the $x$-axis. However, it is also possible, and some times desirable to approximate a line that best fits between the data point in our correlation model. Note that the correlation coefficient does not require a line, nor do the calculations for this coefficient actually define a line. This is in contrast to defining the line of best fit that is required for regression models. As will be discussed in greater detail in Chapter 14, a straight line between our data points can be defined as follows:

$$y = a + bx \qquad \text{Eq. 13.6}$$

where $y$ is a value on the vertical axis, $x$ is a corresponding value on the horizontal axis, $a$ indicates the point where the line crosses the vertical axis, and $b$ represents the amount by which the line rises for each increase in $x$ (the slope of the line). We can define the line that fits best between our data points using the following formulas and data from Table 13.3 for our computational method of determining the correlation coefficient.

$$b = \frac{n\sum xy - (\sum x)(\sum y)}{n\sum x^2 - (\sum x)^2} \qquad \text{Eq. 13.7}$$

$$a = \frac{\sum y - b\sum x}{n} \qquad \text{Eq. 13.8}$$

Such lines are illustrated in Figure 13.1. The correlation coefficient provides an indication of how close the data points are to this line. As mentioned previously, if we produce a correlation coefficient equal to +1.00 or –1.00, then all the data points will fall directly on the straight line. Any value other than a perfect correlation, positive or negative, indicated some deviation from the line. The closer the correlation coefficient is to zero, the greater the deviation from this line.

In our previous example of weight and height for our six subjects, the correlation line that fits based between these points is calculated as follows:

$$b = \frac{(6)(927.76) - (511.1)(10.86)}{(6)(44144.35) - (511.1)^2} = \frac{16.014}{3642.89} = +0.0044$$

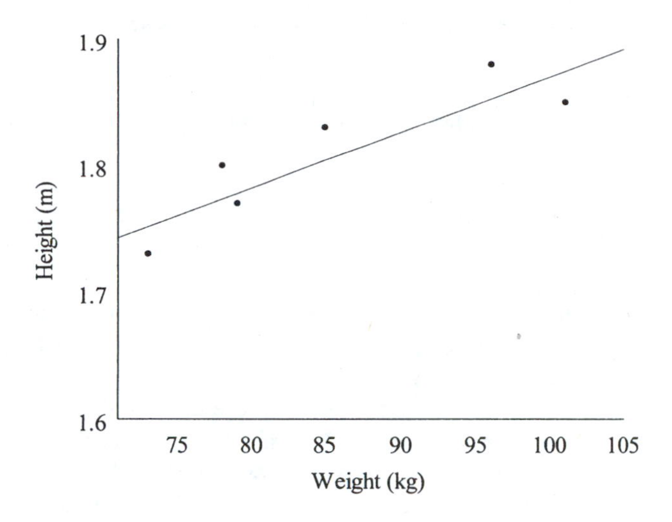


**Figure 13.2** Correlation line representing data presented in Table 13.4.

$$a = \frac{(10.86) - (0.0044)(511.1)}{6} = 1.43$$

The data and resultant line with the slope of +0.044 and *y*-intercept of 1.43 are presented in Figure 13.2. As can be seen data are relatively close to the straight line, indicative of the high correlation value of $r = +0.884$.

**Statistical Significance of a Correlation Coefficient**

A positive or negative correlation between two variables shows that a relationship exists. Whether one considers it as a strong or weak correlation, important or unimportant, is a matter of interpretation. For example in the behavioral sciences a correlation of 0.80 would be considered a high correlation. However, for individuals in the pharmaceutical industry, doing a process validation, they may require a correlation >0.999.

Verbal descriptions of correlations are inconsistent. The simplest might be: less than 0.25 is a "doubtful" correlation; 0.26 to 0.50 represents a "fair" correlation; 0.51 to 0.75 is a "good" correlation, and greater than 0.75 can be considered a "superior" correlation (Kelly et al., 1992). Another rough guide (Guilford, 1956) is as follows:

| | |
|---|---|
| <0.20 | slight; almost negligible relationship |
| 0.20 - 0.40 | low correlation; definite but small relationship |
| 0.40 - 0.70 | moderate correlation; substantial relationship |
| 0.70 - 0.90 | high correlation; marked relationship |
| >0.90 | very high correlation; very dependable relationship |

Similar levels, but slightly different terminology can be seen with yet another guide (Roundtree, 1981):

| | |
|---|---|
| <0.20 | very weak, negligible |
| 0.20 - 0.40 | weak, low |
| 0.40 - 0.70 | moderate |
| 0.70 - 0.90 | strong, high, marked |
| >0.90 | very strong, very high |

The sign (+ or –) would indicate a positive or negative correlation. In the previous example of weight vs. height the result of +0.884 would represent a "high," "strong," or "marked" positive correlation.

The values for correlation coefficients do not represent equal distances along a linear scale. For example, a correlation of 0.50 is not twice as large as $r = 0.25$. Instead, the coefficient is always relative to the conditions under which it was calculated. The larger the $r$, either in the positive or negative direction, the greater the consistency of the two measures.

In addition to identifying the strength and direction of a correlation coefficient, there are statistical methods for testing the significance of a given correlation. Two will be discussed here: 1) use of a Pearson product-moment table and 2) the conversion to a Student $t$-statistic. In both cases, the symbol $r_{yx}$ or $\rho$ (rho) can be used to represent the correlation for the populations from which the samples were randomly selected. The hypotheses being tested are:

$$H_0: \quad r_{yx} = 0 \qquad \text{or} \qquad H_0: \quad \rho = 0$$
$$H_1: \quad r_{yx} \neq 0 \qquad\qquad\quad H_1: \quad \rho \neq 0$$

The null hypothesis indicates that a correlation does not exist between the two continuous variables; the population correlation coefficient is zero. Whereas, the alternative hypothesis states that a significant relationship exists between variables $x$ and $y$. Pearson's correlation coefficient, symbolized by the letter $r$, symbolizes the sample value for the relationship; whereas $\rho$ or $r_{yx}$ represents true population correlation.

Using Table B14 in Appendix B, it is possible to identify a critical r-value and if the correlation coefficient exceeds the critical value, $H_0$ is rejected. The first column in the table represents the degrees of freedom and the remaining columns are the critical values at various allowable levels of Type I error ($\alpha$). For correlation problems the number of degrees of freedom is the number of data points minus two ($n - 2$). The decision rule is to reject $H_0$ (no correlation) if the calculated $r$-value is greater than $r_{n-2}(\alpha)$. In the previous example comparing weights and heights of volunteers in a clinical trial, the decision rule would be with $\alpha = 0.05$, reject $H_0$ if $r > r_4(.05) = 0.8114$. The result of the calculations produce a correlation coefficient of 0.884, which is greater than the critical r-value of 0.8114; therefore, we would reject $H_0$ and conclude that there is a significant correlation with 95% confidence. One might question how well we can trust a correlation coefficient from a sample size of only six to predict the relationship in the population from which the sample is drawn. Two factors will influence this decision: 1) the strength of the correlation (the *r*-value itself); and 2) the sample size. Looking at the table of critical values for the correlation coefficient (Table B14, Appendix B) it is possible to find significance for a relatively small *r*-value, if the result comes from a large sample.

The second method for calculating the level of significance for the sample *r*-value is to enter the results into a special formula for a *t*-test and compare the results to a critical value from a Student *t*-distribution (Table B5, Appendix B). This converted *t*-value, from an *r*-value, is compared to the critical t-value with $n - 2$ degrees of freedom. The decision rule is to reject $H_0$ (no correlation) if $t > t_{n-2}(1 - \alpha/2)$ or $t < -t_{n-2}(1 - \alpha/2)$. The statistical formula is:

$$t = \frac{r\sqrt{n-2}}{\sqrt{1-r^2}} \qquad \text{Eq. 13.9}$$

The correlation coefficient (*r*) incorporates the concept of how scores vary within a given distribution. These potential deviations are considered as a standard error of the correlation coefficient and represent the standard deviation for the theoretical distribution of correlation coefficients for samples from the population with a given size. The closer the correlation coefficient to a perfect result (+1.00 or –1.00), the smaller the standard error (the denominator in Eq. 13.9). Approximately 95% of all possible correlation coefficients will be within two standard deviations of the population $\rho$. Therefore, we can use information from Chapter 9 to create a *t*-statistic to calculate significance of the correlation coefficient.

Using our previous example (weight vs. height) to illustrate the correlation *t*-conversion, the decision rule is with $\alpha = 0.05$, reject $H_0$ if $t > t_4(.975) = 2.776$. The computations are:

$$t = \frac{.884\sqrt{6-2}}{\sqrt{1-(.884)^2}} = \frac{1.768}{0.467} = 3.78$$

In this case the decision, with $t > 2.776$, is to reject $H_0$ and conclude that there is a significant correlation between the volunteers' weight and height. Based on the *t*-conversion, a significant result would indicate that the results could not have occurred by chance alone from a population with a true zero correlation. Note in Table 13.6 that both methods produce identical outcomes.

The *r*-value can be considered a ratio of the actual amount of deviation divided by the total possible deviation. Whereas the square of the *r*-value, is the amount of actual deviation that the two distributions have in common. The interpretation of the correlation between two variables is concerned with the degree to which they **covary**. In other words, how much of the variation in one of the continuous variables can be attributed to variation in the other. This square of the correlation coefficient, $r^2$,

**Table 13.6** Comparison of Critical $r$-Values and $t$-Values

| Table of Critical Values | Statistical Results | $\alpha = 0.05$ | | $\alpha = 0.01$ | |
|---|---|---|---|---|---|
| | | C.V. | Result | C.V. | Result |
| Table B11 | r = 0.884 | 0.8114 | Significant | 0.9172 | NS |
| Table B3 | t = 3.78 | 2.776 | Significant | 4.604 | NS |

indicates the proportion of variance in one of the variables accounted for by the variance of the second variable. The $r^2$ term is sometimes referred to as the "**common variance.**" In the case of $r^2 = 0.49$ (for $r = 0.7$), 49% of the variance in scores for one variable is associated with the variance in scores for the second variable.

**Correlation and Causality**

As a correlation approaches +1.0 or −1.0 there is a tendency for numbers to concentrate closer to a straight line. However, one should not assume that just because correlations come closer to a perfect correlation that they form a straight line. The correlation coefficient says nothing about the percentage of the relationship, only its relative strength. It represents a convenient ratio, not an actual measurement scale. It serves primarily as a data reduction technique and as a descriptive method. Figure 13.3 illustrates this point where four different data sets can produce the same "high" correlation ($r = 0.816$). As discussed in the next chapter, if lines were drawn that best fit between the points in each data set, they would be identical with a slope of 0.5 and a $y$-intercept of 3.0. This figure also shows the advantage of plotting the data on graph paper, or creating a computer-generated visual, to actually observe the distribution of the data points.

The correlation coefficient does not suggest nor prove the reason for this relationship; only that it exists, whether the two variables vary together either positively or negatively and the degree of this relationship. It does not indicate anything about the **causality** of this relationship. Did the $x$-variable cause the result in $y$? Did $y$ affect variable $x$? Could a third variable have affected both $x$ and $y$? There could be many reasons for this relationship.

With correlation the relationship identified between two dependent variables is purely descriptive and no conclusions about causality can be made. By contrast, with experimental or regression studies, where the predictor or independent variable is controlled by the researcher, there is a better likelihood that interpretations about causality can be stated. However, with correlation, this relationship may be due to external variables not controlled for by the experiment. These are called **confounding variables** and represent other unidentified variables that are entwined or confused

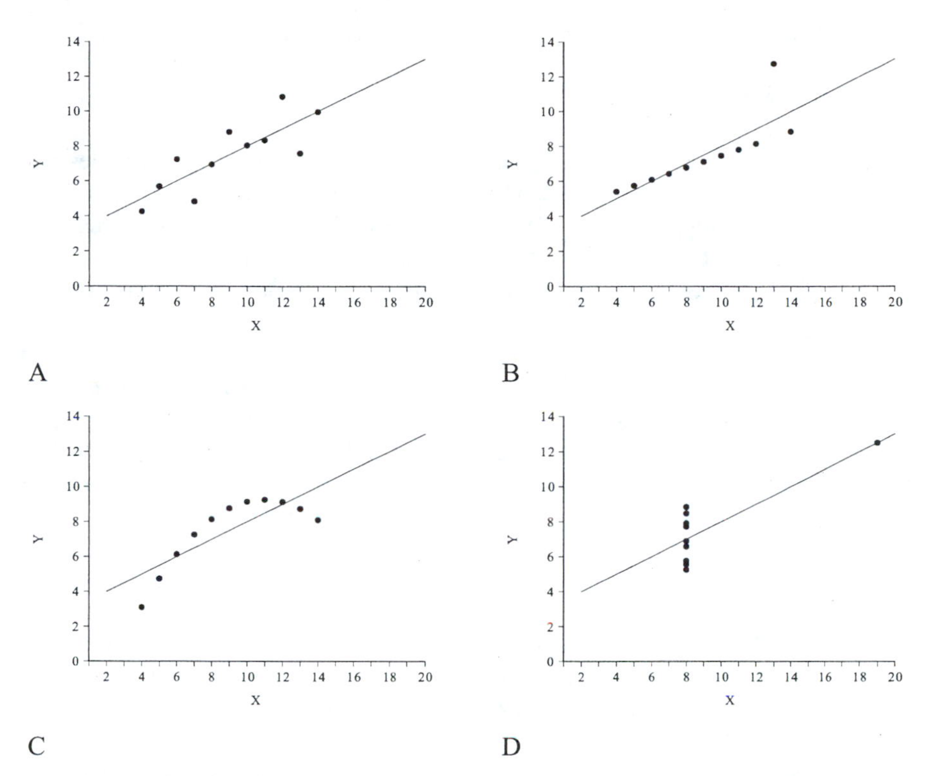


**Figure 13.3** Graphs of four sets of data with identical correlations ($r = 0.816$). From: Anscombe, F.J. (1973). "Graphs in statistical analysis," *American Statistician* 27:17-27.

with the variables being tested. Two factors must be established before the researcher can say that $x$, assumed to be the independent variable, caused the result in $y$. First, $x$ must have preceded $y$ in time. Second, the research design was such that it controlled for other factors that might cause or influence $y$.

Even a significant result from a correlation coefficient does not necessarily represent simply a cause-and-effect relationship between the two variables. In the previous example, does the height of the person directly contribute to his/her weight? Does the weight of the person influence the person's height? The former assumption may be true, but probably not the latter. In this particular case, both variables were influenced by a third factor. The patients volunteering to take part in the study were screened using an inclusion criterion that they must fall within 10% of the ideal height/weight standards established by the Metropolitan Life Insurance Company. Thus, if we approximate ideal weight/height standards, taller volunteers will tend to weigh more and shorter volunteers will weigh less because of the ratio established between these variables based on the standardized tables used by Metropolitan Life.

In some cases causality may not be as important as the strength of the relationship. For example if the researchers were comparing two methods (i.e., analytical assays, cognitive scales, physiological measures), the individual is not interested in whether one method produced a higher mean value than the other, rather they are interested in whether there is a significant correlation between the two methods.

Various types of relationships can exist between two continuous variables and still produce a correlation coefficient. Many are illustrated in Figures 13.1 and 13.3. A **monotonic relationship** is illustrated by Figures 13.1-A, -B, and -D where the relationship is ever-increasing or ever-decreasing. The monotonic relationship could be linear (best represented by a straight line) or **nonlinear** or **curvilinear relationships** where a curved line best fits the data points. In contrast, Figure 13.3-C is an example of a **nonmonotonic relationship**. In this case the relationship is not ever-increasing or ever-decreasing, the points begin as a positive correlation but change near 10 on the *x*-axis and become a negative correlation. This figure represents a nonmonotonic, concave downward relationship. One last type of relationship is a **cyclical relationship** where waves are formed as the correlation continues to change from a positive to a negative to a positive relationship.

## *In vivo–In vitro* Correlation

One example of the use of the correlation coefficient is to establish a relationship between an *in vitro* measure for a pharmaceutical product and an *in vivo* response in living systems. This relationship is referred to as an ***in vivo–in vitro* correlation**, or an **IV/IV correlation.**

In 1977, the Food and Drug Administration issued regulations on bioequivalency and bioavailability, and included a list of drugs described as having "known or potential bioequivalency or bioavailability problems" (*Fed. Reg.*, 1977). In these regulations, it was pointed out that bioequivalence requirement for the majority of products could be the form of an *in vitro* test in which the product is compared to a reference standard. This point will be discussed in greater detail in Chapter 22. Preferably, these *in vitro* tests should be correlated with human *in vivo* data. In most cases the *in vitro* tests are dissolution tests.

Dissolution is a measure of the percent of drug entering a dissolved state over varying periods of time. Tests of dissolution are used to determine if drug products are in compliance with compendia standards in the United States Pharmacopeia (USP) or new drug application (NDA). For example, in USP XXIII there were 532 dissolution tests. Dissolution testing can be performed on a variety of dosage forms including immediate release and extended release solids, transdermal patches, and topical preparations. For immediate release solid dosage forms, one of the most commonly used comparisons for IV/IV correlation are between an *in vivo* parameter (i.e., AUC) and the mean *in vitro* dissolution time (Skelly and Shiu, 1993). If we can establish a strong relationship between this internal response and an equivalent external laboratory measurement we may be able to avoid the risks inherent with human clinical trials. In addition *in vivo* studies can be very expensive and equivalent laboratory results offer a considerable economic advantage.

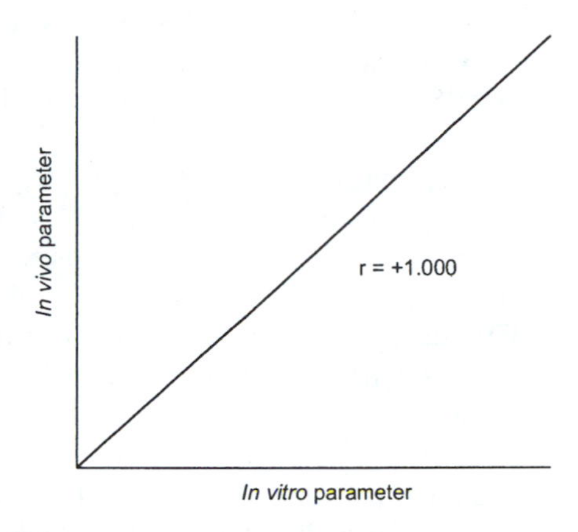


**Figure 13.4** Hypothetical example of a perfect IV/IV correlation.

In an ideal world we would see a correlation of +1.00 relationship between the two parameters. This represents a comparison between single point measures of outcome and rate (Figure 13.4). Using this model it is possible to perform *in vitro* laboratory exercises and predict the response on *in vivo* systems. Unfortunately we do not live in an ideal world and both of these continuous variables will contain some error or variability resulting in an $r < 1.00$. The larger the $r$-value, the more meaningful the predictive abilities. As will be discussed in the next chapter, the strength of a correlation is commonly characterized by $r^2$, the square of the correlation coefficient. The $r^2$ is useful because it indicates the proportion of the variance explained by the line that best fits between the data points in the linear relationship.

In some cases *in vitro* dissolution testing can substitute for bioequivalency testing. This is particularly true for extended-release dosage forms. To use dissolution data as a substitute for bioequivalency testing, one is required to have a very strong correlation. In other words, the IV/IV correlation must be highly predictive of *in vivo* performance. In these cases, *in vitro* dissolution information may be meaningful for predicting an *in vivo* response. However, there is no complete assurance that *in vitro* dissolution equals *in vivo* dissolution. One needs to be confident that for a given product tested that this IV/IV equality exists and that *in vivo* dissolution leads to absorption and absorption results in an *in vivo* response. The processes and potential problems associated with IV/IV correlation are beyond the scope of the book and readers interested in more information are referred to a series of papers in the book edited by Blume and Midha (1995) or the article by Amidon et. al. (1995).

## Other Types of Bivariate Correlations

Illustrated to this point in the chapter are correlations involving two continuous variables (interval or ratio scales). There are other special types of measures of relationships that handle various combinations of variables measured on nominal, ordinal, or interval scales. These are often described as measures of association and are presented in Chapter 17. Correlations involving ordinal scales for both the $x$- and $y$-axis are best evaluated with Spearman's Rho, a nonparametric procedure (Chapter 21).

If at all possible, it is recommended to avoid grouping continuous data into categories that form dichotomous or nominal scale results. This attenuating of the data can lead to an underestimation of the measured effect. Tests for handling this type of edited data are discussed in Chapter 17 as measures of association and the terminology associated with such attenuated data sets is as follows. The **biserial correlation coefficient** is a special type of bivariate correlation coefficient for comparing a continuous normally distributed variable with a dichotomous variable that has an underlying normal distribution (i.e., a continuous variable that has been collapsed to create groups representing "above" and "below" the median result). If comparing two continuous variables that have both been dichotomized this would involve a **tettachoric correlation coefficient**. These are in contrast to a **point biserial correlation coefficient** which involves the correlation between a continuous normally distributed variable with a truly dichotomous variable.

**Pair-wise Correlations Involving More Than Two Variables**

When there are more than just two continuous variables affecting each data point, it is possible to calculate pair-wise correlations. For example if we are evaluating three continuous variables ($X$, $Y$, and $Z$) on the same subjects, we can calculate the correlations ($r_{xy}$, $r_{xz}$, and $r_{yz}$). The simplest way to evaluate the relationship between these variables is to create a table referred to as an **intercorrelation matrix**. Also called a **correlation matrix** it arranges the correlation coefficients in a systematic and orderly fashion represented by a square with an equal number of rows and columns (Table 13.7). The diagonal coefficients have a perfect relationship ($r$ = 1.00) between each variable correlated with itself. The number of cells above or below the diagonal can be calculated using either of the following determinants:

$$C = \frac{k(k-1)}{2} \qquad \text{Eq. 13.10}$$

$$C = \binom{k}{2} = \frac{k!}{2!(k-2)!} \qquad \text{Eq. 13.11}$$

where $k$ equals the number of variables and Eq. 13.11 is simply the combination formula (discussed in Chapter 2) for paired comparisons.

The cells in the lower portion of the correlation matrix are a mirror image of the cells above the diagonal. We could simplify the matrix by discarding the diagonal cells and either the lower or upper portion of the cells and express the matrix as seen in Table 13.8.

**Table 13.7** Example of an Intercorrelation Matrix

| Variables | X | Y | Z |
|---|---|---|---|
| X | $r_{xx}$ | $r_{xy}$ | $r_{xz}$ |
| Y | $r_{xy}$ | $r_{yy}$ | $r_{yz}$ |
| Z | $r_{xz}$ | $r_{yz}$ | $r_{zz}$ |

To illustrate the use of an intercorrelation matrix, consider the data presented in Table 13.9. In this table more information is presented for the volunteer included in the earlier clinical trial. These additional data include: entry laboratory values for blood urea nitrogen (BUN) and serum sodium; and study pharmacokinetic results as represented by the area under the curve (AUC).

Using the data presented in Table 13.9, the intercorrelation matrix is shown in Table 13.10 and the actual pair-wise correlations in Table 13.11. Based on the correlation coefficients presented on this matrix and the descriptive terminology discussed earlier, the results of the multiple correlation would be: 1) a high correlation between weight and height, weight and AUC, and height and AUC; 2) a moderate correlation between weight and BUN, height and BUN, and height and sodium; 3) a low correlation exists between weight and sodium, BUN and sodium, and BUN and AUC; and 4) an almost negligible relationship between sodium and AUC.

This matrix can be extended to include the intercorrelations for any number of continuous variables. Using the correlation matrix it is possible to identify those variables that correlate most highly with each other. Unfortunately, just by inspection of the matrix it is not possible to determine any joint effects of two or more

**Table 13.8** Abbreviated Intercorrelation Matrix

| Variables | Y | Z |
|---|---|---|
| X | $r_{xy}$ | $r_{xz}$ |
| Y | ... | $r_{yz}$ |

**Table 13.9** Leveled Variables from Six Subjects in a Clinical Trial

| | | Entry Lab Values | | Results |
|---|---|---|---|---|
| Weight (kg) | Height (m) | BUN (mg/dl) | Sodium (mmol/l) | AUC (ng/ml) |
| 96 | 1.88 | 22 | 144 | 806 |
| 77.7 | 1.80 | 11 | 141 | 794 |
| 100.9 | 1.85 | 17 | 139 | 815 |
| 79.0 | 1.77 | 14 | 143 | 775 |
| 73.0 | 1.73 | 15 | 137 | 782 |
| 84.5 | 1.83 | 21 | 140 | 786 |

**Table 13.10** Layout of Correlation Matrix for Table 13.8

| Variables | Weight | Height | BUN | Na | AUC |
|---|---|---|---|---|---|
| Weight(A) | 1.00 | $r_{ab}$ | $r_{ac}$ | $r_{ad}$ | $r_{ae}$ |
| Height (B) | $r_{ab}$ | 1.00 | $r_{bc}$ | $r_{bd}$ | $r_{be}$ |
| BUN (C) | $r_{ac}$ | $r_{bc}$ | 1.00 | $r_{cd}$ | $r_{ce}$ |
| Na (D) | $r_{ad}$ | $r_{bd}$ | $r_{cd}$ | 1.00 | $r_{de}$ |
| AUC (E) | $r_{ae}$ | $r_{be}$ | $r_{ce}$ | $r_{de}$ | 1.00 |

**Table 13.11** Correlation Matrix for Table 13.8

| Variables | Height | BUN | Na | AUC |
|---|---|---|---|---|
| Weight(A) | .884 | .598 | .268 | .873 |
| Height(B) | | .665 | .495 | .781 |
| BUN (C) | | | .226 | .334 |
| Na (D) | | | | .051 |

**Table 13.12** Correlation Matrix with Accompanying p-Values

| Variables | Height | BUN | Na | AUC |
|---|---|---|---|---|
| Weight(A) | .884<br>0.019 | .598<br>0.210 | .268<br>0.608 | .873<br>0.023 |
| Height(B) | | .665<br>0.149 | .495<br>0.318 | .781<br>0.067 |
| BUN (C) | | | .226<br>0.667 | .334<br>0.517 |
| Na (D) | | | | .051<br>0.923 |

variables on another variable. Often computer programs will generate such a correlation matrix and include an associated *p*-value for each correlation coefficient (Table 13.12). In this case, statistical significant ($p < 0.05$) positive relationship exist between weight and height ($p = 0.019$) and weight and AUC ($p = 0.023$).

**Multiple Correlations**

Many times when there are multiple concurrent correlations in an experiment, we may be interested in one key variable that has special importance to us and we are interested in determining how other variables influence this factor. This variable is labeled as our **criterion variable**. Other variables assist in the evaluation of this variable. These additional variables are referred to as **predictor variables** because they may have some common variance with the criterion variable; thus information about these latter variables can be used to predict information about our criterion variable. The terms **criterion variable** and **predictor variable** may be used interchangeably with dependent and independent variables, respectively.

In the next chapter we will discuss regression, where the researchers are able to control at least one variable in "controlled experimental studies" and the criterion or dependent variable becomes synonymous with the **experimental variable** or **response variable**. In these experimental studies we will reserve the expression independent variable to variables independent of each other.

In **multiple correlation** we use techniques that allow us to evaluate how much of the variation in our criterion variable is associated with variances in a set of predictor variables. This procedure involves weighing the values associated with our respective predictor variables. The procedures are complex and tedious to compute. However, through the use of computer programs it is possible to derive these weights (usually the higher weights are associated with predictor variables with the higher common variance with our criterion variable).

In a multiple correlation we once again compute a line that fits best between our data points and compute the variability around that line. The formula for a straight line ($y = a + bx$) can be expanded to the following for multiple predictor variables.

$$y_i = \beta_o + \beta_1 x_{1i} + \beta_2 x_{2i} + ... + \beta_k x_{ki} + e_i \qquad \text{Eq. 13.12}$$

In this equation the $e_i$ a common variance associated with the $y$-variable and $\beta_o$ the point where a plane created by the other variables will intercept with the $y$-axis. The remaining $\beta$'s in Eq. 13.12 are weights that are applied to each of the predictor variables, which result in composite scores that correlate most highly with the scores of our criterion variable, are referred to as **beta coefficients** or **beta weights**. These weights are a function of the correlation between the specific predictor variables and the criterion variables, as well as the correlations that exist among all the predictor variables.

The result of the mathematical manipulation, which is beyond the scope of this book, is a **multiple correlation coefficient** ($R$). It is the correlation resulting from the weighted predictor scores. Multiple correlations are closely related to multiple regression models. An excellent source for additional information on multiple correlation is presented by Kachigan (1991, pp. 147-153). Others sources would include Zar (1999, pp. 414-428) and Daniel (1999, pp. 494-503).

## Partial Correlations

An alternative method for the evaluation of multiple correlations is to calculate a **partial correlation coefficient** that shows the correlation between two continuous variables, while removing the effects of any other continuous variables. The simplest type of partial correlation coefficient is to extract the common effects of one variable from the relationship between two other variables of interest:

$$r_{yx,z} = \frac{r_{yx} - (r_{xz})(r_{yz})}{\sqrt{(1 - r_{xz}^2)(1 - r_{yz}^2)}} \qquad \text{Eq. 13.13}$$

where $r_{yx,z}$ is the correlation between variables $x$ and $y$, eliminating the effect of variable $z$. This formula can be slightly modified to evaluate the correlations for the other two combinations (*XZ* and *YZ*). In this formula all three paired correlations must be calculated first and then placed into Equation 13.12.

As an example of a partial correlation for three continuous variables, assume that only the first two columns and fifth column from Table 13.9 were of interest to the principal investigator involved in the clinical trial and that the researcher is interested in the correlation between the AUC and the weight, removing the effect that height might have on the results. The partial correlation coefficient would be as follows:

$$r_{ae,b} = \frac{r_{ae} - (r_{ab})(r_{be})}{\sqrt{(1 - r_{ab}^2)(1 - r_{be}^2)}}$$

$$r_{ae,b} = \frac{.873 - (.884)(.781)}{\sqrt{(1 - (.884)^2)(1 - (.781)^2)}} = \frac{.183}{.292} = +.627$$

Therefore, we see a moderate correlation between AUC and weight when we control the influence of height. In other words, what we have accomplished is to determine the relationship ($r = +0.63$) between our two key variables (AUC and weight) while holding a third variable (height) constant. Is this a significant relationship? We can test the relationship by modifying the t-statistic that was used to compare only two dependent variables.

$$t_{yx.z} = \frac{r_{yx.z}\sqrt{n - k - 1}}{\sqrt{1 - (r_{yx.z})^2}} \qquad \text{Eq. 13.14}$$

In this case, $k$ represents the number of variables being evaluated that might influence the outcome against the $y$-variable. In our example, $k$ equals 2 for variables $x$ and $z$. The decision rule is to reject the null hypotheses of no correlation if $t$ is greater than the critical t-value of the $n - k - 1$ degrees of freedom. In $t$-conversion to evaluate the significance of $r = 0.63$ the critical value would be $t_3(.975) = 2.78$ and the calculations would be as follows:

$$t_{yx.z} = \frac{(.627)\sqrt{6-2-1}}{\sqrt{1-(.627)^2}} = \frac{1.086}{0.779} = 1.394$$

The researcher would fail to reject the null hypothesis and conclude that there is no significant correlation between the AUC and weight excluding the influence of height.

The partial correlation can be expanded to control for more than one additional continuous variable.

### Nonlinear Correlations

For nonlinear correlations the best measure of a relationship is the **correlation ratio**. This **eta-statistic** ($\eta$) can be used when data tend to be curvilinear in their relationship. Based on visual inspection the data, the sample outcomes are divided into categories, at least seven, but no more than 14. These categories represent clusters of data with observable breaking points in the data. If there are fewer than seven categories the eta-statistic may not be sensitive to the curvilinear relationship. The statistic is based on a comparison of the differences, on the $y$-axis, between observed data points and their category mean, as well as a comparison with the total mean for all of the observations:

$$\eta = \sqrt{1 - \frac{\Sigma(y_i - \overline{Y_c})^2}{\Sigma(y_i - \overline{Y_t})^2}} \qquad \text{Eq. 13.15}$$

where $y_i$ represents the data point, $\overline{Y}_c$ is the mean for the category, and $\overline{Y}_t$ is the mean for all of the $y$-observations.

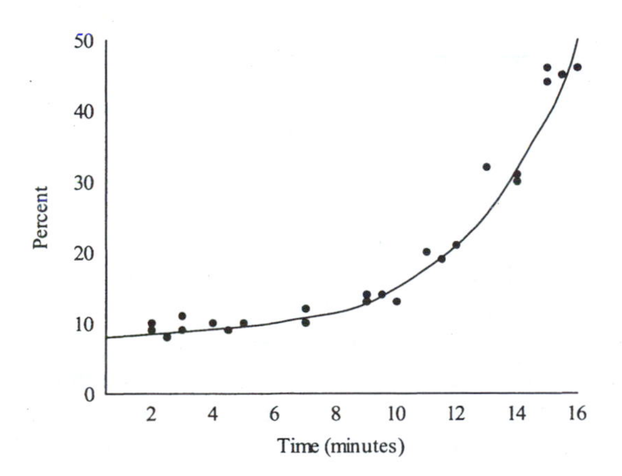


**Figure 13.5** Graphic of a curvilinear relationship.

If there is a nonlinear relationship, the traditional correlation coefficient tends to underestimate the strength of this type of relationship. For example consider the relationship presented in Figure 13.5 where the data appears to curve. Calculation of the traditional correlation coefficient (Eq. 13.15) produces a correlation coefficient of $r = 0.883$. In this case the total mean for all the observations on the $y$-axis is $\overline{Y}_t$ = 20.25. Calculation of the $\eta$ is based on the data in Table 13.13.

$$\eta = \sqrt{1 - \frac{15.6167}{4140.50}} = \sqrt{0.9962} = +0.9981$$

Note that $\eta$ is larger than $r$.

**Assessing Independence and Randomness**

Since this chapter introduced us to correlation and measures of the strength of relationships, two previously discussed topics will be revisited (independence and randomness) and statistical procedures to evaluate these two critical assumptions associated with most inferential statistics.

As mentioned previously, the researcher should be concerned with obtaining an appropriate sample (preferably a random sample) and be comfortable that observations are independent of each other. Assessing independence can be visually determined by graphing how each observation differs from the mean. These differences are sometimes referred to as **residuals**. The residuals are plotted on the $y$-axis of a scatter plot against the $x$-axis, which represents the order in which the sample was collected or recorded. If there is **independence**, a pattern should not appear on the scatter plot. A more formal method for testing independence is to calculate the **Durbin-Watson coefficient**, which uses Studentized residuals:

$$d = \frac{\sum\left[(y_i - \overline{X}_y) - (y_{i-t} - \overline{X}_y)\right]}{\sum(y_i - \overline{X}_y)^2} \qquad \text{Eq. 13.16}$$

where $\overline{X}_y$ is the mean on the $y$-axis, $y_i$ represents each data point and $y_{i-t}$ is the $y$-value for the previous sequential value on the $x$-axis (**serial correlation**). This test is often used for time series correlations where the $x$-axis is time. For serial correlation a $d = 0$ would represent a perfect positive correlation, $d = 2$ no correlation, and $d = 4$ a perfect negative correlation. For testing independence, if the Durbin-Watson coefficient is between 1.5 and 2.5, independence can be assumed.

The second key consideration for inferential tests is randomness in the data. A **runs test** can be used for **assessing randomness**. A "run" is a series of similar responses. For example, 25 true and false questions give the following ordered results:

**Table 13.13** Sample Data Comparing Time and Percent Response

| x (time) | y (%) | $\overline{Y}_c$ | $( - \overline{Y}_c)$ | $(y - \overline{Y}_c)^2$ | $(y - \overline{Y}_t)$ | $(y - \overline{Y}_t)^2$ |
|---|---|---|---|---|---|---|
| 2 | 9 | 9.40 | −0.40 | 0.16 | −11.25 | 126.5625 |
| 2 | 10 | | 0.60 | 0.36 | −10.25 | 105.0625 |
| 2.5 | 8 | | −1.40 | 1.96 | −12.25 | 150.0625 |
| 3 | 9 | | −0.40 | 0.16 | −11.25 | 126.5625 |
| 3 | 11 | | 1.60 | 2.56 | -9.25 | 85.5625 |
| 4 | 10 | 9.67 | 0.33 | 0.1089 | −10.25 | 105.0625 |
| 4.5 | 9 | | −0.67 | 0.4489 | −11.25 | 126.5625 |
| 5 | 10 | | 0.33 | 0.1089 | −10.25 | 105.0625 |
| 7 | 10 | 11.00 | −1.00 | 1.00 | −10.25 | 105.0625 |
| 7 | 12 | | 1.00 | 1.00 | −8.25 | 68.0625 |
| 9 | 13 | 13.50 | −0.50 | 0.25 | −7.25 | 52.5625 |
| 9 | 14 | | 0.50 | 0.25 | −6.25 | 39.0625 |
| 9.5 | 14 | | 0.50 | 0.25 | −6.25 | 39.0625 |
| 10 | 13 | | −0.50 | 0.25 | −7.25 | 52.5625 |
| 11 | 20 | 20.00 | 0.00 | 0.00 | −0.25 | 0.0625 |
| 11.5 | 19 | | −1.00 | 1.00 | −1.25 | 1.5625 |
| 12 | 21 | | 1.00 | 1.00 | 0.75 | 0.5625 |
| 13 | 32 | 31.00 | 1.00 | 1.00 | 11.75 | 138.0625 |
| 14 | 30 | | −1.00 | 1.00 | 9.75 | 95.0625 |
| 14 | 31 | | 0.00 | 0.00 | 10.75 | 115.5625 |
| 15 | 44 | 45.25 | −1.25 | 1.5625 | 23.75 | 564.0625 |
| 15 | 46 | | 0.75 | 0.5625 | 25.75 | 663.0625 |
| 15.5 | 45 | | −0.25 | 0.0625 | 24.75 | 612.5625 |
| 16 | 46 | | 0.75 | 0.5625 | 25.75 | 663.0625 |
| | | $\Sigma =$ | 0 | 15.6167 | 0 | 4140.5000 |

TTFTTFTTTFFFFFTFFTTTFFFFF

This represents ten runs, TT, F, TT, F, TTT, FFFFF, T, FF, TTT, and FFFFF. The following symbols will be used: $u$ = number of runs, $n_1$ = number with the first outcome (T in this case), and $n_2$ = number with the second outcome (F). Tables are available for small samples. For larger samples ($n_1$ or $n_2$ larger than 30) and as approximation for smaller samples, the following equations can be used. As the underlying distribution approaches normality, the mean is:

$$\mu_u = \frac{2n_1n_2}{N} + 1 \qquad \text{Eq. 13.17}$$

The standard deviation would be:

$$\sigma_u = \sqrt{\frac{2n_1n_2(2n_1n_2 - N)}{N^2(N-1)}} \qquad \text{Eq. 13.18}$$

The deviation from expect results would be evaluated using a *z*-statistic:

$$Z = \frac{|u - \mu_u| - 0.5}{\sigma_u} \qquad \text{Eq. 13.19}$$

If the result is less than $Z_{\alpha/2} = 1.96$, the sample can be assumed to be random. In our previous example the approximation would be:

$$n_1 = 11, n_2 = 14, N = 25\ u = 10$$

$$\mu_u = \frac{2(11)(14)}{25} + 1 = 13.32$$

$$\sigma_u = \sqrt{\frac{2(11)(14)[2(11)(14) - 25]}{25^2(24)}} = 2.41$$

$$Z = \frac{|10 - 13.32| - 0.5}{2.41} = 1.17$$

The runs test is a nonparametric procedure (Chapter 21) and thus assumes no specific distribution. In order to do a runs test the variable must have dichotomous results and categories should represent mutually exclusive and exhaustive outcomes. For ordinal or continuous data, the results must be dichotomized into above or below the median

An alternative to the runs test is **autocorrelation**, which also tests for non-randomness in data. It is primarily used for time series tests. It is a correlation coefficient that involves evaluating *y*-values for their corresponding *x*-values arranged sequentially by time. The lag *k* autocorrelation is calculated using the following formula:

$$r_k = \frac{\sum(y_i - \overline{X}_y)(y_{i+k} - \overline{X}_y)}{\sum(y_i - \overline{X}_y)^2} \qquad \text{Eq. 13.20}$$

where $\overline{X}_y$ is the mean on the *y*-axis, $y_i$ represents each data point and $y_{i+k}$ is the *y*-value for the next sequential value on *x*-axis. Additional information about the used of autocorrelation can be found in Box and Jenkins (1976).

**References**

"Bioequivalency requirements and in vivo bioavailability procedures," *Federal Register* 42:1621-1653 (1977).

Amidon, G.L. et al. (1995). "A theoretical basis for a biopharmaceutic drug classification: the correlation of *in vitro* drug product dissolution and *in vivo* bioavailability," Pharmaceutical Research 12:413-420.

Blume, H.H. and Midha, K.K., eds. (1995). *Bio-International 2: Bioavailability, Bioequivalence and Pharmacokinetic Studies*, Medpharm Scientific Publishers, Stuttgart, pp. 247-318.

Box, G.E.P. and Jenkins, G.M. (1976). *Time Series Analysis: Forcasting and Control*, revised edition, Holden-Day, San Francisco, pp. 23-45.

Daniel, W.W. (1999). *Biostatistics: A Foundation for Analysis in the Health Sciences*, Seventh edition, John Wiley and Sons, New York, pp.430,431, 494-503.

Guilford, J.P. (1956). *Fundamental Statistics in Psychology and Education*, McGraw-Hill, New York, p. 145

Kelly, W.D., Ratliff, T.A., and Nenadic, C. *Basic Statistics for Laboratories*, John Wiley and Sons, Hoboken, NJ, 1992, p. 93.

Rowntree, D. (1981). *Statistics Without Tears: A Primer for Non-Mathematicians*, Charles Scribner's Sons, New York, p. 170.

Kachigan, S.K. (1991). *Multivariate Statistical Analysis*, Second edition, Radius Press, New York, pp. 147-153.

Skelly, J.P. and Shiu, G.F. (1993). "*In vitro/in vivo* correlations in biopharmaceutics: scientific and regulatory implications," *European Journal of Drug Metabolism and Pharmacokinetics* 18:121-129.

Zar, J.H. (1999). *Biostatistical Analysis*, Fourth edition, Prentice-Hall, Englewood Cliffs, NJ, pp. 414-428.

**Suggested Supplemental Readings**

Bolton, S. (1997). *Pharmaceutical Statistics: Practical and Clinical Applications*, Third edition, Marcel Dekker, New York, pp. 249-257.

Bradley, James (1968). *Distribution-free Statistical Tests*, Prentice-Hall, Englewood Cliffs, NJ, pp. 255-259.

Cutler, D.J. (1995). "*In Vitro/In Vivo* Correlation and Statistics," *Bio-International 2: Bioavailability, Bioequivalence and Pharmacokinetic Studies*, Blume, H.H. and Midha, K.K., eds., Medpharm Scientific Publishers, Stuttgart, pp. 281-289.

Havilcek, L.L. and Crain, R.D. (1988). *Practical Statistics for the Physical Sciences*, American Chemical Society, Washington, DC, pp. 83-93, 106-108.

**Example Problems**

1. Two different scales are used to measure patient anxiety levels upon admission to a hospital. Method A is an established test instrument, while Method B (which has been developed by the researchers) is a quicker and easier instrument to administer. Is there a correlation between the two measures presented in Table 13.14?

2. Two drugs (A and B) are commonly used together to stabilize patients after stokes and the dosing for each is individualized. Listed in Table 13.15 are the dosages administered to eight patients randomly selected from admission records at a specific hospital over a six month period. Did the dosage of either drug result in a stronger correlation with shortened length of stay (LOS) in the institution?

**Table 13.14** Data for Problem 1

| Method A | Method B |
|---|---|
| 55 | 90 |
| 66 | 117 |
| 46 | 94 |
| 77 | 124 |
| 57 | 105 |
| 59 | 115 |
| 70 | 125 |
| 57 | 97 |
| 52 | 97 |
| 36 | 78 |
| 44 | 84 |
| 55 | 112 |
| 53 | 102 |
| 67 | 112 |
| 72 | 130 |

**Table 13.15** Data for Problem 2

| Patient | LOS (days) | Drug A (mg/kg) | Drug B (mcg/kg) |
|---|---|---|---|
| 1 | 3 | 2.8 | 275 |
| 2 | 2 | 4.0 | 225 |
| 3 | 4 | 1.5 | 250 |
| 4 | 3 | 3.0 | 225 |
| 5 | 2 | 3.7 | 300 |
| 6 | 4 | 2.0 | 225 |
| 7 | 4 | 2.4 | 275 |
| 8 | 3 | 3.5 | 275 |

3. It is believed that two assay methods will produce identical results for analyzing a specific drug. Various dilutions are assayed using both the currently accepted method (GS) and the proposed alternative (ALT). Based on the results listed in Table 13.16, does a high correlation exist?

4. A random sample of twelve students graduating from a school of pharmacy were administered an examination to determine retention of information received during classes. The test contained four sections covering pharmacy law, pharmaceutical calculations (math), pharmacology (p'cology) and medicinal chemistry (medchem). Listed in Table 13.17 are the results of the tests. Create a correlation matrix to compare the results and relationships between the various sections and total test score. Which of the two sections most strongly correlated together? Which section has the greatest correlation with the total test score?

**Answers to Problems**

1. Comparison of two different scales to measure patient anxiety levels.
   Variables: continuous (two measurement scales)

**Table 13.16** Data for Problem 3

| Method GS | Method ALT |
|---|---|
| 90.1 | 89.8 |
| 85.2 | 85.1 |
| 79.7 | 80.2 |
| 74.3 | 75.0 |
| 60.2 | 61.0 |
| 35.5 | 34.8 |
| 24.9 | 24.8 |
| 19.6 | 21.1 |

**Table 13.17** Data for Problem 4

| Student | Law | Math | P'cology | Medchem | Total |
|---|---|---|---|---|---|
| 001 | 23 | 18 | 22 | 20 | 83 |
| 002 | 22 | 20 | 21 | 18 | 81 |
| 003 | 25 | 21 | 25 | 17 | 88 |
| 004 | 20 | 19 | 18 | 20 | 77 |
| 005 | 24 | 23 | 24 | 14 | 85 |
| 006 | 23 | 22 | 22 | 20 | 87 |
| 007 | 24 | 20 | 24 | 15 | 83 |
| 008 | 20 | 17 | 15 | 22 | 74 |
| 009 | 22 | 19 | 21 | 23 | 85 |
| 010 | 24 | 21 | 23 | 19 | 87 |
| 011 | 23 | 20 | 21 | 19 | 83 |
| 012 | 21 | 21 | 20 | 21 | 83 |

a. Pearson Product Moment

Method A - variable $x$ - mean = 57.7
Method B - variable $y$ - mean = 105.5

Calculations (based on summary data in Table 13.18):

$$r = \frac{\Sigma(x-\overline{X})(y-\overline{Y})}{\sqrt{\Sigma(x-\overline{X})^2(y-\overline{Y})^2}} = \frac{2236.85}{\sqrt{(1750.95)(3377.75)}} = 0.92$$

b. Computational formula (based on summary data in Table 13.19):

Calculations:

$$r = \frac{15(93571)-(866)(1582)}{\sqrt{15(51748)-(866)^2}\sqrt{15(170226)-(1582)^2}}$$

$$r = \frac{1403565-1370012}{(162.06)(225.09)} = \frac{33553}{36478.08} = 0.92$$

c. Conversion to $t$-statistic:

Hypothesis: $H_0$: $r_{xy} = 0$
$H_1$: $r_{xy} \neq 0$

**Table 13.18** Data for Problem 1, Definitional Formula

| x | y | $x-\bar{X}$ | $y-\bar{Y}$ | $(x-\bar{X})(y-\bar{Y})$ | $(x-\bar{X})^2$ | $(y-\bar{Y})^2$ |
|---|---|---|---|---|---|---|
| 55 | 90 | −2.7 | −15.5 | 41.85 | 7.29 | 240.25 |
| 66 | 117 | 8.3 | 11.5 | 95.45 | 68.89 | 132.25 |
| 46 | 94 | −11.7 | −11.5 | 134.55 | 136.89 | 132.25 |
| 77 | 124 | 19.3 | 18.5 | 357.05 | 372.49 | 342.25 |
| 57 | 105 | −0.7 | −0.5 | 0.35 | 0.49 | 0.25 |
| 59 | 115 | 1.3 | 9.5 | 12.35 | 1.69 | 90.25 |
| 70 | 125 | 12.3 | 19.5 | 239.85 | 151.29 | 380.25 |
| 57 | 97 | −0.7 | −8.5 | 5.95 | 0.49 | 72.25 |
| 52 | 97 | −5.7 | −8.5 | 48.45 | 32.49 | 72.25 |
| 36 | 78 | −21.7 | −27.5 | 596.75 | 470.89 | 756.25 |
| 44 | 84 | −13.7 | −21.5 | 294.55 | 187.69 | 462.25 |
| 55 | 112 | −2.7 | 6.5 | -17.55 | 7.29 | 42.25 |
| 53 | 102 | −4.7 | −3.5 | 16.45 | 22.09 | 12.25 |
| 67 | 112 | 9.3 | 6.5 | 60.45 | 86.49 | 42.25 |
| 72 | 130 | 14.3 | 24.5 | 350.35 | 204.49 | 600.25 |
| | | | | 2236.85 | 1750.95 | 3377.75 |

**Table 13.19** Data for Problem 1, Computational Formula

| | x | y | $x^2$ | $y^2$ | xy |
|---|---|---|---|---|---|
| | 55 | 90 | 3025 | 8100 | 4950 |
| | 66 | 117 | 4356 | 13689 | 7722 |
| | 46 | 94 | 2116 | 8836 | 4324 |
| | 77 | 124 | 5929 | 15376 | 9548 |
| | 57 | 105 | 3249 | 11025 | 5985 |
| | 59 | 115 | 3481 | 13225 | 6785 |
| | 70 | 125 | 4900 | 15625 | 8750 |
| | 57 | 97 | 3249 | 9409 | 5529 |
| | 52 | 97 | 2704 | 9409 | 5044 |
| | 36 | 78 | 1296 | 6084 | 2808 |
| | 44 | 84 | 1936 | 7056 | 3696 |
| | 55 | 112 | 3025 | 12544 | 6160 |
| | 53 | 102 | 2809 | 10404 | 5406 |
| | 67 | 112 | 4489 | 12544 | 7504 |
| | 72 | 130 | 5184 | 16900 | 9360 |
| $\Sigma =$ | 866 | 1582 | 51748 | 170226 | 93571 |

Decision Rule: With $\alpha = 0.05$, reject $H_0$ if $t > t_{13}(.975) = 2.16$.

Calculations:

$$t = \frac{r\sqrt{n-2}}{\sqrt{1-r^2}} = \frac{.92\sqrt{15-2}}{\sqrt{1-(.92)^2}} = \frac{3.32}{0.39} = 8.51$$

Decision: With $t > 2.16$, is to reject $H_0$ and conclude there is a significant relationship between Method A and Method B.

2. Comparison of two drugs and length of stay at a specific hospital.
Variables: continuous (two measurement scales)

Calculation of the three paired correlations produced the following intercorrelation matrix:

| Variables | LOS | Drug A | Drug B |
|---|---|---|---|
| LOS | ... | –0.923 | –0.184 |
| Drug A | ... | ... | +0.195 |
| Drug B | ... | ... | ... |

The partial correlation for length of stay vs. Drug A is:

$$r_{la,b} = \frac{r_{la} - (r_{lb})(r_{ab})}{\sqrt{(1-r_{lb}^2)(1-r_{ab}^2)}} = \frac{-0.923-(-0.184)(+0.195)}{\sqrt{(1-(-0.184)^2)(1-(0.195)^2)}} = +0.920$$

The partial correlation for length of stay vs. Drug B is:

$$r_{lb,a} = \frac{r_{lb} - (r_{la})(r_{ab})}{\sqrt{(1-r_{la}^2)(1-r_{ab}^2)}} = \frac{-0.184-(-0.923)(+0.195)}{\sqrt{(1-(-0.923)^2)(1-(0.195)^2)}} = -0.011$$

Evaluation of the partial correlation for length of stay vs. Drug A:

Decision rule is with $\alpha = 0.05$, reject $H_0$ if $|t| > t_5(.975) = 2.57$.

$$t_{la.b} = \frac{r_{la.b}\sqrt{n-k-1}}{\sqrt{1-(r_{la.b})^2}}$$

$$t_{yx.z} = \frac{(-0.92)\sqrt{8-2-1}}{\sqrt{1-(-0.92)^2}} = \frac{-2.057}{0.392} = -5.24$$

Decision: There is a strong correlation, statistically significant with 95% confidence, between the length of stay and administration of Drug A, but Drug B has very little influence on the length of stay.

3. Comparison of two analytical procedures on different concentrations of a drug.
   Variables: continuous (two measurement scales)

   Calculations (based on summary data in Table 13.20):

$$r = \frac{n\sum xy - \sum x \sum y}{\sqrt{n\sum x^2 - (\sum x)^2}\sqrt{n\sum y^2 - (\sum y)^2}}$$

$$r = \frac{8(33{,}244.62) - (469.5)(471.8)}{\sqrt{8(33{,}138.09) - (469.5)^2}\sqrt{8(33{,}355.38) - (471.8)^2}}$$

$$r = \frac{265{,}956.96 - 221{,}510.1}{(211.36)(210.35)} = \frac{44{,}446.86}{44{,}459.58} = +0.9997$$

   Conclusion: A very strong correlation between methods GS and ALT.

4. Comparison of multiple test results:
   Variables: continuous (five measurement scales)

**Table 13.20** Data for Problem 3, Computational Formula

| Method GS $x$ | Method ALT $y$ | $x^2$ | $y^2$ | $xy$ |
|---|---|---|---|---|
| 90.1 | 89.8 | 8,118.01 | 8,064.04 | 8,090.98 |
| 85.2 | 85.1 | 7,259.04 | 7,242.01 | 7,250.52 |
| 79.7 | 80.2 | 6,352.09 | 6,432.04 | 6,391.94 |
| 74.3 | 75.0 | 5,520.49 | 5,625.00 | 5,572.50 |
| 60.2 | 61.0 | 3,624.04 | 3,721.00 | 3,672.20 |
| 35.5 | 34.8 | 1,260.25 | 1,211.04 | 1,235.40 |
| 24.9 | 24.8 | 620.01 | 615.04 | 617.52 |
| 19.6 | 21.1 | 384.16 | 445.21 | 413.56 |
| 469.5 | 471.8 | 33,138.09 | 33,355.38 | 33,244.62 |

**Table 13.21** Data for Problem 4, Computational Formula

| Law (x) | Calculations (y) | $x^2$ | $y^2$ | xy |
|---|---|---|---|---|
| 23 | 18 | 529 | 324 | 414 |
| 22 | 20 | 484 | 400 | 440 |
| 25 | 21 | 625 | 441 | 525 |
| 20 | 19 | 400 | 361 | 380 |
| 24 | 23 | 576 | 529 | 552 |
| 23 | 22 | 529 | 484 | 506 |
| 24 | 20 | 576 | 400 | 480 |
| 20 | 17 | 400 | 289 | 340 |
| 22 | 19 | 484 | 361 | 418 |
| 24 | 21 | 576 | 441 | 504 |
| 23 | 20 | 529 | 400 | 460 |
| 21 | 21 | 441 | 441 | 441 |
| 271 | 241 | 6149 | 4871 | 5460 |

Example of correlation coefficient for scores on law and pharmaceutical calculations sections (Table 13.21).

Calculations:

$$r = \frac{n\sum xy - \sum x \sum y}{\sqrt{n\sum x^2 - (\sum x)^2}\sqrt{n\sum y^2 - (\sum y)^2}}$$

$$r = \frac{12(5460) - (271)(241)}{\sqrt{12(6149) - (271)^2}\sqrt{12(4871) - (241)^2}} = \frac{209}{358.8} = +0.582$$

Conclusion: A moderate correlation between law and calculation scores.

Correlation Matrix:

| | Law | Math | P'cology | Medchem | Total |
|---|---|---|---|---|---|
| Law | 1.000 | 0.582 | 0.943 | –0.674 | 0.832 |
| Math | 0.582 | 1.000 | 0.678 | –0.591 | 0.712 |
| P'cology | 0.943 | 0.678 | 1.000 | –0.689 | 0.877 |
| Medchem | –0.674 | –0.591 | –0.689 | 1.000 | –0.324 |
| Total | 0.832 | 0.712 | 0.877 | –0.324 | 1.000 |

Results: Strongest correlation between two sections is +0.943 between law and pharmacology.

# 14

# Linear Regression

Unlike the correlation coefficient, regression analysis requires at least one independent variable. Where correlation describes pair-wise relationships between continuous variables, linear regression is a statistical method to evaluate how one or more independent (predictor) variables influence outcomes for one continuous dependent (response) variable through a linear relationship. A regression line is computed that best fits between the data points. If a linear relationship is established, the magnitude of the effect of the independent variable can be used to predict the corresponding magnitude of the effect on the dependent variable. For example a person's weight can be used to predict body surface area. The strength of the relationship between the two variables can be determined by calculating the amount of the total variability that can be accounted for by the regression line.

Both linear regression and correlation are similar, in that both describe the strength of the relationship between two or more continuous variables. However, with linear regression, also termed **regression analysis**, a relationship is established between the two variables and a response for the dependent variable can be made based on a given value for the independent variable. For correlation, two dependent variables can be compared to determine if a relationship exists between them. Similarly, correlation is concerned with the strength of the relationship between two continuous variables. In regression analysis, or **experimental associations**, researchers control the values of at least one of the variables and assign objects at random to different levels of these variables. Where correlation simply described the strength and direction of the relationship, regression analysis provides a method for describing the nature of the relationship between two or more continuous variables.

The correlation coefficient can be very useful in exploratory research where the investigator is interested in the relationship between two or more continuous variables. One of the disadvantages of the correlation coefficient is that it is not very useful for predicting the value of $y$ from a value of $x$, or vice versa. As seen in the previous chapter, the correlation coefficient ($r$) is the extent of the linear relationship between $x$ and $y$. However, there may be a close correlation between the two variables that are based on a relationship other than a straight line (for example, Figure 13.3). The formulas for correlation and regression are closely related with similar calculations based upon the same sums and sums of squares. Therefore, if an independent variable is involved, calculating both is useful because the correlation coefficient can support the interpretation associated with regression. This chapter will focus primarily on simple regression, where there is only one independent or predictor variable. The adjective *linear* is used to denote that the relationship between the two variables can be described by a straight line.

There are several assumptions associated with the linear regression model. First, values on the $x$-axis, which represent the independent variable are "fixed." This nonrandom variable is predetermined by the researcher so that responses on the $y$-axis are measured at only predetermined points on the $x$-axis. Because the researcher controls the $x$-axis it is assumed that these measures are without error. Second, for each value on the $x$-axis there is a subpopulation of values for the corresponding dependent variable on the $y$-axis. As will be discussed later, for any inferential statistics or tests of hypotheses, it is assumed that these subpopulations are normally distributed. For data that may not be normally distributed, for example, AUC or $C_{max}$ measures in bioavailability studies, log transformations may be required to convert such positively skewed data to a more normally distributed subpopulation. Coupled with the assumption of normality is homogeneity of variance, in that it is assumed that the variances for all the subpopulations are approximately equal. Third, it is assumed that these subpopulations have a linear relationship and that a straight line can be drawn between them. The formula for this line is:

$$\mu_{y/x} = \alpha + \beta x \qquad \text{Eq. 14.1}$$

where $\mu_{y/x}$ is mean for any given subpopulation for an $x$-value for the predictor independent variable. The terms $\alpha$ and $\beta$ represent the true population $y$-intercept and slope for the regression line. Unfortunately, we do not know these population parameters and must estimate these by creating a line, which is our best estimate based on the sample data.

## The Regression Line

As seen above, linear regression is involved with the characteristics of a straight line or **linear function**. This line can be estimated from sample data. Similar to correlation, a scatter plot offers an excellent method for visualizing the relationship between the continuous variables. In the simple regression design there are only two variables ($x$ and $y$). As mentioned in the previous chapter, the $x$-axis, or abscissa, represents the independent variable and the $y$-axis, the ordinate, is the dependent outcome. The scatter plot presented in Figure 14.1 shows a typical representation of these variables with $y$ on the vertical axis and $x$ on the horizontal axis. In this case $x$ is a specific amount of drug (mcg) administered to mice, with $y$ representing some measurable physiological response. The physiological response is obviously not controllable by the researcher and represents the dependent variable. However, prescribed (hopefully exact) doses of the drug are administered and represent the independent, researcher controlled variable.

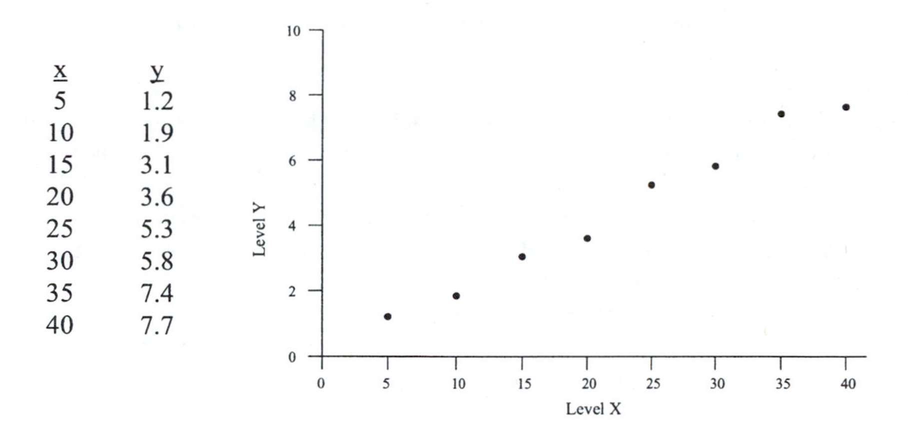

| x | y |
|---|---|
| 5 | 1.2 |
| 10 | 1.9 |
| 15 | 3.1 |
| 20 | 3.6 |
| 25 | 5.3 |
| 30 | 5.8 |
| 35 | 7.4 |
| 40 | 7.7 |



**Figure 14.1** Simple examples of data points for two continuous variables.

The first step in a linear regression analysis is to draw a straight line that best fits between the points. The slope of the line and its intercept of the $y$-axis are then used for the regression calculation. As introduced in the previous chapter, the general equation (Eq. 13.6) for a straight line is:

$$y = a + bx$$

In this formula, $y$ is a value on the vertical axis, $x$ is a corresponding value on the horizontal axis, $a$ is the point where the line crosses the vertical axis, and $b$ represents the amount by which the line rises for each increase in $x$ (the slope of the line). A second method for defining these values is that $a$ is the value on the $y$-axis where $x = 0$ and $b$ is the change in the $y$-value (the response value) for every unit increase in the $x$-value (the predictor variable).

Unfortunately, our estimate of the straight line is based on sample data and therefore subject to random error. Therefore, we need to modify our definition of the regression line to the following, where $e$ is an error term associated with our sampling.

$$y = \alpha + \beta x + e \qquad \text{Eq. 14.2}$$

Once again, it is assumed that the $e$'s associated with each subpopulation are normally distributed with all variances approximately equal.

Our best estimate of the true population regression line, would be the straight line that we can draw through our sample data. However, if asked to draw this line using a straight edge, it is unlikely that any two people, using visual inspection, would draw exactly the same line to fit best among these points. Thus, a variety of slopes and intercepts could be approximated. There are in fact an infinite number of possible lines, $y = a + bx$, which could be drawn between our data points. How can we select the "best" line from all the possible lines that can pass through these data points?

The **least-squares line** is the line that best describes the linear relationship between the independent and dependent variables. The data points are usually scattered on either side of this straight line that fits best between the points on the scatter diagram. Also called the **regression line**, it represents a line from which the smallest sum of squared differences are observed between the observed $(x,y_i)$ coordinates and the line $(x,y_c)$ coordinates along the *y* axis (sum of the squared vertical deviations). This **"best fit" line** represents that line where the sum of squares of the distances from the points in the scatter diagram to the regression line, in the direction of the *y*-variable is smallest. The calculation of the line that best fits between the sample data, is presented below. The slope of this line (Eq. 13.7) is:

$$b = \frac{n\sum xy - (\sum x)(\sum y)}{n\sum x^2 - (\sum x)^2}$$

Data to solve this equation can be generated in a table similar to the one used for the correlation coefficient (Table 13.4). The sample slope ($b$) is our best estimate of the true **regression coefficient** ($\beta$) for the population, but as will be discussed later, it is only an estimate.

The greater the change in *y*, for a constant change in *x*, the steeper the slope of the line. With the calculated slope of the line that best fits the observed points in the scatter diagram, it is possible to calculate an "anchor point" on the *y*-axis (the *y*-intercept) using Eq.13.7 (that point where the *x*-value is zero):

$$a = \frac{\sum y - b\sum x}{n}$$

An alternative approach to the scatter diagram is to display the information in a table. The regression line can be calculated for the data points in Figure 14.1 by arranging the data in tabular format as presented in Table 14.1. Similar to the manipulation of data for the correlation coefficient, each *x*-value and *y*-value are squared, and the product is calculated for the *x*- and *y*-value at each data point. These five columns are then summed to produce a $\Sigma x$, $\Sigma y$, $\Sigma x^2$, $\Sigma y^2$, and $\Sigma xy$. Note that $\Sigma y^2$ is not required for determining the regression line, but will be used later in additional calculations required for the linear regression model. Using the results in Table 14.1, the computations for the slope and *y*-intercept would be as follows:

$$b = \frac{8(1017) - (180)(36)}{8(5100) - (180)^2} = \frac{8136 - 6480}{40800 - 32400} = \frac{1656}{8400} = +0.1971$$

$$a = \frac{36 - 0.1971(180)}{8} = \frac{36 - 35.478}{8} = \frac{0.522}{8} = 0.06725$$

**Table 14.1** Data Manipulation of Regression Line for Figure 14.1

| | x | y | $x^2$ | $y^2$ | xy |
|---|---|---|---|---|---|
| | 5 | 1.2 | 25 | 1.44 | 6.00 |
| | 10 | 1.9 | 100 | 3.61 | 19.00 |
| | 15 | 3.1 | 225 | 9.61 | 46.50 |
| n=8 | 20 | 3.6 | 400 | 12.96 | 72.00 |
| | 25 | 5.3 | 625 | 28.09 | 132.50 |
| | 30 | 5.8 | 900 | 33.64 | 174.00 |
| | 35 | 7.4 | 1225 | 54.76 | 259.00 |
| | 40 | 7.7 | 1600 | 59.29 | 308.00 |
| Σ = | 180 | 36.0 | 5100 | 203.40 | 1017.00 |

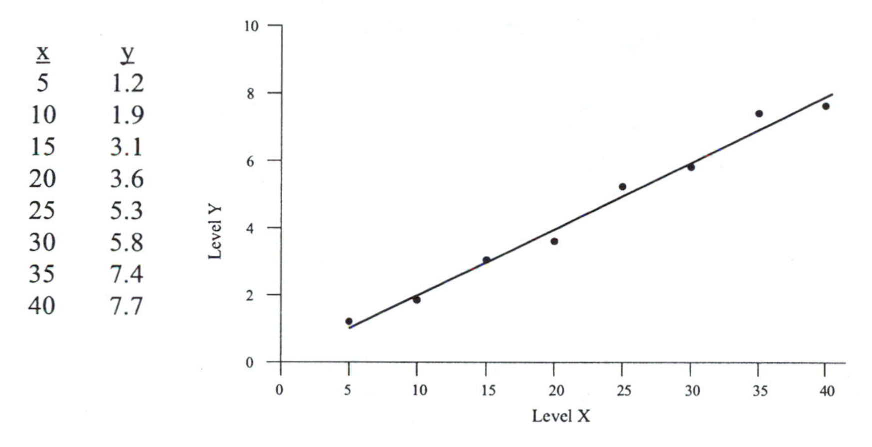


**Figure 14.2** Regression line for two continuous variables.

Based on these data, the regression line is presented in Figure 14.2, where the slope is in a positive direction +0.197 (as values of $x$ increase, values of $y$ will also increase) and the intercept is slightly above zero (0.067).

A quick check of the position of the regression line on the scatter diagram would be to calculate the means for both variables ($\overline{X}_x$, $\overline{X}_y$) and see if the line passes through this point. This can be checked by placing the slope, $y$-intercept, and $\overline{X}_x$ in the straight line equation and then determining if $\overline{X}_y$ equals the $y$-value. In this example, the mean for the abscissa is:

$$\overline{X}_x = \frac{\Sigma x}{n} = \frac{180}{8} = 22.5$$

The mean for the ordinate is:

$$\overline{X}_y = \frac{\Sigma y}{n} = \frac{36}{8} = 4.5$$

and the $y$-value for the mean of $x$ is the same as the mean of $y$:

$$y = a + bx = 0.06725 + 0.1971(22.5) = 0.06725 + 4.43475 = 4.502 \approx 4.5$$

If there is a linear relationship (a statistical procedure will be presented later to prove that a straight line can fit the data), then it is possible to determine any point on the $y$-axis for a given point on the $x$-axis using the formula for a line (Eq. 13.6). Mechanically we could draw a vertical line up from any point on the $x$-axis, where it intercepts our regression line we draw a horizontal line to the $y$-axis and read the value at that point. Mathematically we can accomplish the same result using the formula for a straight line. For example, based on the regression line calculated above, if $x$ = 32 mcg the corresponding physiological response for the $y$-value would be:

$$y = a + bx = 0.06725 + (0.1971)(32) = 0.06725 + 6.3072 = 6.3744$$

If instead the $x$-value is 8 mcg, the expected $y$-value physiological response would be:

$$y = a + bx = 0.06725 + (0.1971)(8) = 0.06725 + 1.5768 = 1.6441$$

Note that both of these results are approximations. As will be discussed later, if we can establish a straight line relationship between the $x$- and $y$-variables, the slope of the line of best fit will itself vary due to random error. Our estimate of the population slope ($\beta$) will be based on our best guess, $b$, plus or minus an amount of uncertainty. This will in fact create a confidence interval around any point on our regression line and provide a range of $y$-values. However, for the present time the use of the straight line equation provides us with a quick estimate of the corresponding $y$-value for any given $x$-value. Conversely, for any given value on the $y$-axis it is possible to estimate a corresponding $x$-value using a modification of the previous formula for a straight line:

$$x = \frac{y - a}{b} \qquad \text{Eq. 14.3}$$

If one wishes to determine, the corresponding $x$-value for a physiological response of 5.0, the calculation for the approximate dose of drug would be:

$$x = \frac{y - a}{b} = \frac{5.0 - 0.06725}{0.1971} = \frac{4.93275}{0.1971} = 25.0266 \ mcg$$

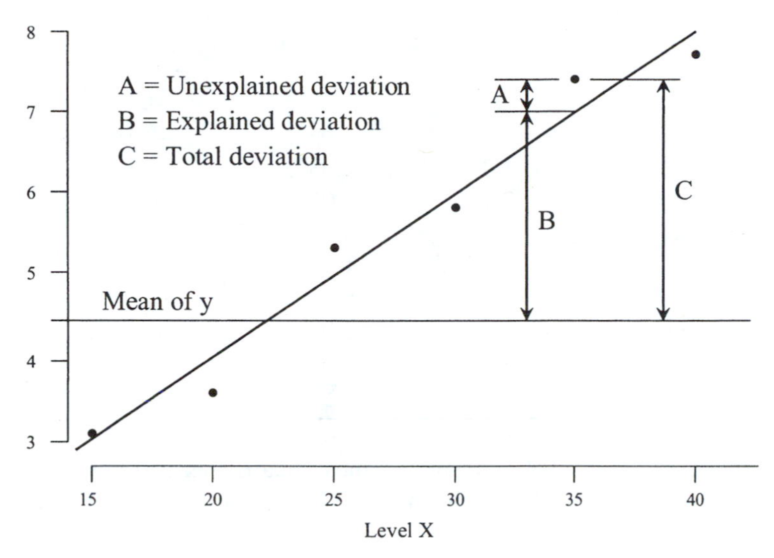


**Figure 14.3** Variability of data points around the mean of the y-variable and the regression line.

A method for calculating whether a relationship between two variables is in fact linear will be discussed subsequently. Many of the relationships that are encountered in research are linear, and those that are not can often be made linear with appropriate data transformation techniques. For example, if a scatter diagram shows that a nonlinear pattern is feasible, it is possible to produce a linear pattern by doing a transformation on one of the variables.

### Coefficient of Determination

As the spread of the scatter dots along the vertical axis ($y$-axis) decreases, the precision of the estimated $\mu_y$ increases. A perfect (100%) estimate is possible only when all the dots (data points) lie on the straight regression line. The **coefficient of determination** offers one method to evaluate if the linear regression equation adequately describes the type of relationship. It compares the scatter of data points about the regression line with the scatter about the mean for the sample values of the dependent $y$-variable. Figure 14.3 shows a scattering of points about both the mean of the $y$-distribution ($\overline{X}_y$) and the regression line itself for part of the data presented in Figure 14.2. As discussed in Chapter 6, in normally distributed data we expect to see data vary around the mean, in this case $\overline{X}_y$. Also, it is possible to measure the deviation of each point ($y_i$) from the mean on the $y$-axis (labeled "$C$" in Figure 14.2). If there were no linear relationship between the $x$- and $y$-variables, we would expect a random distribution of points around the mean on the $y$-axis. However, if the data is truly represented by the straight regression line, then a certain amount of this total variation can be explained by the deviation from the mean to the line ($B$). The point

**Table 14.2** Residuals for Data Points from the Regression Line

| X | y | $y_c$ | Residual |
|---|---|---|---|
| 5 | 1.2 | 1.0525 | −0.1475 |
| 10 | 1.9 | 2.0375 | +0.1375 |
| 15 | 3.1 | 3.0225 | −0.0775 |
| 20 | 3.6 | 4.0075 | +0.4075 |
| 25 | 5.3 | 4.9925 | −0.3075 |
| 30 | 5.8 | 5.9925 | +0.1775 |
| 35 | 7.4 | 6.9625 | −0.4327 |
| 40 | 7.7 | 7.9475 | +0.2475 |
| | | $\Sigma =$ | 0 |

on the straight line is labeled $y_c$. However, most data points will not fall exactly on the regression line and this deviation (*A*) must be caused by other sources (random error).

The coefficient of determination is calculated using the sum of the squared deviations that takes into consideration these deviations (*A*, *B*, and *C*). In this case the total deviation equals the explained deviations (defined by the line) plus the unexplained deviations:

$$\Sigma(y_i - \overline{X}_y)^2 = \Sigma(y_c - \overline{X}_y)^2 + \Sigma(y_i - y_c)^2 \qquad \text{Eq. 14.4}$$

where the total deviation is the vertical difference between the observed data point and the mean for the $y$-axis ($y_i - \overline{X}_y$). The explained deviation is the vertical difference between the point on the regression line and the mean for the $y$-axis ($y_c - \overline{X}_y$). The unexplained deviation is the vertical difference between the observed data point and the corresponding point on the regression line ($y_c - y_i$). These vertical distances between the data points and the regression line are called **residuals**. The residuals for this example are presented in Table 14.2. With the line of best fit between the data points, the sum of the residuals should equal zero, an equal amount of deviation above and below the line. Thus, the best fit line is the line that results in the smallest value for the sum of the squared deviations, $\Sigma(y_c - y_i)^2$. This term is referred to as the **residual sum of squares** or **error sum of squares**.

The computations presented in Eq. 14.4 can be long and cumbersome; involving the calculation of the mean of the $y$-values ($\overline{X}_y$), the $y$-value on the regression line ($y_c$) for each level of the independent $x$-value, various differences between those values, and then summation of the various differences. A more manageable set of formulas use the sums computed in Table 14.1 to calculate the sum of squares due to linear regression:

$$SS_{Total} = SS_{Explained} + SS_{Unexplained} \qquad \text{Eq. 14.5}$$

These will produce the same results as the more time-consuming formula in Equation 14.4. The sum of the total variation between the mean ($\overline{X}_y$) and each observed data point ($y_i$) would be the total sum of squares ($SS_{total}$):

$$SS_{total} = \Sigma(y_i - \overline{X}_y)^2 = \Sigma y^2 - \frac{(\Sigma y)^2}{n} \qquad \text{Eq. 14.6}$$

The variability explained by the regression line of the deviations between the mean ($\overline{X}_y$) and the line ($y_c$) is the explained sum of squares ($SS_{explained}$):

$$SS_{explained} = \Sigma(y_c - \overline{X}_y)^2 = b^2 \cdot \left[\Sigma x^2 - \frac{(\Sigma x)^2}{n}\right] \qquad \text{Eq. 14.7}$$

The remaining, unexplained deviation between the regression line ($y_c$) and the data points ($y_i$) is the unexplained sum of squares ($SS_{unexplained}$). This residual measure can be computed by subtracting the explained variability for the total dispersion:

$$SS_{unexplained} = SS_{total} - SS_{explained} \qquad \text{Eq. 14.8}$$

Calculation for these sums of squares for the previous example (Table 14.1) would be:

$$SS_{total} = \Sigma y^2 - \frac{(\Sigma y)^2}{n} = 203.4 - \frac{(36)^2}{8} = 41.4$$

$$SS_{explained} = b^2 \cdot \left[\Sigma x^2 - \frac{(\Sigma x)^2}{n}\right] = (0.1971)^2\left[5100 - \frac{(180)^2}{8}\right] = 40.79$$

$$SS_{unexplained} = SS_{total} - SS_{explained} = 41.4 - 40.79 = 0.61$$

The sum of squares due to linear regression (**sum of squares regression**) is synonymous with the explained sum of squares and measures the total variability of the observed values that are associated with the linear relationship. The coefficient of determination ($r^2$) is the proportion of variability accounted for by the sum of squares due to linear regression.

$$r^2 = \frac{SS_{explained}}{SS_{total}} = \frac{b^2 \cdot \left[\Sigma x^2 - \frac{(\Sigma x)^2}{n}\right]}{\Sigma y^2 - \frac{(\Sigma y)^2}{n}} \qquad \text{Eq. 14.9}$$

In our previous example the coefficient of determination would be:

$$r^2 = \frac{(0.1971)^2 \cdot \left[5100 - \frac{(180)^2}{8}\right]}{203.4 - \frac{(36)^2}{8}} = \frac{40.79}{41.4} = 0.9853$$

The coefficient of determination measures the exactness of fit of the regression equation to the observed values of $y$. In other words, the coefficient of determination identifies how much variation in one variable can be explained by variations in the second. The rest of the variability ($1 - r^2$) is explained by other factors, most likely unidentifiable, random error unknown to the researcher (**coefficient of nondetermination**). In our example the computed $r^2$ is .9853; this indicates that approximately 98.5% of the total variation is explained by the linear regression model. If the $r^2$ is large, the regression equation accounts for a great proportion of the total variability in the observed values. The coefficient of nondetermination (1 – .9853) represents a random error of approximately 1.15%.

Similar to the correlation coefficient, the coefficient of determination is a measure of how closely the observations fall on a straight line. In fact, the square root of the coefficient of determination is the correlation coefficient:

$$r = \sqrt{r^2} \qquad \text{Eq. 14.10}$$

In this example the correlation coefficient is the square root of 0.9853 or 0.993. As proof of this relationship the correlation coefficient is calculated using Equation 13.4 and the data in Table 14.1:

$$r = \frac{8(1017) - (180)(36)}{\sqrt{8(5100) - (180)^2}\sqrt{8(203.4) - (36)^2}} = \frac{1656}{1667.957} = 0.993$$

This linear correlation (correlation coefficient) can be strongly influenced by a few extreme values. One rule of thumb is to first plot the data points on graph paper and examine the points visually before reporting the linear correlation. An opposite approach would be to consider the correlation coefficient as a measure of the extent of linear correlation. If all the data points fall exactly on a straight line, the two variables would be considered to be perfectly correlated ($r$ = +1.00 or −1.00). Remember that the correlation coefficient measures the extent to which the relationship between two continuous variables and this is not associated with the drawing of a straight line.

Sometimes termed the **common variance**, $r^2$ represents that proportion of variance in the response (dependent) variable that is accounted for by variance in the predictor (independent) variable. As the coefficient of determination increases we are able to account for more of the variation in the dependent variable with values predicted from the regression equation. Obviously, the amount of error associated with the prediction of the response variable from the predictor variable will decrease as the degree of correlation between the two variables increases. Therefore, the $r^2$ is a useful measure when predicting value for one variable from a second variable.

Some computer software packages will list an **adjusted $r^2$** along with the normal coefficient of determination when providing output for linear regression. The $r^2$ calculated previously is an estimate of the population coefficient of determination. $R^2$. Expressed as a percentage, the $r^2$ can be modified from Eq. 14.9 to be expressed as follows:

$$r^2 = \frac{SS_{explained}}{SS_{total}} x\ 100\% \qquad \text{Eq. 14.11}$$

or it can be rewritten in terms of the unexplained sum of squares:

$$r^2 = 1 - \frac{SS_{unexplained}}{SS_{total}} x\ 100\% \qquad \text{Eq. 14.12}$$

Both equations will give the same results. The adjusted coefficient of determination provides an approximate unbiased estimate of the population $R^2$. The formula is a follows:

$$Adj.R^2 = 1 - \frac{\dfrac{SS_{unexplained}}{n-p}}{\dfrac{SS_{total}}{n-1}} x\ 100\% \qquad \text{Eq. 14.13}$$

where $p$ is the number of variables involved in the evaluation (in simple linear regression $p = 2$). As will be seen in for multiple regression models, as the number of independent (predictor) variables increase the $p$ value will increase. For our previous example with the data from Table 14.1, the $r^2$ was 98.5%. The adjusted $R^2$ is:

$$r^2 = 1 - \frac{\dfrac{0.61}{8-2}}{\dfrac{41.4}{8-1}} x\ 100\% = 1 - \frac{0.1016}{5.9143} x\ 100\% = 98.3\%$$

**ANOVA Table**

Once we have established that there is a strong positive or negative relationship between the two continuous variables, we can establish the type of relationship (linear, curvilinear, etc.). This final decision on the acceptability of the linear regression model is based on an objective ANOVA test where a statistical test will determine whether the data is best represented by a straight line:

$H_0$: X and Y are not linearly related
$H_1$: X and Y are linearly related

In this case the ANOVA statistic is:

$$F = \frac{Mean\ Square\ Linear\ Regression}{Mean\ Square\ Residual} \qquad \text{Eq. 14.14}$$

where the amount of variability explained by the regression line is placed in the numerator and the unexplained residual, or error, variability is the denominator. Obviously as the amount of explained variability increases the *F*-value will increase and it becomes more likely that the result will be a rejection of the null hypothesis in favor of the alternative that a straight line relationship exists. The decision rule is, with $\alpha = 0.05$, reject $H_0$ if $F > F_{1,n-2}(1 - \alpha)$. The numerator degrees of freedom is one for the regression line, since the regression line is an estimate of two parameters ($\alpha$ and $\beta$) and degrees of freedom are the number of parameter minus one ($df = 2 - 1$). The denominator degrees of freedom is $n - 2$, where $n$ equals the number of data points. The first page for Table B7 in Appendix B contains the critical values for one as the numerator degrees of freedom and a larger finite set of denominator degrees of freedom. Similar to the one-way ANOVA, the computed $F$ is compared with the critical F-value in Table B7, and if it is greater than the critical value, the null hypothesis that no linear relationship exists between $x$ and $y$ is rejected. The ANOVA table is calculated as follows:

| Source of Variation | df | SS | MS | F |
|---|---|---|---|---|
| Linear Regression | 1 | Explained | $SS_{Explained}/1$ | $MS_{Explained}/$ $MS_{Unexplained}$ |
| Residual | n − 2 | Unexplained | $SS_{Unexplained}/n - 2$ | |
| Total | n − 1 | Total | | |

As an example of linear regression, assume that twelve healthy male volunteers received a single dose of various strengths of an experimental anticoagulant. As the primary investigators, we wish to determine if there is a significant relationship between the dosage and corresponding prothrombin times. In this case the independent variable is the dosage of the drug administered to the volunteers and the dependent variable is their response, measured by their prothrombin times. Results of the study are presented in Table 14.3. The hypotheses in this case are:

$H_0$: Dose ($x$) and pro-time ($y$) are not linearly related
$H_1$: Dose and pro-time are linearly related

**Table 14.3** Prothrombin Times for Volunteers Receiving Various Doses of an Anticoagulant

| Subject | Dose (mg) | Prothrombin Time (seconds) | Subject | Dose (mg) | Prothrombin Time (seconds) |
|---|---|---|---|---|---|
| 1 | 200 | 20 | 7 | 220 | 19 |
| 2 | 180 | 18 | 8 | 175 | 17 |
| 3 | 225 | 20 | 9 | 215 | 20 |
| 4 | 205 | 19 | 10 | 185 | 19 |
| 5 | 190 | 19 | 11 | 210 | 19 |
| 6 | 195 | 18 | 12 | 230 | 20 |

**Table 14.4** Summations of Data Required for Linear Regression

| Subject | Dose (mg) | Time (seconds) | $x^2$ | $y^2$ | xy |
|---|---|---|---|---|---|
| 8 | 175 | 17 | 30625 | 289 | 2975 |
| 2 | 180 | 18 | 32400 | 324 | 3240 |
| 10 | 185 | 19 | 34225 | 361 | 3515 |
| 5 | 190 | 19 | 36100 | 361 | 3610 |
| 6 | 195 | 18 | 38025 | 324 | 3510 |
| 1 | 200 | 20 | 40000 | 400 | 4000 |
| 4 | 205 | 19 | 42025 | 361 | 3895 |
| 11 | 210 | 19 | 44100 | 361 | 3990 |
| 9 | 215 | 20 | 46225 | 400 | 4300 |
| 7 | 220 | 19 | 48400 | 361 | 4180 |
| 3 | 225 | 20 | 50625 | 400 | 4500 |
| 12 | 230 | 20 | 52900 | 400 | 4600 |
| $\Sigma =$ | 2430 | 228 | 495650 | 4342 | 46315 |

and the decision rule with $\alpha = .05$, is to reject $H_0$ if $F > F_{1,10}(.95)$, which is 4.96. The tabular arrangement of the data needed to calculate an ANOVA table is presented in Table 14.4. First the slope and *y*-intercept for the regression line would be:

$$b = \frac{n\sum xy - (\sum x)(\sum y)}{n\sum x^2 - (\sum x)^2}$$

$$b = \frac{12(46315) - (2430)(228)}{12(495650) - (2430)^2} = \frac{1740}{42900} = 0.0406$$

$$a = \frac{\sum y - b\sum x}{n}$$

$$a = \frac{228 - (0.0406)(2430)}{12} = \frac{129.342}{12} = 10.7785$$

In this case there would a gradual positive slope to the line (as dosage increases, the prothrombin time increases) and the predicted *y*-intercept would be 10.78 seconds. The total variability around the mean prothrombin time is:

$$SS_T = \Sigma y^2 - \frac{(\Sigma y)^2}{n}$$

$$SS_T = 4342 - \frac{(228)^2}{12} = 10.0$$

of which the regression line explains a certain amount of variation:

$$SS_E = b^2 \cdot \left[ \Sigma x^2 - \frac{(\Sigma x)^2}{n} \right]$$

$$SS_E = (0.0406)^2 \left[ 495650 - \frac{(2430)^2}{12} \right] = 5.8811$$

However, an additional amount of variation remains unexplained:

$$SS_U = SS_T - SS_E = 10.0 - 5.8811 = 4.1189$$

For this particular example the coefficient of determination is:

$$r^2 = \frac{SS_{explained}}{SS_{total}} = \frac{5.8811}{10} = 0.5881$$

meaning that only approximately 59% of the total variability is explained by the straight line that we drew among the data points. The ANOVA table would be:

| Source | SS | df | MS | F |
|---|---|---|---|---|
| Linear Regression | 5.8811 | 1 | 5.8811 | 14.278 |
| Residual | 4.1189 | 10 | 0.4119 | |
| Total | 10.00 | 11 | | |

The resultant *F*-value is greater than the critical value of 4.96, therefore we would reject $H_0$ and conclude that a linear relationship exists between the dosage of the new anticoagulant and the volunteers' prothrombin times.

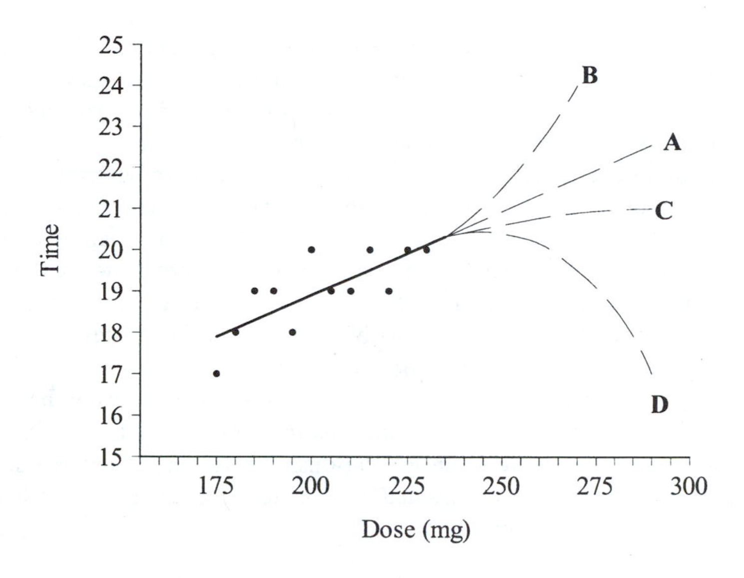


**Figure 14.4** Example of the problems associated with extrapolation.

Once the type of relationship is established, it is possible to predict values for the dependent variable (prothrombin time) based on the corresponding value for the independent variable (dose). Obviously, the accuracy of any prediction, based on a regression line, depends on the strength of the relationship between the two variables (the higher coefficient of determination the better our predictive abilities). Use of the regression analysis enables the researcher to determine the nature (i.e., linear) and strength of the relationship, and allows for predictions to be made.

It is important to realize that the linear regression line, which fit best between our data points, cannot be extrapolated beyond the largest or smallest point for our observations (to predict $y_c$ values for $x_i$ values outside the observed range of $x_i$). For example, in our previous example we identified a linear relationship between the dose of the experimental anticoagulant and volunteer prothrombin times. This linear relationship is illustrated by the solid line in Figure 14.4. What we do not know is what will happen beyond 230 mg, the highest dose. Could a linear relationship continue (*A*), might there be an acceleration in the anticoagulant effect (*B*), a leveling of response (*C*) or an actual decrease in prothromin time with increased doses (*D*)? Correspondingly, we do not know what the relationship is for responses at dosages less than 175 mg of the experimental anticoagulant. If more data were available beyond the last data point, it might be found that the regression line would level out or decrease sharply. Therefore, the regression line and the regression equation apply only within the range of the *x*-values actually observed in the sample data.

### Confidence Intervals and Hypothesis Testing for the Population Slope ($\beta$)

With linear regression we are dealing with sample data and the only way to accurately determine the population parameters of slope ($\beta$) and intercept ($\alpha$) would be to collect all the data for the entire population. Since in most cases this would be impossible, we have to estimate these parameters using our sample data and our best estimates, the sample slope ($b$) and sample intercept ($a$).

The correlation coefficient ($r$) and slope of the line ($b$) are descriptive statistics that define different aspects of the relationship between two continuous variables. When either $r$ or $b$ equal zero, there is no linear correlation and variables $x$ and $y$ can be considered independent of each other, and no mutual interdependence exists. An alternative test to our previously discussed ANOVA test for linearity, is a null hypothesis that no linear relationship exists between the two variables. This is based on the population slope ($\beta$) of the regression line. In general, a positive $\beta$ indicates that $y$ increases as $x$ increases, and represents a direct linear relationship between the two variables. Conversely, a negative $\beta$ indicates that values of $y$ tend to increase as values of $x$ decrease, and an inverse linear relationship between $x$ and y exists.

The hypothesis under test assumes that there is no slope; therefore, a relationship between the variables does not exist:

$$H_0: \beta = 0$$
$$H_1: \beta \neq 0$$

In this case we can either: 1) calculate a $t$-value and compare it to a critical value or 2) compute a confidence interval for all possible slopes for the population ($\beta$). The calculation of the $t$-value is similar to a paired t-test with an observed difference in the numerator and an error term in the denominator:

$$t = \frac{b - \beta_0}{S_b} \qquad \text{Eq. 14.15}$$

Based on the null hypothesis, $\beta_0$ is an expected outcome of zero or no slope and $S_b$ is an error term that is defined below.

Calculation of the error term involves variability about the regression line. The variation in the individual $y_i$ values about the regression line can be estimated by measuring their variation from the regression line for the sample data. The standard deviation for these observed $y_i$ values is termed the **standard error of estimate** ($S_{y/x}$) and is calculated as follows:

$$S_{y/x} = \sqrt{\frac{\Sigma(y_i - y_c)^2}{n-2}} = \sqrt{MS_{residual}} \qquad \text{Eq. 14.16}$$

where the numerator is $SS_{unexplained}$ and the denominator is the degree of freedom associated with the unexplained error. Thus, the standard error of estimate equals the square root of the mean square residual from the ANOVA table. If there is no relationship between the two continuous variables, the slope of the regression equation should be zero. The value $S_{y/x}$ is also referred to as the **residual standard**

**deviation.**

The standard error of the estimate could be used as a measure of precision for the regression line to predict a dependent variable ($y_i$) for a given independent value ($x_i$):

$$y = a + bx \pm S_{y/x} \qquad \text{Eq. 14.17}$$

The magnitude of $S_{y/x}$ is proportional to the magnitude of the $y$-variable and a poor method for comparing different regressions. To standardize this error term, it has been recommend that the standard error of the estimate be divided by the mean of $y$-axis (Dapson, 1980, p. 545). This creates a relative standard deviation for the regression line:

$$RSD_{regression} = \frac{S_{y/x}}{\overline{X}_y} x\ 100\% \qquad \text{Eq. 14.18}$$

For this particular example, the mean on the $y$-axis is 19 (228/12). Therefore, the RSD for the regression line would be:

$$RSD_{regression} = \frac{\sqrt{0.4119}}{19} x\ 100\% = 3.38\%$$

To test the null hypothesis $H_0$: $\beta = 0$, we need to calculate a standard error of the sample slope ($b$), which is our estimate of population slope ($\beta$):

$$S_b = \frac{S_{y/x}}{\sqrt{\Sigma(x_i - \overline{X})^2}} \qquad \text{Eq. 14.19}$$

where the sum of the deviations on the $x$-axis is:

$$\Sigma(x_i - \overline{X})^2 = \Sigma x^2 - \frac{(\Sigma x)^2}{n} \qquad \text{Eq. 14.20}$$

from data collected in tables such as Table 14.3 and the mean square residual from the ANOVA table. The formula can be simplified to:

$$S_b = \sqrt{\frac{MS_{residual}}{\Sigma x^2 - \frac{(\Sigma x)^2}{n}}} \qquad \text{Eq. 14.21}$$

The decision rule is to reject $H_0$ (no slope) if $t$ in Eq. 14.15 is greater than $t_{n-2}(1 - \alpha/2)$ or less than $-t_{n-2}(1 - \alpha/2)$ for a two-tailed test. With regression, we are dealing with sample data that provides the information for the calculation for an intercept ($a$) and slope ($b$), which are estimates of the true population $\alpha$ and $\beta$. Because they are samples, they are subject to random error similar to previously discussed sample statistics. The number of degrees of freedom is $n - 2$. The number two subtracted from the sample size represents the two approximations in our data: 1) the sample slope as an estimate of $\beta$ and 2) the sample $y$-axis intercept as an estimate for $\alpha$.

As noted, a second parallel approach would be to calculate a confidence interval for the possible slopes for the population:

$$\beta = b \pm t_{n-2}(1-\alpha/2) \cdot S_b \qquad \text{Eq. 14.22}$$

In this case the sample slope ($b$) is the best estimate of the population slope ($\beta$) defined in Eq. 14.1:

$$\mu_{y/x} = \alpha + \beta x$$

By creating a confidence interval we can estimate, with 95% confidence, the true population slope ($\beta$). As with previous confidence intervals, if zero falls within the confidence interval the result of no slope is a possible outcome; therefore, one fails to reject the null hypothesis and must assume there is no slope in the true population and thus no relationship between the two continuous variables.

Using our example of the twelve healthy male volunteers who received a single dose of various strengths of an experimental anticoagulant (Tables 14.3 and 14.4), one could determine if there was a significant relationship between the dosage and the corresponding prothrombin time exist by determining if there is a slope to the regression line for the population, based on sample data, has a slope. Once again, the null hypothesis states that there is no slope in the population:

$$H_0: \beta = 0$$
$$H_1: \beta \neq 0$$

The decision rule is, with $\alpha = 0.05$, reject $H_0$ if $|t| > t_{10}(1 - \alpha/2)$ which equals 2.228 (Table B5, Appendix B). The calculation of $S_b$ is:

$$S_b = \sqrt{\frac{MS_{residual}}{\sum x^2 - \frac{(\sum x)^2}{n}}}$$

$$S_b = \sqrt{\frac{0.4119}{495650 - \frac{(2430)^2}{12}}} = \sqrt{\frac{0.4119}{3575}} = 0.0107$$

and the calculation of the $t$-statistics is:

$$t = \frac{b - 0}{S_b} = \frac{0.0406 - 0}{0.0107} = 3.794$$

The decision in this case is, with $t > 2.228$, to reject $H_0$ and conclude that there is a slope, thus a relationship exists between dosage and prothrombin times. Note that the results are identical to those seen in the ANOVA test. In fact, the square of the *t*-statistic equals our previous *F*-value ($3.79^2 \approx 14.27$, with rounding errors).

A possibly more valuable piece of information is obtained by calculating the 95% confidence interval that estimates the true population slope:

$$\beta = b \pm t_{n-2}(1 - \alpha/2) \cdot S_b$$

For our example the estimate on $\beta$ would be:

$$\beta = 0.0406 \pm 2.228(0.0107) = 0.0406 \pm 0.0238$$

$$0.0168 < \beta < 0.0644$$

Since zero does not fall within the confidence interval, $\beta = 0$ is not a possible outcome, therefore $H_0$ is rejected once again and the researcher concludes that a relationship exists between the two variables. It is possible to predict, with 95% confidence, that the true population slope is somewhere between +0.0168 and +0.0644. Figure 14.5 illustrates that even though our sample date provides us with an estimate of the slope ($b = +0.04$), the true slope for the population could range for a +0.0168 to +0.0644 around the mean on the *x*-axis.

$$\overline{X} = \frac{\Sigma x}{n} = \frac{2430}{12} = 202.5$$

If the null hypothesis is rejected in favor of the alternate hypothesis, that $\beta \neq 0$, then higher values of *x* would correspond with higher predicted values of *y*. In this case, there would be a positive correlation.

As mentioned previously, the population slope ($\beta$) is sometimes referred to as the population regression coefficient. An alternative formula for calculating the slope is:

$$b = r \cdot \frac{S_y}{S_x} \qquad \text{Eq. 14.23}$$

where *r* is our correlation coefficient and the standard deviations for each variable are represented by standard deviations for each axis ($S_x$ and $S_y$). In the above example of prothrombin times, the standard deviation of the *x*-variable (dosage) is 18.0278, the standard deviation for the *y*-variable (protime) is 0.9535 and the correlation coefficient is 0.7676 (square root of $r^2 = 0.5893$).

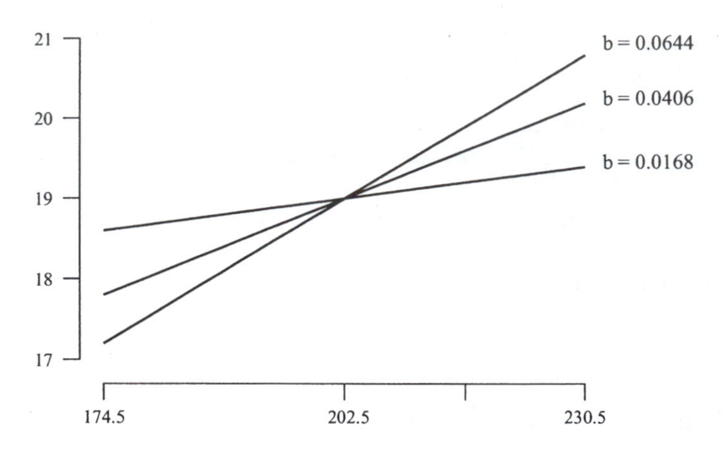


**Figure 14.5** Range of possible population slopes ($\beta$).

$$b = (0.7676)\frac{0.9535}{18.0278} = 0.0406$$

This result is identical to our previous calculation for the slope of the line.

By testing the significance associated with the slope of the regression line we can be certain that the observed linear equation did not represent simply a chance departure from a horizontal line, when there would be no relationship between the two continuous variables. However, using a $t$-test to determine the significance of the relationship, we make additional assumptions that the $y$-values at different levels of $x$ have equal variances and that their distributions are normal in shape.

### Confidence Intervals for the Regression Line

The difference between the observed value and predicted value on our regression line ($y_i - \overline{X}_y$) is our best estimate of the variation of the $y$ population around the true regression line. The variance term $S_{y/x}^2$, or the mean square residual, is an estimate of the variance of the $\overline{Y}$ population about the true population regression line. The **standard deviation about regression** is a third synonym for $S_{y/x}$ and is more meaningful than the variance term and signifies the standard deviation of $y$ at a given $x$-value.

As discussed previously, for a given value on the $x$-axis it is possible to estimate a corresponding $y$-value using $y = a + bx$. Also, because we assume data is normally distributed on the $y$-axis for any point on the $x$-axis, a confidence interval for the expected $y$-value can be computed using a modification of the formula for the hypothesis test of the slope.

$$y = y_c \pm t_{n-2}(1-\alpha/2) \cdot \sqrt{MS_{residual}} \cdot \sqrt{\frac{1}{n} + \frac{(x_i - \overline{X})^2}{\sum x^2 - \frac{(\sum x)^2}{n}}} \qquad \text{Eq. 14.24}$$

where the $MS_{residual}$ is the mean square residual from the ANOVA table in the original regression analysis. Assuming that each point on the regression line ($y_c$) gives the best representation (mean) of the distribution of scores, it is possible to estimate the mean of $y$ for any point on the $x$-axis.

In calculating the 95% confidence interval around the regression line, it is assumed that data are approximately normally distributed in the vertical direction along the $y$-axis (this may require transformation of the data before any of the previous calculations). If we have a large sample size, we would expect that approximately 95% of our prediction errors fall within ± 1.96 $S_{y/x}$. The errors in predicting $y$ for a given value of $x$ are due to several factors. Obviously, there is random variation of $y$ about the true regression line that is expressed as $S_{y/x}$. In addition there is an error in estimating the $y$-axis intercept of the true regression line ($\alpha$) and an error in estimating the slope of the true regression line ($\beta$). Because of the error due to estimating the slope of the line, the error in the estimate of the slope will become more pronounced for values of the independent variable ($x_i$) as those values deviate more from the center (the mean $x$-value, $\overline{X}$). This produces a bowing of the **confidence bands** as seen in Figure 14.6. The point at which the deviation is least, or where the confidence interval is the smallest, is at the mean for the observed $x$-values. This would seem logical since we expect less error as one moves to the middle of the distribution for $x$-values and we expect a larger error as one approaches the extreme areas of the data.

Once again, we will use the previous anticoagulant example to illustrate the determination of confidence intervals. With 95% confidence, what is the expected mean prothrombin time at a dosage of 210 mg of the anticoagulant? Based on the previous data in Table 14.3 we know the following: $\sum x$ = 2,430; $\sum x^2$ = 495,650 and $n$ = 12. The mean for the independent variable is:

$$\overline{X} = \frac{\sum x}{n} = \frac{2430}{12} = 202.5$$

Based on previous calculations the slope ($b$) is 0.04 and the $y$-intercept ($a$) is 10.9. Lastly, from the analysis of variance table, the mean square residual ($S_{x/y}^2$) is 0.4107. Using this data the first step is to calculate the $y_c$ value for each point on the regression line for values of the independent variable ($x_i$). The $y_c$ would be the best estimate of the center for the interval. For example, the expected value on the regression line at 210 mg would be:

$$y_c = a + bx_i = 10.9 + 0.04(210) = 19.3$$

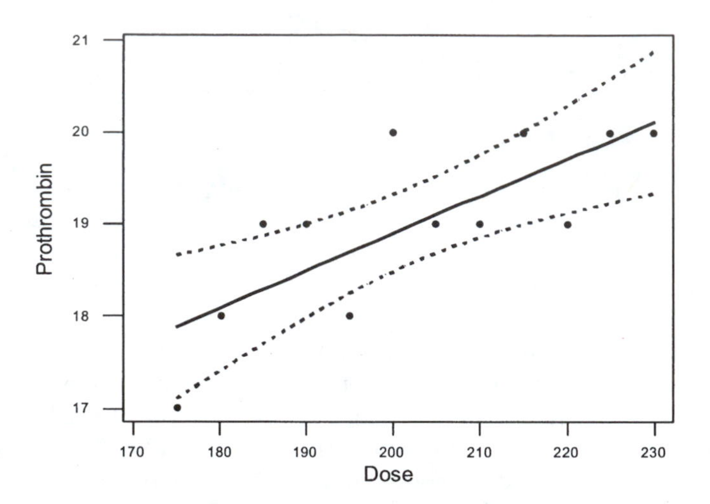


**Figure 14.6** Graphic illustration of 95% confidence intervals (created using Minitab® Release 12.21).

The calculation of the confidence interval around the regression line at 210 mg of drug would be:

$$\bar{y} = 19.3 \pm 2.228\sqrt{0.4107}\sqrt{\frac{1}{12} + \frac{(210 - 202.5)^2}{495650 - \frac{(2430)^2}{12}}}$$

$$\bar{y} = 19.3 \pm 2.228(0.6409)\sqrt{0.0833 + \frac{56.25}{3575}} = 19.3 \pm 0.449$$

$$18.851 < \bar{y} < 19.749$$

Thus, based on sample data and the regression line that fits best between the data points, the researcher could conclude with 95% confidence that the true population mean for a dosage of 210 mg would be between 18.85 and 19.75 seconds. Results from the calculation of the confidence intervals at the various levels of drug used are presented in Table 14.5 and is graphically represented in Figure 14.6.

**Inverse Prediction**

As seen in the previous section, the original prediction of $y$ for any given $x$ using the straight line equation is:

$$y = a + bx$$

**Table 14.5** 95% Confidence Intervals at Selected Dosages

| Dose (mg) | Time (seconds) | $y_c$ | Lower Limit | Upper Limit | Range |
|---|---|---|---|---|---|
| 175 | 17 | 17.9 | 17.10 | 18.70 | 1.60 |
| 180 | 18 | 18.1 | 17.40 | 18.80 | 1.40 |
| 190 | 19 | 18.5 | 17.98 | 19.02 | 1.04 |
| 200 | 20 | 18.9 | 18.47 | 19.33 | 0.86 |
| 210 | 19 | 19.3 | 18.85 | 19.75 | 0.90 |
| 220 | 19 | 19.7 | 19.10 | 20.30 | 1.20 |
| 230 | 20 | 20.1 | 19.31 | 20.89 | 1.58 |

This offers a quick estimate, but a more exact estimate is the confidence interval (Eq. 14.24) at any point on the independent variable, the $x$-axis. Similarly, Eq. 14.3 is only a quick estimate of a possible value of the $x$-axis for any given value of the dependent ($y$-axis) variable. Following the same logic as the previous calculations (Eq. 14.24), a 95% confidence interval can be created on the $x$-axis around the value $x_i$ determined by Eq. 14.3.

$$x = x_i + \frac{b(y_i - \bar{y})}{K} \pm \frac{t}{K}\sqrt{MS_{residual}}\sqrt{\frac{(y_i - \bar{y})^2}{\sum x^2 - \frac{(\sum x)^2}{n}} + K\left(1 + \frac{1}{n}\right)} \qquad \text{Eq. 14.25}$$

where the intermediate $K$ is based on the slope, the critical t-value and standard deviation about the line $S_b$:

$$K = b^2 - t^2 S_b^2 \qquad \text{Eq. 14.26}$$

For example, assume we want to predict a dosage that would be required to produce a prothrombin time of 20. In this case the $y$-value was 195, $\bar{y}$ was 19 (228/12) and the slope was calculated to be 0.04. The t-value remains the same for a 95% confidence interval (2.228) and the $S_b$ was previously calculated. The best estimate of $x$ , with 95% confidence, would be:

$$x = \frac{y - a}{b} = \frac{20 - 10.7785}{0.0406} = 227.13\ mg$$

The 95% confidence interval around that best estimate would be:

$$K = (0.0406)^2 - (2.228)^2(0.0107)^2 = 0.00108$$

$$x = 227.13 + \frac{0.0406(20-19)}{0.00108} \pm \frac{2.228}{0.00108}\sqrt{0.4119} \cdot \sqrt{\frac{(20-19)^2}{495650 - \frac{(2430)^2}{12}} + 0.00108\left(1+\frac{1}{12}\right)}$$

$$x = 264.7226 \pm 1323.9980\sqrt{0.00145} = 264.7226 \pm 50.4163$$

$$214.31 < x < 315.14$$

Thus, with 95% confidence, the true dosage to obtain a prothrombin time of 20 is somewhere between 214.31 and 315.14 mg of drug. This computation is sometimes referred to as **inverse prediction.** Note in the previously worked out example that the confidence interval is asymmetric around the estimated $x$-value. The inverse prediction interval is symmetrical only at the mean for sample data on the $y$-axis. The interval becomes more asymmetrical as $y$-values become more distant from the mean.

## Multiple Data at Various Points on the Independent Variable

What if the data represents multiple (i.e., duplicate, triplicate) measures at the same points for the independent variable? Obviously, more data at each point on the $x$-axis, will provide a better estimate of the true population values and should create a smaller confidence interval for both the estimate of $\beta$ and the intervals around the line of least-squares. For illustrative purposes, let us use the previous example of doses for an experimental anticoagulant vs. the resultant pro-time. In an alternative Scenario A, let us assume these represent the results for three different patients at each dose and by chance each patient presented with the exact same results (i.e., in Table 14.3 three subjects received 175 mg of drug and all three responded with pro-times of 17 seconds). In Scenario B, again there are three patients but by chance the patients at each dosage varies by one second around the mean seen in the original data (i.e., in Table 14.3 three subjects receiving 180 mg of the drug and their responses were pro-times of 17, 18, and 19 seconds). In Scenario A we would expect the data to produce a much tighter estimate of $\beta$ and confidence interval around the line. Because of variability in the results in Scenario B we would again expect tighter estimates due to the fact that our sample size has increased three-fold, but because of increased variability estimates should not be as tight as those seen in Scenario A.

The calculations would be the same as those originally used for the data in Table 14.3, but now the number of data points will increase from 12 to 36. Results of the three outcomes are presented in Table 14.6. Results are as expected due to the greater sample size and more information about the population.

**Table 14.6** Scenarios, Results with Triplicate Measures

| | Original Data | Scenario A | Scenario B |
|---|---|---|---|
| n | 12 | 36 | 36 |
| Slope | 0.0406 | 0.0406 | 0.0406 |
| Intercept | 10.78 | 10.78 | 10.78 |
| Coefficient of Determination | 0.5881 | 0.5881 | 0.3267 |
| F (p) | 14.27 (0.0036) | 48.55 (<0.0001) | 16.50 (0.0003) |
| β | 0.0166<<0.0645 | 0.0287<<0.0524 | 0.0203<<0.0609 |
| β range | 0.479 | 0.0237 | 0.0406 |
| CI at 210 | 18.851<<19.749 | 19.082<<19.527 | 18.922<<19.686 |
| Range at 210 | 0.898 | 0.445 | 0.764 |
| CI at 175 | 17.108<<18.661 | 17.501<<18.269 | 17.226<<18.544 |
| Range at 175 | 1.553 | 0.768 | 1.318 |

**Assessing Parallelism of the Slopes of Two Samples**

At times the researcher may wish to compare the linear regression lines from two different samples to determine if there are any statistical differences between the two slopes or distance between the lines (i.e., *y*-intercepts are different). When comparing the slopes for two samples to determine if the slopes for their respective populations are the same, the hypotheses being tested are as follows:

$$H_0: \beta_1 = \beta_2$$
$$H_1: \beta_1 \neq \beta_2$$

If the null hypothesis is rejected, the two population slopes are different. The best estimate for the population slopes would be the sample slopes, $b_1$ and $b_2$. The evaluation of parallelism is handled similarly to the ratio method for dealing with a two-sample t-test (Chapter 9); where the numerator is the best guess of the difference $(b_1 - b_2)$ and the denominator contains an error term (as will be seen in Eq.14.28). The first step is to create a weighted average deviation term, analogous to the pooled variance in the two-sample t-test (Eq. 9.3). In this case we create what is called a **pooled residual mean square,** a term that represents the addition of the two sum of squares residuals ($SS_R$) for each slope (this involves calculating an ANOVA table for each regression line) divided by their respective degrees of freedom ($n - 2$):

$$(S^2_{x/y})_p = \frac{SS_{R1}}{n_1 - 2} + \frac{SS_{R2}}{n_2 - 2} = \frac{SS_{R1} + SS_{R2}}{n_1 + n_2 - 4} \qquad \text{Eq. 14.27}$$

This pooled residual mean square then becomes part of the denominator in the calculation of the *t*-statistic. Notice the similarities between this equation and the two-sample t-test (Eq. 9.6):

$$t = \frac{b_1 - b_2}{\sqrt{\dfrac{(S^2_{x/y})_p}{\sum x_1^2 - \dfrac{(\sum x_1)^2}{n_1}} + \dfrac{(S^2_{x/y})_p}{\sum x_2^2 - \dfrac{(\sum x_2)^2}{n_2}}}} \qquad \text{Eq. 14.28}$$

Assessment of significance is determined by comparing the calculated *t*-value with the critical value off a t-table (Table B5 in Appendix B) for $1 - \alpha/2$ level of significance and the appropriate degrees of freedom ($n_1 + n_2 - 4$).

A confidence interval can be used also to assess parallelism, by creating the interval and determining if zero falls within the interval. Once again, this interval is analogous to the interval created for the two-sample t-test (Eq. 9.4):

$$\beta_1 - \beta_2 = (b_1 - b_2) \pm$$

$$t_{n_1-n_2-4}(1-\alpha/2)\sqrt{\frac{(S^2_{x/y})_p}{\sum x_1^2 - \dfrac{(\sum x_1)^2}{n_1}} + \frac{(S^2_{x/y})_p}{\sum x_2^2 - \dfrac{(\sum x_2)^2}{n_2}}} \qquad \text{Eq. 14.29}$$

If the null hypothesis is rejected ($t > t_{critical}$ or $t < -t_{critical}$) we can assume that the two lines do not have the same slopes and are not parallel to each other.

As an example, assume the following data has been collected at a pharmacy department in a large Eastern hospital for two different suspensions of a carbonic anhydrase inhibitor. Table 14.7 lists the results for the two formulations (Suspension B involving a sugar-free vehicle). Results of the various calculations are presented in Table 14.8. The null hypothesis would be that both suspensions degrade at the same rate, illustrated by the fact that the slopes of the two regression lines are equal:

$$H_0: \beta_A = \beta_B$$
$$H_1: \beta_A \neq \beta_B$$

Additional information needed to evaluate the results of the study is presented in Table 14.9. The calculation to assess parallelism (using the t-ratio approach) would be as follows:

$$(S^2_{x/y})_p = \frac{0.408 + 0.275}{8} = 0.085$$

**Table 14.7** Stability Data for Suspensions

| | % Labeled Amount | |
|---|---|---|
| Time (months) | Suspension A | Suspension B |
| 0 | 99.2 | 99.50 |
| 1 | 98.7 | 98.80 |
| 2 | 96.9 | 97.10 |
| 2.5 | - | 96.50 |
| 3 | 96.1 | 95.90 |
| 3.5 | - | 95.40 |
| 4 | 95.5 | 95.10 |

**Table 14.8** Summary Results for Suspensions

| | Suspension A | Suspension B |
|---|---|---|
| $n$ | 5 | 7 |
| $\Sigma x$ | 10 | 16 |
| $\Sigma y$ | 486.4 | 678.3 |
| $\Sigma x^2$ | 30 | 48.50 |
| $\Sigma y^2$ | 47327.40 | 65744.33 |
| $\Sigma xy$ | 962.8 | 1536.25 |
| $b$ | −1.000 | −1.186 |
| $a$ | 99.28 | 99.61 |
| $SS_T$ | 10.408 | 17.060 |
| $SS_E$ | 10.0 | 16.785 |
| $SS_R$ | 0.408 | 0.275 |
| $F$ $(p)$ | 73.5 (p=0.003) | 305.3 (p<0.001) |

**Table 14.9** Additional Summary Results for Suspensions

| | Suspension A | Suspension B |
|---|---|---|
| $n$ | 5 | 7 |
| $df$ | 3 | 5 |
| $\Sigma x$ | 10 | 16 |
| $\Sigma x^2$ | 30 | 48.50 |
| $b$ | −1.000 | −1.186 |
| $SS_R$ | 0.408 | 0.275 |

$$t = \frac{-1.000 - (-1.186)}{\sqrt{\dfrac{0.085}{30 - \dfrac{(10)^2}{5}} + \dfrac{0.085}{48.5 - \dfrac{(16)^2}{7}}}} = \frac{0.186}{0.125} = 1.488$$

The decision rule would be, with $\alpha$ = .05, reject $H_0$ if $t > t_8(.975)$ or $t < t_8(.975)$, which is 2.306 from Table B5 for $n_1 + n_2 - 4$ degrees of freedom. With 1.488 < 2.306, we fail to reject the null hypothesis and cannot identify a significant difference between the slopes for the two carbonic anhydrase inhibitor suspensions. Creation of a confidence interval confirms that the difference of

$$H_0:\ \beta_1 - \beta_2 = 0$$

is a possible outcome that falls within the interval:

$$\beta_1 - \beta_2 = (-1-(-1.186)) \pm 2.306\sqrt{\frac{0.085}{30-\frac{(10)^2}{5}}+\frac{0.085}{48.5-\frac{(16)^2}{7}}}$$

$$\beta_1 - \beta_2 = (+0.186) \pm (2.306)(0.125) = +0.186 \pm 0.288$$

$$-0.102 < \beta_1 - \beta_2 < 0.474$$

As seen in Figure 14.7, the two slopes are in identical, but relatively close, especially considering the results are based on only a total of 12 data points. Unfortunately, if we fail to reject the null hypothesis we do not prove that the two lines are parallel, we simply fail to identify a difference. Problems with this approach to assessing parallelism have been discussed by Hauck (Hauck, 2005).

## Multiple Linear Regression Models

**Multiple regression** is a logical extension of the concepts illustrated for a simple regression model where one is dealing with only two continuous variables. With simple regression analysis, we were concerned with identifying the line which best fits between our data points (Eq. 14.2):

$$y = a + \beta x + e$$

Rather than using values on one predictor or independent variable, as we did with the simple regression analysis (to estimate values on a criterion or dependent variable), with multiple regression we can control for several independent variables. By using many predictor variables, we will hopefully reduce our error of prediction even further, by accounting for more of the variance. Multiple linear regression is a powerful multivariate statistical technique for controlling any number of confounding variables:

$$y_j = a + \beta_1 x_1 + \beta_2 x_2 + \beta_2 x_2 + \ldots + \beta_j x_j + e_j \qquad \text{Eq. 14.30}$$

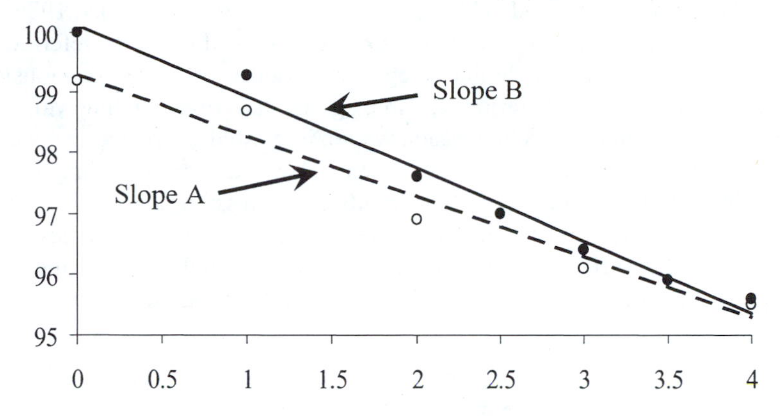


**Figure 14.7** Graphic illustration of two similar slopes.

where $y_j$ is the value of the independent variable and $j$ is the number of independent variables. The values of $\beta_1$, $\beta_2$ ... $\beta_k$ in the equation are referred by several synonyms including **beta coefficients**, **beta weights**, and **regression coefficients**.

The beta coefficients indicate the relative importance of the various independent predictor variables and are based on their standardized $z$ score. The prediction equation can be written as:

$$z_y = \beta_1 z_1 + \beta_2 z_2 + \beta_3 z_3 + \ldots \beta_k z_k \qquad \text{Eq. 14.31}$$

These beta weights are estimates of their corresponding coefficients for the population equation in standardized $z$ score form. These beta coefficients are also referred to as **partial regression coefficients**, because these regression coefficients are related to the partial correlation coefficients, which were discussed in Chapter 13.

As seen in the previous chapter, the multiple correlation coefficient ($R$) indicates the correlation for a weighted sum of the predictor variables and the criterion variable. The squared multiple correlation coefficient ($R^2$) will indicate the proportion of the variance for the dependent criterion variable, which is accounted for by combining the various predictor variables.

Unlike simple regression analysis, which was represented by a straight line, multiple regression represents "planes in multidimensional space, a concept admittedly difficult to conceive and virtually impossible to portray graphically" (Kachigan, 1991). Instead of thinking of a least-squares line to fit our data, we must think of a least-squares solution based on weighted values for each of the various predictor variables. Using computer software it is possible to calculate the appropriate beta weights to create the least-squares solution, with those having the greatest correlation having the largest weight.

The calculations for multiple linear regression analysis are extensive, complex, and fall beyond the scope of this book. Excellent references for additional information on this topic include Zar (1999), Snedecor and Cochran (1989), and the

Sage University series (Berry and Feldman, 1985; Achen, 1982; Schroeder, 1986).

Regression analysis allows us to make **predictions**, and could be referred to as **prediction analysis**. In the simple linear regression model, discussed previously, we can predict a value on the criterion variable, given its corresponding value on a predictor variable. With multiple regression we are interested in predicting a value for the criterion variable given the value on each of several corresponding predictor variables. The primary objectives of a multiple regression analysis are to: 1) determine whether a relationship exists between two continuous variables; 2) if a relationship exists, describe the nature of the relationship; and 3) assess the relative importance of the various predictor variables to contribute variation in the criterion variable.

## References

Achen, C.H. (1982). *Interpreting and Using Regression* (paper 29), Sage University Series on Quantitative Applications in the Social Sciences, Sage Publications, Newbury Park, CA.

Berry, W.D. and Feldman, S. (1985). *Multiple Regression in Practice* (paper 50), Sage University Series on Quantitative Applications in the Social Sciences, Sage Publications, Newbury Park, CA.

Dapson, R.W. (1980). "Guidelines for Statistical Usage in Age-Estimation Technics," *Journal of Wildlife Management* 44:541-548.

Hauck, W.W. et al. (2005). "Assessing Parallelism Prior to Determining Relative Potency," *PDA Journal of Pharmaceutical Science and Technology* 59:127-137.

Kachigan, S.K. (1991). *Multivariate Statistical Analysis*, Second edition, Radius Press, New York, p. 181.

Schroeder, L.D. et al. (1986). *Understanding Regression Analysis: An Introductory Guide* (paper 57), Sage University Series on Quantitative Applications in the Social Sciences, Sage Publications, Newbury Park, CA.

Snedecor, G.W. and Cochran, W.G. (1989). *Statistical Methods*, Eighth edition, Iowa State University Press, Ames, IA, pp. 333-365.

Zar, J.H. (1999). *Biostatistical Analysis*, Fourth edition, Prentice-Hall, Englewood Cliffs, NJ, pp. 413-450.

## Suggested Supplemental Readings

Bolton, S. (1997). *Pharmaceutical Statistics: Practical and Clinical Applications*, Marcel Dekker, Inc., New York, pp. 216-241.

Daniel, W.W. (1999). *Biostatistics: A Foundation for Analysis in the Health Sciences*, Seventh edition, John Wiley and Sons, New York, pp. 401-429, 474-493.

**Example Problems**

1. Samples of a drug product are stored in their original containers under normal conditions and sampled periodically to analyze the content of the medication.

| Time (months) | Assay (mg) |
|---|---|
| 6 | 995 |
| 12 | 984 |
| 18 | 973 |
| 24 | 960 |
| 36 | 952 |
| 48 | 948 |

Does a linear relationship exist between the two variables? If such a relation exists, what is the slope, *y*-intercept, and 95% confidence interval?

2. Acme Chemical is testing various concentrations of a test solution and the effect the concentration has on the optical density of each concentration.

| Concentration (%) | Optical Density |
|---|---|
| 1 | 0.24 |
| 2 | 0.66 |
| 4 | 1.15 |
| 8 | 2.34 |

Is there a significant linear relationship between the concentration and optical density. If there is a relationship, create a plot representing this relationship and 95% confidence intervals.

3. Acme Chemical reassesses the previous results by comparing the data against a reference standard solution at the same concentrations and found the following results:

| | Optical Density | |
|---|---|---|
| Concentration (%) | Test | Standard |
| 1 | 0.24 | 0.22 |
| 2 | 0.66 | 0.74 |
| 4 | 1.15 | 1.41 |
| 8 | 2.34 | 2.76 |

Were the slopes of the test solution and reference standard parallel?

**Answers to Problems**

1. Comparison of content of a medication at different time periods.
   Variables: continuous independent variable (time in months)
   continuous dependent variable (amount of drug in mg)

   Hypothesis: $H_0$: Time ($x$) and assay results ($y$) are not linearly related
   $H_1$: Time and assay results are linearly related

   Decision Rule: With $\alpha = .05$, reject $H_0$ if $F > F_{1,4}(.95) = 7.71$

   x = time (months) y = assay (mg)

| | x | y | $x^2$ | $y^2$ | xy |
|---|---|---|---|---|---|
| | 6 | 995 | 36 | 990025 | 5970 |
| | 12 | 984 | 144 | 968256 | 11808 |
| | 18 | 973 | 324 | 946729 | 17514 |
| n = 6 | 24 | 960 | 576 | 921600 | 23040 |
| | 36 | 952 | 1296 | 906304 | 34272 |
| | 48 | 948 | 2304 | 898704 | 45504 |
| Σ = | 144 | 5812 | 4680 | 5631618 | 138108 |

Calculations:

Slope and intercept:

$$b = \frac{n\sum xy - (\sum x)(\sum y)}{n\sum x^2 - (\sum x)^2} = \frac{6(138108) - (144)(5812)}{6(4680) - (144)^2} = -1.13$$

$$a = \frac{\sum y - b\sum x}{n} = \frac{5812 - (-1.13)(144)}{6} = 995.78$$

Coefficient of determination:

$$SS_{explained} = b^2\left[\sum x^2 - \frac{(\sum x)^2}{n}\right] = (1.13)^2\left[4680 - \frac{(144)^2}{6}\right] = 1562.93$$

$$SS_{total} = \sum y^2 - \frac{(\sum y)^2}{n} = 5631618 - \frac{(5812)^2}{6} = 1727.33$$

$$SS_{unexplained} = SS_{total} - SS_{explained} = 1727.33 - 1562.93 = 164.40$$

$$r^2 = \frac{SS_{explained}}{SS_{total}} = \frac{1562.93}{1727.33} = 0.905$$

ANOVA Table:

| Source | SS | df | MS | F |
|---|---|---|---|---|
| Linear Regression | 1562.93 | 1 | 1562.93 | 38.03 |
| Residual | 164.40 | 4 | 41.10 | |
| Total | 1727.33 | 5 | | |

Decision: With $F > 7.71$, reject $H_0$ and conclude that a linear relationship exists between the storage time and the assayed amount of drug.

Slope of the population:

Hypotheses: $H_0$: $\beta = 0$
$H_1$: $\beta \neq 0$

Decision Rule: With $\alpha = .05$, reject $H_0$ if $t > |t_4(1 - \alpha/2)| = 2.776$

Calculations:

$$S_b = \sqrt{\frac{MS_{residual}}{\sum x^2 - \frac{(\sum x)^2}{n}}}$$

$$S_b = \sqrt{\frac{41.10}{4680 - \frac{(144)^2}{6}}} = 0.183$$

$$t = \frac{b - 0}{S_b} = \frac{-1.13 - 0}{0.183} = -6.17$$

Decision: With $t < -2.776$, reject $H_0$, conclude that there is a slope and thus a relationship between time and assay results.

95% C.I. for the slope:

$$\beta = b \pm t_{n-1}(1 - \alpha/2) \cdot S_b$$

$$\beta = -1.13 \pm 2.776(0.183) = -1.13 \pm 0.51$$

$$-1.64 < \beta < -0.62$$

Decision: Since zero does not fall within the confidence interval, reject $H_0$ and conclude that a relationship exists. With 95% confidence the slope of the line ($\beta$) is between −1.64 and −0.62.

Confidence interval around the regression line:

Example at 48 months, where $\overline{X} = 24$

$$\overline{y} = y_c \pm t_{n-2}(1-\alpha/2) \cdot \sqrt{MS_{residual}} \cdot \sqrt{\frac{1}{n} + \frac{(x_i - \overline{X})^2}{\sum x^2 - \frac{(\sum x)^2}{n}}}$$

$$\overline{y} = 941.54 \pm 2.776\sqrt{41.102}\sqrt{\frac{1}{6} + \frac{(48-24)^2}{4680 - \frac{(144)^2}{6}}}$$

$$\overline{y} = 941.54 \pm 14.20$$

$$927.34 < \overline{y} < 955.74$$

Results (Figure 14.8):

95% Confidence Intervals

| Time (months) | Sample (mg) | $y_c$ | Lower Limit | Upper Limit | Range |
|---|---|---|---|---|---|
| 6 | 995 | 989.00 | 977.40 | 1000.60 | 23.20 |
| 12 | 984 | 982.22 | 972.84 | 991.60 | 18.76 |
| 18 | 973 | 975.44 | 967.69 | 983.19 | 15.50 |
| 24 | 960 | 968.66 | 961.54 | 975.78 | 14.24 |
| 36 | 952 | 955.10 | 945.72 | 964.48 | 18.75 |
| 48 | 948 | 941.54 | 927.34 | 955.74 | 28.40 |

2. Comparison of various concentrations to effect on the optical density
   Variables: continuous independent variable (concentration)
   continuous dependent variable (optical density)

   Hypotheses: $H_0$: Concentration and density are not linearly related
   $H_1$: Concentration and density are linearly related

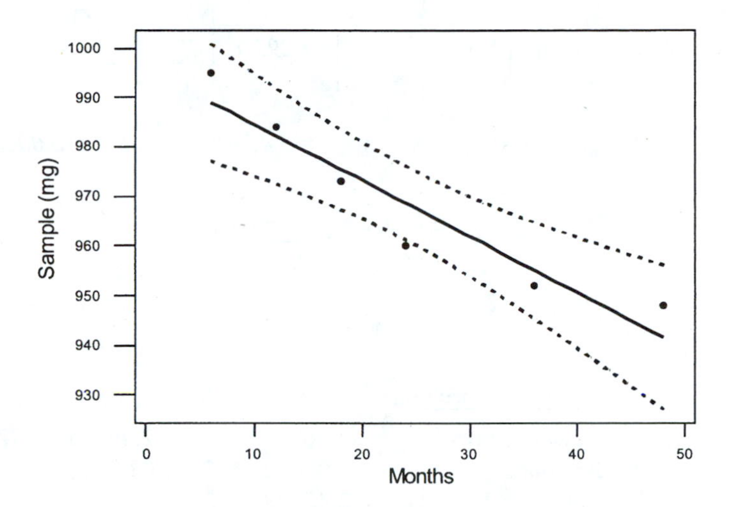


**Figure 14.8** Confidence bands for results of question 1 (created using Minitab® Release 12.21).

Decision Rule: With $\alpha = 0.05$, reject $H_0$ if $F > F_{1,2}(1-\alpha) = 18.5$

| | Concentration x | Density y | $x^2$ | $y^2$ | xy |
|---|---|---|---|---|---|
| | 1 | 0.24 | 1 | 0.058 | 0.24 |
| | 2 | 0.66 | 4 | 0.436 | 1.32 |
| n = 4 | 4 | 1.15 | 16 | 1.323 | 4.60 |
| | 8 | 2.34 | 64 | 5.476 | 18.72 |
| $\Sigma =$ | 15 | 4.39 | 85 | 7.293 | 24.88 |

Calculations:

Slope and $y$-intercept:

$$b = \frac{4(24.88) - (15)(4.39)}{4(85) - (15)^2} = 0.293$$

$$a = \frac{4.39 - 0.293(15)}{4} = -0.00125$$

Coefficient of determination:

$$SS_{total} = \sum y^2 - \frac{(\sum y)^2}{n} = 7.293 - \frac{(4.39)^2}{4} = 2.47498$$

$$SS_{explained} = b^2 \cdot \left[ \sum x^2 - \frac{(\sum x)^2}{n} \right] = (.293)^2 \left[ 85 - \frac{(15)^2}{4} \right] = 2.46816$$

$$SS_{unexplained} = SS_{total} - SS_{explained} = 2.47498 - 2.46816 = 0.00682$$

$$r^2 = \frac{SS_{explained}}{SS_{total}} = \frac{2.46816}{2.47498} = .997$$

ANOVA table:

| Source of Variation | SS | df | MS | F |
|---|---|---|---|---|
| Linear Regression | 2.46816 | 1 | 2.46816 | 723.80 |
| Residual | 0.00682 | 2 | 0.00341 | |
| Total | 2.47498 | 3 | | |

Decision: With $F > 18.5$, reject $H_0$ and conclude that a linear relationship exists between the concentration and amount of optical density.

Slope of the population:

Hypotheses: $H_0$: $\beta = 0$
$H_1$: $\beta \neq 0$

Decision Rule: With $\alpha = .05$, reject $H_0$ if $t > |t_2(1 - \alpha/2)| = 4.302$

Calculations:

$$S_b = \sqrt{\frac{MS_{residual}}{\sum x^2 - \frac{(\sum x)^2}{n}}}$$

$$S_b = \sqrt{\frac{0.00341}{85 - \frac{(15)^2}{4}}} = 0.0109$$

$$t = \frac{b - 0}{S_b} = \frac{0.293 - 0}{0.0109} = 26.88$$

Decision: With $t > 4.302$, reject $H_0$, conclude that there is a slope and thus a relationship between concentration and density.

95% C.I. for the slope:

$$\beta = b \pm t_{n-1}(1-\alpha/2) \cdot S_b$$

$$\beta = 0.23 \pm 4.302(0.0109) = 0.293 \pm 0.047$$

$$0.246 < \beta < 0.340$$

Decision: Since zero does not fall within the confidence interval, reject $H_0$ and conclude that a relationship exists. With 95% confidence the slope of the line ($\beta$) is between +0.246 and +0.340.

Confidence interval around the regression line:

Example at 4% concentration, where $\overline{X} = 3.75$

$$\overline{y} = y_c \pm t_{n-2}(1-\alpha/2) \cdot \sqrt{MS_{residual}} \cdot \sqrt{\frac{1}{n} + \frac{(x_i - \overline{X})^2}{\sum x^2 - \frac{(\sum x)^2}{n}}}$$

$$\overline{y} = 1.17 \pm 4.302\sqrt{0.00341}\sqrt{\frac{1}{4} + \frac{(4-3.75)^2}{85 - \frac{(15)^2}{4}}}$$

$$\overline{y} = 1.17 \pm 0.13$$

$$1.04 < \overline{y} < 1.30$$

Results (Figure 14.9):

95% Confidence Intervals

| Concentration | Density | $y_c$ | Lower Limit | Upper Limit | Range |
|---|---|---|---|---|---|
| 1 | 0.24 | 0.29 | 0.11 | 0.47 | 0.36 |
| 2 | 0.66 | 0.58 | 0.43 | 0.73 | 0.30 |
| 4 | 1.15 | 1.17 | 1.04 | 1.30 | 0.26 |
| 8 | 2.34 | 2.34 | 2.11 | 2.57 | 0.46 |

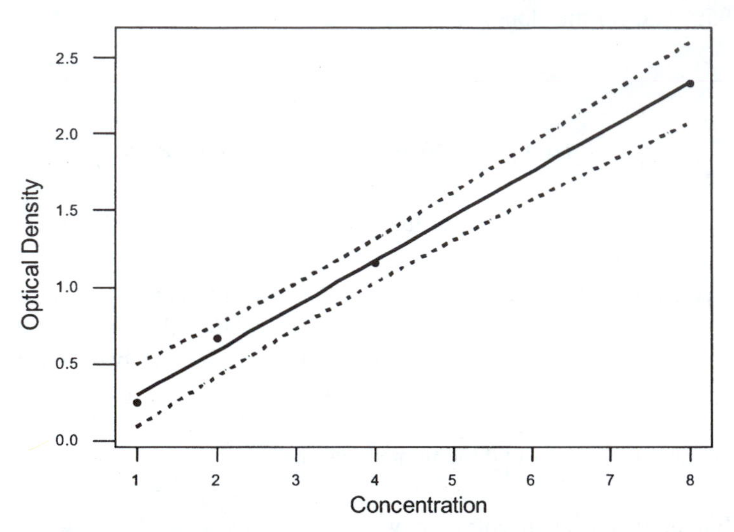


**Figure 14.9** Confidence bands for results of question 2 (created using Minitab® Release 12.21).

3. Comparison of various concentrations to affect the optical density for two solutions (test vs. reference standard) and evaluating if the two results produce parallel lines.

Variables: continuous independent variables (concentrations for the test solution and the reference standard )
continuous dependent variable (optical density )

Hypotheses:

$$H_0: \beta_T = \beta_S$$
$$H_1: \beta_T \neq \beta_S$$

Decision Rule: With $\alpha = 0.05$, reject $H_0$ if $t > t_{4+4-4}(1 - \alpha/2) = 2.777$

Much of the information needed about the test solution was calculated in question 2 and will be presented below. Information needed for the reference standard solution is as follows:

| | Concentration x | Density y | $x^2$ | $y^2$ | xy |
|---|---|---|---|---|---|
| | 1 | 0.22 | 1 | 0.0484 | 0.22 |
| | 2 | 0.74 | 4 | 0.5476 | 1.48 |
| n=4 | 4 | 1.41 | 16 | 1.9881 | 5.64 |
| | 8 | 2.76 | 64 | 7.6176 | 22.08 |
| $\Sigma =$ | 15 | 5.13 | 85 | 10.2017 | 29.42 |

Calculations:

Slope and y-intercept:

$$b = \frac{4(29.42) - (15)(5.13)}{4(85) - (15)^2} = 0.354$$

$$a = \frac{5.13 - 0.354(15)}{4} = -0.0450$$

Coefficient of determination:

$$SS_{total} = \sum y^2 - \frac{(\sum y)^2}{n} = 10.2017 - \frac{(5.13)^2}{4} = 3.62248$$

$$SS_{explained} = b^2 \cdot \left[\sum x^2 - \frac{(\sum x)^2}{n}\right] = (.354)^2 \left[85 - \frac{(15)^2}{4}\right] = 3.60284$$

$$SS_{unexplained} = SS_{total} - SS_{explained} = 3.62248 - 3.60284 = 0.01964$$

ANOVA table:

| Source of Variation | SS | df | MS | F |
|---|---|---|---|---|
| Linear Regression | 3.60284 | 1 | 3.60284 | 366.89 |
| Residual | 0.01964 | 2 | 0.00982 | |
| Total | 3.62248 | 3 | | |

Information required for a comparison of parallelism:

| | Test | Standard |
|---|---|---|
| $n$ | 4 | 4 |
| $df$ | 2 | 2 |
| $\Sigma x$ | 15 | 15 |
| $\Sigma x^2$ | 85 | 85 |
| $b$ | 0.293 | 0.354 |
| $SS_R$ | 0.00682 | 0.01964 |

$$(S^2_{x/y})_p = \frac{0.00682 + 0.01964}{4 + 4 - 4} = 0.00662$$

$$t = \frac{0.293 - 0.354}{\sqrt{\frac{0.00662}{85 - \frac{(15)^2}{4}} + \frac{0.00662}{85 - \frac{(15)^2}{4}}}} = \frac{-0.061}{0.0215} = -2.84$$

Decision: With $t < -2.777$, reject $H_0$, conclude that the data have slopes that are not parallel.

95% C.I. for the difference between the two slopes:

$$\beta_1 - \beta_2 = (0.293 - .0354) \pm (2.777)\sqrt{\frac{0.00662}{85 - \frac{(15)^2}{4}} + \frac{0.00662}{85 - \frac{(15)^2}{4}}}$$

$$\beta_1 - \beta_2 = (-0.061) \pm (0.0597)$$

$$-0.1207 < \beta_1 - \beta_2 < -0.0013$$

Decision: Since zero does not fall within the confidence interval, reject $H_0$ and conclude that two lines are not parallel. With 95% confidence the difference between the two slopes is between –0.121 and –0.001.

# 15

# z-Tests of Proportions

As an introduction to this new set of z-tests, consider the following two problems. First, we are presented with a coin and we wish to determine if the coin is "fair" (an equal likelihood of tossing a head or a tail). To test the assumption of fairness, we toss the coin 20 times and find that we have 13 heads and only 7 tails. Is the coin unfair, loaded in such a way that heads occur more often, or could the outcome be the result of chance error? In a second situation, 50 patients are randomly divided into two groups each receiving a different treatment for their condition. In one group 75% show improvement and in the second group only 52% improve. Do the results prove that the first therapy results in a significantly greater therapeutic response, or is this difference due to chance alone?

Z-tests of proportions can address each of these examples, when comparisons are made between proportions or percentages for one or two levels of a discrete independent variable. They are useful when comparing proportions of two discrete levels of an independent variable or when comparing a sample proportion to a known population proportion. The formula and procedures are similar to those used for the t-tests.

## z-Test of Proportions – One-Sample Case

The z-tests of proportions involve a dependent variable that has only two discrete possible outcomes (i.e., pass or fail, live or die). These outcomes should be mutually exclusive and exhaustive. Similar to the statistics used for t- and F-tests, this *z*-statistic involves the following ratio:

$$z = \frac{\textit{difference between proportions}}{\begin{array}{c}\textit{standard error of the}\\ \textit{difference of the proportions}\end{array}} \qquad \text{Eq. 15.1}$$

The simplest example would be the tossing of a fair coin. We would expect the proportion of heads to be equal to the proportion of tails. Therefore, we would expect a head to occur 50% of the time, or have a proportion of 0.50. Our null hypothesis is that we are presented with a fair coin:

$$H_0: P_{heads} = 0.50$$

The only alternative is that the likelihood of tossing a head is something other than 50%.

$$H_1: P_{heads} \neq 0.50$$

If we toss the coin 100 times and this results in 50 heads and 50 tails, the numerator of the above ratio (Eq. 15.1) would be zero, resulting in a $z = 0$. As the discrepancy between what we observe and what we expect (50% heads) increases, the resultant $z$-value will increase until it eventually becomes large enough to be significant. Significance is determined using the critical z-values for a normalized distribution previously discussed in Chapter 6. For example, from Table B2 in Appendix B, +1.96 or −1.96 are the critical values in the case of a 95% level of confidence. For a 99% level of confidence the critical z-values would be +2.57 or −2.57.

In the one sample case the proportions found for a single sample are compared to a theoretical population to determine if the sample is selected from that same population.

$$H_0: \hat{p} = P_0$$
$$H_1: \hat{p} \neq P_0$$

The test statistic is as follows:

$$z = \frac{\hat{p} - P_0}{\sqrt{\frac{P_0(1 - P_0)}{n}}} \qquad \text{Eq. 15.2}$$

where $P_0$ is the expected proportion for the outcome, $1 - P_0$ is the complement proportion for the "not" outcome, $\hat{p}$ is the observed proportion of outcomes in the sample, and $n$ is the number of observations (sample size). The decision rule is, with a certain $\alpha$, reject $H_0$ if $z > z_{(1-\alpha/2)}$ or $z < -z_{(1-\alpha/2)}$ (where $z_{(1-\alpha/2)} = 1.96$ for $\alpha = 0.05$ or 2.57 for $\alpha = 0.01$). Like the t-test, this is a two-tailed test and modifications can be made in the decision rule to test directional hypotheses with a one-tailed test.

The one-sample case can be used to test the previous question about fairness of a particular coin. If a coin is tossed 20 times and 13 heads are the result, is it a fair coin? As seen earlier the hypotheses are:

$$H_0: P_{heads} = 0.50$$
$$H_1: P_{heads} \neq 0.50$$

In this case the $\hat{p}$ is 13/20 or 0.65, $P_0$ equals 0.50 and $n$ is 20. The calculation would be as follows:

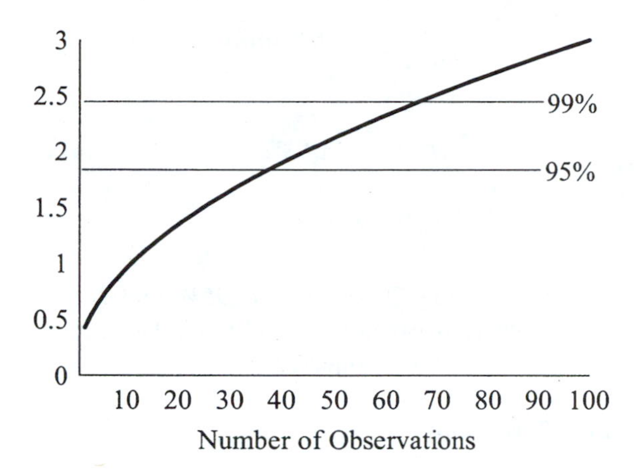


**Figure 15.1** Effects of sample size on z-test results.

$$z = \frac{0.65 - 0.50}{\sqrt{\frac{(0.50)(0.50)}{20}}} = \frac{0.15}{0.11} = 1.36$$

Because the calculated $z$-value is less than the critical value of 1.96, we fail to reject the hypothesis, and we assume that the coin is fair and the difference between the observed 0.65 and expected 0.50 was due to random error. What if we had more data and the results were still the same? The z-test is an excellent example of the importance of sample size. Figure 15.1 shows the same proportional differences with an increasing number of observations. Note that if these results appeared with more than 47 or 48 tosses the results would be significant at 95% confidence and the null hypothesis would be rejected. If the same proportional difference exists with over 75 tosses $H_0$ can be rejected with 99% confidence.

Similar to one-sample t-tests, confidence intervals can also be created for the z-test of proportions:

$$P_0 = \hat{p} \pm Z_{(1-\alpha/2)} \sqrt{\frac{P_0(1-P_0)}{n}} \qquad \text{Eq. 15.3}$$

The interval indicates the possible range of results, with 95% confidence. With the above example, the hypotheses would continue to be:

$$H_0: \ \hat{p} = 0.50$$
$$H_1: \ \hat{p} \neq 0.50$$

and the interval would be:

$$P_0 = 0.65 \pm 1.96\sqrt{\frac{(0.50)(0.50)}{20}}$$

$$P_0 = 0.65 \pm 0.22$$

$$0.43 < P_0 < 0.87$$

Therefore, based on a sample of only 20 tosses, with 95% confidence, the probability of tossing a head is somewhere between 0.43 and 0.87. The outcome of 0.50 is a possible outcome, therefore $H_0$ cannot be rejected.

**z-Test of Proportions – Two-Sample Case**

In the two-sample case, proportions from two levels of a discrete independent variable are compared and the hypothesis under test is that the two proportions for the population are equal.

$$H_0: \quad P_1 = P_2$$
$$H_1: \quad P_1 \neq P_2$$

If the two populations ($P_1$ and $P_2$) are equal, then the best estimation of that population proportion would be the weighted average of the sample proportions:

$$\hat{p}_0 = \frac{n_1 \hat{p}_1 + n_2 \hat{p}_2}{n_1 + n_2} \qquad \text{Eq. 15.4}$$

This estimate of the population proportion is then used in the denominator of the z-ratio (Eq. 15.1) and the numerator is the difference between the two sample proportions:

$$z = \frac{\hat{p}_1 - \hat{p}_2}{\sqrt{\frac{\hat{p}_0(1-\hat{p}_0)}{n_1} + \frac{\hat{p}_0(1-\hat{p}_0)}{n_2}}} \qquad \text{Eq. 15.5}$$

In these two equations, $\hat{p}_1$, $\hat{p}_2$ are sample proportions and $n_1$, $n_2$ are the sample sizes. The decision rule for a two-tailed z-test would be, with $\alpha = 0.05$, reject $H_0$, if $z > z_{(1-\alpha/2)} = 1.96$ or $z < -1.96$.

To illustrate this test assume the following fictitious clinical trial. To possibly improve the survival rate for protozoal infections in AIDS patients, individuals with newly diagnosed infections were randomly assigned to treatment with either zidovudine alone or a combination of zidovudine and trimethoprim. Based on the following results did either therapy show a significantly better survival rate?

Zidovudine alone, 23 out of 94 patients survived, $\hat{p}_Z = 0.245$

Zidovudine with trimethoprim, 42 out of 98 patients survived, $\hat{p}_{Z\&T} = 0.429$

Is there a significant difference between 0.245 and 0.429 based on less than 200 patients? The best estimate of the population proportion, if there is no difference between the two samples, is calculated from the two weighted average for the sample proportions:

$$\hat{p}_0 = \frac{94(0.245) + 98(0.429)}{94 + 98} = 0.339$$

The null hypothesis would be that there was not a significant difference between the two groups of patients in the proportion of patients surviving.

$$H_0: \; P_Z = P_{Z\&T}$$
$$H_1: \; P_Z \neq P_{Z\&T}$$

If the $z$-statistic is greater than +1.96 or less than −1.96, the researcher should reject the null hypothesis and conclude that there is a significant difference between the two groups. The computations would be:

$$z = \frac{0.245 - 0.429}{\sqrt{\dfrac{0.339(0.661)}{94} + \dfrac{0.339(0.661)}{98}}}$$

$$z = \frac{-0.184}{\sqrt{0.00467}} = \frac{-0.184}{0.068} = -2.71$$

With $z = -2.71$ (which is smaller than the critical value of −1.96) the decision would be to reject $H_0$ and conclude that there was a significant difference in the results for the two treatments. In this case the patients receiving both zidovudine and trimethoprim have a significantly better survival rate.

**Estimating Power and Desired Sample Size for Two-Sample Z-Test of Proportions**

To calculate the power for a two-sample $z$-test of proportions it is the sum of two probabilities associated with $z$-values:

$$power = p[z \le Z_1] + p[z \ge Z_2] \qquad \text{Eq. 15.6}$$

where:

$$Z_1 = \frac{-Z_{1-\alpha/2}(SE)-(\hat{p}_1-\hat{p}_2)}{\sqrt{\frac{\hat{p}_1\hat{q}_1}{n_1}+\frac{\hat{p}_2\hat{q}_2}{n_2}}} \quad \text{Eq. 15.7}$$

$$Z_2 = \frac{+Z_{1-\alpha/2}(SE)-(\hat{p}_1-\hat{p}_2)}{\sqrt{\frac{\hat{p}_1\hat{q}_2}{n_1}+\frac{\hat{p}_1\hat{q}_2}{n_2}}} \quad \text{Eq. 15.8}$$

with the *SE* term being the standard error in the denominator of the original *z*-ratio:

$$SE = \sqrt{\frac{p_O(1-p_O)}{n_1}+\frac{p_O(1-p_O)}{n_2}} \quad \text{Eq. 15.9}$$

These are modified from Zar's equations (1999) to be consistent with the symbols used previously in this chapter. With a desired $\alpha$ of 0.05, the $Z_{1-\alpha/2}$ would be 1.96 (for 99% confidence the value would be 2.58). Using the previous example of the two HIV therapeutic approaches the power based on 192 patients would be:

$$SE = \sqrt{\frac{(0.323)(0.677)}{94}+\frac{(0.323)(0.677)}{98}} = 0.067$$

$$Z_1 = \frac{-1.96(0.068)-(0.245-0.429)}{\sqrt{\frac{(0.245)(.755)}{94}+\frac{(0.429)(0.571)}{98}}} = \frac{0.0501}{0.0668} = +0.75$$

$$Z_2 = \frac{+1.96(0.068)-(0.245-0.429)}{\sqrt{\frac{(0.245)(0.755)}{94}+\frac{(0.429)(0.571)}{98}}} = \frac{+0.3173}{0.0668} = +4.75$$

$$power = p[Z < +0.75] + p[Z > +4.75]$$

Using the area under the curve in Table B2, the probability of $z < +0.75$ is 1) 0.50 for the area below the mean; and 2) the probability of $z$ at +0.75, which equals 0.2743, (sum = 0.7743). Similarly the probability of being >+4.75 is outside the table values, thus $p = 0$. The combined probability for the power equation is:

$$power = 0.7743 + 0.0000 \approx 0.7743$$

**Table 15.1** Various Power and Sample Size Determinations*

| For a Power of 80% | | For a Difference of 20% | |
|---|---|---|---|
| δ | n | n | 1 − β |
| 0.05 | 1,390 | 30 | 0.323 |
| 0.10 | 348 | 50 | 0.495 |
| 0.15 | 155 | 96 | 0.774 |
| 0.18 | 108 | 100 | 0.791 |
| 0.20 | 87 | 150 | 0.925 |

* Using the previous data comparing the two HIV therapies.

In designing a study, sample sized for each level of the discrete independent variable should be equal. The appropriate sample size per group for a given power ($1 - \beta$) can be estimated using the following formulas:

$$n = \frac{\left[\left(Z_{1-\alpha/2} \cdot \sqrt{2\hat{p}_0(1-\hat{p}_0)}\right) + \left(Z_\beta \cdot \sqrt{\hat{p}_1\hat{q}_1 + \hat{p}_2\hat{q}_2}\right)\right]^2}{\delta^2} \qquad \text{Eq. 15.10}$$

where $\hat{p}_0$ is the average of the two sample probabilities

$$p_0 = \frac{p_1 + p_2}{2} \qquad \text{Eq. 15.11}$$

and δ is the desired proportional difference we would like to be able to identify. Using the previous example with the estimated sample size to be able to identify a 20% difference ($\delta = 0.20$) with 80% power and a Type I error rate of 0.05, where $Z_{1-\alpha/2}$ is 1.96 and $Z_\beta = 0.84$.

$$p_0 = \frac{0.245 + 0.429}{2} = 0.337$$

$$n = \frac{\left[\left(1.96 \cdot \sqrt{2(0.337)(0.663)}\right) + \left(0.84 \cdot \sqrt{(0.245)(0.755) + (0.429)(0.571)}\right)\right]^2}{(0.20)^2}$$

$$n = \frac{[1.3102 + 0.5508]^2}{(0.20)^2} = 86.6 \approx 87 \text{ volunteers}$$

Using these formula for power and sample size it is possible to create different scenarios (Table 15.1). Notice that the results are similar to what would be expected based on the discussion in Chapter 8. As the differences increases the power increases. As the sample size increases the power increases.

**z-Tests for Proportions – Yates' Correction for Continuity**

In performing a z-test of proportions, the calculated $z$-value is based upon discrete, or discontinuous data, but as discussed in Chapter 6 the normal standardized distribution is based on a continuous distribution. Therefore, the calculated $z$-values are only an approximation of the theoretical z-distribution. Therefore, Frank Yates (1934) argued that a more conservative approach was needed to estimate the $z$-statistic, which is more appropriate with the standardized normal distribution. In the two-sample case, the Yates' correction for continuity is:

$$z = \frac{|\hat{p}_1 - \hat{p}_2| - \frac{1}{2}\left(\frac{1}{n_1} - \frac{1}{n_2}\right)}{\sqrt{\frac{\hat{p}_0(1-\hat{p}_0)}{n_1} + \frac{\hat{p}_0(1-\hat{p}_0)}{n_2}}} \qquad \text{Eq. 15.12}$$

Because of the smaller numerator, this will result in a slightly smaller calculated $z$-value, and a more conservative estimate. Obviously, as the sample sizes become smaller and we know less about the true population, there will be a decrease in the calculated $z$-value and an even more conservative answer.

Using this correction for continuity, we can recalculate the previous AIDS treatment example, where we were able to reject the null hypothesis and assumed that there was a better survival rate with the combination therapy. However, with Yates' correction:

$$z = \frac{|0.245 - 0.429| - \frac{1}{2}\left(\frac{1}{94} + \frac{1}{98}\right)}{\sqrt{\frac{0.339(0.661)}{94} + \frac{0.339(0.661)}{98}}}$$

$$z = \frac{0.184 - 0.010}{\sqrt{0.00467}} = \frac{0.174}{0.068} = 2.56$$

We again reject $H_0$ and 95% confidence assume that there is a significant difference between the two therapeutic approaches. However, what we want is to be 99% confident in our decision ($|z| > 2.576$)? In this case we would reject the null hypothesis with the first z-score, but fail to reject it with the Yates' correction.

Similarly, Yates' correction can be applied to the one-sample case (i.e., the previous example of tossing a fair coin):

$$z = \frac{|p - P_0| - \frac{1}{n}}{\sqrt{\frac{(P_0)(1 - P_0)}{n}}} \qquad \text{Eq. 15.13}$$

Obviously the larger the amount of information ($n$), the smaller the correction factor. Recalculation of our previous example gives:

$$z = \frac{|0.65 - 0.50| - \frac{1}{20}}{\sqrt{\frac{(0.50)(0.50)}{20}}} = \frac{0.10}{0.11} = 0.91$$

We still fail to reject $H_0$, but the calculated $z$-value is much smaller (0.91 compared to 1.36).

## Proportion Testing for More Than Two Levels of a Discrete Independent Variable

What if there are more than two levels of the discrete independent variable? Could the z-test of proportions be expanded beyond only two levels of the discrete independent variable? In these cases, it is best to establish a **contingency table** based on the frequency associated with each outcome. For example, assume in the previous zidovudine/trimethoprim study that there were actually four levels of treatment. The frequencies could be presented as a contingency table (Table 15.2). In this case a more appropriate test would be a chi square test of independence, where the interrelationship is measured between the survival rate and type of drug therapy received to determine if the two variables are independent of each other. This test will be discussed in the next chapter.

**Table 15.2** Comparison of Survival and Various Treatment Strategies

| | Zidovudine alone | Zidovudine/ Trimethoprim | Zidovudine/ Drug A | Zidovudine/ Drug B |
|---|---|---|---|---|
| Lived | 24 | 38 | 24 | 6 |
| Died | 70 | 60 | 86 | 51 |

## References

Yates, F. (1934). "Contingency tables involving small numbers and the $\chi^2$ test," *Royal Statistical Society Supplement* 1(series B):217-235.

Zar JH. (1999). *Biostatistical Analysis*, Fourth edition, Prentice-Hall, Englewood Cliffs, NJ, pp.558-562.

## Suggested Supplemental Readings

Bolton, S. (1997). *Pharmaceutical Statistics: Practical and Clinical Applications*, Third edition, Marcel Dekker, Inc., New York, pp. 162-168.

Daniel, W.W. (1999). *Biostatistics: A Foundation for Analysis in the Health Sciences*, Seventh edition, John Wiley and Sons, New York, pp. 211-218, 228-230.

Glantz, S.A. (1987). *Primer of Biostatistics*, McGraw-Hill, New York, pp. 111-119.

## Example Problems

1. During production runs, historically a specific dosage form is expected to have a defect rate of 1.5%. During one specific run, a sample of 100 tablets was found to have a defect rate of 5%. Does this differ significantly from what would normally be expected?

2. During initial Phase I and II studies, the incidence of nausea and vomiting of a new cancer chemotherapeutic agent was 36% for 190 patients, while 75 control patients receiving conventional therapy experience nausea and vomiting at a rate of 55%.

    a. Is there a significant difference between the incidence of nausea and vomiting between these two drug therapies?

    b. Did the new agent produce a significantly lower incidence of nausea and vomiting?

3. During the development of a final dosage form, the frequency of defects were analyzed to determine the effect of the speed of the tablet press. Samples were collected at 80,000 (lower) and 120,000 (higher) units per hour. Initially 500 tablets were to be collected at each speed; unfortunately due to an accident only 460 tablets were retrieved at the higher speed. Based on the following results were there any significant differences between the two tablet press speeds?

| Speed | n | # of defects |
|---|---|---|
| Low | 500 | 11 |
| High | 460 | 17 |

4. During preapproval clinical trials with a specific agent, it was found that the incidence of blood dyscrasia was 2.5%. In a later Phase IV study involving 28 patients, two developed blood dyscrasia. Is this outcome possible or is there something unique about the population from which the sample was taken for this last clinical trial?

**Answers to Problems**

1. Production was run with an expected defect rate of 1.5%, but a rate of 5% for 100 tablets was found.

Hypotheses: $H_0$: $\hat{p} = 0.015$
$H_1$: $\hat{p} \neq 0.015$

Decision rule: With $\alpha = 0.05$, reject $H_0$, if $z > z_{(1-\alpha/2)} = 1.96$ or $z < -1.96$.

Data: $P_0 = 0.015$; $\hat{p} = 0.05$; $n = 100$

Calculations:

$$z = \frac{\hat{p} - P_0}{\sqrt{\frac{P_0(1-P_0)}{n}}}$$

$$z = \frac{0.05 - 0.015}{\sqrt{\frac{(0.015)(0.985)}{100}}} = \frac{0.035}{0.012} = 2.92$$

Decision: With $z > 1.96$, reject $H_0$, conclude that there is a significant difference between the sample and the expected proportion of defects.

Alternative confidence interval approach:

$$P_0 = \hat{p} \pm Z_{(1-\alpha/2)} \sqrt{\frac{P_0(1-P_0)}{n}}$$

$$P_0 = 0.05 \pm 1.96 \sqrt{\frac{(0.015)(0.985)}{100}} = 0.05 \pm 0.024$$

$$+0.026 < P_0 < +0.074$$

Decision: The outcome 0.015 does not fall within the interval, therefore reject $H_0$.

2. Incidence of nausea and vomiting between two therapies.

   a. Two-tailed, not predicting direction:

   Hypotheses: $H_0$: $P_N = P_T$
   $H_0$: $P_N \neq P_T$

   Decision rule: With $\alpha = 0.05$, reject $H_0$, if $z > z_{(1-\alpha/2)} = 1.96$ or $z < -1.96$.

   Calculations:

$$\hat{p}_0 = \frac{n_F \hat{N}_N + n_T \hat{p}_T}{n_N + n_T} = \frac{(190)(0.36) + (75)(0.55)}{190 + 75} = 0.413$$

$$1 - \hat{p}_0 = 1.00 - 0.413 = 0.587$$

$$z = \frac{0.36 - 0.55}{\sqrt{\frac{(0.413)(0.587)}{190} + \frac{(0.413)(0.587)}{75}}} = \frac{-0.19}{0.067} = -2.83$$

   Decision: With $z < -1.96$ reject $H_0$, and conclude there is a significant difference between the incidence of nausea and vomiting between the new drug and traditional therapy.

   b. One-tailed, predicting lower incidence with a new agent:

   Hypotheses: $H_0$: $P_N \geq P_T$
   $H_0$: $P_N < P_T$

   Decision rule: With $\alpha = 0.05$, reject $H_0$, if $z < z_{(1-\alpha)} = -1.64$.

   Decision: The computed z-value was –2.83. With $z < -1.64$ reject $H_0$, and conclude that the newer agent causes a significant decrease in the incidence of nausea and vomiting compared to traditional therapy.

3. Defects at two different speeds for a tablet press.

| Speed | n | # of defects |
|---|---|---|
| Low | 500 | 11 |
| High | 460 | 17 |

$\hat{p}_L = 11/500 = 0.022$ $\hat{p}_H = 17/460 = 0.037$

Hypotheses: $H_0$: $P_L = P_H$
$H_1$: $P_L \neq P_H$

Decision rule: With $\alpha = 0.05$, reject $H_0$, if $z > z_{(1-\alpha/2)} = 1.96$ or $z < -1.96$.

Calculations:

$$\hat{p}_0 = \frac{n_L \hat{p}_L + n_H \hat{p}_H}{n_L + n_H} = \frac{(500)(0.022) + (460)(0.037)}{500 + 460} = 0.029$$

$$1 - \hat{p}_0 = 1.00 - 0.029 = 0.971$$

$$z = \frac{\hat{p}_L - \hat{p}_H}{\sqrt{\frac{\hat{p}_0(1-\hat{p}_0)}{n_L} + \frac{\hat{p}_0(1-\hat{p}_0)}{n_H}}}$$

$$z = \frac{0.022 - 0.037}{\sqrt{\frac{0.029(0.971)}{500} + \frac{0.029(0.971)}{460}}} = \frac{-0.015}{0.011} = -1.36$$

Decision: With the $z > -1.96$, fail to reject $H_0$, conclude that there is no significant difference in the defect rate based on the tablet press speed.

Yates' correction for continuity:

$$z = \frac{|\hat{p}_1 - \hat{p}_2| - \frac{1}{2}(\frac{1}{n_1} + \frac{1}{n_2})}{\sqrt{\frac{\hat{p}_0(1-\hat{p}_0)}{n_1} + \frac{\hat{p}_0(1-\hat{p}_0)}{n_2}}}$$

$$z = \frac{|0.022 - 0.037| - \frac{1}{2}(\frac{1}{500} + \frac{1}{460})}{\sqrt{\frac{0.029(0.971)}{500} + \frac{0.029(0.971)}{460}}}$$

$$z = \frac{0.015 - 0.002}{0.011} = \frac{0.013}{0.011} = 1.18$$

Decision: With the $z < 1.96$, fail to reject $H_0$.

4. Incidence of a blood dyscrasia in a Phase IV clinical trail.

Hypotheses: $H_0$: $\hat{p} = 0.025$
$H_1$: $\hat{p} \neq 0.025$

Decision rule: With $\alpha = 0.05$, reject $H_0$, if $z > z_{(1-\alpha/2)} = 1.96$ or $z < -1.96$.

Data: $P_0 = 0.025$; $\hat{p} = 2/28 = 0.071$; $n = 28$

Calculations:

$$z = \frac{\hat{p} - p_0}{\sqrt{\frac{p_0(1-p_0)}{n}}} \frac{0.071 - 0.025}{\sqrt{\frac{(0.025)(0.975)}{28}}} = \frac{0.046}{0.029} = 1.59$$

Decision: With $z < 1.96$, fail to reject $H_0$,and cannot conclude that the sample results are different from what was found with the original clinical trials.

Alternative confidence interval approach:

$$P_0 = \hat{p} \pm Z_{(1-\alpha/2)} \sqrt{\frac{P_0(1-P_0)}{n}}$$

$$P_0 = 0.071 \pm 1.96 \sqrt{\frac{(0.025)(0.975)}{28}} = 0.071 \pm 0.057$$

$$+0.014 < P_0 < +0.128$$

Decision: The outcome 0.025 falls within the interval, therefore $H_0$ cannot be rejected.

# 16

# Chi Square Tests

The chi square tests are used when only discrete variables are involved. In the goodness-of-fit test there is one discrete variable. For the test of independence, two discrete variables are compared: one is usually independent (i.e., experimental vs. control group) and the other variable is dependent upon the first (i.e., cured vs. died). The chi square test, sometimes referred to as **Pearson's chi square**, evaluates the importance of the difference between what is expected (under given conditions) and what is actually observed. When criteria are not met for the chi square test of independence, the Fisher's exact test may be used. Pairing of dichotomous outcomes is possible using the McNemar test and the effects of a third possible confounding variable can be addressed using the Mantel-Haenszel test.

## Chi Square Statistic

The chi square ($\chi^2$) can best be thought of as a discrepancy statistic. It analyzes the difference between observed values and those values that one would normally expect to occur. It is calculated by determining the difference between the frequencies actually observed in a sample data set and the expected frequencies based on probability. Some textbooks classify $\chi^2$ as a nonparametric procedure because it is not concerned with distributions about a central point and does not require assumptions of homogeneity or normality.

In the previous chapter, the z-tests of proportion evaluated the results of a coin toss. This one-sample case was a measure of discrepancy, with the numerator representing the difference between the observed frequency ($p$) and the expected population results for a fair coin ($P_O$) (Eq. 15.2). With the z-tests in Chapter 15, we were concerned with proportions, or percents, and these were used with the appropriate formulas. With the chi square statistics, the frequencies are evaluated. The calculation involves squaring the differences between the observed and expected frequencies divided by the expected frequency. These results are summed for each cell in a contingency table or for each level of the discrete variable.

$$\chi^2 = \sum \frac{(f_O - f_E)^2}{f_E} \qquad \text{Eq. 16.1}$$

This formula can be slightly rewritten as follows:

$$\chi^2 = \sum \left[ \frac{(Observed - Expected)^2}{Expected} \right]$$

or

$$\chi^2 = \sum \frac{(O - E)^2}{E} \qquad \text{Eq. 16.2}$$

Obviously, if all of the observed and expected values are equal for each level of the discrete variable the numerator is zero and the $\chi^2$-statistic will be zero. Similar to the *z*-test, as the differences between the observed and expected frequencies increase, the numerator will increase and the resultant $\chi^2$-value will increase. Because the numerator is squared, the resultant value must be equal to or greater than zero. Therefore at a certain point in the continuum from zero to positive infinity, the calculated $\chi^2$-value will be large enough to indicate that the difference cannot be due to chance alone. Like the *z*-, *t*-, and *F*-tests, critical values for the chi square distribution are presented in tabular form (Table B15, Appendix B). Like the *t*- and *F*-distributions, there is not one single $\chi^2$ distribution, but a set of distributions. The characteristics of each distribution are dependent on the number of degrees of freedom (Figure 16.1). As the number of degrees of freedom increases, the skew in the distribution decreases and the curve approaches a normal distribution. The first column on the left side of Table B15 indicates the number of degrees of freedom (determination of which will be discussed later) and the remaining columns are the critical chi square values at different acceptable levels of a Type I error ($\alpha$).

The decision rule is written similarly to previous tests. For example, assume we are dealing with four degrees of freedom and wish to have a 95% level of confidence. The decision rule would be: with $\alpha = 0.05$, reject $H_0$ if $\chi^2 > \chi^2_4(0.05) = 9.448$. If the calculated statistic derived from the formula (Eq. 16.2) is larger than the critical (9.448), the null hypothesis (the observed and expected values are the same) is rejected.

**Chi Square for One Discrete Independent Variable**

As seen in the previous chapter, the *z*-tests of proportions were limited to only one or two levels of a discrete independent variable. If the frequency counts are used (instead of proportions), the chi square test can be used and expanded to more than two levels. For example, assume that we wish to compare four lots of a particular

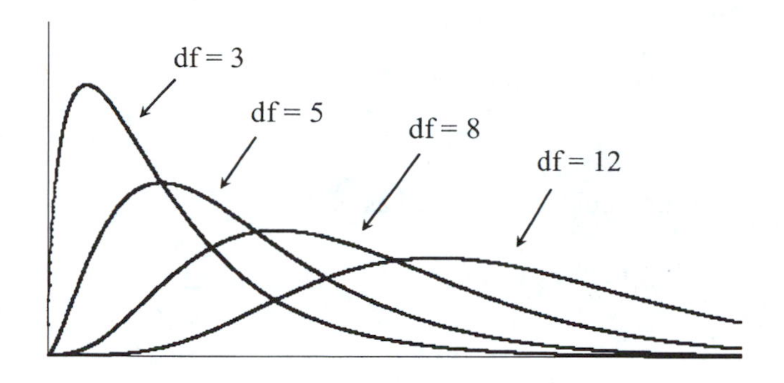


**Figure 16.1** Various chi square distributions.

drug for some minor undesirable trait (i.e., a blemish on the tablet coating). We randomly sample 1000 tablets from each batch and examine the tables for that trait. The results of the experiment are as follows:

| | Number of Tablets with Blemishes |
|---|---|
| Batch A | 12 |
| Batch B | 15 |
| Batch C | 10 |
| Batch D | 9 |

A simple hypothesis to evaluate this data could be as follows:

$H_0$: The samples are selected from the same population
$H_1$: The samples are from different populations

The null hypothesis states that there is no significant difference between the four batches of drug based on the criteria tested. If there is no difference then they must be from the same population. In selecting the appropriate critical $\chi^2$-value, the number of degrees of freedom is one less than number of levels of the discrete variable. Once again the $K - 1$ levels are selected to correct for bias. In this example, since there are four batches being tested, the number of degrees of freedom is four minus one, or three. The decision rule, assuming 95% confidence is: with $\alpha = 0.05$, reject $H_0$ if $\chi^2 > \chi^2_3(0.05) = 7.8147$. The value 7.8147 is found in Table B15 at the intercept of the third row (degrees of freedom equal to three) and the second column of critical values ($\alpha = 0.05$). If there were no differences among the batches, we would expect to see the same results. Our best estimate of expected frequency is the average of the sample frequencies:

$$f_E = \frac{\sum \textit{frequencies per level}}{\textit{number of levels}} = \frac{\sum f_i}{k_i} \qquad \text{Eq. 16.3}$$

In this particular case:

$$f_E = \frac{12+15+10+9}{4} = 11.5$$

Therefore the $\chi^2$ statistic would be calculated as follows:

| | Observed | Expected | O – E | $(O-E)^2/E$ |
|---|---|---|---|---|
| Batch A | 12 | 11.5 | +0.5 | 0.02 |
| Batch B | 15 | 11.5 | +3.5 | 1.07 |
| Batch C | 10 | 11.5 | –1.5 | 0.20 |
| Batch D | 9 | 11.5 | –2.5 | 0.54 |
| | | | $\chi^2 =$ | 1.83 |

Based on the results of the chi square test, with the calculated $\chi^2$ less than 7.8147, we fail to reject the null hypothesis. Therefore, our best guess is that they are from the same population; in other words, that there is no difference among the four batches.

**Chi Square Goodness-of-Fit Test**

All chi square tests can be thought of as goodness-of-fit procedures because they compare what is observed to what is expected in the hypothesized distribution. However, the term goodness-of-fit is reserved for comparisons of a sample distribution to determine if the observed set of data is distributed as expected by a preconceived distribution. It is assumed that the sample distribution is representative of the population from which it is sampled. Sample observations are placed into mutually exclusive and exhaustive categories, and the frequencies of each category are noted and compared to expected frequencies in the hypothetical distribution. The following are examples of the use of this method for both normal and binomial distributions.

**Goodness-of-Fit for a Normal Distribution.** The chi square goodness-of-fit test, can be used to determine if a sample is selected from a population that is normally distributed. The underlying assumption is that the sample distribution, because of random sampling, is reflective of the population from which it is sampled. Therefore, if the sample has characteristics similar to what is expected for a normal distribution, one cannot reject the hypothesis that the population is normally distributed.

$H_0$: Population is normally distributed
$H_1$: $H_0$ is false

Since many statistical procedures assume that sample data are drawn from normally distributed populations it is useful to have a method to evaluate this assumption. The chi squared test provides an excellent method, but should be restricted to sample sets

**Table 16.1** Determination of Expected Values

| Interval Range | Expected Values below the Largest Value in Each Class Interval | | Expect Values within Range |
|---|---|---|---|
| 705.5-716.5 | 1.74 | | 1.74 |
| 716.5-727.5 | 7.57 | | 5.83 |
| 727.5-738.5 | 23.01 | | 15.44 |
| 738.5-749.5 | 52.59 | | 29.58 |
| 759.5-760.5 | 84.20 | | 31.61 |
| 760.5-771.5 | 109.36 | | 25.16 |
| 771.5-782.5 | 120.51 | | 11.15 |
| 782.5-793.5 | 125.00 | | 4.49 |
| | | Σ = | 125 |

with 50 or more observations. For example, using Sturges' Rule the distribution presented in Table 16.1 is created from the data presented and discussed in Chapter 4. If this sample distribution is the best estimation of the population from which it was sampled, is the population in question normally distributed? Obviously, the greater the discrepancy between what is expected and what is actually observed, the less likely the difference is attributed to chance alone and the greater the likelihood that the sample is not from a normally distributed population. The test statistic would be Eq. 15.2:

$$\chi^2 = \Sigma\left[\frac{(O-E)^2}{E}\right]$$

Degrees of freedom are based on the number of categories or class intervals and a number of estimated values. In order to calculate areas within a normal distribution, and by extension the frequencies, one needs to know both the population mean and population standard deviation (Eq. 6.3):

$$z = \frac{x-\mu}{\sigma}$$

Calculation of $z$-values provides probabilities associated with the dividing points (boundaries) for our class intervals. The sample mean and standard deviation are the best available estimates of the population:

$$\bar{X} \approx \mu$$
$$S \approx \sigma$$

Therefore our best estimate of $z$-values would be an approximation based on our sample measurements:

$$z = \frac{x - \overline{X}}{S}$$ Eq. 16.4

These estimates will affect the degrees of freedom associated with the critical value in Table B15. Because we are estimating two population parameters, each is subtracted from the number of levels of the independent discrete variable. One additional degree is subtracted to control for bias. Thus, the degrees of freedom equals the number of levels minus three; one for the estimate of the population mean; one for the estimate of the population standard deviation and one for bias. In the above example, degrees of freedom equals eight levels minus three, or five degrees of freedom. The decision rule is: with $\alpha = 0.05$, reject $H_0$ if $\chi^2 > \chi^2_{v=5}(.05) = 11.070$.

Based on the discussion in Chapter 6, we can use the information presented about areas under the curve of a normal distribution to estimate the expected frequencies in each interval of this sample distribution, if the population is normally distributed. For example, with a sample of 125 observations; if normally distributed, how many observations would be expected below 716.5 mg? The first step is to determine the z-value on a normal distribution representing 716.5 mg.

$$Z = \frac{x - \overline{X}}{S} = \frac{716.5 - 752.9}{16.5} = \frac{-36.4}{16.5} = -2.20$$

where 752.9 was the sample mean for the 125 data points and 16.5 was the sample standard deviation. Looking at the standardized normal distribution (Table B2, Appendix B) the area under the curve between the mean (0) and $z = -2.20$ is 0.4861. The proportion, or area under the curve, falling below the $z$-value is calculated by subtracting the area between the center and $z$-value from 0.5000, which represents all the area below the mean.

$$p(< 2.20) = 0.5000 - 0.4861 = 0.0139$$

The expected number of observations is the total number of observations multiplied by the proportion of the curve falling below $z = -2.20$:

$$E(< 716.5) = 125(0.0139) = 1.74$$

Using this same method, it is possible to estimate the number of observations expected to be below 727.5 in a normal distribution (the greatest value in the second class interval).

$$Z = \frac{x - \overline{X}}{S} = \frac{727.5 - 752.9}{16.5} = \frac{-25.4}{16.5} = -1.54$$

**Table 16.2** Comparison of Observed and Expected Data

| Interval | Observed | Expected | (O – E) | $(O-E)^2/E$ |
|---|---|---|---|---|
| 705.5-716.5 | 2 | 1.74 | 0.26 | 0.039 |
| 716.5-727.5 | 6 | 5.83 | 0.17 | 0.005 |
| 727.5-738.5 | 18 | 15.44 | 2.56 | 0.424 |
| 738.5-749.5 | 22 | 29.58 | –7.58 | 1.942 |
| 759.5-760.5 | 35 | 31.61 | 3.39 | 0.364 |
| 760.5-771.5 | 28 | 25.16 | 2.84 | 0.321 |
| 771.5-782.5 | 10 | 11.15 | –1.15 | 0.119 |
| 782.5-793.5 | 4 | 4.49 | –0.49 | 0.053 |
| | | | $\chi^2 = \Sigma =$ | 3.267 |

$$p(<-1.54) = 0.5000 - 0.4394 = 0.0606$$

$$E(<727.5) = 125(0.0606) = 7.57$$

Continuing this procedure it is possible to calculate all areas below given points in the proposed normal distribution (Table 16.1, second column). By default, if all the observations are represented under the area of the curve, then the expected number of observations below the upper value of the highest interval must include all of the observations (in this case 125).

Unfortunately, we are interested in not only the areas below given points on the distribution, but also areas between the boundaries of the class intervals. Therefore, the number of observations expected between 716.5 and 727.5 is the difference between the areas below each point:

$$\text{Expected (Range 716.5-727.5)} = E(<727.5) - E(<716.5)$$
$$\text{Expected (Range 716.5-727.5)} = 7.57 - 1.74 = 5.83$$

$$\text{Expected (Range 727.5-738.5)} = E(<738.5) - E(<727.5)$$
$$\text{Expected (Range 727.5-738.5)} = 23.01 - 7.57 = 15.44$$

Using this same procedure it is possible to determine the expected results for the remaining categories and create a table (Table 16.1, third column). The expected amounts reflect a normal distribution. The chi square statistic is then computed comparing what is expected if the population distribution is normal to what was actually observed in the sample distribution. The greater the difference, the more likely one is to reject the hypothesis that the population represented by the sample is normally distributed. The chi square is a calculation using the data presented in Table 16.2. The decision is, with $\chi^2 < 11.070$, to not reject $H_0$ and conclude that we are unable to reject the hypothesis that the population is normally distributed. This process is laborious, but useful when evaluating data where it is important to determine if the population is normally distributed. Similar to previous tests, we cannot prove the null hypothesis, we simply cannot reject the possibility that the population from which our data were selected might be normally distributed.

**Goodness-of-Fit for a Binomial Distribution.** To illustrate the use of the chi square goodness-of-fit test for a binomial distribution, assume that four coins are tossed at the same time. This procedure is repeated 100 times. Based on the following results, are these "fair" coins?

| | |
|---|---|
| 0 heads | 15 times |
| 1 head | 30 times |
| 2 heads | 32 times |
| 3 heads | 17 times |
| 4 heads | 6 times |

From the discussion of probability in Chapter 2, using factorials, combinations, and the binomial equation (Eq. 2.12), it is possible to produce the theoretical binomial distribution given the coins are fair, $p$(head) = .50. For example, the probability of tossing only one head is:

$$p(x) = \binom{n}{x} p^x q^{n-x}$$

$$p(1) = \binom{4}{1} (0.5)^1 (0.5)^3 = 0.25$$

A table can be produced for the probability of all possible outcomes. If the four coins are fair these would produce the expected outcomes displayed in Table 16.3. The comparison is made for the discrepancy between what was actually observed with 100 coin tosses and what was expected to occur if the $p$(head) was in fact .50. Is the discrepancy just due to change error or large enough to be significant? The hypotheses would be:

$H_0$: Population is a binomial distribution with $p = 0.50$
$H_1$: $H_0$ is false

The test statistic remains the same (Eq. 16.2):

$$\chi^2 = \Sigma \left[ \frac{(O-E)^2}{E} \right]$$

The decision rule is: with $\alpha = 0.05$, reject $H_0$ if $\chi^2 > \chi^2_{v=5-2}(0.05) = 7.8147$. Here the degrees of freedom is based upon the number of discrete intervals minus two; one degree of freedom is subtracted because we are estimating the population proportions ($p$) and one is subtracted to prevent bias. The data required for computing the $\chi^2$-

**Table 16.3** Expected Outcomes from Tossing Four Coins

| Outcome | p(x) | Frequency for 100 Times |
|---|---|---|
| 0 heads | 0.0625 | 6.25 |
| 1 head | 0.2500 | 25.00 |
| 2 heads | 0.3750 | 37.50 |
| 3 heads | 0.2500 | 25.00 |
| 4 heads | 0.0625 | 6.25 |

**Table 16.4** Data for Comparing Observed and Expected Results for Four Tossed Coins

| | Observed | Expected | (O-E) | $(O-E)^2/E$ |
|---|---|---|---|---|
| 0 heads | 15 | 6.25 | 8.75 | 12.25 |
| 1 head | 30 | 25.00 | 5.00 | 1.00 |
| 2 heads | 32 | 37.50 | –5.50 | 0.81 |
| 3 heads | 17 | 25.00 | –8.00 | 2.56 |
| 4 heads | 6 | 6.25 | –0.25 | 0.01 |
| | | | $\chi^2 =$ | 16.63 |

statistic is presented in Table 16.4. Based on 100 coin tosses, the decision is with $\chi^2 > 7.8147$, reject $H_0$, conclude that the sample does not come from a binomial distribution with *p*(head) = 0.50. The coins are not fair.

## Chi Square Test of Independence

The most common use of the chi square test is to determine if two discrete variables are independent of each other. With this test we are concerned with conditional probability; what the probability is for some level of variable *A* given a certain level of variable *B* (Eq. 2.6)

$$p(A)\ given\ B = p(A \mid B) = \frac{p(A \cap B)}{p(B)}$$

If the two discrete variables are independent of each other, then the probability of each level should be the same regardless of which level of the *B* characteristic it contains.

$$p(A_1|B_1) = p(A_1|B_2) = ...p(A_1|B_k) = p(A_1) \qquad \text{Eq. 16.5}$$

A contingency table is created where frequency of occurrences are listed for the various levels of each variable. This **contingency table** is used to determine whether

| | | Levels of the First Variable | | | | |
|---|---|---|---|---|---|---|
| | | $A_1$ | $A_2$ | $A_3$ | ... | $A_K$ |
| Levels of the Second Variable | $B_1$ | | | | ... | |
| | $B_2$ | | | | ... | |
| | ... | ... | ... | ... | ... | |
| | $B_K$ | | | | ... | |

**Figure 16.2** Design of the contingency table, chi square test of independence.

two discrete variables are contingent or dependent on each other. The table has a finite number of mutually exclusive and exhaustive categories in the rows and columns (Figure 16.2). Such a design is a "*K x J*" contingency with *K* rows, *J* columns, and *K* x *J* cells. This bivariate table can be used to predict if two variables are independent of each other or if an association exists. The hypothesis under test implies that there is no relationship (complete independence) between the two variables and that each is independent of the other.

$$H_0: \quad P(B_1|A_1) = P(B_1|A_2) = P(B_1|A_3) \ldots = P(B_1|A_K) = P(B_1)$$
$$P(B_2|A_1) = P(B_2|A_2) = P(B_2|A_3) \ldots = P(B_2|A_K) = P(B_2)$$
$$\ldots$$
$$P(B_K|A_1) = P(B_K|A_2) = P(B_K|A_3) \ldots = P(B_K|A_K) = P(B_K)$$

$H_1$: $H_0$ is false

The chi square test of independence tests the hypothesis that two variables are related only by chance. A simpler terminology for the two previous hypotheses is:

$H_0$: Factor *B* is independent of Factor *A*
$H_1$: Factor *B* is not independent of Factor *A*

Thus, in the null hypothesis, the probability of $B_1$ (or $B_2$ ... or $B_M$) remains the same regardless of the level of the second variable, *A*. If we fail to reject $H_0$, the two variables have no systematic association and could also be referred to as **unrelated, uncorrelated**, or **orthogonal variables.** Once again the test statistic (Eq. 16.2) is:

$$\chi^2 = \Sigma\left[\frac{(O-E)^2}{E}\right]$$

Much like the goodness-of-fit model, if there is complete independence the difference between the observed and expected outcomes will be zero. As the difference in the numerator increases the calculated $\chi^2$-value will increase and eventually exceed a critical value; past that point the difference cannot be attributed to chance or random variability. To determine the critical value, the degrees of freedom are based on the number of rows minus one $(K-1)$ times the number of columns minus one $(J-1)$. This is based on the fact that if we had a contingency table such as the following:

| | $A_1$ | $A_2$ | $A_3$ | $A_4$ | |
|---|---|---|---|---|---|
| $B_1$ | | | | | 100 |
| $B_2$ | | | | | 200 |
| $B_3$ | | | | | 100 |
| | 100 | 100 | 100 | 100 | 400 |

If we know the information for any six cells $[(J-1)(K-1)]$ the remaining cells within the table would become automatically know; thus having no freedom to vary. With the following information for six cells (example bolded) the remaining cells could be easily determined and these last six cells have no freedom to change once the first six are identified.

| | $A_1$ | $A_2$ | $A_3$ | $A_4$ | |
|---|---|---|---|---|---|
| $B_1$ | **26** | **18** | 10 | 46 | 100 |
| $B_2$ | 43 | **56** | **68** | 33 | 200 |
| $B_3$ | **31** | 26 | 22 | **21** | 100 |
| | 100 | 100 | 100 | 100 | 400 |

The decision rule is: with $\alpha = 0.05$, reject $H_0$ if $\chi^2$ is greater than $\chi^2_{(J-1)(K-1)}(\alpha)$. In the case of four columns and three rows, the critical chi square value with $\alpha = 0.05$ from Table B15 is:

$$\chi^2_{(3)(2)}(\alpha) = \chi^2_6(\alpha) = 12.592$$

The expected value for any cell is calculated by multiplying its respective row sum times its respective column sum and dividing by the total number or the grand sum.

$$E = \frac{\sum C \cdot \sum R}{\sum Total} \qquad \text{Eq. 16.6}$$

To illustrate this, the calculations for the expected values for a three by two contingency table would be:

| | | | |
|---|---|---|---|
| (C1 x R1)/T | (C2 x R1)/T | (C3 x R1)/T | $\Sigma$ = R1 |
| (C1 x R2)/T | (C2 x R2)/T | (C3 x R2)/T | $\Sigma$ = R2 |
| $\Sigma$ = C1 | $\Sigma$ = C2 | $\Sigma$ = C3 | $\Sigma\Sigma$ = T |

For example, in a pharmacology study mice of various age groups are administered a chemical proposed to induce sleep. After 30 minutes the animals are assessed to determine if they are asleep or awake (based on some predetermined criteria). The purpose of the study is to determine if the particular agent is more likely to induce sleep in different age groups. The study results are as follows:

| | Asleep ($C_1$) | Awake ($C_2$) |
|---|---|---|
| 3 months ($R_1$) | 7 | 13 |
| 10 months ($R_2$) | 9 | 11 |
| 26 months ($R_3$) | 15 | 5 |

Simply stated, the hypothesis under test is that age does not influence sleep induction by the proposed agent being tested.

$H_0$: $P(C_1|R_1) = P(C_1|R_2) = P(C_1|R_3) = P(C_1)$
$P(C_2|R_1) = P(C_2|R_2) = P(C_2|R_3) = P(C_2)$
$H_1$: $H_0$ is false

Or simply stated:

$H_0$: Sleep is independent of the age of the mice
$H_1$: $H_0$ is false, a relationship exists

The decision rule is, with $\alpha = 0.05$, reject $H_0$ if $\chi^2 > \chi^2_{v=2}(0.05) = 5.99$. A comparison of the observed and expected values are as follows:

Observed

| | $C_1$ | $C_2$ | $\Sigma$ |
|---|---|---|---|
| $R_1$ | 7 | 13 | 20 |
| $R_2$ | 9 | 11 | 20 |
| $R_3$ | 15 | 5 | 20 |
| $\Sigma$ | 31 | 29 | 60 |

Expected

| | $C_1$ | $C_2$ |
|---|---|---|
| $R_1$ | 10.3 | 9.7 |
| $R_2$ | 10.3 | 9.7 |
| $R_3$ | 10.3 | 9.7 |

Calculation of the chi square statistic is:

$$\chi^2 = \frac{(7-10.3)^2}{10.3} + \frac{(13-9.7)^2}{9.7} + \frac{(9-10.3)^2}{10.3} + \ldots \frac{(5-9.7)^2}{9.7} = 6.94$$

The decision based on a sample of 60 mice is that with $\chi^2 > 5.99$, is to reject $H_0$ and conclude that age does influence the induction of sleep by this particular chemical. It appears that the agent has the greatest effect on the older animals.

For the chi square test of independence there are two general rules: 1) there must be at least one observation in every cell, no empty cells and 2) the expected value for each cell must be equal to or greater than five. The chi square formula is theoretically

**Table 16.5** Original Data for Example Comparing Age Groups and Incidence of Side Effects

| | Age in Years | | | | |
|---|---|---|---|---|---|
| Side Effects | <18 | 18-45 | 46-65 | >65 | |
| None | 80 | 473 | 231 | 112 | 896 |
| Mild | 9 | 68 | 43 | 27 | 147 |
| Moderate | 2 | 24 | 8 | 8 | 42 |
| Severe | 1 | 5 | 3 | 6 | 15 |
| Total | 92 | 570 | 285 | 153 | 1100 |

**Table 16.6** Original Expected Values for Age Groups and Incidence of Side Effects

| | Age in Years | | | | |
|---|---|---|---|---|---|
| Side Effects | <18 | 18-45 | 46-65 | >65 | |
| None | 74.94 | 464.29 | 232.15 | 124.62 | 896 |
| Mild | 12.30 | 76.17 | 38.08 | 20.45 | 147 |
| Moderate | 3.51 | 21.77 | 10.88 | 5.84 | 42 |
| Severe | 1.25 | 7.77 | 3.89 | 2.09 | 15 |
| Total | 92 | 570 | 285 | 153 | 1100 |

valid only when the expected values are sufficiently large. If these criteria are not met, adjacent rows or columns should be combined so that cells with extremely small values or empty cells are combined to form cells large enough to meet the criteria. To illustrate this consider the following example of a multicenter study where patients were administered an experimental aminoglycoside for gram negative infections. The incidences of side effects are reported in Table 16.5. Is there a significant difference in the incidence of side effects based upon the age of the patients involved in the study?

Unfortunately, an examination of the expected values indicates that four cells fall below the required criteria of an expected value of at least five (Table 16.6). One method for correcting this problem would be to combine the last two rows (moderate and severe side effects) and create a 3 x 4 contingency table (Table 16.7). This combination is more logical than combining the severe side effects with either the mild side effects or the absence of side effects. However, one cell still has an expected value less than five. The next logical combination would be the first two columns (ages <18 and 18-45 years old) as presented in Table 16.8. This 3 x 3 design meets all of the criteria for performing a chi square analysis. Adjusting the initial observed data to the new 3 x 3 design is presented in Table 16.9. It should be noted that the number of data points is the same as those in the original 4 x 4 design and we have not sacrificed any of our information by collapsing the cells. The new hypotheses would be:

**Table 16.7** Expected Values Resulting from Collapsing Side Effects

| | Age in Years | | | | |
|---|---|---|---|---|---|
| Side Effects | <18 | 18-45 | 46-65 | >65 | |
| None | 74.94 | 464.29 | 232.15 | 124.62 | 896 |
| Mild | 12.30 | 76.17 | 38.08 | 20.45 | 147 |
| Moderate/Severe | 4.76 | 29.54 | 14.77 | 7.93 | 57 |
| Total | 92 | 570 | 285 | 153 | 1100 |

**Table 16.8** Expected Values Resulting from Collapsing Both Age Groups and Side Effects

| | Age in Years | | | |
|---|---|---|---|---|
| Side Effects | 18-45 | 46-65 | >65 | |
| None | 539.23 | 232.15 | 124.62 | 896 |
| Mild | 88.47 | 38.08 | 20.45 | 147 |
| Moderate/Severe | 34.30 | 14.77 | 7.93 | 57 |
| Total | 662 | 285 | 153 | 1100 |

**Table 16.9** Observed Outcomes with Collapsing Both Age Groups and Side Effects

| | Age in Years | | | |
|---|---|---|---|---|
| Side Effects | <46 | 46-65 | >65 | |
| None | 553 | 231 | 112 | 896 |
| Mild | 77 | 43 | 27 | 147 |
| Moderate/Severe | 32 | 11 | 14 | 57 |
| Total | 662 | 285 | 153 | 1100 |

$H_0$: $P(S_1 \mid A_1) = P(S_1 \mid A_2) = P(S_1 \mid A_3) = P(S_1)$
$P(S_2 \mid A_1) = P(S_2 \mid A_2) = P(S_2 \mid A_3) = P(S_2)$
$P(S_3 \mid A_1) = P(S_3 \mid A_2) = P(S_3 \mid A_3) = P(S_3)$

$H_1$: $H_0$ is false

or:

$H_0$: Severity of side effects is independent of age group

$H_1$: $H_0$ is false, a relationship exists

and the decision rule would be: with $\alpha = 0.05$, reject $H_0$ if $\chi^2 > \chi_4^2\,(0.05) = 9.4877$. Note the decrease from the original nine degrees of freedom (4 – 1 rows time 4 – 1 columns) to the new four degrees of freedom. The calculation for the chi square statistic would be:

$$\chi^2 = \frac{(553 - 539.23)^2}{539.23} + \frac{(231 - 232.15)^2}{232.15} + \ldots \frac{(14 - 7.93)^2}{7.93}$$

$$\chi^2 = 11.62$$

The decision is with $\chi^2 > 9.4877$ reject $H_0$, conclude that there is a significant difference in side effects based on age.

If the chi square data for the test of independence is reduced to the smallest possible design, a 2 x 2 contingency table, and the expected values are still too small to meet the requirements (no empty cells and every expected value ≥5 per cell), then the **Fisher's exact test** should be considered (below).

The chi square test of independence provides little information about the strength or type of relationship between the two variables. Means of assessing such associations are discussed in Chapter 17.

### Yates' Correction for a 2 x 2 Contingency Table

A 2 row by 2 column (2 x 2) contingency table also could be set up by designating the four cells as *a*, *b*, *c*, and *d* (Figure 16.3). This particular format will be used for several tests in this and the following three chapters. Using these letters, another way to calculate $\chi^2$ for a 2 x 2 design (which would produce the identical same results as Equation 15.2), is:

$$\chi^2 = \frac{n(ad - bc)^2}{(a+c)(b+d)(a+b)(c+d)} \qquad \text{Eq. 16.7}$$

As an example, consider the following data. A new design in shipping containers for ampules is compared to the existing one to determine if the number of broken units can be reduced. One hundred shipping containers of each design are subjected to identical rigorous abuse and failures are defined as broken ampules in excess of 1%. The results of the study are presented in Table 16.10. Notice the exact percent of breakage is ignored in favor of a success/failure criteria. Do the data suggest the new

| | | |
|---|---|---|
| a | b | a + b |
| c | d | c + d |
| a + c | b + d | n |

**Figure 16.3** Format for defining the contents of a 2 x 2 contingency table.

**Table 16.10** Data Comparing Tow Container Designs

| Results | New Container | Old Container | Total |
|---|---|---|---|
| Success | 97 | 88 | 185 |
| Failure | 3 | 12 | 15 |
| Totals | 100 | 100 | 200 |

design is an improvement over the one currently used? In this case the expected values would be:

| | |
|---|---|
| 92.5 | 92.5 |
| 7.5 | 7.5 |

and the definitional calculation for the chi square statistic (Eq. 16.2) would be:

$$\chi^2 = \sum \frac{(O-E)^2}{E}$$

$$\chi^2 = \frac{(97-92.5)^2}{92.5} + \frac{(88-92.5)^2}{92.5} + \frac{(3-7.5)}{7.5} + \frac{(12-7.5)^2}{7.5} = 5.84$$

Using the alternate formula (Eq. 16.7), the same results are obtained:

$$\chi^2 = \frac{n(ad-bc)^2}{(a+b)(c+d)(a+c)(b+d)}$$

$$\chi^2 = \frac{200(97(12)-3(88))^2}{(100)(100)(185)(15)} = \frac{162{,}000{,}000}{27{,}750{,}000} = 5.84$$

In this particular example the hypotheses would be:

$H_0$: Success or failure is independent of container style
$H_1$: $H_0$ is false

or more accurately:

$H_0$: $P(S_1 | C_1) = P(S_1 | C_2) = P(S_1)$
$P(S_2 | C_1) = P(S_2 | C_2) = P(S_2)$
$H_1$: $H_0$ is false

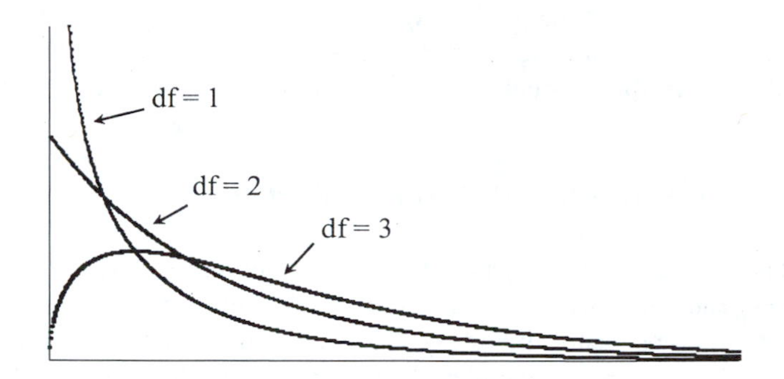


**Figure 16.4** Chi square distributions for less than four degrees of freedom.

and the decision rule is: with $\alpha$ = 0.05, reject $H_0$ if $\chi^2 > \chi_1^2$ (0.05) = 3.8415. Therefore, based on either formula the decision, since $\chi^2 > 3.8415$ we would reject $H_0$, conclude that the rate of damage is not independent of the type of container used.

Similar to the discussion of the *z*-test for proportions, the calculated chi square value is based upon discrete, discontinuous data, but the chi square critical value is based on a continuous distribution (Figure 16.1). Therefore, the calculated chi square value is only an approximation of the theoretical chi square distribution and these approximations are good for larger numbers of degrees of freedom, but not as accurate for only one degree. Also, since there is a decrease to the smallest possible degrees of freedom, the distribution no longer resembles a normal distribution (Figure 16.4). Therefore, we must once again use a correction to produce a more conservative estimate. Using the symbols in Figure 16.3, Yates' modification of Eq. 16.7 produces a smaller numerator and a more conservative estimate for the chi square statistic.

$$\chi^2_{corrected} = \frac{n(|ad - bc| - .5n)^2}{(a+c)(b+d)(a+b)(c+d)} \qquad \text{Eq. 16.8}$$

Recalculating the chi square statistic for data from the above example using Yates' correction for continuity, the results are:

$$\chi^2_{corrected} = \frac{n(|ad - bc| - .5n)^2}{(a+b)(c+d)(a+c)(a+d)}$$

$$\chi^2_{corrected} = \frac{200[\,|(97)(12) - (3)(88)| - (.5)(200)\,]^2}{(100)(100)(185)(15)}$$

$$\chi^2_{corrected} = \frac{128000000}{27750000} = 4.61$$

Yates' correction provides a more conservative, harder to reject, chi square value. If the above example were computed without Yates' correction the resulting $\chi^2$ would have equaled 6.88. In this particular case either finding would have resulted in the rejection of $H_0$.

**Comparison of Chi Square to the Z-Test of Proportions**

In the case of a 2 x 2 contingency table, one could either perform a chi square test of independence or a two-sample z-test of proportions on the same information and the results would be identical. For example, consider our previous example of the shipping containers and broken ampules. The exact *p*-value for a $\chi^2 = 5.84$ is 0.0157 (determined using the Excel® function CHIDIST). One could also present this same data in the format seen in Table 16.10. The proportion of failures, 0.03 (3/100) for the new design and 0.12 (12/100) for the old design are presented in the table. Using Eq. 15.5 to determine if there is a significant difference between the two proportions, the resulting *z*-value would 2.416, which represents a *p*-value of 0.0157 (determined using the Excel® function [1-NORMSDIST(z)]*2). Similarly, using Yates' correction for either of the tests (Eq. 15.11 or Eq. 16.8) produces the same results, both *p*-values equal to 0.032. Thus, either test can be performed for data appearing in a 2 x 2 contingency table.

**Fisher's Exact Test**

If data for a chi square test of independence is reduced to a 2 x 2 contingency table and the expected values are still too small to meet the requirements (at least five per cell) or have a zero in one or more of the four cells, the Fisher's exact test can be employed (Fisher, 1936). The term "exact" is used because the result of the calculations produces the exact probabilities of obtaining the observed results if the two variables are independent. This test is sometimes referred to as **Fisher's four-fold test** because of the four cells of frequency data. The test used the previously described *a-b-c-d* four cell format (Figure 16.3). The formula involves the factorials for the cells and margins:

$$p = \frac{(a+b)!\,(c+d)!\,(a+c)!\,(b+d)!}{n!\,a!\,b!\,c!\,d!} \qquad \text{Eq. 16.9}$$

An alternative formula, using possible combinations (Chapter 2), produces the exact same results:

$$p = \frac{\binom{a+b}{a}\binom{c+d}{c}}{\binom{n}{a+c}} \qquad \text{Eq. 16.10}$$

The first formula is identical to the nonparametric median test that will be discussed in Chapter 21. However, in this test, cells are based on the evaluation of two independent variables and not on estimating a midpoint based on the sample data.

Multiple tests are performed to determine the probability of not only the research data, but also the probabilities for each possible combination to the extreme of the observed data. These probabilities are summed to determine the exact probability of the outcome observed given complete independence. For example, assume the following data is collected:

| | | |
|---|---|---|
| 3 | 7 | 10 |
| 7 | 3 | 10 |
| 10 | 10 | 20 |

The *p*-value is calculated for this one particular outcome; however, *p*-values are also calculated for the possible outcomes that are even more extreme with the *same fixed margins*:

| | |
|---|---|
| 2 | 8 |
| 8 | 2 |

| | |
|---|---|
| 1 | 9 |
| 9 | 1 |

| | |
|---|---|
| 0 | 10 |
| 10 | 0 |

Then the probabilities of all four possibilities are summed.

The decision rule compares this exact probability to a $p_{critical}$ (for example, 0.05). If it is smaller than the $p_{critical}$, reject $H_0$ and conclude that the rows and columns are not independent.

To illustrate the use of this test, assume the following example. Twelve laboratory rats are randomly assigned to two equal-sized groups. One group serves as a control, while the experimental group is administered a proposed carcinogenic agent. The rats are observed for the development of tumors. The following results are observed:

| | Tumor | No Tumor | |
|---|---|---|---|
| Experimental | 4 | 2 | 6 |
| Control | 1 | 5 | 6 |
| | 5 | 7 | 12 |

Is the likelihood of developing a tumor the same for both groups? The hypotheses are:

$H_0$: The group and appearance of a tumor are independent

$H_1$: The two variables are not independent

The decision rule is, with $\alpha = 0.05$, reject $H_0$ if $p < 0.05$. The computation for the probability of four tumors in the experimental group is:

$$p = \frac{(a+b)!(c+d)!(a+c)!(b+d)!}{n!\,a!\,b!\,c!\,d!}$$

$$p = \frac{6!\,6!\,5!\,7!}{12!\,4!\,1!\,2!\,5!} = 0.1136$$

For five tumors in the experimental group:

$$p = \frac{6!\,6!\,5!\,7!}{12!\,5!\,0!\,1!\,6!} = 0.0076$$

The probability of four or more experimental mice developing a tumor:

$$\begin{aligned} p(5) &= .0076 \\ p(4) &= \underline{.1136} \\ &\phantom{=}\ .1212 \end{aligned}$$

Therefore the decision, with $p > 0.05$, is that $H_0$ cannot be rejected. It is assumed that the two variables are independent and that the incidence of tumor production is independent of the agent's administration.

### McNemar's Test

The McNemar test can be used to evaluate the relationship or independence of paired discrete variables. The test involves dichotomous measurements (i.e., pass/fail, yes/no, present/absent) that are paired. The paired responses are constructed into a fourfold, or 2 x 2 contingency table and outcomes are tallied into the appropriate cell. Measurement can be paired on the same individuals or samples over two different time periods (similar to our previous use of the paired t-test in Chapter 9) and the layout for the contingency table is presented in Figure 16.5. Alternatively subjects can be paired based on some predetermined and defined characteristic (replacing First Measurement and Second Measurement with the two characteristics in Figure 16.5.

For example, if it were based on a yes/no response over two time periods, those individuals responding “yes” at both time periods would be counted in the upper left corner (cell *a*) and those answering “no” on both occasions are counted in the lower right corner (cell *d*). Mixed answers, indicating changes in responses, would be counted in the other two diagonal cells (*b* and c). If there was absolutely no change over the two time periods, we would expect that 100% of the results would appear in cells *a* and *d*. Those falling in cells *c* and *b* represent changes between the two measurements periods and are of primary interest to the researcher.

| | | First Measurement | |
|---|---|---|---|
| | | Outcome 1 | Outcome 2 |
| Second Measurement | Outcome 1 | a | b |
| | Outcome 2 | c | d |

**Figure 16.5** Design for a McNemar test for paired data.

For the McNemar's test the statistic is as follows:

$$\chi^2_{McNemar} = \frac{(b-c)^2}{b+c} \qquad \text{Eq. 16.11}$$

As with the previous Yates' correction of continuity, a similar correction can be made to produce a more conservative approximation for the McNemar test:

$$\chi^2_{McNemar} = \frac{(|b-c|-1)^2}{b+c} \qquad \text{Eq. 16.12}$$

In either case, the null hypothesis would be that there is no significant change between the two times or characteristics. Because we are dealing with a 2 x 2 contingency table, the number of degrees of freedom is one (rows – 1 x columns – 1). Thus we will compare our calculated statistic to a critical $\chi^2$ with one degree of freedom or 3.8415, (Appendix B, Table B15). If the $\chi^2_{McNemar}$ exceeds 3.8415 we reject $H_0$ and assume a significant change between the two measurements (similar to our previous $H_0$: $\mu \neq 0$ in the paired t-test).

As an example, assume that 100 patients are randomly selected based on visits to a local clinic and assessed for specific behavior that is classified as a risk factor for colon cancer. The risk factor is classified as either present or absent. During the course of their visit and with a follow-up clinic newsletter, they are educated about the incidence and associated risks for a variety of cancers. Six months after the initial assessment patients are evaluated with respect to the presence or absence of the same risk factor. The following table represents the results of the study:

| | | Risk Factor Before Instruction | | |
|---|---|---|---|---|
| | | Present | Absent | |
| Risk Factor After Instruction | Present | 40 | 5 | 45 |
| | Absent | 20 | 35 | 55 |
| | | 60 | 40 | 100 |

The null hypothesis would be that the instructional efforts had no effect.

$H_0$: Instruction did not influence presence of the risk factor
$H_1$: $H_0$ is false

The decision rule would be to reject $H_0$, of independence, if $\chi^2_{McNemar}$ greater than $\chi^2_1(1-\alpha) = 3.8415$. The calculations would be:

$$\chi^2_{McNemar} = \frac{(b-c)^2}{b+c} = \frac{(5-20)^2}{5+20} = \frac{225}{25} = 9.0$$

Yates' correction of continuity would produce a more conservative estimation:

$$\chi^2_{McNemar} = \frac{(|b-c|-1)^2}{b+c} = \frac{(|5-20|-1)^2}{5+20} = \frac{196}{25} = 7.84$$

Either method would result in the rejection of $H_0$ and the decision that the instruction of patients resulted in a change in risk taking behavior.

Another way to think of McNemar's procedure is as a test of proportions, based on samples that are related or correlated in some way. The McNemar's test does not require the computation of the standard error for the correlation coefficient. The computation, using the previous notations for a 2 x 2 contingency table is:

$$z = \frac{a-d}{\sqrt{a+d}} \qquad \text{Eq. 16.13}$$

where in large samples $\chi^2 = z^2$.

## Cochran's Q Test

Cochran's Q test can be thought of as a complement to the complete randomized block design, discussed in Chapter 10, when dealing with discrete data. It is an extension of the McNemar's test to three or more levels of the independent variable. Similar to the randomized complete block design, subjects or observations are assigned to blocks to reduce variability within each level of the independent variable. The design is used to create homogenous blocks. The data is set up so that each level of the independent variable represents a column and each row represents a homogeneous block. Subjects within each block are more homogeneous than subjects within the different blocks. As seen in Table 16.11, the blocking effect is represented by the row and each block contains results for each level of the independent variable. There is still only one observation per cell and this is reported as a pass (coded as 1) or fail (coded as 0) result. Each of the columns are summed ($C$) and the sum squared ($C^2$). Also, each block is summed ($R$) and the sum squared ($R^2$). Lastly, both the $R$ and $R^2$ are summed producing $\Sigma R$ and $\Sigma R^2$. The formula for Cochran's Q is:

**TABLE 16.11** General Structure of a Randomized Block Design

| | Levels of the Independent Variable | | | | | |
|---|---|---|---|---|---|---|
| | $C_1$ | $C_2$ | | $C_k$ | R | $R^2$ |
| Block $b_1$ | $x_{11}$ | $x_{12}$ | ... | $x_{1k}$ | $\Sigma x_{1k}$ | $\Sigma x_{1k}^2$ |
| Block $b_2$ | $x_{21}$ | $x_{22}$ | ... | $x_{2k}$ | $\Sigma x_{2k}$ | $\Sigma x_{2k}^2$ |
| Block $b_3$ | $x_{31}$ | $x_{32}$ | ... | $x_{3k}$ | $\Sigma x_{3k}$ | $\Sigma x_{3k}^2$ |
| ... | ... | ... | ... | ... | ... | ... |
| Block $b_j$ | $x_{j1}$ | $x_{j2}$ | ... | $x_{jk}$ | $\Sigma x_{jk}$ | $\Sigma x_{jk}^2$ |
| C | $\Sigma x_{j1}$ | $\Sigma x_{j2}$ | | $\Sigma x_{jk}$ | | |
| $C^2$ | $\Sigma x_{j1}^2$ | $\Sigma x_{j2}^2$ | ... | $\Sigma x_{jk}^2$ | | |
| | | | | $\Sigma R =$ | $\Sigma\Sigma x_k$ | |
| | | | | $\Sigma R^2 =$ | | $\Sigma\Sigma x_k^2$ |

$$Q = \frac{(k-1)\,[(k\Sigma C^2) - (\Sigma R)^2]}{k(\Sigma R) - \Sigma R^2} \qquad \text{Eq. 16.14}$$

where $k$ is the number of levels of the discrete independent variable. The resultant $Q$-value is compared to the chi square critical value with $k-1$ degrees of freedom. If the $Q$-value exceeds the critical value there is a significant difference among the various levels of the independent variable.

As an example, a pharmaceutical company is trying to decide among four different types of gas chromatographs produced by four different manufacturers. To evaluate the performance of these types of equipment, ten laboratory technicians are asked to run samples and evaluate the use of each piece of equipment. They are instructed to respond as either acceptable (coded 1) or unacceptable (coded 0) for the analysis performed by the equipment. The results of their evaluations appear in Table 16.12. Is there a significant relationship between the pieces of equipment and technicians' evaluations? The hypotheses being tested are:

$H_0$: Technician evaluations are independent of the equipment tested
$H_1$: $H_0$ is false

The decision rule is, with 95% confidence or $\alpha$ equal less than 0.05, reject $H_0$ if $Q$ is greater than $\chi^2_{(k-1)}(1-\alpha)$, which is 7.8147 ($k-1=3$). The sum of columns and rows are presented in Table 16.13 and the calculation of Cochran's Q is as follows:

$$Q = \frac{(k-1)\,[(k\Sigma C^2) - (\Sigma R)^2]}{k(\Sigma R) - \Sigma R^2}$$

**Table 16.12** Evaluations for Various Types of Equipment

| | Manufacturer | | | |
|---|---|---|---|---|
| Technician | A | B | C | D |
| 1 | 0 | 1 | 0 | 1 |
| 2 | 0 | 0 | 0 | 1 |
| 3 | 1 | 0 | 0 | 1 |
| 4 | 0 | 1 | 0 | 1 |
| 5 | 0 | 0 | 1 | 0 |
| 6 | 0 | 0 | 1 | 1 |
| 7 | 0 | 0 | 0 | 1 |
| 8 | 0 | 1 | 1 | 1 |
| 9 | 0 | 0 | 0 | 1 |
| 10 | 1 | 0 | 0 | 1 |

**Table 16.13** Example of Cochran's Q Test

| | Manufacturer | | | | | |
|---|---|---|---|---|---|---|
| Technician | A | B | C | D | R | $R^2$ |
| 1 | 0 | 1 | 0 | 1 | 2 | 4 |
| 2 | 0 | 0 | 0 | 1 | 1 | 1 |
| 3 | 1 | 0 | 0 | 1 | 2 | 4 |
| 4 | 0 | 1 | 0 | 1 | 2 | 4 |
| 5 | 0 | 0 | 1 | 0 | 1 | 1 |
| 6 | 0 | 0 | 1 | 1 | 2 | 4 |
| 7 | 0 | 0 | 0 | 1 | 1 | 1 |
| 8 | 0 | 1 | 1 | 1 | 3 | 9 |
| 9 | 0 | 0 | 0 | 1 | 1 | 1 |
| 10 | 1 | 0 | 0 | 1 | 2 | 4 |
| C = | 2 | 3 | 3 | 9 | | |
| $C^2$ = | 4 | 9 | 9 | 81 | | |
| | | | | $\Sigma R$ = | 17 | |
| | $\Sigma C^2$ = 103 | | | $\Sigma R^2$ = | | 33 |

$$Q = \frac{(3)[(4)(103) - (17)^2]}{(4)(17) - 33} = \frac{369}{35} = 10.54$$

With Q greater than the critical value of 7.8147, the decision is to reject the hypothesis of independence and assume that the type of equipment tested did influence the technicians' responses. Based on the *C's* presented in Tables 16.12 and 16.13, manufacturer *D*'s product appears to be preferred.

**Mantel-Haenszel Test**

The Mantel-Haenszel test sometimes referred to as the **Cochran-Mantel-Haenszel test**, can be thought of as a three-dimensional chi square test, where a 2 x 2 contingency table is associated with main factors in the row and column dimensions. However a third, possibly confounding variable, is added as a depth dimension in our design. This third extraneous factor may have *k*-levels and the resultant design would be 2 x 2 x k levels of three discrete variables. In other words, we are comparing *k* different 2 x 2 contingency tables. Using the *a,b,c,d* labels as in the previous 2 x 2 designs, the Mantel-Haenszel compares each $a_i$ ($a_1$ through $a_k$) with its corresponding expected value. The $a_i$ is the observed value for any one level of the possible confounding variable. The statistic is:

$$\chi^2_{MH} = \frac{\left[\sum \frac{a_i d_i - b_i c_i}{n_i}\right]^2}{\sum \frac{(a+b)_i(c+d)_i(a+c)_i(b+d)_i}{(n_i - 1)(n_i^2)}} \qquad \text{Eq. 16.15}$$

This can be modified to create a numerator that compares the observed and expected values for one cell of the 2 x 2 matrix and sums this comparison for each level of the confounding variable.

$$\chi^2_{MH} = \frac{\left[\Sigma( a_i - \frac{(a_i + b_i)(a_i + c_i)}{n_i}\right]^2}{\sum \frac{(a+b)_i(c+d)_i(a+c)_i(b+d)_i}{n_i^2(n_i - 1)}} \qquad \text{Eq. 16.16}$$

The null hypothesis reflects independence between the row and column variable, correcting for the third extraneous factor. The calculated $\chi^2_{MH}$ is compared to the critical value $\chi^2_1(1-\alpha)$. If that value exceeds the critical value, the row and column factors are not independent and there is a significant relationship between the two factors.

For example, consider a study of smoking and the presence or absence of chronic lung disease. Assume that we are concerned that the subjects' environment might confound the finding. We decide to also evaluate the data based on home setting (i.e., urban, suburb, rural). The results of the data collection are presented in Table 16.14.

Equation 16.16 can be simplified by modifying certain parts of the equation. For example the $e_i$ (the expected value) for each confounding level of $a_i$ is:

$$e_i = \frac{(a_i + b_i)(a_i + c_i)}{n_i} \qquad \text{Eq. 16.17}$$

**Table 16.14** Evaluation of Setting as a Possible Confounding Factor

| Site | Chronic Lung Disease | Smoker | Nonsmoker | Totals |
|---|---|---|---|---|
| Urban | Yes | 45 | 7 | 52 |
| | No | 16 | 80 | 96 |
| | | 61 | 87 | 148 |
| Suburban | Yes | 29 | 10 | 39 |
| | No | 19 | 182 | 201 |
| | | 48 | 192 | 240 |
| Rural | Yes | 27 | 18 | 45 |
| | No | 16 | 51 | 67 |
| | | 43 | 69 | 112 |

This is equivalent to stating that the sum of the margin for the row multiplied by the margin for the column divided by the total number of observations associated with the *i*th level is the expected value. This is the same way we calculated the expected value in the contingency table for a chi square test of independence. For example, for the suburban level the $e_i$ is:

$$e_2 = \frac{(39)(48)}{240} = 7.8$$

This will be compared to the observed result ($a_2 = 29$) to create part of the numerator for Eq. 16.17. In a similar manner, a $v_i$ can be calculated for the denominator at each level of the confounding variable:

$$v_i = \frac{(a_i + b_i)(c_i + d_i)(a_i + c_i)(b_i + d_i)}{n_i^2 (n_i - 1)} \qquad \text{Eq. 16.18}$$

The $v_i$ for the rural level is:

$$v_3 = \frac{(45)(67)(43)(69)}{(112)^2(112 - 1)} = 6.425$$

These intermediate results can be expressed in a table format:

| | Urban | Suburban | Rural |
|---|---|---|---|
| $a_i$ | 45 | 29 | 27 |
| $e_i$ | 21.43 | 7.80 | 17.28 |
| $v_i$ | 8.23 | 5.25 | 6.42 |

and entered into the following equation:

$$\chi^2_{MH} = \frac{[\Sigma(a_i - e_i)]^2}{\Sigma v_i} \qquad \text{Eq. 16.19}$$

The results are

$$\chi^2_{MH} = \frac{[(45-21.43)+(29-7.80)+(27-17.28)]^2}{(8.23+5.25+6.42)} = \frac{(54.49)^2}{19.90} = 149.20$$

With the $\chi^2_{MH}$ greater than $\chi^2_i(1-\alpha)$ we reject the null hypothesis of no association between the two main factors controlling for the potentially confounding environmental factor. If the value would have been less than the critical $\chi^2$ value we would have failed to reject the null hypothesis and assumed that the confounding variable affected the initial $\chi^2$ results for the 2 x 2 contingency table.

A correction for continuity can also be made with the Mantel-Haenszel procedure:

$$\chi^2_{MH} = \frac{[\Sigma(a_i - e_i) - 0.5]^2}{\Sigma v_i} \qquad \text{Eq. 16.20}$$

In the previous example this correction would produce the expected, more conservative result:

$$\chi^2_{MH} = \frac{(54.49 - 0.5)^2}{19.90} = 146.47$$

In this case, either the Mantel-Haenszel test or the corrected version would produce a statistically significant result and rejection of the null hypothesis.

**Reference**

Fisher, R.A. (1936). *Statistical Methods for Research Workers*, Oliver and Boyd, London, pp. 100-102.

**Suggested Supplemental Readings**

Agresti, A. (2002). *Categorical Data Analysis*, Second edition, John Wiley and Sons, Inc., New York, pp. 36-101.

Bolton, S. (1997). *Pharmaceutical Statistics: Practical and Clinical Applications*, Third edition, Marcel Dekker, Inc., New York, pp. 570-578.

Daniel, W.W. (1999). *Biostatistics: A Foundation for Analysis in the Health Sciences*, Seventh edition, John Wiley and Sons, New York, pp. 571-599.

Havilcek, L.L. and Crain, R.D. (1988). *Practical Statistics for the Physical Sciences*, American Chemical Society, Washington, DC, pp. 212-221.

**Example Problems**

1. A medication, known to cause severe irritation to stomach mucosa, is tested with a series of special tablet coatings to prevent release until after the tablet has passed through the stomach. Three variations of the coating formula are tested on 150 fasted volunteers, randomly assigned to each group. The presence or absence of irritation, through endoscopic examination, is noted for each subject.

| | GI Irritation | |
|---|---|---|
| | Present($P_1$) | Absent($P_2$) |
| Formula A | 10 | 40 |
| Formula B | 8 | 42 |
| Formula C | 7 | 43 |

   Was there a significant difference in the likelihood of irritation based on the coating formulas?

2. A pharmacist is evaluating the amount of time needed for nurse surveyors to observe drug delivery in 70 long-term care facilities. The median time required by the surveyors is 2.5 hours. The researcher wishes to know if the type of delivery system (unit dose vs. traditional) influences the amount of survey time required.

| | Unit Dose | Traditional | Total |
|---|---|---|---|
| 2.5 hours or less | 26 | 10 | 36 |
| More than 2.5 hours | 14 | 20 | 34 |
| Total | 40 | 30 | 70 |

3. Immediately after training on a new analytical method, technicians were asked their preference between the new method and a previously used, "old" method. Six months later, after the technicians had experience with the new method, they were resurveyed with respect to their preference. The results of the two surveys are presented below. Did experience with the new method significantly change their preferences?

| | | Preferred Method before Experience | | |
|---|---|---|---|---|
| | | New | Old | |
| Preferred Method After Experience | New | 12 | 8 | 20 |
| | Old | 3 | 7 | 10 |
| | | 15 | 15 | 30 |

4. In preparing to market an approved tablet in a new package design, the manufacturer tests two different blister packs to determine the rates of failure (separation of the adhesive seal) when stored at various temperatures and humidities. One thousand tablets in each of two conditions were stored for three months and the number of failures were observed:

| | 40 degrees 50% relative humidity | 60 degrees 50% relative humidity |
|---|---|---|
| Blister pack A | 2 | 5 |
| Blister pack B | 6 | 6 |

Is there a significant relationship between the storage conditions and the frequency of failures based on the blister pack used?

5. A manufacturer is experimenting with a new 50-mm diameter screw-type container using various amounts of torque for closure. The tightness of the containers are tested based on moisture permeability. From the data reported below, is there any significant difference in moisture level based on the torque used to tighten the cap?

| | Torque (inch-pounds) | | | | |
|---|---|---|---|---|---|
| Moisture | 21 | 24 | 27 | 30 | |
| $< 2000$ | 26 | 31 | 36 | 45 | 138 |
| $\geq 2000$ | 24 | 19 | 14 | 5 | 62 |
| Total | 50 | 50 | 50 | 50 | 200 |

6. Twenty volunteers were randomly assigned to a randomized three-way cross-over clinical trial involving the same topical medication presented in three different formulations (A, B, and C). During each phase of the study volunteers were assessed for the presence or absence of erythema (redness) at the site of application. Was there any significant difference among the formulation for the incidence of erythema?

| Volunteer | Formulation A | B | C | Volunteer | Formulation A | B | C |
|---|---|---|---|---|---|---|---|
| 001 | 0 | 1 | 0 | 011 | 0 | 0 | 1 |
| 002 | 1 | 0 | 1 | 012 | 0 | 0 | 0 |
| 003 | 0 | 0 | 0 | 013 | 1 | 0 | 1 |
| 004 | 0 | 0 | 0 | 014 | 0 | 0 | 0 |
| 005 | 0 | 1 | 1 | 015 | 0 | 0 | 0 |
| 006 | 0 | 0 | 0 | 016 | 0 | 0 | 0 |
| 007 | 0 | 0 | 0 | 017 | 1 | 1 | 0 |
| 008 | 0 | 0 | 0 | 018 | 0 | 0 | 0 |
| 009 | 0 | 0 | 0 | 019 | 1 | 0 | 1 |
| 010 | 1 | 1 | 0 | 020 | 1 | 1 | 1 |

(code: 1 = erythema)

7. In one of the example problems in Chapter 15, an instrument manufacturer ran a series of disintegration tests to compare the pass/fail rate of a new piece of equipment at two extreme temperatures. The manufacturer decided to also evaluate the influence of paddle speed as a possible confounding factor. The test was designed to collect results at two speeds, defined as fast and slow. The results were as follows:

| Speed of Paddle | Temperature | Test Results Pass | Fail | Totals |
|---|---|---|---|---|
| Fast | 39°C | 48 | 2 | 50 |
| | 35°C | 47 | 3 | 50 |
| | | 95 | 5 | 100 |
| Slow | 39°C | 48 | 2 | 50 |
| | 35°C | 45 | 5 | 50 |
| | | 93 | 7 | 100 |

Without Yate's correction for continuity there is a significant relationship between the temperature and proportion of test failures ($\chi^2$ = 4.35). Could the paddle speed be a confounding factor in the design?

**Answers to Problems**

1. Severe irritation to stomach mucosa compared with special tablet coatings.

| | GI Irritation Present($P_1$) | Absent($P_2$) |
|---|---|---|
| Formula A | 10 | 40 |
| Formula B | 8 | 42 |
| Formula C | 7 | 43 |

Hypotheses: $H_0$: $P(P_1|F_A) = P(P_1|F_B) = P(P_1|F_C) = P(P_1)$
$P(P_2|F_A) = P(P_2|F_B) = P(P_2|F_C) = P(P_2)$

$H_1$: $H_0$ is false

Decision rule: With $\alpha = 0.05$, reject $H_0$ if $\chi^2 > \chi_2^2\ (0.05) = 5.99$

Observed

| | | |
|---|---|---|
| 10 | 40 | 50 |
| 8 | 42 | 50 |
| 7 | 43 | 50 |
| 25 | 125 | 150 |

Expected

| | | |
|---|---|---|
| 8.33 | 41.67 | 50 |
| 8.33 | 41.67 | 50 |
| 8.33 | 41.67 | 50 |
| 25 | 125 | 150 |

Calculations:

$$\chi^2 = \sum \frac{(O-E)^2}{E}$$

$$\chi^2 = \frac{(10-8.33)^2}{8.33} + \frac{(40-41.67)^2}{41.67} + \ldots \frac{(43-41.67)^2}{41.67} = 0.66$$

Decision: With $\chi^2 < 5.99$, cannot reject $H_0$.

2. Above and below the median time needed for nurse surveyors to observe drug deliveries.

Hypotheses: $H_0$: P(2.5 or less|UD) = P(2.5 or less|Trad) = P(2.5 or less)
P(>2.5|UD) = P(>2.5|Trad) = P(>2.5)
(time required is not influenced by the delivery system)
$H_1$: $H_0$ is false

Decision rule: With $\alpha = 0.05$, reject $H_0$ if $\chi^2 > \chi_1^2\ (0.05) = 3.84$

Test statistic: (because of only one degree of freedom, use Yates' correction)

$$\chi^2_{corrected} = \frac{n(|ad-bc|-.5n)^2}{(a+b)(b+d)(a+b)(c+d)}$$

Data:

| | Unit Dose | Traditional | Total |
|---|---|---|---|
| 2.5 hours or less | 26 | 10 | 36 |
| More than 2.5 hours | 14 | 20 | 34 |
| Total | 40 | 30 | 70 |

Calculations:

$$\chi^2_{corrected} = \frac{70(\,|(26)(20)-(14)(10)|-.5(70)\,)^2}{(40)(30)(36)(34)}$$

$$\chi^2_{corrected} = \frac{70(\,|520-140|-35\,)^2}{1468800} = \frac{70(345\,)^2}{1468800} = \frac{8331750}{1468800} = 5.67$$

Decision: With $\chi^2 > 3.84$, reject $H_0$ and conclude that the time required to do the nursing home surveys is dependent on the type of delivery system used in the facility.

3. Paired comparison between technicians' evaluations at two times: McNemar's test.

Hypotheses: $H_0$: Experience did not influence opinion of equipment
$H_1$: $H_0$ is false

Decision rule: With $\alpha = 0.05$, reject $H_0$, if $\chi^2_{McNemar} > \chi^2_1(1-\alpha) = 3.84$.

Calculations:

| | | Preferred Method Before Experience | | |
|---|---|---|---|---|
| | | New | Old | |
| Preferred Method After Experience | New | 12 | 8 | 20 |
| | Old | 3 | 7 | 10 |
| | | 15 | 15 | 30 |

$$\chi^2_{McNemar} = \frac{(b-c\,)^2}{b+c} = \frac{(8-3)^2}{8+3} = \frac{25}{11} = 2.27$$

Correction of continuity:

$$\chi^2_{McNemar} = \frac{(\,|b-c|-1\,)^2}{b+c} = \frac{(\,|8-3|-1\,)^2}{8+3} = \frac{16}{11} = 1.45$$

Decision: Fail to reject $H_0$, conclude there was no significant change in method preference over the six-month period.

4. Comparisons of two blister packs stored under different conditions.
Independent variable: Storage conditions (discrete)
Dependent variable: Type of blister pack (discrete)
Test statistic: Fisher exact test (cell A has an expected value <5)

| | 40 degrees 50% relative humidity | 60 degrees 50% relative humidity | |
|---|---|---|---|
| Blister pack A | 2 | 5 | 7 |
| Blister pack B | 6 | 6 | 12 |
| | 8 | 11 | 19 |

Hypothesis: $H_0$: Blister pack and storage conditions are independent
$H_1$: The two variables are not independent

Decision rule: With $\alpha = 0.05$, reject $H_0$ if $p(>2) > 0.05$.

Calculations:

a. $p(2)$ of two failures with blister pack A

$$p = \frac{(a+b)!(c+d)!(a+c)!(b+d)!}{n!a!b!c!d!}$$

$$p = \frac{7!12!8!11!}{19!2!5!6!6!} = 0.256$$

b. $p(1)$ of one failure with blister pack A

$$p = \frac{7!12!8!11!}{19!1!6!7!5!} = 0.073$$

c. $p(0)$ of no failures with blister pack A

$$p = \frac{7!12!8!11!}{19!0!7!8!4!} = 0.006$$

Decision: The probability of two or less failures with blister pack A under independent conditions is 0.335 (0.256 + 0.073 + 0.006), therefore we cannot reject $H_0$ and assume that the frequency of failures by blister pack is independent of the storage conditions.

5. Experiment with different amounts of torque and resulting moisture content in a pharmaceutical product.

| Moisture | Torque (inch-pounds) 21 | 24 | 27 | 30 | |
|---|---|---|---|---|---|
| <2000 | 26 | 31 | 36 | 45 | 138 |
| ≥2000 | 24 | 19 | 14 | 5 | 62 |
| Total | 50 | 50 | 50 | 50 | 200 |

Hypotheses:

$H_0$: $P(M_1|T_1) = P(M_1|T_2) = P(M_1|T_3) = P(M_1|T_4) = P(M_1)$
$P(M_2|T_1) = P(M_2|T_2) = P(M_2|T_3) = P(M_2|T_4) = P(M_2)$
$H_1$: $H_0$ is false
(The null hypothesis stating that there the moisture observed is independent of the torque place upon the lid.)

Decision rule: With $\alpha = 0.05$, reject $H_0$ if $\chi^2 > \chi_3^2\ (0.05) = 7.81$

Expected values:

| Moisture | Torque (inch-pounds) 21 | 24 | 27 | 30 | |
|---|---|---|---|---|---|
| <2000 | 34.5 | 34.5 | 34.5 | 34.5 | 138 |
| ≥2000 | 15.5 | 15.5 | 15.5 | 15.5 | 62 |
| Total | 50 | 50 | 50 | 50 | 200 |

Computation:

$$\chi^2 = \frac{(26-34.5)^2}{34.5} + \frac{(31-34.5)^2}{34.5} + \ldots \frac{(5-15.5)^2}{15.5}$$

$$\chi^2 = 18.43$$

Decision: With $\chi^2 > 7.81$ reject $H_0$, conclude that there is a significant difference in moisture level based on the amount of torque applied during closure.

6. Comparison of three topical formulations: Cochran's Q.

Hypotheses: $H_0$: Development of erythema is independent of formulation used
$H_1$: $H_0$ is false

Decision rule: With $\alpha = 0.05$, reject $H_0$ if $Q > \chi^2_2(1-\alpha) = 5.99$.

Data: Table 16.15

Computations:

$$Q = \frac{(k-1)[(k\Sigma C^2) - (\Sigma R)^2]}{k(\Sigma R) - \Sigma R^2} = \frac{(2)[(3)(97) - (17)^2]}{(3)(17) - 35} = \frac{4}{16} = 0.25$$

Decision: With $Q < 5.99$, fail to reject $H_0$ and conclude that erythema is independent of the formulation.

**Table 16.15** Data for Question 6

| | Formulation (1 = erythema) | | | | |
|---|---|---|---|---|---|
| Volunteer | A | B | C | R | $R^2$ |
| 001 | 0 | 1 | 0 | 1 | 1 |
| 002 | 1 | 0 | 1 | 2 | 4 |
| 003 | 0 | 0 | 0 | 0 | 0 |
| 004 | 0 | 0 | 0 | 0 | 0 |
| 005 | 0 | 1 | 1 | 2 | 4 |
| 006 | 0 | 0 | 0 | 0 | 0 |
| 007 | 0 | 0 | 0 | 0 | 0 |
| 008 | 0 | 0 | 0 | 0 | 0 |
| 009 | 0 | 0 | 0 | 0 | 0 |
| 010 | 1 | 1 | 0 | 2 | 4 |
| 011 | 0 | 0 | 1 | 1 | 1 |
| 012 | 0 | 0 | 0 | 0 | 0 |
| 013 | 1 | 0 | 1 | 2 | 4 |
| 014 | 0 | 0 | 0 | 0 | 0 |
| 015 | 0 | 0 | 0 | 0 | 0 |
| 016 | 0 | 0 | 0 | 0 | 0 |
| 017 | 1 | 1 | 0 | 2 | 4 |
| 018 | 0 | 0 | 0 | 0 | 0 |
| 019 | 1 | 0 | 1 | 2 | 4 |
| 020 | 1 | 1 | 1 | 3 | 9 |
| C = | 6 | 5 | 6 | | |
| $C^2$ = | 36 | 25 | 36 | | |
| | | | $\Sigma R$ = | 17 | |
| | $\Sigma C^2$ = 97 | | $\Sigma R^2$ = | | 35 |

7. Comparison of pass/fail rate with a piece of disintegration equipment at different temperatures, controlling for paddle speed: Mantel-Haenszel chi square.

Hypotheses: $H_0$: Temperature and failure rate are independent (controlling for paddle speed)

$H_1$: $H_0$ is false

Decision rule: With $\alpha = 0.05$, reject $H_0$ if $\chi^2_{MH} > \chi^2_1(1-\alpha) = 3.84$.

Data: disintegration test

| Speed of Paddle | Temperature | Test Results Pass | Fail | Totals |
|---|---|---|---|---|
| Fast | 39°C | 48 | 2 | 50 |
| | 35°C | 47 | 3 | 50 |
| | | 95 | 5 | 100 |
| Slow | 39°C | 48 | 2 | 50 |
| | 35°C | 45 | 5 | 50 |
| | | 93 | 7 | 100 |

Intermediate steps for fast speed:

$$e_1 = \frac{(a_1+b_1)(a_1+c_1)}{n_1} = \frac{(50)(95)}{100} = 47.5$$

$$v_1 = \frac{(a_1+b_1)(c_1+d_1)(a_1+c_1)(b_1+d_1)}{n_1^2(n_1-1)} = \frac{(50)(50)(95)(5)}{100^2(99)} = 1.199$$

| | Fast | Slow |
|---|---|---|
| $a_i$ | 48 | 48 |
| $e_i$ | 47.5 | 46.5 |
| $v_i$ | 1.2 | 1.6 |

Mantel-Haenszel chi square:

$$\chi^2_{MH} = \frac{[\Sigma(a_i-e_i)]^2}{\Sigma v_i} = \frac{[(48-47.5)+(48-46.5)]^2}{1.2+1.6} = 1.43$$

Decision: Fail to reject $H_0$, conclude that the temperature and failure rates are independent.

# 17

# Measures of Association

To this point, most of this book has dealt with tests of differences (i.e., t-tests, F-tests, z-tests of proportions). Other tests have dealt with relationships (i.e., chi-square test of independence, correlation). This chapter focuses on other types of relationships with tests that can measure the degree of association between different types of variables. As will be seen the term "measures of association" refers to a wide variety of procedures used to evaluate the strengths of various types of relationships. One type of measure of association has already been discussed in Chapter 13 where the correlation coefficient measured the association, or strength of the relationship between two or more variables where those variables involve interval or ratio data. This chapter will focus primarily on measures of association for nominal and ordinal types of data scales (Chapter 1 defined these types of scales).

## Introduction

These measures of association require that at least one of the variables presented in a nominal or ordinal scale and can be applied only to data from a contingency table reporting frequencies (or counts). Basically, there is a significant relationship, if the magnitude of the observed relationship is different than what one would expect due to chance produced from random sampling. If there is no association, the two variables are independent and there is an absence of any predictable relationship between the variables tested. Data will be presented in contingency tables similar to those used for the chi square test of independence (Chapter 16). Chi square itself is not a measure of association, but a test of the null hypothesis that two nominal or ordinal variables are unrelated.

The strengths of the various measures of association are evaluated by their **coefficients of association**. Most coefficients of association vary from 0 (indicating no relationship) to +1.0 (a perfect positive relationship) or −1.0 (a perfect negative relationship). This is similar to the type of association for continuous data was seen with the correlation coefficient (Chapter 13). As discussed in the following sections, there are various types of "perfect relationships" and "null relationships." When these specific coefficients of associate are discussed, their definitions of perfect and no relationships will be cited and this is an important criterion for choosing among the available tests. Most coefficients of association define "perfect relationship" as monotonicity (discussed below) and consider the null relationship as statistical independence.

There are four type of "perfect linear" relationship when dealing with nominal and ordinal data (and their respective measures of association) and these are based on **monotonicity**. These types of perfect linear relationship are defined as those where there is: 1) strict monotonicity; 2) ordered monotonicity; 3) predictive monotonicity; and 4) weak monotonicity. These terms are defined below. If there is perfect strict monotonicity all other three monotonic states will also be perfect. If either the ordered monotonicity or predictive monotonicity is perfect, there will be perfect weak monotonicity. However, it is impossible to have perfect ordered monotonicity and perfect predictive monotonicity at the same time unless there is perfect strict monotonicity. None of the definitions for monotonicity are appropriate for a curvilinear relationship which is beyond the scope of this book.

Monotonicity is based on the possible pairs of cells within a contingency table. Seen below is a three by four contingency table with the cells labeled *a* to *l*.

| | | Factor X | | | |
|---|---|---|---|---|---|
| | | 1 | 2 | 3 | 4 |
| Factor Y | 1 | a | b | c | d |
| | 2 | e | f | g | h |
| | 3 | i | j | k | l |

Data for the *X*-factor (the *X* variable) contain four levels and the *Y*-factor (*Y* variable) contains three levels of a nominal or ordinal variable. Based on possible various combinations (discussed in Chapter 2, Eq. 2.12) there should be 66 different pairs of cells in this contingency table (twelve cells taken two at a time).

$$\binom{12}{2} = \frac{12!}{2!10!} = \frac{12 \times 11 \times 10!}{2 \times 1 \times 10!} = 66$$

These pairs can be identified by combining cells across rows, down columns or across diagonals to identify all 66 possible pair. The symbol $X_0$ represents the pairs moving down the columns (*X*-factor). For the first column they would be *ae*, *ai* and *ei*. Which can be written *ae* + *ai* + *ei or a(e* + *i)* +*ei*. Expanding this for all columns there are:

$$X_0 = ae + ai + bf + bj + cg + ck + dh + dl + ei + fj + gk + hl$$

pairs and this formula can be simplified and written as follows:

$$X_0 = a(e + i) + b(f + j) + c(g + k) + d(h + l) + ei + fj + gk + hl$$

Using this same nomenclature the $Y_0$ is the pairs moving across each row (*Y*-factor):

$$Y_0 = a(b{+}c{+}d) + e(f{+}g{+}h) + i(j{+}k{+}l) + b(c{+}d) + f(g{+}h) + j(k{+}l) + cd + gh + kl$$

Thus, the columns account for 12 pairs and the rows for 18 pairs. These are also referred to as "ties by row" or "ties by column." The remaining 36 possible pairs (66–30) can be identified moving diagonally through the table. **Concordant pairs** (*P*) are those moving diagonally from upper left to lower right (this is based on the assumption that for ordinal data, values will nominally increase moving from left to right in the columns and from top to bottom on the rows):

$$P = a(f + g + h + j + k + l) + b(g + h + k + l) + c(h + l) + e(j + k + l) + f(k + l) + gl$$

Concordant pairs represent an additional 18 pairs. The discordant pairs must account for the remaining 18 pairs. **Discordant pairs** (*Q*) are those moving from upper right to lower left:

$$Q = d(e + f + g + I + j + k) + c(e + f + I + j) + b(e + i) + h( i + j + k) + g(I + j) + fi$$

A parallel terminology is to refer to the concordant pairs as the pairing of values along the "diagonal" (i.e., cells *af, ak, al*) and the term "off-diagonal" (i.e., cells *dg, di, dj*) for discordant pairs. Thus, as summarized in Table 17.1, all possible results presented in the previous contingency table we observe are as follows:

| | |
|---|---|
| Pairs by row ($Y_0$) | 18 |
| Pairs by column ($X_0$) | 12 |
| Concordant pairs (*P*) | 18 |
| Discordant pairs (*Q*) | 18 |
| Total possible pairs | 66 |

The use of concordant and discordant pairs will be needed for many of the tests of association discussed in this chapter.

This simplest matrix for a contingency table would be the 2 x 2 design (read two by two) and used in dichotomous tests of association, Figure 16.3. We have already seen the use of all possible pairs in the second formula (Eq. 16.5) presented for calculating the 2 x 2 chi square test of independence.

$$\chi^2 = \frac{n(ad - bc)^2}{(a+c)(b+d)(a+b)(c+d)}$$

Note that the numerator contains the only possible concordant and discordant pairs and the denominator is the product of the pairs by row and pairs by column:

**Table 17.1** Summary of all Possible Pairs for a 4 x 3 Table

| Type of Pair | Symbol | Possible Pairs | Numbers of pairs |
|---|---|---|---|
| Concordant | P | a(f+g+h+j+k+l) + b(g+h+k+l) + c(h+l) + e(j+k+l) + f(k+l) + gl | 18 |
| Discordant | Q | d(e+f+g+i+j+k) + c(e+f+i+j) + b(e+i) + h(i+j+k) + g(i+j) + fi | 18 |
| Pairs by Columns | $X_0$ | a(e+i) + b(f+j) + c(g+k) + d(h+l) + ei + fj + gk + hl | 12 |
| Pairs by Rows | $Y_0$ | a(b+c+d) + e(f+g+h) + i(j+k+l) + b(c+d) + f(g+h) +j(k+l) + cd + gh + kl | 18 |

$$\chi^2 = \frac{n(ad - bc)^2}{(a+c)(b+d)(a+b)(c+d)} = \frac{n(P-Q)}{X_0 Y_0} \qquad \text{Eq. 17.1}$$

In this case the diagonal pairing is cells *a* and *d*, and the off-diagonal is cells *b* and *c*. Unfortunately, this same logic cannot be expanded for tables larger than a 2 x 2 scenario.

Recall that the chi square test of independence (Chapter 16) indicates if a significant relationship exists (rejection of the null hypothesis of independence).

Failure to reject the null hypothesis resulted in the failure to reject the assumption of statistical independence between the row and column variables. The tests in this chapter will provide a measure of the strength of the relationship between the variables, expressed as the coefficient of association. Consider the following perfect linear relationship.

| | | Factor X | | |
|---|---|---|---|---|
| | | A | B | C |
| | A | 25 | 0 | 0 |
| Factor Y | B | 0 | 25 | 0 |
| | C | 0 | 0 | 25 |

In this example, there is a perfect positive **strict monotonicity** (by definition the $Q$, $X_0$ and $Y_0$ each equal 0); a perfect **ordered monotonicity** (defined as both $Q$ and $Y_0$ equal 0); a perfect **predictive monotonicity** (defined as both $Q$ and $X_0$ equal 0); and a perfect **weak monotonicity** (defined as $Q$ equals 0). If this data were evaluated for a chi square test of independence there would be a statistically significant relationship ($\chi^2 = 150$, $p < 0.0001$). As seen later, measures of association (such as Cramer's V for nominal data or *gamma* for ordinal data) would both produce a coefficient of association equal to 1.0. Thus, the following measures of association can be thought of as determinations of how close (or far) the relationships are to a perfect linear relationship.

In addition, some of the tests discussed in this chapter are **symmetric**, meaning that not only can values be predicted for *Y*-factor from *X*-factor, but values for the *X*-factor can be predicted from *Y*-factor. In contrast **asymmetric** test cannot be used to predict the *X*-factor from the *Y*-factor. Thus, care must be taken in the selection of the row and column variables. For consistency, if an independent variable exists, it will always be used as the columns variable.

A second reason for the use of measures of association is that the chi square test of independence is very sensitive to the sample size. When a sample size is too small, the chi square value may represent an overestimate. However, if the sample size is too large, the chi square values could be an underestimate. The use of tests such as the phi, contingency coefficient, Cramer's $V$ or *gamma*, in general overcome this problem.

**Dichotomous Associations**

As discussed in Chapter 2, a dichotomous variable is a discrete, nominal variable with only two possible levels (i.e., control-experimental, live-die). Therefore, coefficients of association used for these tests employ 2 x 2 contingency tables. Measures of association for larger contingency tables will be presented under nominal and ordinal associations. Another term used to generically label measures of association involving two dichotomous variables in a **fourfold point correlation coefficient**.

A chi square test of independence with one degree of freedom (discussed in Chapter 16) is an example of a dichotomous test of association and employs the traditional 2 x 2 matrix (Figure 16.3). As mentioned previously, if there is an independent variable it will be presented as the column factor.

For descriptive statistics involving dichotomous data the reporting of **percent difference** is the most common and simplest to use. The percent difference (*%d*) is computed by subtracting the difference (measured in percent) between the columns in either row. Using the previous layout, *%d* would equal $a - b$ or $b - a$, and $c - d$ or $d - c$. Consider the following example:

Example 1:

| Hospitalization Required | | Initial Outpatient Therapy | | |
|---|---|---|---|---|
| | | Treatment A | Treatment B | %d |
| | Yes | 20 (50%) | 10 (25%) | -25% (b – a) |
| | No | 20 (50%) | 30 (75%) | +25% (d – c) |

In this case there was a 25% difference in the incidence of hospitalization depending upon which treatment was selected. With Treatment B there appeared to be 25% fewer hospital admissions. In this type of association *%d* would define the "perfect association" as strictly monotonic and "null relation" is statistical independence between the two treatments.

Note that in a 2 x 2 table the *%d*'s are asymmetric. If number were changes the *%d* would still be the same. Adjusting the data:

Example 2:

| Hospitalization Required | | Initial Outpatient Therapy | | |
|---|---|---|---|---|
| | | Treatment A | Treatment B | %d |
| | Yes | 18 (45%) | 14 (35%) | –10% (b – a) |
| | No | 22 (55%) | 26 (65%) | +10% (d – c) |

As noted, if the independent variable is always represented by the column percentages, the sum for each column will be 100%. If independent and dependent variables were reversed the columns would not add up to 100% (80% and 120% in Example 2).

In additional, the percent difference allows one to state whether the independent variable makes a difference in predicting values for the dependent variable. In Example 1, if *d%* equals 25%, then knowing the independent variable (i.e., which treatment) makes a 25% difference in predicting the outcome for the dependent variable (i.e., hospitalization).

As seen in Chapter 16, evaluation of the significance for a 2 x 2 contingency table could be evaluated using either Pearson's or Yate's chi square, both using the traditional *a,b,c,d*-matrix presented earlier. Three measures of association can be used to evaluate this data: 1) the *phi*-coefficient; 2) Yule's $Q$ test; and 3) Yule's $Y$ test.

The **phi-statistic** ($\phi$) is a chi square-based measure of association for 2 x 2 tables involving nominal or ordinal dichotomous data. Phi eliminates the impact of sample size by dividing chi square by *n* (the sample size) and taking the square root of the results:

$$\phi = \sqrt{\frac{\chi^2}{n}} \qquad \text{Eq. 17.2}$$

The chi square used in the calculation should be the Pearson's chi square (Eq. 16.5), not the Yate's correction for continuity formula (Eq. 16.6). The phi-value measures the strength of the relationship based on the number of cases in the discordant pair minus the number of cases in the concordant pair, adjusted for by the sample size. An equivalent formula is:

$$\phi = \frac{|(B)(C) - (A)(D)|}{\sqrt{(A+B)(C+D)(A+C)(B+D)}} \qquad \text{Eq. 17.3}$$

Phi represents the mean percent difference between the column variable and row variable where either can be considered to cause the other. Thus, the $\phi$-statistic is symmetrical and it does not matter if the column is an independent or dependent variable. The $\phi$-statistic defines perfect association as a perfect predictive monotonicity and the null hypothesis is statistical independence. This test is sometime referred to as a **fourfold point correlation.**

For the previous example (Example 2) for hospitalization following treatment with Treatments A and B the chi square value would be:

$$\chi^2 = \frac{n(ad - bc)^2}{(a+c)(b+d)(a+b)(c+d)} = \frac{80((18)(26)-(14)(22))^2}{(40)(40)(32)(48)}$$

$$\chi^2 = \frac{2048000}{2457600} = 0.83$$

The phi-value would be:

$$\phi = \sqrt{\frac{\chi^2}{n}} = \sqrt{\frac{0.83}{80}} = 0.102$$

The alternative formula produces the same results:

$$\phi = \frac{|(B)(C) - (A)(D)|}{\sqrt{(A+B)(C+D)(A+C)(B+D)}} = \frac{|(14)(22)-(18)(26)|}{\sqrt{(40)(40)(32)(48)}}$$

$$\phi = \frac{160}{1567.67} = 0.1202$$

The results make sense, since the coefficient of association (in this case $\phi$) should show a weak relationship since the chi square value was not significant (critical value for rejecting the null hypothesis of independence is 3.84). If there was a significant chi square, resulting in the rejection of the null hypothesis of independent, we would expect a stronger measure of association. For example, if the chi square (for the same sample size) were 9.00 the resulting phi statistic would be much closer to 1.0:

$$\phi = \sqrt{\frac{\chi^2}{n}} = \sqrt{\frac{9.00}{80}} = 0.335$$

The resultant $\varphi$ can be viewed as a symmetric percent difference (*%d*), measuring the percent of results seen on the diagonal. In the 2 x 2 table, the φ-value is identical to a correlation coefficient for the same data. It is possible to dichotomize continuous data (i.e., above and below the median value for the row variable and column variable). This type of comparison is referred to as a **tetrachoric correlation**. Phi is also referred to as the **Pearson's coefficient of mean-square contingency.** Unfortunately this same name is sometimes also applied to the Pearson's contingency coefficient, which is a modification of the phi-statistic. For tables larger than a 2 x 2 design the maximum value for phi depends on the size of the table and can exceed 1.0. Thus, even though phi can handle larger tables, it is not practical to use for such situations. Other tests discussed in the next sessions are appropriate for a larger table involving nominal or ordinal data.

The **Yule's Q** is another symmetric measure of association based on the difference between the concordant ($P = ad$) and discordant ($Q = bc$) data pairings. Yule's Q is recommended for situations where at least one variable is ordinal and is calculated as follows:

$$Q = \frac{(ad - bc)}{(ad + bc)} = \frac{P - Q}{P + Q} \qquad \text{Eq. 17.4}$$

This represents the difference ($P - Q$) as a percentage of all nontied (column or row) pairs ($P + Q$). Once again using the example cited above for hospitalizations (Example 2), the Yule's Q would be:

$$Q = \frac{(18)(26) - (14)(22)}{(18)(26) + (14)(22)} = \frac{160}{776} = 0.206$$

Thus, the surplus of consistent data pairs over inconsistent pairs is 20.6% of all the nontied data pairs. In this case, consistent implies consistent with the null hypothesis of independence between treatment choices and hospitalization. The $Q$-value approaches 1.0 under perfect weak monotonicity. Interpretation of the results can be difficult and arbitrary with measures of association and there are various ways to verbally describe the magnitude of the association. One rule of thumb (Knoke and Bohrnstedt, 1991) goes as follows:

| | |
|---|---|
| 0 – 0.249 | virtually no relationship |
| 0.25 – 0.49 | weak relationship |
| 0.50 – 0.75 | moderate relationship |
| 0.75 - 1.00 | strong relationship |

This same terminology could serve for other measures of association presented in this chapter. As will be seen later, the *gamma* statistic is used as a measure of association involving tables larger than 2 x 2. The resultant $Q$-value is equal to *gamma* for a 2 x 2 table. However, the $Q$-value will often be higher than *gamma* for the dichotomized data since the process of dichotomization will tend to mask small differences that in turn lead to inconsistent pairs in *gamma*. Therefore it is not recommended to take ordinal or nominal data and force it into a dichotomous situation. It is better to evaluate the data in its original larger format (larger than a 2 x 2 configuration). Also, Yule's Q should not be used if there is a zero in any of the cells.

The **Yule's Y test** is a modification of the Yule's $Q$. It is also called **Yule's coefficient of colligation**, and uses the geometric mean of diagonal and off-diagonal pairs rather than the number of pairs seen in the $Q$-statistic.

$$Y = \frac{(\sqrt{ad} - \sqrt{bc})}{(\sqrt{ad} + \sqrt{bc})} = \frac{\sqrt{P} - \sqrt{Q}}{\sqrt{P} + \sqrt{Q}} \qquad \text{Eq. 17.5}$$

Yule's $Y$ is rarely used, because there is no easily expressible interpretation. Yule's $Y$ tends to estimate associations more conservatively than Yule's $Q$. Unfortunately, this measure of association has little substantive or theoretical meaning.

Also associated with the results with a dichotomous independent variable are odds ratios and relative risk ratios. These two measures will be discussed separately and in greater detail in the next chapter.

### Nominal Associations

This portion of the chapter will consider a test of association where the nominal data exceed the 2 x 2 contingency table. These nominal coefficients of association may be computed for ordinal or higher levels of data, but tests designed specifically for higher types of scales have more power and are preferred to these tests. The tests presented in this section include: 1) Pearson's C: 2) Cramer's V; 3) Tschuprow's T; 4) the lambda statistic; and 5) the uncertainty coefficient. These procedures adjust the chi square statistic to remove the effect of sample size. Unfortunately they are not easily interpretable, but provide an index regarding the strength of the association between nominal variables.

As seen in Chapter 1, a nominal variable consists of a set of unique categories in no specific order (i.e., males-females, treatments A-B-C-D). Tests in this section measure the strength of association between variables; however, they cannot indicate a direction or describe the nature of relationship. Each measure of association for nominal data attempts to modify the chi square statistic to reduce the influence of sample size and degrees of freedom (shape of the table). These tests also restrict the range of possible outcome to values between 0 and 1 (with zero indicating no association linking the two variables0.

**Pearson's C** or the **contingency coefficient** is a modification of the phi-statistic for contingency tables that are larger than two rows by two columns. The formula is as follows:

$$C = \sqrt{\frac{\chi^2}{\chi^2 + N}} \qquad \text{Eq. 17.6}$$

The *C*-statistic will approach a maximum of 1.0 only for large tables (i.e., 5 x 5 or larger contingency tables). Unfortunately, the *C*-statistic is influenced by the size and shape of the contingency table. In larger nonsquare tables, the *C*-value will never reach 1.0 and for smaller tables the *C*-value will underestimate the level of association. To correct for this underestimation there is **Sakoda's adjusted Pearson's C** (*C**). Regardless of the size of the table the *C** will vary between 0 and 1. *C** is calculated using the following modification on Pearson's *C*:

$$C^* = \frac{C}{\sqrt{\frac{k-1}{k}}} \qquad \text{Eq. 17.7}$$

where *k* equals the number of rows or columns (whichever is smaller).

As an example, let us expand on the previous problem to four different treatment levels. Notice that the treatments represent nominal categories with no particular order. Once again, for consistency, the independent variable is presented as the column factor.

| | Initial Outpatient Therapy | | | | |
|---|---|---|---|---|---|
| Hospitalization Required | Rx A | Rx B | Rx C | Rx D | |
| Yes | 22 | 14 | 10 | 14 | 60 |
| No | 18 | 26 | 30 | 26 | 100 |
| | 40 | 40 | 40 | 40 | 160 |

The chi square value (Eq. 16.2) for this example would be 8.11. With three degrees of freedom (critical value = 7.815, $p < 0.05$) the result for the chi square would be statistically significant and we would reject the null hypothesis of independence between the two variables. But how strong is the relationship between the therapy and hospitalization? The resultant $C$ and $C^*$ values are:

$$C = \sqrt{\frac{\chi^2}{\chi^2 + N}} = \sqrt{\frac{8.11}{168.11}} = 0.220$$

$$C^* = \frac{C}{\sqrt{\frac{k-1}{k}}} = \frac{0.220}{\sqrt{\frac{2-1}{2}}} = \frac{0.220}{0.707} = 0.311$$

Neither $C$ nor $C^*$ are easily interpreted. It is possible to view $C$ as a nominal approximation of the correlation coefficient ($r$). Both $C$ and $C^*$ define a perfect relationship as a perfect weak monotonic, and view the null hypothesis as statistical independence. For smaller the tables, it is more likely that $C$ (but not $C^*$) will be less than 1.0 regardless of monotonicity. Therefore, Pearson's C is recommended for tables smaller than a 5 x 5 design. As with the $\phi$-statistic, both $C$ and $C^*$ are symmetrical and either variable (row or column) can be the independent variable.

An alternative for tables equal to or larger than a 5 x 5 design, is **Tshuprow's T**, which is another chi square-based measure of association. It approaches 1.0 in square contingency tables (equal number of rows and columns) where the row marginal values are identical to column marginal values. The greater the deviation from a square table or the more unequal the marginal values, the more $T$ will be less than 1.0. Tshuprow's T is the square root of chi square value divided by sample size $n$ times the square root of the number of degrees of freedom (rows minus one times columns minus one):

$$T = \sqrt{\frac{\chi^2}{n\sqrt{(r-1)(c-1)}}} \qquad \text{Eq. 17.8}$$

Since the $T$-value is less than 1.0 for nonsquare tables, it is recommended for square tables. For 2 x 2 tables, $T$ equals the phi-statistics, since the square root of $(r-1)(c-1)$ is the one.

$$T = \sqrt{\frac{\chi^2}{N\sqrt{1*1}}} = \sqrt{\frac{\chi^2}{N}} = \phi$$

$T$-statistic defines a perfect linear relationship for weak monotonicity and defines a null relationship as statistical independence. As with previous tests, Tshuprow's $T$ is symmetrical. Using the previous example ($\chi^2 = 8.11$) Tshuprow's $T$-value would be:

$$T = \sqrt{\frac{8.11}{160\sqrt{(3)(1)}}} = \sqrt{\frac{8.11}{277.13}} = 0.171$$

Of all the tests for nominal associations, **Cramer's V** is the most popular. Also a chi square-based measure, it has the best 0-to-1 association when row marginal values equal column marginal values (regardless of table size). Cramer's V test is used when one or both of the variables are nominally scaled. The formula is:

$$V = \sqrt{\frac{\chi^2}{Nm}} \qquad \text{Eq. 17.9}$$

where $N$ is the total sample size and $m$ is either $(r - 1)$ or $(c - 1)$, whichever is smaller. Cramer's $V$ can be considered as a test of association between two variables measuring the percentage of their maximum possible variation. Squaring the $V$-value is the mean square canonical correlation between the variables. If either the rows or columns are equal to two categories Cramer's $V$ equals the phi-statistic.

$$V = \sqrt{\frac{\chi^2}{N(1)}} = \phi$$

The $V$-statistic defines a perfect linear relationship as one that has either predictive or ordered monotonicity and the null relationship is defined as statistical independence. As with previous tests, Cramer's $V$ is symmetrical and either variable can be the independent (column) variable.

Using the previous example ($\chi^2 = 8.11$) Cramer's $V$ is:

$$V = \sqrt{\frac{\chi^2}{Nm}} = \sqrt{\frac{8.11}{(160)(1)}} = 0.225$$

Note that each measure of association gave a slightly different value ($T = 0.171 < C = 0.220 < V = 0.225 < C^* = 0.311$).

Another type of measure of association deals with the **proportionate reduction of error** (*PRE*). *PRE* measures are generally used only when both an independent and dependent variable are present. For nominal data a *PRE* measure of association is *lambda*; for ordinal data *PRE* measurements include *gamma* and Somer's *d*. *Lambda* is discussed below and *gamma* and Somer's *d* will be discussed in the next section. Values for all three tests range between 0 and 1. They can be interpreted as follows: if for example, we have a *PRE* value equal to 0.47; by knowing the values represented by the independent variable, we are able to reduce our errors of predicting values for the dependent variable by 47%. In other words, we reduced our amount of error by 47%. *PRE* reflects the percentage reduction in errors in predicting the dependent variable given knowledge about the independent variable. With *PRE* measurements you are trying to assess whether knowing the distribution of the dependent variable, in relationship to the categories for the independent variable, will enable you to reduce the amount of error in predicting the distribution of the dependent variable.

The **lambda** test, also referred to as the **Goodman-Kruskal lambda**, is the first *PRE* measurement to be discussed. *Lambda* ($\lambda$) can be used for both nominal or ordinal data (two nominal variables, one nominal and one ordinal variable, or two ordinal variables). This probabilistic measurement is defined as the probability that an observation is in a category other than the most common category (the modal category). In other words, with no knowledge of the independent variable, the researcher could guess that each observation of the dependent variable will have the same value as the most frequent level. Therefore, the marginal value for this modal category is the number of correct guesses by chance alone. This creates the denominator of the lambda equation.

$$\lambda = \frac{\sum f_i - f_d}{N - f_d} \qquad \text{Eq. 17.10}$$

where $N$ is the total sample size, $f_d$ is marginal total of the modal category for the dependent variable, and $f_i$ is largest frequency for each level of the $i$ categories of the independent variable. For the example we have used in this section (hospitalization for four different therapies), the $N$=160, $f_d$ = 100, and the $f_i$'s are 22, 26, 30, and 26 for treatments A, B, C, and D, respectively. The lambda is:

$$\lambda = \frac{\sum f_i - f_d}{N - f_d} = \frac{(22 + 26 + 30 + 26) - 100}{160 - 100} = \frac{4}{60} = 0.067$$

In this example, knowing the drug therapy reduces errors in guessing the hospitalizations by 6.7%. The denominator represents the errors made not knowing which is subtracting the modal category of the dependent variable ($f_d$) from the total number of observations. In other words, if the researcher did not know the distribution of the drug therapies used, then she would guess at the likelihood of hospitalization, and she would be right 100 (($f_d$)) times and wrong 60 ($N - f_d$) times.

*Lambda* can be used when both variables are dependent variables. Lambda ranges between 0 and 1. A value of 0 means the independent variable offers no value in predicting the dependent variable. However, it does not necessarily imply statistical independence. *Lambda* reflects the reduction in error when the value for one of the variables is used to predict values of the other variable. With a 1.0, the independent variable perfectly predicts the categories of the dependent variable. For example, a lambda value of 0.65 indicates that the independent variable predicts 65% of the variation of the dependent variable.

The final measure of association for nominal data is the **uncertainty coefficient (UC)**, which is also referred to as **Theil's U**. The *UC* represents a percent reduction in error that accounts for the variance in the dependent variable. This variance is defined in terms of the logarithm of the ratios, thus the *UC* is sometimes referred to as the **entropy coefficient**. Both lambda and *UC* are *PRE* measures of nominal association, but *UC* is different because the formula takes into account the entire distribution rather than just the modal distribution. Therefore, it is often preferred over lambda. The *UC* can vary from 0 to 1. The formula for *UC(R|C)*, is the uncertainty coefficient for predicting the dependent variable (row) based on independent variable (column):

$$UC(R|C)=\frac{\left[\sum\left(\frac{r_j}{N}\cdot ln\frac{r_j}{N}\right)+\sum\left(\frac{c_k}{N}\cdot ln\frac{c_k}{N}\right)-\sum\sum\left(\frac{n_{ij}}{N}\cdot ln\frac{n_{ij}}{N}\right)\right]}{\sum\left(\frac{c_k}{N}\cdot ln\frac{c_k}{N}\right)} \quad \text{Eq. 17.11}$$

where $r_j$ is the margin total for each row, $c_j$ is the margin totals for each column, and $n_{ij}$ is the frequency within each cell. This test also could be used for ordinal data. When the *U* is 0, the independent variable is of no value in predicting the dependent variable. The uncertainty coefficient is an asymmetric measure and requires that the independent variable be placed in the columns. The "uncertainty coefficient" also has a proportionate reduction in error but the formula accounts for the entire distribution not just the mode (which is used for lambda). Therefore the uncertainty coefficient is preferred over the lambda-statistic.

As seen, the adjusted contingency coefficient ($C$*) and Cramer's *V* will vary between 0 and 1.0 regardless of sample size. However, the phi-, *C*-, and *T*-statistic do not. All measures that define a perfect linear relationship as strict monotonicity, require that the distribution of the marginal values be equal for the coefficient to reach 1.0. Also, note that measures of association do not assume randomly sampled data.

## Ordinal Associations

Looking at higher types of measurement scales, this section focuses on ordinal data and presents four different tests for measuring the association between two variables (*gamma*, Kendall's *tau-b*, Kendall's *tau-c*, and Somer'*d*). With ordinal measurements there are two or more categories and there is some inherent order among them (i.e., a five-point Likert scale ranging from strong disagreement to strong agreement with a statement). For *PRE* measurements, lambda can be used for both nominal and ordinal data (two nominal variables, one nominal and one ordinal variable, or two ordinal variables), but *gamma*, the Kendall taus and Somer's *d* are recommended only for two ordinal variables.

The **Goodman and Kruskal's gamma**, also simply referred to as **gamma**, is a symmetric measure based on the difference between concordant pairs (*P*) and discordant pairs (*Q*). The results can range from –1 to +1. As discussed previously concordant pairs are all possible pair going diagonally from the upper left to lower right and discordant pairs are diagonal pairs from the upper right to lower left. *Gamma* is 0 in the case of independence and is +1 if all the observations are concentrated in the upper-left to lower-right diagonal of the contingency table. *Gamma* is calculated as follows:

$$\Gamma = \frac{P-Q}{P+Q} \qquad \text{Eq. 17.12}$$

The sampling distribution for *gamma* is approximating normal for large samples and it is possible to compute its standard error and significance. *Gamma* can be thought of as the surplus of concordant pairs over discordant pairs. It is a percentage of all pairs ignoring ties (by row pairs and by column pairs). The *gamma* defines a perfect association as weak monotonicity. With statistical independence, *gamma* will be 0. However, *gamma* can also be 0 whenever the concordant pairs minus discordant pairs are 0. The strength of the association would commonly be verbally described; for example, a *gamma* of +0.65 would indicate a moderate, positive association between the two variables.

For 2 x 2 contingency tables, *gamma* will equals Yule's *Q*-statistic. If ordinal or higher data is dichotomized into two levels, *Q* will usually be lower than *gamma* for the original nondichotomized data. This is because the act of dichotomizing results in the loss of information since levels of one variable are being combined. Obviously, *gamma* cannot be computed when there is only one row or one column. However, it can be computed even when cell(s) frequencies are small or zero.

There are two Kendall tau tests: Kendall's *tau-b* and Kendall's *tau-c*. Kendall's *tau-b* and *tau-c* should be used when both variables are on ordinal scales. The range of possible outcomes varies from –1 to +1. The tests differ in the manner in which the concordant pairs minus discordant pairs are normalized. As a measure of association the **Kendall's tau-b** is often used for 2 x 2 contingency tables, but also may be used for larger matrices associated with ordinal data. Where *gamma* was concerned with the concordant and discordant pairs, Kendall's measures of association are based on the comparison of all possible pairs for both variables for all possible pairs of cases. It evaluates the excess of concordant over discordant pairs in the numerator and uses a term in the denominator that measures the geometric mean between the number of row pairs and column pairs. Theses terms were defined at the beginning of this chapter. The formula for Kendall's tau-b is:

$$\tau_b = \frac{P-Q}{\sqrt{(P+Q+X_0)(P+Q+Y_0)}} \qquad \text{Eq. 17.13}$$

Kendall's tau-b will reach either +1.0 or –1.0 for square tables only (equal number of rows and columns). However, *tau-b* is 0 under statistical independence for both square and nonsquare tables. It is recommended to use *tau-c* for tables that are not square.

**Kendall's tau-c** (also referred to as **Stuart's tau-c** or **Kendall-Stuart tau-c**) is a modification of the *tau-b* for large tables and specifically for nonsquare contingency tables (the number of rows and columns are not equal). *Tau-c* is an excess of concordant pairs over discordant pairs, times an adjustment factor for the size of the contingency table:

$$\tau_c = (P-Q)\left(\frac{2m}{n^2(m-1)}\right) \qquad \text{Eq. 17.14}$$

where $n$ is the total sample size and $m$ is the number of row or columns, whichever is smaller. *Tau-c* is a symmetrical test and can vary from −1 (for negative relationships) to +1. Neither *tau-b* nor *tau-c* are easy to interpret; they are simply an index of the strength of the association (somewhere between −1 and +1).

The **Somers' d** is a modified *gamma* statistic that penalizes for tied pairs on independent variable only, for hypotheses that are directional, where $x$ causes of predicts $y$; and to penalize for pairs tied on $y$ only, in hypotheses in which $y$ causes of predicts $x$. Somers' $d$ is used with ordinal data. The formula for the hypothesis that the column variable ($y$) causes or can predict the row variable ($x$) is:

$$d_{yx} = \frac{(P-Q)}{(P+Q+Y_0)} \qquad \text{Eq. 17.15}$$

If the hypothesis is that the row variable ($x$) causes or predicts the column variable ($y$), the formula is:

$$d_{xy} = \frac{(P-Q)}{(P+Q+X_0)} \qquad \text{Eq. 17.16}$$

Somers' $d$ is an asymmetric statistic, but by averaging $d_{xy}$ and $d_{yx}$ it can be made symmetrical. The symmetric $d$-value will be 1.0 only when both variables have strict monotonicity. Somer's $d$ result can be similar to the findings for other measures of association. For example, for 2 x 2 table, Somers' d will be equivalent to percent difference. For square tables, *tau-b* is the geometric mean between $d_{xy}$ and $d_{yx}$. An asymmetric Somers' $d$ will be less than or equal to *gamma* or *tau-c* for the same table.

To illustrate these ordinal measures of association, the following are data associated with two ordinal sets of data. In a study, pharmacists are asked their agreement with a statement using the Likert Scale. At the same time, the years of pharmacy practice for the respondents is divided into four ordinal categories. The results are listed in Table 17.2. What is the strength of the association between these two variables? The first task would be to calculate the impact of the concordant ($P$) and discordant pairs ($Q$):

$$P = (2)(3)+(2)(3)+(2)(2)+\ldots(4)(15)+(8)(15) = 3257$$

$$Q = (1)(3)+(1)(3)+(1)(2)+\ldots(8)(25)+(4)(8) = 2747$$

**Table 17.2** Evaluation Results from Pharmacist Survey

| | Year of Practice | | | |
|---|---|---|---|---|
| Evaluation | 10 or less | 11-20 | 21-30 | 31 or more |
| 5 "strongly agree" | 2 | 3 | 2 | 1 |
| 4 "agree" | 2 | 3 | 3 | 2 |
| 3 "uncertain" | 8 | 6 | 7 | 4 |
| 2 "disagree" | 12 | 4 | 8 | 18 |
| 1 "strongly disagree" | 8 | 25 | 17 | 15 |
| | 32 | 41 | 37 | 40 |

The Goodman and Kruskal's *gamma* would be:

$$\Gamma = \frac{P-Q}{P+Q} = \frac{3257-2747}{3257+2747} = \frac{510}{6004} = 0.085$$

In this example, by knowing the pharmacists' years of practice, we can reduce the error in predicting the rank (not value) of the Likert scale response by 8.5%. The *gamma* value tells us that we can reduce our predictive error by 8.5% when we use the independent variable to predict the dependent variable. Since the $\chi^2$ statistic was not significant (failure to reject the null hypothesis) it is not surprising that the measure of association is so small.

Even though the contingency table is not square, we will still calculate both Kandall's taus. For *tau-b* we need also to calculate the pairs for tie on the columns and ties on the rows. Continuing with the same example, there are 40 pairs for the columns and 30 pairs for the rows:

$$Y_0 = (2)(2) + (2)(8) + (2)(8) + \ldots (4)(15) + (18)(15) = 1857$$

$$X_0 = (2)(3) + (2)(3) + (8)(6) + \ldots (8)(18) + (17)(15) = 2409$$

Calculated earlier there were 60 pairs each for the concordant and discordant pairs. Note that the total number of pairs is 190 (60 concordant, 60 discordant, 40 ties for columns and 30 ties for rows) which is the combination of 20 cells taken two at a time.

$$\binom{20}{2} = \frac{20!}{2! \cdot 18!} = 190$$

The *tau-b* value is:

$$\tau_b = \frac{(3257 - 2747)}{\sqrt{(3257 + 2747 + 2409)(3257 + 2747 + 1857)}} = \frac{510}{8132.32} = 0.063$$

Because the table is not square, the more appropriate statistic would be *tau-c*. In this example the $N$ is 150 and $m$ equals 4 (the smaller value for the number of columns or rows). The *tau-c* is:

$$\tau_c = (3257 - 2747)\left(\frac{2(4)}{(150)^2(3)}\right) = (510)(0.000119) = 0.060$$

Continuing with this same example, Somers' d for the ability to predict an evaluation response ($y$) based on years of practice experience ($x$) would be:

$$d_{yx} = \frac{(P-Q)}{(P+Q+Y_0)} = \frac{(3257 - 2747)}{(3257 + 2747 + 1857)} = \frac{510}{7861} = 0.065$$

Conversely, if we were to use the evaluation response ($y$) as a predictor of the years of practice ($x$), the Somers' d would be:

$$d_{xy} = \frac{(P-Q)}{(P+Q+X_0)} = \frac{(3257 - 2747)}{(3257 + 2747 + 2409)} = \frac{510}{8413} = 0.061$$

All three tests produce similar, although not identical, results.

With Goodman and Kruskal's *gamma tau-b*, *tab-c*, and Somers'*d* it is assumed that the data are on ordinal scales. It is possible to used interval data for these tests; however some information is lost use the ordinal process and a better assessment have already been discussed in Chapter 13 (i.e., Pearson's correlation). Once again with these tests of association, one does not need to assume that the data is randomly sampled.

### Nominal-by-Interval Associations

In Chapter 10 we saw that the analysis of variance typically focuses on significance differences, not associations or relationships among variables. However, with large sample sizes, levels of the discrete independent variable may be found to be significantly different on a dependent variable, but the differences may be small. In these cases researchers may wish to use the ANOVA to report the strength of association effects.

**Eta (E)**, or the **correlation ratio**, is a coefficient for nonlinear association. As seen in Chapters 13 and 14, for linear relationships the more appropriate test is the correlation coefficient ($r$) or linear regression. For a linear relationship *eta* will equal $r$, but for nonlinear relationships *eta* will be larger. Therefore, the difference between *eta* and $r$ can be used as a measure of the extent to which the relationship between two variables is nonlinear.

When discussing a nominal or ordinal independent variable and a interval (continuous) dependent variable, the first test that should come to mind is a one-way analysis of variance (Chapter 10). *Eta* measures of strength of relationship between these two variables based on sums of squares presented in the ANOVA table. Therefore, the ANOVA must be computed first, before the *eta*-statistic can be determined.

$$E = \sqrt{\frac{SS_B}{SS_T}} \qquad \text{Eq. 17.17}$$

Where $SS_B$ and $SS_T$ are taken directly from the one-way ANOVA table. Eta may be a useful coefficient outside the context of an analysis of variance. Although the numerator and denominator in Eq. 17.17 have meanings as in the *F*-statistics for the analysis of variance, they also measure the extent to which the $x$ and $y$ variables are linearly or nonlinearly related. The numerator will approach the value in the denominator as *eta* will approach 1.0.

The **coefficient of nonlinear correlation** (**$E^2$**) is the percent of total variance in the dependent variable that is accounted for by the variance between levels of the independent variable(*s*). This is calculated by dividing the between-groups sum of squares by the total sum of squares.

$$E^2 = \frac{SS_B}{SS_T} \qquad \text{Eq. 17.18}$$

For linear relationships, *eta* is equal to the Pearson correlation coefficient. Also, just as $r^2$ can be described as the percent of in the dependent variance that can be accounted for by the linear relationship, $E^2$ is the percent of variance explained linearly or nonlinearly by the independent variable. Thus, $E^2$ is analogous to $r^2$ in linear regression (Eq. 14.9). *Eta* defines "perfect relationship" as curvilinear and uses statistical independence as the null hypothesis. Also, by defining the perfect association as curvilinear, *eta* is not sensitive to the order of the categories in the ordinal or nominal variable.

Similar to the ANOVA, one variable must be on the interval or ratio scale (usually but not always the dependent variable). *Eta* can be computed with either variable considered the dependent variable. The second variable must be categorical (nominal or ordinal). The frequencies of each level of the nominal or ordinal variable should be large enough to give stability to the sample means for each category.

A second measure of association, where there is nominal data (independent variable) and interval/ratio data, is **omega-squared (**$\omega^2$**)**; some times referred to as the **coefficient of determination**. This is the proportion of variance in the dependent variable that is accounted for by the independent variable. It is interpreted similarly to $r^2$ in Chapter 14 (also called the coefficient of determination) in the linear regression model:

$$\omega^2 = \frac{SS_B - (k-1)MS_W}{SS_T + MS_W} \qquad \text{Eq. 17.19}$$

where *SS*, *MS*, and *k* are taken from the ANOVA table. *Omega-square* usually varies from 0 to 1, but may have negative values when the *F*-ratio is less than 1. *Omega-square* is a common measure for the magnitude of the effect for an independent variable. An $\omega^2$ is considered large when the value is over 0.15, a medium effect if between 0.06 and 0.15, and a small effect if less than 0.06 (based on a conversion by Cohen, 1988). *Omega-square* is not used for random effects models. Also, due to large variability, $\omega^2$ is not used for two-way or higher repeated measures designs.

To illustrate the use of these tests, consider the following data for patients randomly assigned to receive different doses for a specific analgesic and the patients' responses to a 100-point scale for pain relief (100 = complete pain relief, 0 = no change in pain).

Patient responses to different amounts of analgesic

| | 5 mg | 10 mg | 12.5 mg | 15 mg |
|---|---|---|---|---|
| | 9 | 19 | 29 | 49 |
| | 0 | 15 | 39 | 29 |
| | 35 | 26 | 37 | 35 |
| | 21 | 22 | 23 | 19 |
| | 19 | 36 | 55 | 40 |
| | 10 | 47 | 39 | 33 |
| | 24 | 36 | 45 | 19 |
| | 16 | 26 | 51 | 39 |
| Mean = | 16.75 | 28.38 | 39.75 | 32.88 |
| SD = | 10.66 | 10.57 | 10.63 | 10.37 |

The analysis of variance table for this data would be:

| Source | DF | SS | MS | F |
|---|---|---|---|---|
| Between | 3 | 2242 | 747.3 | 6.70 |
| Within | 28 | 3122 | 111.5 | |
| Total | 31 | 5364 | | |

There is a significant difference in the patients responses ($p < 0.001$); is there a curve linear relationship? The *eta* and *omega square* would be as follows:

$$E = \sqrt{\frac{SS_B}{SS_T}} = \sqrt{\frac{2242}{5364}} = \sqrt{0.418} = 0.647$$

$$\omega^2 = \frac{SS_B - (k-1)MS_W}{SS_T + MS_W} = \frac{2242 - (3)(111.5)}{5364 + 111.5} = \frac{1907.5}{5475.5} = 0.348$$

If a Pearson's correlation coefficient were run on the same data, $r$ would equal 0.556. Thus, in this example, *eta* is 0.647, which compares with a Pearson's $r$ correlation of .556 for the *grouped* data. Squaring each value, we find that linear relationship (reflected in $r^2$) accounts for about 30.9% of the variance, whereas the nonlinear relationship (reflected in $\omega^2$) accounts for 41.9% of the variance.

**Reliability Measurements**

The last part of the chapter will be of interest to pharmacy educators and those involved with cognitive testing and/or survey research; primarily, the researcher concerned that results from such instruments are stable and have a certain degree of consistence when administered to different groups of individuals. **Reliability** is the extent to which the measurements from the entire survey instrument and those from each item within the instrument, yield the same results when administered at different times, in different locations, or to different populations. Reliability coefficients, which can be calculated, are special types of correlation coefficients. For example, consider a test instrument being used to collect information about a study participant (i.e., survey questionnaire). The observed results or scores can be divided into the true score and the error score (the total score = true score + error score). The error score, or deviation from the true score, can be due to either systematic error (bias) or random error. The larger the error component associated with the scores, the lesser the reliability of the instrument. As described in the following paragraphs, there are several types of reliability, each measuring a different dimension of reliability.

The assumptions associated with tests for reliability are the same as those required for the correlation coefficient; the tests involve interval/ratio scales, and the data are derived from a normally distributed population. It is also desirable that the test instrument have **validity** (measures what it is intended to measure). Reliability and validity are related, but not the same. An instrument can be reliable but not valid, but it cannot be valid without being reliable. In other word, reliability is essential, but not enough to prove validity. Reliability can refer to test stability, internal consistency, or equivalency.

**Test stability** means that the same results will be obtained over repeated administration of the instrument. Stability is assessed by the process of test-retest reliability or parallel forms reliability. The **test-retest reliability** involves the administration of the same test to the same subjects at two or more different points in time. The appropriate length of the interval will vary based on the specific instrument and the stability of the information being evaluated. The scores for each subject are compared using a correlation coefficient (Chapter 13). In general, an $r \geq 0.70$ is acceptable. **Parallel forms reliability** is where two or more equivalent series of items or test questions are used. These parallel sets of questions are administered to the same people and the scores are compared using a correlation coefficient. The disadvantage with the parallel forms approach is that administration of two tests are required. However it offers an advantage for the researcher who feels that repeated administration of the same instrument (i.e. test-retest reliability) may result in "test-wiseness" on the part of the individuals taking the tests (they will perform better the second time simply because of repeated exposure to the same question).

The homogeneity of the items is a measure of the **internal consistency reliability** of the test instrument. Such measures determine the extent to which the items in the instrument are measuring the desired skill or knowledge. In other words, is the instrument consistently measuring the same skill or knowledge? The advantage is that only one administration of the instrument is required. Sometime referred to as **split-form reliability**, these measures of internal consistency include: 1) item-total correlations; 2) split-half reliability; 3) Kuder-Richardson coefficients; and 4) Cronbach's alpha. These tests will be illustrated below. The closer these various correlations are to 1.0, the greater the reliability and certainty that the two forms are equivalent.

The simplest measure of internal consistency is an **item-total correlation**, where each item in the instrument is correlated to the total score. If used as a pretest to develop an instrument, those items with low correlations should be deleted from the final instrument. This type of correlation is only important if the researcher wants homogeneity of items. The **split-half method** for measuring internal consistency involves dividing the instrument into two halves (usually odd items vs. even items, or first half vs. second half). The scores for each split-half are calculated and differences between each half-test for each individual subject are computed. Specific methods for evaluating this type of reliability are the Spearman-Brown conversion of the correlation coefficient and Rulon's split-half method. The **Spearman-Brown formula** is applied to the correlation coefficient comparing each half:

$$\rho = \frac{2r_{xy}}{1 + r_{xy}} \quad \text{Eq. 17.20}$$

where $r_{xy}$ is the Pearson correlation coefficient. With **Rulon's split-half method**, the variance of the differences is compared to the variance for the total scores:

$$\rho = 1 - \frac{S_d^2}{S^2} \quad \text{Eq. 17.21}$$

where $S_d^2$ is the variance for the difference between each split half and $S^2$ is the total variance to the test instrument. Obviously, if each half produces the exact same results the $S_d^2$ will be 0 and $\rho = 1$. Both Spearman-Brown and Rulon's method will give similar results.

To illustrate these two tests, consider the data presented in Table 17.3, which evaluates student responses to the odd and even questions on a final examination. The correlation comparing the two sets of questions is very positive ($r = 0.933$). The mean and standard deviation for the entire test for these ten students are 76.5 and 17.42, respectively. Using the approach for calculating the variance for the paired t-test (Eq.

9.10), the variance for the differences between the odd and even questions is 15.57. The calculations for the two methods of internal consistency are:

$$\rho = \frac{2r_{xy}}{1 + r_{xy}} = \frac{2(0.933)}{1 + 0.933} = \frac{1.866}{1.933} = 0.965$$

$$\rho = 1 - \frac{S_d^2}{S^2} = 1 - \frac{15.57}{(17.42)^2} = 0.949$$

The most commonly used measures of internal consistency involving dichotomous results (yes/no, true/false), are two methods developed by G.F. Kuder and M.W. Richardson at the University of Chicago in the late 1930s: the Kuder-Richardson 20 (*KR20*) and Kuder-Richardson 21 (*KR21*). The *KR20* and *KR21* are calculated as follows:

$$\rho_{KR20} = \left(\frac{k}{k-1}\right)\left(1 - \frac{\sum pq}{S^2}\right) \qquad \text{Eq. 17.22}$$

$$\rho_{KR21} = \left(\frac{k}{k-1}\right)\left(1 - \frac{\overline{X}(k - \overline{X})}{k \cdot S^2}\right) \qquad \text{Eq. 17.23}$$

where $k$ is the number of test items (i.e., questions), $p$ is the proportion of correct responses per question for each individual, $\overline{X}$ is the mean score for all persons tested and $S^2$ is the total variance to the test instrument. The higher the *KR* value, the stronger the relationship between the individual items in the instrument. The *KR21* is similar to the *KR20*, but easier to compute; unfortunately the *KR20* is considered a more accurate measure. The *KR21* is a rough approximation because it involves the mean for all subjects rather than the proportion of successes and failures for each individual. The *KR21* is always less than the *KR20* unless the items are all equal in difficulty, in which case the *KR20* will equal *KR21*. Both methods are based on the consistency of responses to all the items in a single instrument.

Examples of the use of *KR20* and *KR21* are presented below using the data in Table 17.4. The table presents the results for 20 students completing a ten-item test and each item is scored as a correct or incorrect response. Listed in the lower section of the table are the $p$ (proportion of correct answers), $q$ (proportion of incorrect answers), and their product ($pq$). The sum of these products ($\Sigma pq$) is 1.57. The mean for the test scores is 7.25, with a variance of 5.88. Thus, the calculations for both Kuder-Richardson measures of reliability are:

$$\rho_{KR20} = \left(\frac{10}{10-1}\right)\left(1 - \frac{1.57}{5.88}\right) = (1.111)(0.733) = 0.814$$

**Table 17.3** Original Data for Measures of Internal Consistency (scores for the even-numbered and odd-numbered questions)

| Student | Odd | Even | d |
|---|---|---|---|
| 1 | 44 | 46 | 2 |
| 2 | 35 | 36 | 1 |
| 3 | 47 | 50 | 3 |
| 4 | 43 | 39 | –4 |
| 5 | 33 | 39 | 6 |
| 6 | 25 | 32 | 7 |
| 7 | 39 | 40 | 1 |
| 8 | 44 | 40 | –4 |
| 9 | 17 | 23 | 6 |
| 10 | 47 | 46 | –1 |

$$\rho_{KR21} = \left(\frac{10}{10-1}\right)\left(1-\frac{(7.25)(10-7.25)}{(10)(5.88)}\right) = (1.111)(0.661) = 0.734$$

The reason for this high reliability becomes visually obvious if the students are ranked in order of the scores and the questions are ranked in order of their difficulty (Table 17.5). Note the clustering of correct answer in the upper left and incorrect answers (0) in the lower left. In this example, the more difficult the question, the more likely that the poorer students will respond with incorrect answers.

Another commonly used measure of reliability is **Cronbach's alpha**. It measures how consistently individuals respond to the items within an instrument and can be used for nondichotomous responses (i.e., Likert scales). Cronbach's alpha, also called the **reliability coefficient**, measures the extent to which responses to items, obtained at the same time, correlate highly with each other. It is a measure of the level of mean intercorrelation weighted by the variances and can be thought of as the average of all possible split-half estimates. In addition to estimating the reliability of the items for the average correlation, the Cronbach's alpha also takes into account the number of questions in the instrument. The general theory is that the larger the number of questions, the more reliable the instrument. Cronbach's alpha makes no assumptions about what one would obtain at a different point in time (i.e., test-retest reliability). The Cronbach's alpha formula is:

$$\rho_\alpha = \left(\frac{k}{k-1}\right)\left(1-\frac{\sum S_i^2}{S^2}\right) \qquad \text{Eq. 17.24}$$

where $k$ is the total number of questions or items in the instrument, $S_i^2$ is the variance

**Table 17.4** Original Data for Example Problem for KR-20 and KR-21

| | Instrument Items* | | | | | | | | | | |
|---|---|---|---|---|---|---|---|---|---|---|---|
| Student | A | B | C | D | E | F | G | H | I | J | Score |
| 1 | 1 | 1 | 1 | 1 | 1 | 1 | 1 | 1 | 1 | 0 | 9 |
| 2 | 1 | 1 | 1 | 1 | 0 | 0 | 1 | 1 | 1 | 0 | 7 |
| 3 | 1 | 1 | 0 | 0 | 0 | 0 | 1 | 1 | 0 | 0 | 4 |
| 4 | 0 | 1 | 1 | 1 | 1 | 1 | 1 | 1 | 1 | 1 | 9 |
| 5 | 1 | 1 | 1 | 1 | 1 | 0 | 1 | 1 | 1 | 1 | 9 |
| 6 | 1 | 1 | 1 | 1 | 1 | 1 | 1 | 1 | 1 | 1 | 10 |
| 7 | 1 | 0 | 0 | 0 | 0 | 0 | 1 | 0 | 1 | 0 | 3 |
| 8 | 1 | 1 | 1 | 1 | 1 | 0 | 1 | 1 | 1 | 1 | 9 |
| 9 | 1 | 1 | 1 | 1 | 1 | 0 | 1 | 0 | 0 | 1 | 7 |
| 10 | 1 | 1 | 1 | 1 | 1 | 1 | 1 | 1 | 1 | 1 | 10 |
| 11 | 1 | 1 | 0 | 1 | 0 | 0 | 1 | 1 | 0 | 0 | 5 |
| 12 | 1 | 0 | 0 | 0 | 0 | 0 | 1 | 1 | 0 | 0 | 3 |
| 13 | 1 | 1 | 1 | 1 | 1 | 1 | 1 | 1 | 1 | 1 | 10 |
| 14 | 0 | 1 | 1 | 1 | 1 | 1 | 1 | 1 | 1 | 1 | 9 |
| 15 | 1 | 1 | 1 | 1 | 0 | 0 | 1 | 1 | 1 | 0 | 7 |
| 16 | 1 | 1 | 0 | 1 | 0 | 0 | 1 | 1 | 0 | 0 | 5 |
| 17 | 1 | 1 | 0 | 1 | 1 | 0 | 1 | 1 | 1 | 0 | 7 |
| 18 | 1 | 1 | 1 | 1 | 1 | 0 | 1 | 1 | 1 | 1 | 9 |
| 19 | 1 | 1 | 1 | 1 | 1 | 0 | 1 | 1 | 1 | 1 | 9 |
| 20 | 1 | 0 | 0 | 1 | 0 | 0 | 1 | 1 | 0 | 0 | 4 |
| Σ = | 18 | 17 | 13 | 17 | 12 | 6 | 20 | 18 | 14 | 10 | |
| p = | .90 | .85 | .65 | .85 | .60 | .30 | 1.0 | .90 | .70 | .50 | |
| q = | .10 | .15 | .35 | .15 | .40 | .70 | 0 | .10 | .30 | .50 | |
| pq = | .09 | .13 | .23 | .13 | .24 | .21 | 0 | .09 | .21 | .25 | |
| $S^2$ = | .09 | .13 | .24 | .13 | .25 | .22 | .00 | .09 | .22 | .26 | |

* Code: 1 – correct answer; 0 – incorrect answer.

for each individual item and $S^2$ is the variance for the total score. Thus, the more consistent within-subject responses (individual variances), the greater the variability between subjects (total variance), the larger the Cronbach's alpha . Also, alpha will be higher if there is homogeneity of variances among questions. The generally accepted cut-off for Cronbach's alpha is 0.70 or greater for an item to be considered in the instrument. To illustrate Cronbach's alpha, we can use the same data from the *KR20* and *KR21* example. Note that the last row in Table 17.4 is the variance for each test item, the sum of which is 1.655 ($\Sigma S_i^2$) and as noted previously the variance for the test scores in 5.88. For this example the Cronbach's alpha is:

**Table 17.5** Sorted Data for Example Problem for KR-20 and KR-21

| | Instrument Items* | | | | | | | | | | |
|---|---|---|---|---|---|---|---|---|---|---|---|
| Student | G | A | H | D | B | I | C | E | J | F | Score |
| 10 | 1 | 1 | 1 | 1 | 1 | 1 | 1 | 1 | 1 | 1 | 10 |
| 6 | 1 | 1 | 1 | 1 | 1 | 1 | 1 | 1 | 1 | 1 | 10 |
| 13 | 1 | 1 | 1 | 1 | 1 | 1 | 1 | 1 | 1 | 1 | 10 |
| 4 | 1 | 0 | 1 | 1 | 1 | 1 | 1 | 1 | 1 | 1 | 9 |
| 19 | 1 | 1 | 1 | 1 | 1 | 1 | 1 | 1 | 1 | 0 | 9 |
| 8 | 1 | 1 | 1 | 1 | 1 | 1 | 1 | 1 | 1 | 0 | 9 |
| 5 | 1 | 1 | 1 | 1 | 1 | 1 | 1 | 1 | 1 | 0 | 9 |
| 14 | 1 | 0 | 1 | 1 | 1 | 1 | 1 | 1 | 1 | 1 | 9 |
| 18 | 1 | 1 | 1 | 1 | 1 | 1 | 1 | 1 | 1 | 0 | 9 |
| 1 | 1 | 1 | 1 | 1 | 1 | 1 | 1 | 1 | 0 | 1 | 9 |
| 9 | 1 | 1 | 0 | 1 | 1 | 0 | 1 | 1 | 1 | 0 | 7 |
| 15 | 1 | 1 | 1 | 1 | 1 | 1 | 1 | 0 | 0 | 0 | 7 |
| 17 | 1 | 1 | 1 | 1 | 1 | 1 | 0 | 1 | 0 | 0 | 7 |
| 2 | 1 | 1 | 1 | 1 | 1 | 1 | 1 | 0 | 0 | 0 | 7 |
| 11 | 1 | 1 | 1 | 1 | 1 | 0 | 0 | 0 | 0 | 0 | 5 |
| 16 | 1 | 1 | 1 | 1 | 1 | 0 | 0 | 0 | 0 | 0 | 5 |
| 3 | 1 | 1 | 1 | 0 | 1 | 0 | 0 | 0 | 0 | 0 | 4 |
| 20 | 1 | 1 | 1 | 1 | 0 | 0 | 0 | 0 | 0 | 0 | 4 |
| 12 | 1 | 1 | 1 | 0 | 0 | 0 | 0 | 0 | 0 | 0 | 3 |
| 7 | 1 | 1 | 0 | 0 | 0 | 1 | 0 | 0 | 0 | 0 | 3 |
| Σ = | 20 | 18 | 18 | 17 | 17 | 14 | 13 | 12 | 10 | 6 | |

* Code: 1 – correct answer; 0 – incorrect answer.

$$\rho_\alpha = \left(\frac{10}{10-1}\right)\left(1-\frac{1.655}{5.88}\right) = (1.111)(0.719) = 0.799$$

**Test equivalence** is the last measure of reliability for a test or survey instrument. It is the consistency of the agreement among various observers, or data collectors, using the same measurement or among alternative forms of the instrument. One measure is the parallel forms approach previously discussed. The second is **interrater reliability**, which requires the administration of the same instrument to the same people by two or more raters (interviewers or observed) to establish the extent of consensus between the various raters. If nominal or ordinal data, this consensus is measured as the number of agreements divided by total number of observations. Consensus for interval or ratio scales is measured using the correlation coefficient between the scores for pairs of raters. Because reliability coefficient makes no assumptions about mean scores for the individual raters, a *t*-test of the significance of *r* (Eq. 13.8) can be used to determine if interrater means are significantly different.

Thus, for data involving interval or ratio, a Pearson's correlation coefficient can be employed. **Intraclass correlation (ICC)** can be used to measure interrater reliability. Even though the correlation coefficient can be use to measure the test-retest reliability, the ICC is recommended when sample size is small (<15) or when there are more than two tests being evaluated. It is the ratio of between-groups variance to total variance. The ICC process is described by Shrout and Fleiss (1979) and Ebel (1951).

For nominal or ordinal data one would use a different measure of agreement between two raters, **Cohen's kappa**. The two variables that contain the ratings must have the same range of values (creating a matrix with an even number of rows and columns). The *kappa* statistic normalizes the difference between the observed proportion of cases where both raters agree with the expected proportion by chance alone. This is accomplished by dividing it by the maximum difference possible for the marginal totals. The *t*-value is the ratio of the value of *kappa* to its asymptotic standard error when the null hypothesis (i.e., $kappa = 0$) is true. Obviously, if there are an equal number of categories for both raters, the contingency table will always be square. Consider the example of raters classifying an outcome into one of three possible categories (either nominal or ordinal). If the raters were in perfect agreement all results would fall on the diagonal.

| | | Rater One | | | |
|---|---|---|---|---|---|
| | | A | B | C | |
| | A | **30** | 0 | 0 | 30 |
| Rater Two | B | 0 | **25** | 0 | 25 |
| | C | 0 | 0 | **15** | 15 |
| | | 30 | 25 | 15 | 70 |

Realistically there would probably be some differences between the observer responses:

| | | Rater One | | | |
|---|---|---|---|---|---|
| | | A | B | C | |
| | A | **20** | 5 | 5 | 30 |
| Rater Two | B | 6 | **18** | 5 | 25 |
| | C | 4 | 4 | **7** | 15 |
| | | 30 | 25 | 15 | 70 |

Using the method described in Chapter 16 for the chi square test of independence, it is possible to calculate the expected values for each cell if the two rater's responses are independent of each other.

| | | Rater One | | | |
|---|---|---|---|---|---|
| | | A | B | C | |
| Rater Two | A | **12.9** | 10.7 | 6.4 | 30 |
| | B | 10.7 | **8.9** | 5.4 | 25 |
| | C | 6.4 | 5.4 | **3.2** | 15 |
| | | 30 | 25 | 15 | 70 |

The chi square for this particular set of data is 22.01, which would result in the rejection of the null hypothesis of independence between the two raters. The follow-up questions might be, how strong is the relationship between these two observers? Is there reliability between the two individuals raters?

Since the diagonal values indicate the strength of the agreement we use the diagonal values (or concordant items) in calculating Cohen's *kappa.* In this example, the observed data for the concordant items ($f_O$) sum up to 45 (20+18+7) and the sum of the concordant items by chance alone ($f_C$) or for the expected results under independence is 25 (12.9+8.9+3.2). The excess in observed results compared to the number of chance occurrences as 45 – 25 = 20. Similarly, the expected number of nonconcordant numbers is $N$ minus the expected concordant items ($f_C$), which is 70 – 25 = 45. Cohen's kappa is simply the ratio of the two differences:

$$\kappa = \frac{f_O - f_C}{N - f_C} \qquad \text{Eq. 17.25}$$

Note that the actual frequency counts, not proportions, are used for the Cohen's *kappa.* For this example the results would be:

$$\kappa = \frac{45 - 25}{70 - 25} = \frac{20}{45} = 0.444$$

In other words, 44.4% of the results are concordant or the judges are in agreement 44.4% of the time. If there were perfect agreement between the two observers (first table), the results would be:

$$\kappa = \frac{70 - 25}{70 - 25} = \frac{45}{45} = 1.0$$

Thus, similar to other "coefficients of association" the measure of association is the proximity of the *kappa* to a perfect association of 1.0.

## Summary

Measures of association are used to estimate both the strength (strong/moderate/weak) and the direction (positive/negative) of the relationship. The selection of the appropriate test is based on the type of data, hypothesis being tested ,and the properties of the various measures (nominal, ordinal, or index/ratio). Various textbooks provide rules interpreting for strength of the coefficient of association. A general rule of thumb for nominal and ordinal measures of association is: 0.30 or greater represents a strong relationship; 0.20 to 0.29 a moderately strong relationship; 0.10 to 0.19 a moderate relationship and less than 0.10 a weak relationship. Table 17.6 presents a summary of the tests presented above and the types of variables for which each is most appropriate.

## References

Cohen, J. (1988). *Statistical Power Analysis for the Behavioral Sciences*, Second edition, L. Erlbaum Associated, Hillsdale, NJ, pp. 284-288.

Ebel, R.L. (1951). “Estimation of the reliability of ratings,” *Psychometrika* 16:407-424.

Knoke, D. and Bohrnstedt, G.W (1991). *Basic Social Statistics*, F.E. Peacock Publishers, p. 126.

Kuder G.F. and Richardson, M.W. (1937). “The theory of the estimation of test reliability,” *Psychometrika* 2:151-160.

Shrout, P.E. and Fleiss, J.L. (1979). “Intraclass correlations: Uses in assessing rater reliability,” *Psychological Bulletin* 86:420-428.

## Suggested Supplemental Readings

Bohrnstedt, G.W. and Knoke, D. (1982). *Statistics for Social Data Analysis*, F.E. Peacock Publishers, Inc., Itasca, IL, pp. 283-314.

Goodman, L.A. (1979). *Measures of Association for Cross Classifications*, Springer-Verlag, New York.

Liebetrau, A.M. (1983). *Measures of Association*, Sage Publications. Newbury Park, CA.

Miller, M.B. (1995). “Coefficient alpha: A basic introduction from the perspectives of classical test theory and structural equation modeling,” *Structural Equation Modeling* 2(3):255-273.

**Table 17.6** Summary of Measures of Association by Type of Scale

| Dependent Variable | Second or Independent Variable | 2 x 2 Table | Table Larger than 2 x 2: Square | Table Larger than 2 x 2: Not Square |
|---|---|---|---|---|
| Nominal | Nominal | Phi | Pearson C (≤ 4 x 4)<br>Pearson C*<br>Tshuprow's (> 4 x 4) | Cramer's V<br>Theil's U<br>Lambda* |
| | Ordinal | Yule's Q | Cramer's V<br>Lambda* | Cramer's V<br>Lambda* |
| Ordinal | Nominal | Yule's Q | Tau-c<br>Lambda* | Tau-c<br>Lambda* |
| | Ordinal | Tau-b | Tau-b<br>Somer's d<br>gamma | Tau-c<br>gamma<br>Lambda*<br>Somer's d |
| Interval or ratio | Nominal or ordinal | Eta<br>$Eta^2$ | | |
| | Interval or ratio | Correlation coefficient | | |

* No independent variable.

Reynolds, H.T. (1977). *The Analysis of Cross-Classifications*. The Free Press, New York, pp. 34-61.

**Example Problems**

1. Using the following information: a) calculate the various measures of association for a 2 x 2 design; and b) indicate which results are best, given the types of variables involved.

   Assume an equal number of males and females are treated with the same medication for a specific illness and the outcome is either success or failure. Is there a relationship between patient gender and therapeutic outcome?

| | Females | Males | |
|---|---|---|---|
| Success | 45 | 30 | 75 |
| Failure | 5 | 20 | 25 |
| | 50 | 50 | 100 |

2. Using the following information: a) calculate the various measures of association for a 3 x 3 design; and b) indicate which results are best, given the types of variables involved.

   Patients are randomly divided into three groups and treated with one of three medications for high cholesterol. After six months of therapy they are assessed to determine if they met their desired cholesterol goal, did not meet goal, or were changed to a different treatment regimen. Is there a relationship between treatment and therapeutic outcome?

| | Treatment A | Treatment B | Treatment C | |
|---|---|---|---|---|
| At goal | 56 | 46 | 35 | 137 |
| Not at goal | 30 | 18 | 18 | 66 |
| Discontinued | 13 | 20 | 37 | 70 |
| | 99 | 84 | 90 | 273 |

3. Using the following information: a) calculate the various measures of association for a 3 x 5 design; and b) indicate which results are best, given the types of variables involved.

   A survey of pharmacists in different practice settings asks their level of agreement with a series of questions. Listed below is their response to one question. Is there an association between practice setting and response to the question?

| | Practice Setting | | | |
|---|---|---|---|---|
| Evaluation | Retail | Hospital | Long-Term Care | |
| 5 "strongly agree" | 10 | 2 | 4 | 16 |
| 4 "agree" | 12 | 2 | 6 | 20 |
| 3 "uncertain" | 24 | 12 | 14 | 50 |
| 2 "disagree" | 36 | 20 | 28 | 84 |
| 1 "strongly disagree" | 18 | 64 | 48 | 130 |
| | 100 | 100 | 100 | 300 |

**Answers to Problems**

1. Measures of association between patient gender and outcome.

| | Males | Females | |
|---|---|---|---|
| Success | 45 | 30 | 75 |
| Failure | 5 | 20 | 25 |
| | 50 | 50 | 100 |

Several tests can be run on dichotomous data, including the phi statistic, including the phi statistic, Yule's Q, Yule's Y, and tau-b:

Preliminary information: $\chi^2 = 12.00$
$P = 900$ (45 x 20)
$Q = 150$ (5 x 30)
$X_0 = 825$ (45·5 + 30·20)
$Y_0 = 1450$ (45·30 + 5·20)

Phi statistic:

$$\phi = \sqrt{\frac{\chi^2}{n}} = \sqrt{\frac{12}{100}} = 0.346$$

Yule's Q:

$$Q = \frac{P-Q}{P+Q} = \frac{900-150}{900+150} = 0.714$$

Yule's Y:

$$Y = \frac{\sqrt{P}-\sqrt{Q}}{\sqrt{P}+\sqrt{Q}} = \frac{\sqrt{900}-\sqrt{150}}{\sqrt{900}+\sqrt{150}} = 0.420$$

Tau-b :

$$\tau_b = \frac{P-Q}{\sqrt{(P+Q+X_O)(P+Q+Y_O)}}$$

$$\tau_b = \frac{900-150}{\sqrt{(900+150+825)(900+150+1450)}} = 0.346$$

The most appropriate would be the phi statistic since both variables are nominal (see Table 17.6). However, if one considers "success/failure" an ordinal variable with success being better than failure, then Yule's Q could be used.

2. Measures of association comparing three therapies and three possible outcomes.

| | Treatment A | Treatment B | Treatment C | |
|---|---|---|---|---|
| At goal | 56 | 46 | 35 | 137 |
| Not at goal | 30 | 18 | 18 | 66 |
| Discontinued | 13 | 20 | 37 | 70 |
| | 99 | 84 | 90 | 273 |

Various tests could be run on this contingency table, including Pearson $C$, $C^*$, Tshuprow's $T$, Cramer's $V$, *lamdba*, *tau-c*, *tau-b*, Somer's $d$, and *gamma*.

Preliminary information: $\chi^2 = 20.44$ $\quad X_0 = 7497$
$P = 10114$ $\quad Y_0 = 9031$
$Q = 5641$

Pearson $C$:

$$C = \sqrt{\frac{\chi^2}{\chi^2 + N}} = \sqrt{\frac{20.44}{20.44 + 273}} = 0.264$$

Pearson $C^*$:

$$C^* = \frac{C}{\sqrt{\frac{k-1}{k}}} = \frac{0.264}{\sqrt{\frac{3-1}{3}}} = 0.323$$

Tshuprow's $T$:

$$T = \sqrt{\frac{\chi^2}{n\sqrt{(r-1)(c-1)}}} = \sqrt{\frac{20.44}{273\sqrt{(2)(2)}}} = 0.193$$

Cramer's $V$:

$$V = \sqrt{\frac{\chi^2}{Nm}} = \sqrt{\frac{20.44}{(273)(2)}} = 0.193$$

Note in a square table that T = V.

*Lamdba*:

$$\lambda = \frac{\sum f_i - f_d}{N - f_d} = \frac{(56 + 46 + 37) - 137}{273 - 137} = 0.015$$

*Tau-c*:

$$\tau_c = (P - Q)\left(\frac{2m}{n^2(m-1)}\right)$$

$$\tau_c = (10114 - 5641)\left(\frac{2(3)}{(273)^2 \cdot (2)}\right) = 0.180$$

*Tau-b*:

$$\tau_b = \frac{P - Q}{\sqrt{(P + Q + X_O)(P + Q + Y_O)}}$$

$$\tau_b = \frac{10114 - 5641}{\sqrt{(10114 + 5641 + 7497)(10114 + 5641 + 9031)}} = 0.186$$

Somer's *d*:

$$d_{yx} = \frac{(P - Q)}{(P + Q + Y_0)} = \frac{10114 - 5641}{10114 + 5641 + 9031} = 0.180$$

*Gamma*:

$$\Gamma = \frac{P - Q}{P + Q} = \frac{10114 - 5641}{10114 + 5641} = 0.284$$

Pearson $C$ or $C^*$ would seem appropriate since both variables are nominal and the table is square and less than a 5 x 5 configuration.

3. Association between practice setting and response on a Likert scale.

| | Practice Setting | | | |
|---|---|---|---|---|
| Evaluation | Retail | Hospital | Long-Term Care | |
| 5 "strongly agree" | 10 | 2 | 4 | 16 |
| 4 "agree" | 12 | 2 | 6 | 20 |
| 3 "uncertain" | 24 | 12 | 14 | 50 |
| 2 "disagree" | 36 | 20 | 28 | 84 |
| 1 "strongly disagree" | 18 | 64 | 48 | 130 |
| | 100 | 100 | 100 | 300 |

Several tests can be run on dichotomous data, including the phi statistic, including *tau-c*, *lambda*, *eta*, *omega*.

Preliminary information: $\chi^2 = 48.8$; $P = 14288$; $Q = 7368$

ANOVA Table:

| Source | df | SS | MS | F |
|---|---|---|---|---|
| Between | 2 | 54.43 | 27.21 | 23.13 |
| Within | 297 | 349.36 | 1.18 | |
| Total | 299 | 403.79 | | |

*Tau-c:*

$$\tau_c = (P - Q)\left(\frac{2m}{n^2(m-1)}\right)$$

$$\tau_c = (14288 - 7368)\left(\frac{2(3)}{300^2(2)}\right) = 0.231$$

*Lamdba*:

$$\lambda = \frac{\sum f_i - f_d}{N - f_d} = \frac{(36 + 64 + 48) - 130}{300 - 130} = 0.106$$

*Eta*:

$$E = \sqrt{\frac{SS_B}{SS_T}} = \sqrt{\frac{54.43}{403.79}} = 0.367$$

*Omega*:

$$\omega^2 = \frac{SS_B - (k-1)MS_W}{SS_T + MS_W} = \frac{54.43 - (2)(1.18)}{403.79 + 1.18} = 0.129$$

*Tau-c*: Use if the researcher considers setting as an independent variable, if not, then *lambda*. However, if the Likert scale is considered an interval scale, *eta* or *omega* could be used.

# 18

# Odds Ratios and Relative Risk Ratios

The previous three chapters have focused on discrete results and this chapter will continue our discussion of such outcomes. The last two chapters have focused on descriptive statistics presented in contingency tables and inferentially evaluated using a variety of tests, both looking for statistical independence and measures of association. This chapter will focus on ratio measures, which have become increasingly more common in the literature over the last few decades, odds ratios and risk ratios. The chapter will conclude with similar procedures looking at Mantel-Haenszel relative risk ratio and logistic regression.

## Probability, Odds, and Risk

Commonly used methods for evaluating the importance of observed dichotomous outcomes (i.e., success/failure, live/die) are odds ratios and relative risk ratios. As discussed in Chapter 2, **probability** is the chance that something will occur (i.e., tossing a fair coin once, the probability of a head is 0.50). In contrast, **odds** for a given outcome is the ratio of the probability of a specific outcome occurring divided by the probability of that same outcome not occurring (i.e., tossing a fair, the odds of a head occurring is 1 = 0.5/0.5 or an even odds of 1). **Risk** is more closely associated with probability, in that risk is the number of a negative (or positive) outcomes divided by the total number of possible outcomes (i.e., a coin is tossed 100 times and a tail occurs 60 times, the risk of a tail is 0.60 = 60/100). It is important to understand which of these outcomes to report under given situations and conditions.

Odds and relative risks are most commonly used as ratios when comparing two levels of an independent variable (i.e., treatment group vs. control group). Both the odds ratio and the relative risk compare the likelihood of an event between two groups. The odds ratio compares the relative odds of two different events occurring. The relative risk compares the probability of two different events occurring. The relative risk is closer to what most individuals think of when they think of the relative likelihood of two events. As discussed in the following sections, ratios are created between the two groups. Both the odds ratio estimator and relative risk estimator employ a 2 x 2 contingency table (similar to the layouts seen in the previous two chapters, Figure 16.3), usually with the ratio between the two outcomes in each column. Some research designs, for example the case-control design, prevents computing a relative risk because the design involves the selection of research subjects based on outcome measurements rather than exposure. However, with retrospective case control studies it is possible to calculate and interpret an odds ratio.

## Odds Ratio

An odds ratio is used when retrospective data is being analyzed and involves unpaired samples. Because the data are gathered after the fact, meaningful calculations between the proportions is not possible, as will be described later when discussing relative risk. The best summary of such data is to calculate the odds ratio, which is an approximate risk.

Calculation of odds and odds ratio involve a binary dependent variable with two possible outcomes (i.e., success or failure, positive or negative results). For example, assume that an event has a 75% chance of occurring (success) and a 25% chance of not occurring (failure). The probabilities of success and failure are $p = 0.75$ and $q = 1 - p = 0.25$, respectively. Thus the odds of observing or not observing the specific event are calculated as follows:

$$odds(success) = \frac{p}{q} \qquad \text{Eq. 18.1}$$

$$odds(failure) = \frac{q}{p} \qquad \text{Eq. 18.2}$$

With this particular example the odds of success or failure are:

$$odds(success) = \frac{0.75}{0.25} = 3.00$$

$$odds(failure) = \frac{0.25}{0.75} = 0.33$$

As noted in the chapter introduction, odds and probability are not the same. In this example the probability of a success is 0.75, but the of odds of success are 3 to 1 and the odds of failure are 0.33 to 1. This makes sense; if we randomly select one sample from all possible outcomes there is a three times greater chance of selecting a "success" than a failure.

In the search for causes of specific diseases, epidemiologists are interested in the risks of certain behaviors or characteristics on the causes of these diseases. Outcomes (i.e., yes or no for a specific disease, disability, or death) are compared against potential risk factors (i.e., predisposing characteristics, exposure to disease or pollutants, risk-taking behavior). The design of such comparisons is presented below:

| | | Exposure | | |
|---|---|---|---|---|
| | | Yes (+) | No (−) | |
| Outcome | Yes (+) | a | b | a + b |
| | No (−) | c | d | c + d |
| | | a + c | b + d | n |

Using this design, a cross-sectional study can be undertaken where an overall sample of the population is collected regardless of the outcomes or factors involved. For example, a cross-section of individuals living in the Midwest are compared for the incidence of chronic lung disease and compared to the individual smoking histories. The previous 2 x 2 model can be employed, then two levels of a criterion variable are compared with two possible outcomes. Results of the hypothetical study of chronic lung disease found the results presented in Table 18.1.

The odds of developing an outcome (i.e., disease) in the group exposed to the risk factor is referred to as the experimental event odds (*EEO*). The odds of developing chronic lung disease for smokers would be the odds of the outcome of interest being present (chronic lung disease) in those with the risk factor present (smokers):

$$EEO = \frac{a}{c} \qquad \text{Eq. 18.3}$$

The odds of developing the outcome in the nonexposed (or control) group is the control event odds (*CEO*). In this case, the odds of developing chronic lung disease without the risk factor (smoking) present would be:

$$CEO = \frac{b}{d} \qquad \text{Eq. 18.4}$$

The odds ratio for developing the outcome in the experimental group is the experimental event odds divided by the control event odds, or the ratio of the odds for the risk factor present divided by the odds for the risk factor being absent:

$$OR = \frac{EEO}{CEO} = \frac{a/c}{b/d} \qquad \text{Eq. 18.5}$$

The results would indicate the number of times the experimental groups is more likely to develop the disease. For the data presented in Table 18.1 the odds of developing chronic lung disease for smokers and nonsmokers is as follows:

$$odds(\,present\,) = \frac{a}{c} = \frac{84}{68} = 1.235$$

**Table 18.1** Example of Odds Ratio Data

| | | Risk Factor | | |
|---|---|---|---|---|
| | | Smoker | Nonsmoker | |
| Chronic Lung Disease | Present | 84 | 133 | 217 |
| | Absent | 68 | 215 | 283 |
| | | 152 | 348 | 500 |

The odds of developing chronic lung disease for a nonsmoker is:

$$odds(absent) = \frac{b}{d} = \frac{133}{215} = 0.619$$

The odds ratio ($OR$) for developing chronic lung disease, comparing smokers to nonsmokers is:

$$OR = \frac{a/b}{c/d} = \frac{1.235}{0.619} = 1.995$$

Thus, based on the results of this retrospective study, the odd of developing chronic lung disease in smokers is approximately two times greater than not developing the disease.

When analyzing a case-control retrospective clinical trial, there are no differences between the proportion of outcomes of interest or their relative risk. Thus, the best way to summarize the data is to report the odds ratio. When the event rate is small, odds ratios are very similar to relative risks.

An odds ratio with a numeric value of one indicates no difference between the two outcomes. Thus, if the population odds ratio ($\theta$) has an outcome of one, there is no significant relationship between the independent variable and the outcome.

$$H_0: \theta = 1$$
$$H_1: \theta \neq 1$$

An outcome with an odds ratio less than *one* indicates that the factor was effective in reducing the odds of a negative outcome. When the odds ratio is greater than one, there is an increase in the likelihood of the negative outcome occurring. To test the null hypothesis, it is possible to create a confidence interval, similar to previous intervals, using the best estimate (based on the sample) plus or minus a reliability coefficient times an error term. To calculate the standard error term, data is converted to the natural logarithm, because the distribution of the natural logarithm of $\theta$ ($ln\ \theta$) converts to the normal distribution for smaller sample sizes than the distribution of $\theta$. After finding the confidence interval for $ln\ \theta$, data can be transformed back to a confidence interval for $\theta$. The estimated error term for the sample based on of $ln\ \theta$ is:

$$\hat{\sigma}_{ln(OR)} = \sqrt{\frac{1}{a} + \frac{1}{b} + \frac{1}{c} + \frac{1}{d}} \qquad \text{Eq. 18.6}$$

Using this **log-odds ratio** is more convenient than trying to work with the odds ratio itself. The confidence interval for $ln\ \theta$ is:

$$ln\,\theta = ln_{(OR)} \pm Z_{1-\alpha/2}(\hat{\sigma}_{ln(OR)}) \qquad \text{Eq. 18.7}$$

Each $ln\ \theta$ is converted back to $\theta$ by

$$\theta = e^{ln\,\theta} \qquad \text{Eq. 18.8}$$

Where $e$ is the base of the natural logarithm and equals 2.718281828. Using the previous example we can test the significance of chronic lung disease with the associated risk factor of smoking:

$$\hat{\sigma}_{ln(OR)} = \sqrt{\frac{1}{84} + \frac{1}{133} + \frac{1}{68} + \frac{1}{215}} = 0.197$$

The $ln$ of 1.995 is 0.691:

$$ln\,\theta = 0.691 \pm 1.96(0.197)$$

$$0.305 < ln\,\theta < 1.077$$

$$e^{0.305} = 1.357 \quad and \quad e^{1.077} = 2.936$$

Thus, since *one* is not within the interval, there is a significant difference in odds ratios, with smokers at 1.36 to 2.94 times more likely than nonsmokers to develop chronic lung disease.

Alternatively, it is possible to establish a ratio between the *ln OR* and error term and refer to a table for the normal standardized distribution (Appendix B, Table B2) to determine the $p$-value associated with the $z$-value from the ratio.

$$z = \frac{ln\frac{(ad)}{(cb)}}{\sqrt{\frac{1}{a} + \frac{1}{b} + \frac{1}{c} + \frac{1}{d}}} = \frac{ln\ OR}{\sigma_{log(OR)}} \qquad \text{Eq. 18.9}$$

In the previous example this would result in the following:

$$z = \frac{0.691}{0.197} = 3.51$$

with a $z$-value of 3.51 is not listed on Table B2, but can be calculated using Excel command *fx=(1–NORMSDIST(x))*2*. In this case $p = 0.00045$.

The odds ratio also can be useful in the interpretation of the results of logistic regression analysis, which will be discussed later in this chapter. Odds ratio can also be used in making covariate adjustment. It is relatively easy to adjust an odds ratio for potentially confounding variables. Such adjustments are more difficult with relative risk ratios.

## Relative Risk

A second type of ratio is the risk ratio or **relative risk ratio** (*RR*). For prospective studies, the *RR* involves sampling subjects with and without the risk factor (or experimental condition) and to evaluate the development of a certain condition or outcome over a period of time. Where the term "odds" was associated with the ratio of the number of success in an outcome with an event to the number of failures, the term "risk" is the ratio of people experience negative outcomes compared to the total number within the group. With respect to proportions, odds equal $np/nq$ or $p/q$, whereas risk is $np/np+nq$ or $p/p+q$, which equals $p$. Where odds was calculated as the number of positive outcomes divided by the number of negative outcomes, risk is the number of negative outcomes divided by the total number of outcomes.

One could think of an odds ratio as a measure of the odds of suffering some fate or outcome. Whereas the risk ratio gives you the percentage difference in outcomes between two groups or conditions. These two ratios (*OR* and *RR*) can be compared; however, the risk ratio is easier to interpret. One can think of an odds ratio as an approximate relative risk. However, an odds ratio is used more commonly because an odds ratio is more closely related to logistic regression and linked to other procedures. Also, relative risk requires that the contingency table have a specific orientation (factors in the columns and outcomes in the rows), an odds ratio offers more flexibility because the results will be the same even if the table is rotated by 90 degrees.

Using the same 2 x 2 matrix seen with odds ratios, the **experimental event rate** (*EER*) is the risk associated with developing a specific outcome for the group exposed to the risk factor:

$$EER = \frac{a}{a+c} \qquad \text{Eq. 18.10}$$

and the **control event rate** (*CER*) is the risk associated with the outcome for the unexposed control group:

$$CER = \frac{b}{b+d} \qquad \text{Eq. 18.11}$$

The relative risk (*RR*) is the experimental event rate divided by the control event rate:

$$Relative\ Risk = \frac{EER}{CER} = \frac{a/(a+c)}{b/(b+d)} \qquad \text{Eq. 18.12}$$

Algebraically this can be simplified to:

$$Relative\ Risk = \frac{ab+ad}{ab+bc} \qquad \text{Eq. 18.13}$$

The relative risk predicts the likelihood of a given outcome associated with the experimental factor (i.e., there is a 1.5 greater probability of cancer is individuals exposed to a given risk factor). Relative risk can be any value greater than or equal to zero. If the $RR = 1$ there is no association between the factor and the outcome (independence). If the *RR* is greater than one this indicates a positive association or an increased risk that the outcome will occur with exposure to that factor. If *RR* is less than one there is a negative association, or protection against the outcome. The relative risk is our best estimate of the strength of the factor-outcome association.

The complement of the risk ratio is the **relative risk reduction** (*RRR*).

$$RRR = 1 - RR \qquad \text{Eq. 18.14}$$

It can also be defined as the risk rate in the treatment group minus the risk rate in the control group, divided by the risk rate in the control group.

$$RRR = \frac{\left(\frac{a}{a+c}\right)-\left(\frac{b}{b+d}\right)}{\left(\frac{b}{b+d}\right)} \qquad \text{Eq. 18.15}$$

Relative risk means that the treatment group has a certain percentage of the risk compared to the control group. Relative risk reduction indicated that treatment reduces risk by a certain percentage compared to the control group.

In a prospective study, cases or patients are allocated to two groups and the relative risk is the ratio of the proportion of cases having a positive outcome in the two groups. For example, workers in a chemical production facility are divided into two groups: one group working unprotected in the existing conditions and the other group required to wear protective masks. After a period of time, workers in such a follow-up or longitudinal study would be evaluated on respiratory function tests. After two years the respiratory function tests are compared to baseline (values at the beginning of the study). The results are either positive (no change or an improvement in test results) or negative (a decrease in scores on the respiratory function tests). This results are seen in Table 18.2. The relative risk for developing poorer (negative)

**Table 18.2** Example of Relative Risk

| | | Risk Factor | | |
|---|---|---|---|---|
| | | Mask | No Mask | |
| Respiratory Function | Negative | 6 | 12 | 18 |
| | Positive | 19 | 13 | 32 |
| | | 25 | 25 | 50 |

respiratory function results for those wearing a mask is compared to those without the mask would be calculated as follows:

$$EER = \frac{a}{a+c} = \frac{6}{25} = 0.24$$

$$CER = \frac{b}{b+d} = \frac{12}{25} = 0.48$$

$$Relative\ Risk = \frac{a/(a+c)}{b/(b+d)} = \frac{0.24}{0.48} = 0.5$$

or:

$$RR = \frac{ab+ad}{ab+bc} = \frac{(6)(12)+(6)(13)}{(6)(12)+(12)(19)} = 0.5$$

As indicated earlier, a relative risk of less than one indicates that the intervention (in this example wearing a protective mask) was effective in reducing the risk of the outcome (decreased respiratory function). But how does one evaluate the significance of the relative risk ratio? Two methods are available, either a confidence interval or chi square test of independence. The hypotheses associated with determining the relative risk is:

$H_0$: $RR_{Population} = 1$
$H_1$: $RR_{Population} \neq 1$

Similar to previous tests, a confidence interval is constructed and if 1 is within the interval, the researcher cannot reject the null hypothesis. If however, 1 is not within the interval, the null hypothesis can be rejected and one can conclude that the relative risk is significant. The interval is constructed as follows:

$$RR_{Population} = RR_{Sample}\left(e^{\pm Z_{RR}}\right) \qquad \text{Eq. 18.16}$$

where: $e = 2.718$ and

$$Z_{RR} = Z_{1-\alpha/2}\sqrt{\frac{1}{a} - \frac{1}{a+c} + \frac{1}{b} - \frac{1}{b+d}} \qquad \text{Eq. 18.17}$$

For the previous example involving protective masks, the 95% confidence interval is calculated as follows:

$$Z_{RR} = (1.96)\sqrt{\frac{1}{6} - \frac{1}{25} + \frac{1}{12} - \frac{1}{25}} = (1.96)(0.41) = 0.80$$

$$RR_{Population} = 0.5(2.7183)^{\pm 0.80}$$

$$0.5(2.7183)^{-0.80} < RR_{Population} < 0.5(2.7183)^{+0.80}$$

$$0.22 < RR_{Population} < 1.11$$

Since one is within the confidence interval it can be concluded that working with or without the protective masks does not appear to significantly influence respiratory function.

A second way to test for significance is to perform a chi square analysis for our 2 x 2 table, with one degree of freedom, using the same hypotheses associated with risk:

$$H_0: \; RR_{Population} = 1$$
$$H_1: \; RR_{Population} \neq 1$$

The null hypothesis is independence between the factor and the outcome. As they become closely related, the *RR* will increase and there is a greater likelihood that the difference is not due to chance alone and $H_0$ is rejected. For this test we will employ the Yates' correction for continuity equation. In this example (Eq. 14.5):

$$\chi^2 = \frac{n(|ad - bc| - .5n)^2}{(a+b)(c+d)(a+c)(b+d)}$$

$$\chi^2 = \frac{50[|(6)(13) - (12)(19)| - (0.5)(50)]^2}{(18)(32)(25)(25)} = 2.17$$

**Table 18.3** Modified Results for Previous Example

| | | Risk Factor | | |
|---|---|---|---|---|
| | | Mask | No Mask | |
| Respiratory | Negative | 6 | 14 | 18 |
| Function | Positive | 19 | 11 | 32 |
| | | 25 | 25 | 50 |

With a chi square less than $\chi^2_1 = 3.84$, we fail to reject $H_0$ and assume that there is not a significant association between wearing a mask (as a risk factor) and decreased pulmonary function test results (the outcome).

To prove that the statistical results are the same, let us slightly modify the results, so the results are just barely significant at 95% confidence. Consider the alternative results presented in Table 18.3, where the *RR* is 0.571. In this scenario the relative risk ratio confidence would be significant, because the value of one is not within the possible confidence interval (with 95% confidence):

$$0.197 < RR_{Population} < 0.934$$

The chi square test of independence would be significant because the calculated value is greater than the critical value of 3.84:

$$\chi^2 = \frac{50[|(6)(11)-(14)(19)|-(0.5)(50)]^2}{(18)(32)(25)(25)} = 4.25$$

In this particular case the Yates' correction for continuity was used since it gives a better approximation of the confidence interval calculated with the relative risk (Table 18.4).

As we have seen, in the case of a simple clinical trial comparing a treatment group to a control group, the relative risk ratio is the probability of an event in the experimental group divided by the probability of the event in the control group. Subtracting the relative risk for the experimental group from the relative risk for the control group produced the **absolute risk reduction** (*ARR*).

$$ARR = CER - EER \qquad \text{Eq. 18.18}$$

If the *ARR* is zero, the treatment is neither beneficial nor harmful. If the *ARR* is positive the intervention has had an advantageous effect on the outcome. Often the *ARR* is stated as the inverse of the decimal. This is termed the "**number needed to treat**" (*NNT*) and represents the number needed to prevent one adverse event.

$$NNT = \frac{1}{ARR} \qquad \text{Eq. 18.19}$$

**Table 18.4** Comparison of Chi Square Results with Relative Risk

| Matrix (a,b,c,d) | Relative Risk CI | Yates' Chi Square | Pearson Chi Square |
|---|---|---|---|
| 12,6,13,19 | 0.89 < RR < 4.48 | 2.17 | 3.13 |
| 13,6,12,19 | 0.98 < RR < 4.79 | 3.06 | 4.16* |
| 14,6,11,19 | 1.07 < RR < 5.09* | 4.08* | 5.33* |
| 12,6,13,19 | 0.89 < RR < 4.48 | 2.17 | 3.13 |
| 12,5,13,20 | 0.99 < RR < 5.81 | 3.21 | 4.37* |
| 12,4,13,21 | 1.12 < RR < 8.05* | 4.50* | 5.88* |

* Significant with $p < 0.05$.

In our previous example of chemical workers, the absolute risk reduction is:

$$ARR = 0.48 - 0.24 = 0.24$$

And the number needed to treat is:

$$NNT = \frac{1}{0.24} = 4.2 \approx 5$$

For every 5 chemical workers using protective face masks, prevention of one case of decreased respiratory function is possible.

## Graphic Displays for Odds Ratios and Relative Risk Ratios

Often graphics are used to illustrated results from either odds ratios or relative risk ratios. These are used when evaluating multiple predictor variables or when comparing multiple studies, for example, in a meta analysis. The estimate of the *OR* or *RR* is denoted by a circle (sometimes a square or diamond) and horizontal lines to each side of the circle represent the confidence interval for the population $\theta$ or $RR_{Population}$ (Figure 18.1). In this illustration, Factor A, B, and D are not significant because one is a possible outcome (within the confidence intervals. Factor C is the only significant predictor variable and represents the results seen earlier in the chapter with the *OR* for smoking and developing chronic lung disease.

## Mantel-Haenszel Estimate of Relative Risk

In Chapter 16 we discussed the Mantel-Haenszel test for evaluating a potential confounding third variable for a 2 x 2 chi square test of independence. This procedure can be modified for dealing with odds and risk ratios. The **Mantel-Haenszel relative risk ratio**, some times referred to as the **Mantel-Haenszel common odds ratio,** is a method for calculating relative risk while controlling for a third potentially

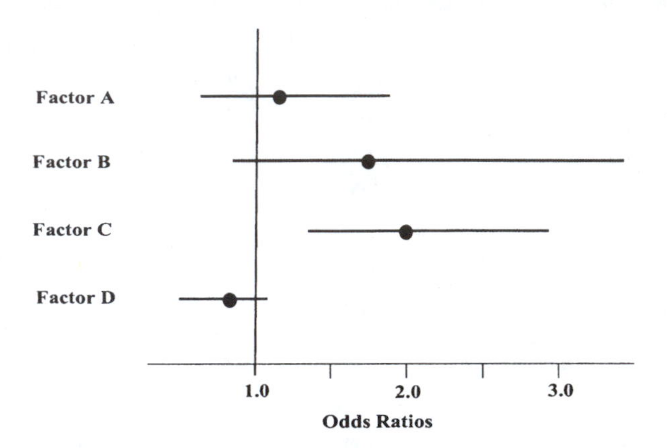


**Figure 18.1** Example of graphic illustration for odds ratios.

confounding variable. It removes the confounding that can result from a possible second independent variable and estimated the *RR* without the effect of a third variable. It involves stratification of our original data into levels for the third variable. The Mantel-Haenszel relative risk ($RR_{MH}$) is calculated as follows:

$$RR_{MH} = \frac{\sum \frac{a_i(c_i + d_i)}{N_i}}{\sum \frac{c_i(a_i + b_i)}{N_i}} \qquad \text{Eq. 18.20}$$

where $a_i$, $b_i$, ... $N_i$ represent results at each individual strata or level. The test statistic produces an overall risk ratio controlling for the third variable. For example, consider gender as a possible confounding variable for a study comparing the incidence of Type II diabetes in "overweight" volunteers vs. normal weight volunteers. After ten years of following initially healthy volunteers, the results presented in Table 18.5 were observed. For this example the relative risk of developing Type II diabetes in overweight and normal weight volunteers, controlling for gender is:

$$RR_{MH} = \frac{\frac{4(46+36)}{100} + \frac{22(28+48)}{100}}{\frac{46(4+14)}{100} + \frac{28(22+2)}{100}} = \frac{20.00}{15.00} = 1.333$$

The results are interpreted similar to the *RR* discussed in the previous section. Without controlling for gender, the *RR* would have equaled 1.625 and is not statistically significant with a 95% confidence interval of 0.940 to 2.838. It is possible

**Table 18.5** Relative Risk of Diabetes between Two Weight Categories and Controlling for Gender

| Gender | Developed Diabetes | Over-Weight | Normal Weight | Totals |
|---|---|---|---|---|
| Male | Yes | 4 | 14 | 18 |
| | No | 46 | 36 | 82 |
| | | 50 | 50 | 100 |
| Female | Yes | 22 | 2 | 24 |
| | No | 28 | 48 | 76 |
| | | 50 | 50 | 100 |

to test the null hypothesis that these is no association between the exposed and unexposed groups using the following formula.

$$\chi^2_{MH} = \frac{\left(\sum a_i - \sum \frac{a_i(c_i+d_i)}{N_i}\right)^2}{\sum \frac{(a_i+b_i)(c_i+d_i)(a_i+c_i)(b_i+d_i)}{N_i^2\,(N_i-1)}} \qquad \text{Eq. 18.21}$$

The resulting statistic is compared to the critical $\chi^2$ with one degree of freedom (3.8415). If the calculated statistic is greater than 3.8415 the null hypothesis is rejected and there is a significant association between the exposure and resultant outcome. For the example presented above, the Mantel-Haenszel relative risk may have been closer to one, but the chi square results indicate that there is a significant difference when gender is considered as a confounding variable.

$$\chi^2_{MH} = \frac{\left((4+22)-\left[\frac{4(82)}{100}+\frac{22(76)}{100}\right]\right)^2}{\frac{18\cdot 82\cdot 50\cdot 50}{100^2(99)}+\frac{24\cdot 76\cdot 50\cdot 50}{100^2(99)}} = \frac{36.00}{8.33} = 4.32$$

## Logistic Regression

Logistic regression is the appropriate regression model to use when the dependent variable is a dichotomous outcome (i.e., live or die, pass or fail a criteria). This binary logistic regression can be thought of as a regression analysis where the dependent variable response is a so-called dummy variable (coded *zero* or *one*). The dummy variable is used in mathematical manipulation and result in means and standard deviation that are meaningless in terms of quantifiable measures. In the traditional least squares model in regression and the formula for linearity (Eq. 14.2) was:

$$y = a + \beta x + e$$

where $y$ is the dependent variable, $x$ is the independent variable, $a$ is the coefficient for the constant, $\beta$ is the coefficient on the independent variable(s), and $e$ is the random error term. This might be extended to logistic regression by making $y$ the dummy dependent variable (one if the outcome occurs, zero if it does not), However there are several problems with this model, including: $e$ is not normally distributed when there is a dichotomous outcome; homogeneity of variance does not exist among different levels of the independent variable; and the predictive probability associated with the independent variable($s$) can be greater than one or less than zero. Use of the logit model solves these problems.

Logistic regression analysis allows us to examine the relationship between a dependent discrete variable with two possible outcomes, and one or more independent variables. In logistic regression the independent variable(s) may be continuous or discrete. Also, unlike regression analysis, it may not be possible to order the levels of the independent variable. This method is especially useful in epidemiological studies involving a binary dependent variable, where we wish to determine the relationship between outcomes and exposure variables (i.e., age, smoking history, obesity, presence or absence of given pathologies). Such binary outcomes include the presence or absence of a disease state or survival given a particular disease state. The use of odds and odds ratios, for the evaluation of outcomes is one of the major advantages of logistic regression analysis.
Logistic regression can involve a single independent variable or several different predictor variable. To begin with a simple analogy to a simple regression model, with only one independent variable and one dichotomous dependent variable, consider the following example. Assume 156 patients undergoing endoscopy examinations, and based on predefined criteria, are classified into two groups based on the presence or absence of gastric ulcer(s). For this specific dichotomous outcome the majority of patients (105) are found to have gastric ulcers present and the remaining 51 are diagnosed as ulcer free. Researchers are concerned that smoking may be associated with the presence of gastric ulcers, through the swallowing of chemicals found in smoking products. These same individuals are further classified as either smokers or nonsmokers. The results of the endoscopic examinations, based on the two variables, are presented in Table 18.6. The odds ratio (Eq. 18.5) for having a gastric ulcer given that the person was a smoker is:

$$OR = \frac{a/c}{b/d} = \frac{60/23}{45/28} = 1.623$$

Thus, the odds are 1.6 times greater for a smoker to exhibit a gastric ulcer ($EEO$ = 2.609) than a nonsmoker (CEO = 1.607). The 95% confidence interval for the

**Table 18.6** Outcomes from Endoscopic Examinations

| | Risk Factor | | |
|---|---|---|---|
| Gastric Ulcer(s) | Smokers | Nonsmokers | |
| Present | 60 | 45 | 105 |
| Absent | 23 | 28 | 51 |
| | 83 | 73 | 156 |

population, based on these results (Eq. 18.7) would be 0.828 to 3.183 (not significant because the value one does not fall within the interval). The outcomes seen in Table 18.6 represent a 2 x 2 contingency table similar to ones previously discussed in Chapters 16 and 17 and for which we already have several tests to analyze the data (i.e., chi square and measures of association). Where the chi square tested the relationship between the two discrete variables, the odds ratio focuses on the likelihood that the act of smoking can be used as a predictor of an outcome of gastric ulcers. Unfortunately odds ratio are only concerned with 2 x 2 contingency tables and only one dependent, or predictor, variable. Logistic regression can be used when there are two or more levels of the independent variable.

If regression analysis were used on scores of one for success and zero for failure using a fitted process, the resultant value would be interpreted as the predicted probability of a successful outcome. However, as indicated above, with dichotomous outcomes the outcomes or predicted probabilities could exceed one or fall below zero (as discussed in Chapter 2, $0 \leq p(E) \leq 1$). In logistic regression, the equations involve the natural logarithm (*ln*) of the probabilities associated with the possible outcomes. These logarithms associated with the probabilites are referred to as the **log odds** or **logit**.

$$logit = ln\frac{\pi_{i1}}{\pi_{i2}} \qquad \text{Eq. 18.22}$$

Where $\pi_{i1}$ is the probability of the first possible outcome of the dichotomous outcome (presence), $\pi_{i2}$ is the probability of the second outcome (absence) at *i*th lead level of the predictor variable (smoking). These odds are based on the probabilities of being in any given cell of the matrix based on the total number of observations. The probability ($\pi_{11}$) of the presence of a gastric ulcer and being a heavy smoker is 60/156 = 0.385 and the second possible outcome for heavy smokers ($\pi_{12}$ – absence of ulcer) is 23/156 = 0.147. The result would be the following probabilities, where the sum of all possible outcomes is one ($\Sigma p$=1.00):

| | Risk Factor | |
|---|---|---|
| Gastric Ulcer(s) | Smoker | Nonsmoker |
| Present | 0.385 | 0.288 |
| Absent | 0.147 | 0.179 |

Therefore, for smokers the logit would be:

$$logit(S) = ln\frac{0.385}{0.147} = ln(2.62) = 0.96$$

and for nonsmokers:

$$logit(\overline{S}) = ln\frac{0.288}{0.179} = ln(1.61) = 0.48$$

By using the logit transformation the transformed proportion values can range from minus infinity and plus infinity (logit(1) = +∞, logit(.5) = 0, and logit(0) = −∞). In this particular example, the larger the logit value the greater the likelihood that the action (smoking) will serve as a predictor of the outcome (gastric ulcer).

| | Risk Factor | |
|---|---|---|
| Gastric Ulcer(s) | Smoker | Nonsmoker |
| Present | 60 | 45 |
| Absent | 23 | 28 |
| Logit | 0.96 | 0.48 |

A second way to express the logit model is a modification of Eq. 18.22:

$$logit = ln\frac{\pi_{i1}}{\pi_{i2}} = \mu + \alpha_i \qquad \text{Eq. 18.23}$$

where $\mu$ is a constant and $\alpha_i$ is the effect at the $i$th level. In our previous example of smoker vs. nonsmokers the effect could be defined as the difference between the two logits:

$$\alpha = ln\frac{\pi_{11}}{\pi_{12}} - ln\frac{\pi_{21}}{\pi_{22}}$$

The difference of two logarithms is the logarithm of the ratio:

$$\alpha = ln\frac{\pi_{11}}{\pi_{12}} - ln\frac{\pi_{21}}{\pi_{22}} = ln\left(\frac{\pi_{11}\cdot\pi_{22}}{\pi_{12}\cdot\pi_{21}}\right) \qquad \text{Eq. 18.24}$$

In this case $\alpha$ is also the natural logarithm of the odds ratio:

$$OR = \frac{\pi_{11} \cdot \pi_{22}}{\pi_{12} \cdot \pi_{21}} \quad \text{Eq. 18.25}$$

In this example the odds ratio is:

$$OR = \frac{\pi_{11} \cdot \pi_{22}}{\pi_{12} \cdot \pi_{21}} = \frac{(0.385)(0.179)}{(0.288)(0.147)} = 1.63$$

The advantage of using the logistic regression analysis is we can expand the number of our levels of the independent variable to more than just two. Using the above example, assume that the researcher instead classified the smokers as light and heavy smokers and found the results in Table 18.7. Logits can be calculated for each of the levels seen in Table 18.7. For example the logit for heavy smokers would be:

$$logit(HS) = ln\frac{19/156}{7/156} = ln\frac{0.122}{0.045} = ln(2.711) = 0.997$$

In this particular example, the larger the logit value the greater likelihood that the action (smoking) will serve as a predictor of the outcome (gastric ulcer). Listed below are the logit numbers for all three levels of smokers:

| | Gastric Ulcer(s) | | |
|---|---|---|---|
| | Present | Absent | Logit |
| Heavy smokers | 19 | 7 | 0.997 |
| Light smokers | 41 | 16 | 0.937 |
| Nonsmokers | 45 | 28 | 0.476 |

An advantage with logistic regression is that it does not require the assumption of normality or homogeneity of variance.

What if the researchers are interested in a possible third confound variable, such as stress, alcohol intak,e or socioeconomic class? Multiple logistic regression offers procedures and interpretations similar to those found with multiple linear regression, except the transformed scale is based on the probability of success of a particular outcome. Also, many of the procedures used for multiple linear regression can be adapted for logistic regression analysis. In Chapter 14 the plane for multiple regression was defined as follows (Eq. 14.30):

$$y_j = a + \beta_1 x_1 + \beta_2 x_2 + \beta_2 x_2 + \ldots + \beta_j x_j + e_j$$

and the regression model could measure the effects of one or more predictor variables ($x_i$) on a single dependent continuous outcome ($y_i$). Logistic regression analysis allows us to examine the relationship between a dependent discrete variable

**Table 18.7** Outcomes from Endoscopic Examinations with Three Levels of Smokers

| | Gastric Ulcer(s) | | |
|---|---|---|---|
| | Present | Absent | |
| Heavy smokers | 19 | 7 | 26 |
| Light smokers | 41 | 16 | 57 |
| Nonsmokers | 45 | 28 | 73 |
| | 105 | 51 | 156 |

with two possible outcomes, and one or more independent variables (continuous or discrete). The logit model can be described by either of the two following equivalent formulas:

$$ln\left(\frac{p}{1-p}\right) = ln\,OR = a + \beta x + e \qquad \text{Eq. 18.26}$$

$$\frac{p}{1-p} = OR = exp(a + \beta x + e) \qquad \text{Eq. 18.27}$$

where *ln* is the natural logarithm and *exp* is the natural exponential function (2.718). Thus, logistic regression can be thought of a nonlinear transformation of the linear regression model. The "logistic" distribution will be s-shaped similar to the cumulative frequency polygon (Figure 4.13) and similar to other probability outcomes ($0 \leq p \leq 1$). This probability can be calculated modifying Eq. 18.27:

$$p = \frac{1}{1 + exp-(a + \beta x)} \qquad \text{Eq. 18.28}$$

The functional form defined in the previous equation is the logistic function, thus the term logistic model.

The coefficient $\beta$ is approximated by the coefficient from our sample data *b*. Note in linear regression the *b*-values represent slope coefficients and indicate the rate of change in *y* as *x* changes. However, in logistic regression the *b*-values represent the rate of change in the "log odds" as *x* changes. The formula Eq. 18.28 can be expanded for multiple independent variables:

$$p = \frac{1}{1 + exp^{[-(a+\beta_1 x_1+\beta_2 x_2+...+\beta_k x_k)]}} \qquad \text{Eq. 18.29}$$

where $a$ is the intercept or constant coefficient, $b_1$ through $b_k$ are the regression coefficients. In this case the chi square test (instread of the ANOVA) will determine the significance of the predicted outcome. Other variables that can be dichotomized (such as gender, race, age groupings) can use this coding system. Using this zero or one coding system it is possible to use odds and odds ratios for the evaluation of outcomes and this is one of the major advantages of logistic regression.

The **maximum likelihood estimation** (MLE) is a statistical method for determining the slope coefficients ($b$) and is a nonlinear least squares determination for nonlinear equations. Its determination is well beyond the scope of this book and involves computer iterations. Results of computer manipulation are presented in output tables similar to Table 18.8. The $b$-values (approximations of the $\beta$s) are in the "Coefficient" column and their associated error terms in the "Standard Error" column. The "intercept," sometime referred to as the constant, is the point where the plane crosses the $y$-axis for the dependent variable. In Table 18.8, a chi square and its associated $p$-value are calculated for each of the specific independent variables (factors). The chi square indicates the significant association of the factor to the prediction of the binary outcome. Some computer software will also generate the odds ratio and 95% confidence interval for each factor. Using Eq. 18.27, it is possible to estimate the odds ratio by using the sample logistic coefficient:

$$OR = exp(a + bx) \qquad \text{Eq. 18.30}$$

and calculate the odds ratio by raising the *exp* to the power of the logistic coefficient:

$$OR = exp^{b} \qquad \text{Eq. 18.31}$$

In the previous example in Table 18.8, the individual OR can be calculated for each of the four factors. For example, Factor C would have an odds ratio of

$$OR_C = exp^{-1.567} = 0.209$$

For illustrative purposes, let us assume that Table 18.8 represents risk factors associated with patients seen in the emergency room and being admitted to the hospital. Let us assume that a patient is seen in the ER and has Factors A, C, and D, but not Factor B in the table. What is the probability of admission for this patient? In this case our estimate of the constant ($a$) would be the intercept of 0.601. Using the Eq. 18.30, the estimated prediction of admission would be:

$$p = \frac{1}{1 + exp^{[-\{0.601+(0.835)(1)+(-0.284)(0)+(-1.567)(1)+(+0.307)(1)\}]}}$$

$$p = \frac{1}{1 + exp^{[-0.176]}} = \frac{1}{1 + 1.192} = \frac{1}{2.192} = 0.456$$

**Table 18.8** Example of a Computer Output for Logistic Regression

| Variable | Coefficient | Standard Error | Chi Square | Probability |
|---|---|---|---|---|
| Intercept | +0.601 | 0.955 | 6.443 | 0.011 |
| Factor A ($\beta_1$) | +0.835 | 0.125 | 10.486 | 0.001 |
| Factor B ($\beta_2$) | −0.284 | 0.103 | 2.667 | 0.102 |
| Factor C ($\beta_3$) | −1.567 | 0.870 | 36.244 | <0.0001 |
| Factor D ($\beta_k$) | +0.307 | 0.942 | 3.128 | 0.077 |

In this example the patient would have a probability of 0.456 of being admitted based on the factors presented. As will be seen in Chapter 19, this regression model can be used as part of evidence-based medicine.

If the dependent variable has more than two possible outcomes it is termed a **multinominal logistic regression** and when the multiple levels can be presented in a rank order it becomes an **ordinal logistical regression**. Application usually requires significant computer manipulation of the data to calculate the regression coefficients and goes beyond the scope of this book. A more extensive introduction to the topic of multiple logistic regression can be found in Forthofer and Lee (1995), Agresti (2002), or Kleinbaum et. al. (1982).

## References

Agresti, A. (2002). *Categorical Data Analysis*, Wiley-Interscience, New York, pp. 182-191.

Forthofer, R.N. and Lee, E.S. (1995). *Introduction to Biostatistics: A Guide to Design, Analysis and Discovery*, Academic Press, San Diego, pp. 440-444.

Kleinbaum, D.G., Kupper, L.L., and Morgenstern, H. (1982). *Epidemiologic Research: Principles and Quantitative Methods*, Lifetime Learning Publications, Belmont, CA, pp. 448-456.

## Suggested Supplemental Readings

Agresti, A. (2002). *Categorical Data Analysis*, Wiley-Interscience, New York.

Fisher, L.D. and van Belle, G. (1993). *Biostatistics: A Methodology for the Health Sciences*, John Wiley and Sons, Inc., New York, pp. 631-647.

Forthofer, R.N. and Lee, E.S. (1995). *Introduction to Biostatistics: A Guide to Design, Analysis and Discovery*, Academic Press, San Diego, pp. 440-444.

Kleinbaum, D.G. (2002). *Logistic Regression: A Self-Learning Text*, Springer, New York.

**Example Problems**

1. In a retrospective study of 170 randomly selected patients, the researcher is interested in determining if several factors (family history of hyperlipidemia, presence of hypertension, presence of diabetes, and smoking) might significantly influence the odds of meeting the cholesterol level goal set for them by their physician based on institutional standards. The evaluation for patients with and without hypertension were as follows:

| | | Hypertension | | |
|---|---|---|---|---|
| | | Yes | No | |
| Met goal | Yes | 60 | 24 | 84 |
| | No | 57 | 29 | 86 |
| | | 117 | 53 | 170 |

2. A total of 750 women were followed for a period of ten years following radical mastectomy. A comparison of their survival rates versus whether there was axial node involvement at the time of the surgery is presented below:

| | | Nodal Involvement | | |
|---|---|---|---|---|
| | | Yes | No | |
| Outcome in 10 years | Dead | 299 | 107 | 406 |
| | Alive | 126 | 218 | 344 |
| | | 425 | 325 | 750 |

   a. Based on this one study, what is the relative risk of death within ten years following a mastectomy and positive nodes? Is the relationship between survival and node involvement statistically significant?

   b. The researchers are concerned that the presence of estrogen receptors, because this factor (estrogen positive or estrogen negative patients) may have confounded the results of the study. Based on the following outcomes, what is the relative risk of death within 10 years and does estrogen receptor status appear to confound the results?

| Estrogen Receptors | Outcome | Node(+) | Node(−) | Totals |
|---|---|---|---|---|
| Positive | Dead | 179 | 26 | 205 |
| | Alive | 100 | 148 | 248 |
| | | 279 | 174 | 453 |
| Negative | Dead | 120 | 81 | 201 |
| | Alive | 26 | 70 | 96 |
| | | 146 | 151 | 297 |

3. Modifying question 5 in Chapter 16, assume that containers that contained a moisture level <2000 are defined as “success.” Using logistic regression, identify which amount of torque applied to the container closures would have the greatest likelihood of success?

| Torque (inch-pounds): | Success (<2000) | Failure (≥2000) | |
|---|---|---|---|
| 21 | 26 | 24 | 50 |
| 24 | 31 | 19 | 50 |
| 27 | 36 | 14 | 50 |
| 30 | 45 | 5 | 50 |
| | 138 | 62 | 200 |

**Answers to Problems**

1. Results of an odds ratio evaluation

| | | Hypertension Yes (+) | Hypertension No (−) | |
|---|---|---|---|---|
| Met goal | Yes (+) | 60 | 24 | 84 |
| | No (−) | 57 | 29 | 86 |
| | | 117 | 53 | 170 |

The odds of meeting goal with hypertension:

$$a/c = 60/57 = 1.053$$

Whereas, the odds of meeting goal without hypertension:

$$b/d = 24/29 = 0.828$$

The odds ration for the factor of hypertension is:

$$OR = \frac{a/c}{b/d} = \frac{1.053}{0.828} = 1.272$$

Thus, a patient with hypertension is 1.272 times more likely to meet the established goal than one without hypertension. Is this statistically significant?

$$\ln\theta = \ln_{(OR)} \pm Z_{1-\alpha/2}\sqrt{\frac{1}{a}+\frac{1}{b}+\frac{1}{c}+\frac{1}{d}}$$

$$\ln\theta = \ln(1.272) \pm 1.96\sqrt{\frac{1}{60}+\frac{1}{57}+\frac{1}{24}+\frac{1}{29}}$$

$$\ln\theta = 0.241 \pm 0.651$$

$$0 - 0.410 < \ln\theta < +0.892$$

$$e^{-0.410} = 0.664 \quad \text{and} \quad e^{+0.892} = 2.439$$

$$0.664 < OR_{Population} < 2.439$$

Since one is within the interval, we fail to reject the null hypothesis that OR = 1, therefore, even though hypertensive patients are 1.27 more likely to meet their goal, this is not significantly better than nonhypertensive counterparts.

2. Survival ten years following radical mastectomy.

   a. Relative risk of death with positive node involvement:

| | | Nodal Involvement | | |
|---|---|---|---|---|
| | | Yes (+) | No (−) | |
| Outcome in 10 years | Dead (+) | 299 | 107 | 406 |
| | Alive (−) | 126 | 218 | 344 |
| | | 425 | 325 | 750 |

$$RR = \frac{ab+ad}{ab+bc} = \frac{(299)(107)+(299)(218)}{(299)(107)+(107)(126)} = 2.136$$

$$Z_{RR} = Z_{1-\alpha/2}\sqrt{\frac{1}{a}-\frac{1}{a+c}+\frac{1}{b}-\frac{1}{b+d}}$$

$$Z_{RR} = 1.96\sqrt{\frac{1}{299}-\frac{1}{425}+\frac{1}{107}-\frac{1}{325}} = 0.264$$

$$RR_{Population} = RR_{Sample}\left(e^{\pm Z_{RR}}\right)$$

$$RR_{Population} = 2.136\left(e^{\pm 0.264}\right)$$

$$1.640 < RR_{Population} < 2.781$$

Decision: The risk of death is 2.136 time greater in patients with positive node involvement and this difference is significant since the calculated confidence interval for the population does not include the value one.

Chi square test of significance:

Hypotheses: $H_0$: RR = 1
$H_1$: RR ≠ 1

Decision rule: With $\alpha = 0.05$, reject $H_0$, if $\chi^2 > \chi^2_1(1-\alpha) = 3.84$.

Computations:

$$\chi^2 = \frac{n(|ad - bc| - .5n)^2}{(a+b)(c+d)(a+c)(b+d)}$$

$$\chi^2 = \frac{750[|(299)(218)-(126)(107)|-(0.5)(750)]^2}{(406)(344)(425)(325)} = 102.41$$

Decision: With $\chi^2 > 3.84$, reject $H_0$, conclude there is a significant relationship between survival and presence or absence of positive nodes.

b. Relative risk of death with positive node involvement controlling for estrogen receptors:

$$RR_{MH} = \frac{\sum \frac{a_i(c_i+d_i)}{N_i}}{\sum \frac{c_i(a_i+b_i)}{N_i}}$$

$$RR_{MH} = \frac{\frac{179(100+148)}{453} + \frac{120(26+70)}{297}}{\frac{100(179+26)}{453} + \frac{26(120+81)}{297}} = \frac{136.783}{62.850} = 2.176$$

Significance of nodal involvement and death as an outcome controlling for the possible confounding factor of estrogen receptors.

Hypotheses: $H_0$: Nodal involvement and survival are independent (controlling for estrogen receptors)
$H_1$: $H_0$ is false

Decision rule: With $\alpha = 0.05$, reject $H_0$ if $\chi^2_{MH} > \chi^2_1(1-\alpha) = 3.84$.

Calculations:

$$\chi^2_{MH} = \frac{\left(\sum a_i - \sum \frac{a_i(c_i+d_i)}{N_i}\right)^2}{\sum \frac{(a_i+b_i)(c_i+d_i)(a_i+c_i)(b_i+d_i)}{N_i^2(N_i-1)}}$$

$$\chi^2_{MH} = \frac{(179+120)-\left(\frac{179\cdot 248}{453}+\frac{120\cdot 96}{297}\right)^2}{\left(\frac{205\cdot 248\cdot 279\cdot 174}{(453)^2\cdot 452}\right)+\left(\frac{201\cdot 96\cdot 146\cdot 151}{(297)^2\cdot 296}\right)} = \frac{26315.33}{42.906} = 613.33$$

Decision: Reject $H_0$, conclude that survival and nodal involvement are related, controlling for estrogen receptors.

3. Logistic regression on four levels of torque:

| Torque (inch-pounds): | Success (<2000) | Failure (≥2000) | |
|---|---|---|---|
| 21 | 26 | 24 | 50 |
| 24 | 31 | 19 | 50 |
| 27 | 36 | 14 | 50 |
| 30 | 45 | 5 | 50 |
| | 138 | 62 | 200 |

Probabilities associated with each outcome:

| Torque (inch-pounds): | Success (<2000) | Failure (≥2000) |
|---|---|---|
| 21 | .130 | .120 |
| 24 | .155 | .095 |
| 27 | .180 | .070 |
| 30 | .225 | .025 |

Calculation of the logit for the 21 inch-pounds of pressure would be:

$$log\,it = ln\frac{\pi_{i1}}{\pi_{i2}}$$

$$logit(21) = ln\frac{.130}{.120} = ln(1.083) = 0.080$$

The logit for 30 inch-pounds would be:

$$logit(30) = ln\frac{.225}{.025} = ln(9.000) = 2.197$$

The results for all the logit calculations would be:

| Torque (inch-pounds): | Success (<2000) | Failure (≥2000) | Logit |
|---|---|---|---|
| 21 | 26 | 24 | 0.080 |
| 24 | 31 | 19 | 0.490 |
| 27 | 36 | 14 | 0.944 |
| 30 | 45 | 5 | 2.197 |

Based on the data available, it appears that there is an increasing likelihood of success as the torque increases during the sealing process.

# 19

# Evidence-Based Practice: An Introduction

The chapter will introduce the topic of evidence-based practice, which involves estimating the probability of a specific outcome. This determination involves historical data and information about the "goodness" of diagnostic tests or procedures. Having this information the clinician can estimate the probability of certain outcomes based on positive or negative diagnostic test results.

Determining whether a patient is likely to have a specific disease or condition, usually begins with a prior probability for an occurrence. This is often the prevalence (or pretest probability) of the disease in a specific population. Most diagnostic tests are not perfect, but the results of the test(s) will be used to increase or decrease our estimate of the likelihood (posttest probability) of the disease. This process is sometime referred to as the **refining probability.** The most important reason physicians and other health professionals order a test is to help refine probability and make a decision about the best approach to treating the patient. This refining probability is the process of modifying our estimate of the probability that a disease or condition is present through the results observed on some diagnostic test(s). As will be developed in this chapter, probabilities are critical in predicting the likelihood for a particular disease in a given patient. This prediction will be based on the prevalence of the disease and the likelihood ratio associated or a modification of conditional probability resulting from a diagnostic test, which is affected by the test's sensitivity and specificity.

## Sensitivity and Specificity

Conditional probability was important when we discussed the chi square test of independence. Based on Equation 2.6 the probability of some level of variable *A* given a certain level of variable *B* was defined as

$$p(A)\ given\ B = p(A \mid B) = \frac{p(A \cap B)}{p(B)}$$

| | | The Real World | |
|---|---|---|---|
| | | Positive | Negative |
| Test Results | Positive | Sensitivity | False Positive |
| | Negative | False Negative | Specificity |

**Figure 19.1** Contingency table for determining sensitivity and specificity.

and if the two discrete variables are independent of each other, then the probability of each level of $A$ should be the same regardless of which $B$ characteristic it contains.

$$P(A_1/B_1) = P(A_1/B_2) = P(A_1/B_3) \ldots = P(A_1/B_K) = P(A_1)$$

These points will be revisited in this chapter where more complex tests involving frequency data are discussed.

If we develop a specific test or procedure to identify a certain characteristic or attribute (i.e., presence or absence of a disease), it is important that such a test produces the correct results. **Sensitivity** is defined as the probability that the test we use to identify a specific outcome will identify that outcome when it is truly present. If we are evaluating a diagnostic test for a specific disease, it will produce a **true positive result** given the patient actually has the disease. In the case of chemical analysis, a method will detect a specific compound if that material is present. In contrast, **specificity** is the probability that the test or method will produce a negative result when the given outcome is not present. Once again, using the example of a diagnostic test, the test will present a **true negative result** when the patient does not have the specific condition that the test is designed to detect. We can depict these results in Figure 19.1. This is similar to the figure seen in Chapter 8 for hypothesis testing where potential errors exist in the lower left and upper right quadrants. In a "perfect" world we would expect sensitivity and specificity to both have a probability of 1.00 (with all the outcomes in the upper left and lower right quadrants. Unfortunately in the real world sensitivity and specificity will usually have probabilities less than 1.00. Just like hypotheses testing, errors can occur. Continuing with our example of a diagnostic test, if administered to a "healthy" person it is possible that a positive result might occur. This would be called a **false positive result**. If the test were administered to a patient known to have the disease, but it fails to detect the condition, it would be deemed a **false negative result**. Obviously, we want our test to have high sensitivity and specificity; resulting in a low probability of either false positive or false negative results.

Before a diagnostic or analytical test is used in practice, it is important to evaluate these rates of error (false positives and false negatives) that are possible with the test. In the case of an analytical procedure, mixtures can be produced with and without the material that we wish to detect and then tested to determine whether the material is identified by the test.

| | | Study Volunteers | | |
|---|---|---|---|---|
| | | HIV(+)($D$) | HIV(−)($\overline{D}$) | |
| Results of Diagnostic Procedure | Positive ($T$) | 97 | 40 | 137 |
| | Negative ($\overline{T}$) | 3 | 360 | 363 |
| | | 100 | 400 | 500 |

**Figure 19.2** Results of testing with a new HIV diagnostic.

Using a medical diagnostic test we will illustrate this process. Assume we have developed a simple procedure for identifying individuals with HIV antibodies. Obviously we want our test to have a high probability of producing positive results if the person has the HIV infection (sensitivity). However, we want to avoid producing extreme anxiety, insurance complications, or even the potential for suicide, from a false positive result (1.0 – $p$ (specificity)). Therefore we pretest on a random sample of patients who have the presence or absence of HIV antibodies based on the current gold standard for this diagnostic procedure. Assume we start with 500 volunteers with 100 determined to be HIV-positive and the remaining 400 test as HIV-negative based on currently available procedures. We administer our diagnostic procedure and find the results presented in Figure 19.2.

Similar to the symbols used in Chapter 2, let us identify the true diagnostic status of the patient with the letter $D$ (disease) for the volunteers who are HIV(+) and $\overline{D}$ (no disease) for volunteers who are HIV(−). We will use the letter $T$ to indicate the results from our new diagnostic procedure: $T$ for a positive test result and $\overline{T}$ for a negative test result.

Suppose we randomly sample one of the 100 HIV(+) volunteers, what is the probability that the person will have a positive diagnostic result from our test? Using conditional probability (Eq. 2.6) and the outcomes expressed as proportions (Figure 19.3) we calculate the results to be:

$$p(T \mid D) = \frac{p(T \cap D)}{p(D)} = \frac{.194}{.200} = .970$$

This meets our definition of sensitivity, the probability that a person will give a positive test result given they have the disease. Thus, the sensitivity for a diagnostic test is 97%. In a similar manner, if we sample one patient from our 400 HIV(−) patients, what is the probability that our test result will be negative?

$$p(\overline{T} \mid \overline{D}) = \frac{p(\overline{T} \cap \overline{D})}{p(\overline{D})} = \frac{.720}{.800} = .900$$

| | | Study Volunteers | | |
|---|---|---|---|---|
| | | HIV(+)($D$) | HIV(−)($\overline{D}$) | |
| Results of Diagnostic Procedure | Positive ($T$) | 0.194 | 0.080 | 0.274 |
| | Negative ($\overline{T}$) | 0.006 | 0.720 | 0.726 |
| | | 0.200 | 0.800 | 1.000 |

**Figure 19.3** Results for Figure 19.2 expressed as proportions.

In this example the result is 90% and meets our definition of specificity as the probability that a person will give a negative test result given they do not have the disease. Identical results can be obtained if we work vertically within our table by dividing the frequency within each cell by the sum of the respective column.

$$Sensitivity = \frac{97}{100} = .970$$

$$Specificity = \frac{360}{400} = .900$$

Conditional probabilities can be used to calculate the probability of a false negative rate (probability of a negative result given the disease):

$$False\ negative = p(\overline{T} \mid D) = \frac{p(\overline{T} \cap D)}{p(D)} = \frac{.006}{.200} = .030$$

or a false positive rate (probability of a positive result given no disease):

$$False\ positive = p(T \mid \overline{D}) = \frac{p(T \cap \overline{D})}{p(\overline{D})} = \frac{.080}{.800} = .100$$

Because they are complementary, the same results can be obtained by subtracting the results for sensitivity and specificity from the total for all possible outcomes (1.00):

$$False\ negative = 1 - p(sensitivity) = 1.000 - .970 = .030$$

$$False\ positive = 1 - p(specificity) = 1.000 - .900 = .100$$

| | | Real World | | |
|---|---|---|---|---|
| | | Present | Absent | |
| Test Results | Present | a | b | a + b |
| | Absent | c | d | c + d |
| | | a + c | b + d | n |

**Figure 19.4** Modification of a two-by-two contingency table for sensitivity and specificity.

### Two-by-Two Contingency Table

As seen previously, the sensitivity is the ability of a test (diagnostic or analytical) to detect a condition for which it is testing. For example, as a diagnostic test, if sensitive, it will give a positive result for a patient who actually has the given disease or condition. Using our previous layout for a two-by-two chi square design (Figure 16.3), it is possible to label a similar table for outcomes from a diagnostic test (Figure 19.4). In this model we would hope most of the test results fall in either the *a* or *d* cells of the table. Similar to conditional probability, the upper left cell (*a*) represents the frequency of **true positives** (*TP*). The lower right cell (*d*) represents the frequency of **true negatives** (*TN*). Both are desirable outcomes; unfortunately some patients may test which are **false positives** (*PF*, cell *b*) or **false negatives** (*FN*, cell *c*). Ideally, there would be a low false positive rate and low false negative rate, meaning a low incidence of incorrect results. An alternative to the calculations for conditional probability, the frequency counts from the contingency table can be used to calculate the sensitivity and specificity of a test using the following formula:

$$sensitivity = \frac{TP}{TP + FN} = \frac{a}{a + c} \qquad \text{Eq. 19.1}$$

$$specificity = \frac{TN}{TN + FP} = \frac{d}{d + b} \qquad \text{Eq. 19.2}$$

In addition the probability of a false positive or false negative result can also be calculated directly from a two-by-two contingency table:

$$p(false\ positive\ results) = \frac{FP}{FP + TN} = \frac{b}{b + d} \qquad \text{Eq. 19.3}$$

$$p(false\ negative\ results) = \frac{FN}{FN + TP} = \frac{c}{c + a} \qquad \text{Eq. 19.4}$$

Notice in Figure 19.4, for sensitivity and specificity, we are dealing once again with information vertically in our two-by-two contingency table. Using the previous example we get the exact same results employing this method:

$$Sensitivity = \frac{97}{97+3} = .970$$

$$Specificity = \frac{360}{40+360} = 0.900$$

$$p(false\ positive\ results) = \frac{40}{40+360} = .100$$

$$p(false\ negative\ results) = \frac{3}{97+3} = .030$$

For this example, the probability that the diagnostic test will indicate the presence of disease, when the disease is actually present (sensitivity or a true positive rate) is .970 or 97%. The probability that the diagnostic test will indicate an absence of the disease when the disease is actually absent (specificity or a true negative rate) is .900 or 90%.

The sensitivity and specificity of diagnostic procedures or commercially available tests are often available through medical literature or the manufacturer's product information.

**Defining Evidence-Based Practice**

Also referred to as **evidence-based medicine,** evidence-based decision making or evidence-based analysis; a simple definition for this process is the use of the best evidence in the literature to provide the best care for an individual patient.. With evidence-based practice, instead of making predictions about a population, we use statistics to apply population information to decisions about individual patients. What the practitioner is attempting to do is update his or her information about a specific patient; based on previous knowledge plus diagnostic test information.

Using sensitivity and specificity alone, one cannot determine the value of a diagnostic test for a specific patient. It also requires the practitioner's index of suspicion (or the pretest probability) that the patient might have the disease. Used together, these facts can provide an estimate of the probability of disease (or absence of disease) for a specific patient. The pretest (or *a priori*) probability is the probability that a patient has the disease before undergoing a test. The best estimate of this probability is the **prevalence** of the disease or condition in that specific population. To estimate prevalence we need an understanding of the historical probability of a particular condition.

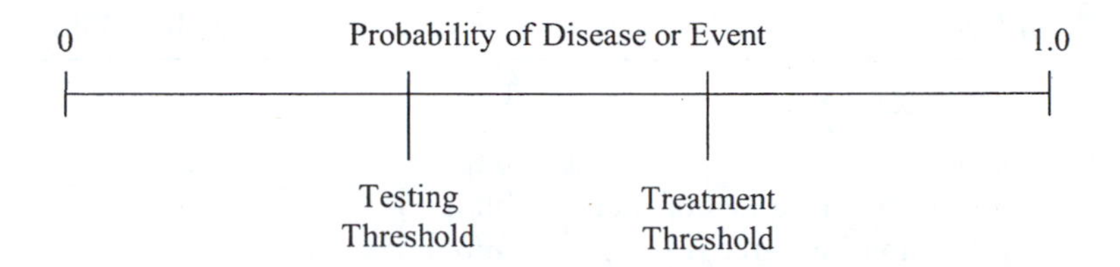


**Figure 19.5** The threshold model.

The pretest probability can be estimated by either professional experience or published scientific studies. The latter is probably more reliable, but the value of the former cannot be overlooked. Published studies in the medical and pharmacy literature are invaluable in therapeutic decision making. One of the commonly used hierarchical structures for information used for evidence-based practice is the "4S" model. This is usually represented as a pyramid or triangle with four subdivisions. The first, at the widest base portion of the triangle is "studies," followed by "syntheses," "synopses," and the top of the pyramid "systems" (Brian, 2001). The "studies" level represents original studies and clinical trials. These studies are primary literature sources and, in ascending order of importance, include: 1) case studies; 2) cases series; 3) retrospective and prospective cohort studies; 4) clinical trials; 5) randomized clinical trials; and 6) blinded randomized clinical trails. The "syntheses" level involves systematic reviews or meta analyses of relevant studies. The "synopses" level includes resources that evaluate and discuss the implications of selected studies or reviews. They are usually brief abstracts reviewing important study findings. Finally, the highest level in this hierarchy is the "systems" level; this is pre-evaluated evidence-based practice information with clinical advice on relevance of the information. With the Internet and electronic retrieval sources for these types of information, searching for information has become much easier for the practitioner. Some currently electronic resources and their URLs are listed in Table 19.1.

Using the information that can be obtained from the references sources listed in the previous paragraph, coupled with the tests described below, can result in a posttest probability. This posterior probability is the probability that a patient has the disease, given the results of the diagnostic procedure.

The threshold model can be used to estimate the probability of a patient having a disease and the value of treatment. The model is based on a continuous probability line from 0 to 1 (Figure 19.5). The testing threshold is that point on this continuum where no difference exists between the value of not treating the patient and performing a diagnostic test. The treatment threshold is that point on the continuum where no difference exists between the value of performing the test and treating the patient without doing the diagnostic test. This model was originally proposed by Pauker and Kassirer (1980). This model can be used to assist practitioners in making decisions based on the risks and benefits associated with ordering tests and therapeutic interventions. The questions that must be answered are: 1) what is the

**Table 19.1** Information Sources for Decision Making with Evidence-based Practice

| Level | Resource | URL |
|---|---|---|
| Systems | UptoDate | http://www.uptodate.com |
| | Physicians' Information and Education Resource (PIER) | http://pier.acponline.org/info/index.htm |
| | FIRSTConsult | http://www.firstconsult.com/home/framework/fs_main.htm |
| Synopses | Database of Abstracts of Reviews of Effectiveness (DARE) | http://www.york.ac.uk/inst/crd/index.htm |
| | Bondolier | http://www.jr2.ox.ac.uk/bandolier/index.html |
| | ACP Journal Club | http://www.acpjc.org/ |
| Syntheses | Cochrane DSR (Database of Systematic Reviews) | http://www3.interscience.wiley.com/cgi-bin/mrhome/10658754/HOME |
| | Ovid Medline | http://www.ovid.com |
| Studies | PubMed/MEDLINE | http://www.ncbi.nlm.nih.gov/PubMed/ |
| | CINAHL | http://www.cinahl.com/index.html |
| | OTSeeker | http://www.otseeker.com/ |
| | PEDro | http://www.pedro.fhs.usyd.edu.au/index.html |
| | WebMD | http://webmd.com |

probability that a given patient has the disease; and 2) where on this continuum that probability lies. The diagnostic test results may have varying effects on our estimate of the probability of disease. Clinicians will make choices on whether to treat or not treat a disease by considering if the results have crossed a treatment threshold.

As seen in the previous section, in order to calculate of sensitivity and specificity for a test, the information in the columns require that we already knew who had the disease or condition. However, in day-to-day clinical decision making what we really are interested in is what a positive or negative test result will mean to an individual patient being tested and the probability (given a positive or negative test result) that he or she will have the disease or condition. Using the test sensitivity and specificity, along with the estimated prevalence of the disease or condition, the calculation of a refined probability of a specific outcome can be accomplished by different methods: 1) Bayes' theorem; 2) a two-by-two contingency table and application of the likelihood ratio; or 3) a decision tree. This chapter will focus first the two approaches; discussion of the decision tree approach is discussed in Shlipak (1998).

**Frequentist versus Bayesian Approaches to Probability**

As discussed in previous chapters, probability theory is the body of knowledge that enables us to make determinations about uncertain events. The populist, or **frequentist approach**, was presented in Chapter 2 where the probability $p$ of an uncertain event $A$, written $p(A)$, is defined by the frequency of that event based on *previous* observations. As seen in Chapter 2, using a fair deck of cards, the probability of drawing a queen at random is .077 (four queens out of 52 cards). In health care, based on prior knowledge of a disease state, one could estimate the probability that an individual will develop that disease. This is based on the prevalence of the particular disease.

This frequentist approach to the probability of an uncertain event is helpful, if we have accurate information about past instances of that event or disease. However, what if no historical database exists? In these situations we need to consider an alternative approach. Using our previous example of a new HIV diagnostic test, since there is no previous experience with this kit, we cannot use the frequentist approach to define our degree of confidence in correct test results for this uncertain event.

As seen in the beginning of this chapter, conditional probability was defined with respect to joint probability (Eq. 2.6):

$$p(A) \text{ given } B = p(A \mid B) = \frac{p(A \cap B)}{p(B)}$$

Conditional probability $p(A|B)$ can also be calculated without reference to the joint probability $p(A \cap B)$. Rearranging the previous formula we can calculate $p(A \cap B)$:

$$p(A \cap B) = p(A|B) \cdot p(B) \qquad \text{Eq. 19.5}$$

because of symmetry we can also create:

$$p(A \cap B) = p(B|A) \cdot p(A) \qquad \text{Eq. 19.6}$$

Substituting for $p(A \cap B)$ we remove the need for the information about this intercept term and create what is called **Bayes' rule or Bayes' theorem**:

$$p(A|B) = \frac{p(B|A) \cdot p(A)}{p(B)} \qquad \text{Eq. 19.7}$$

Bayes' rule (British clergyman, Thomas Bayes, 1702-1761) provides a mechanism for updating our estimate of the probability of $A$ based on evidence provided by $B$. Our final estimate $p(A/B)$ is calculated by multiplying our prior estimate $p(A)$ and the likelihood $p(B/A)$ that $B$ will occur if $A$ is true. In many situations computing $p(A|B)$ is difficult to do directly. However, we might have direct information about $p(B|A)$.

One of the strengths of Bayes' rule is that it enables us to compute $p(A|B)$ in terms of $p(B|A)$. Bayes' theorem has become the basis for **Bayesian statistics**. This evaluation of data involves using a utility function (which is probability-based) and then maximizing expected utility.

With the frequentist approach, statistical methods attempt to provide information about outcomes or effects through the use of easily computed *p*-values. However, as seen in previous chapters there are problems surrounding the use of *p*–values, including statistical vs. clinical significance, one–tailed versus two–tailed tests, and difficulty in interpreting confidence intervals and null hypotheses associated with Type I and II errors. In contrast, the Bayesian approach can provide probabilities that are often of greater interest to clinicians. For example, the probability that treatment X is similar to treatment Y or the probability that treatment Y is at least 10% better than treatment X. These methods may be simpler to use and understand in monitoring ongoing trials. However, at the same time, Bayesian methods are controversial in that they require assumptions about prior probabilities and sometimes the calculations are more complex, even though the concepts are simpler. Good sources of information about Bayesian statistics include Lee (1997) and Press (1989). These are listed in the suggested readings at the end of this chapter.

## Predictive Values

Using the previous example of our HIV diagnostic test, let us apply Bayes' theorem. Based on the initial trial results with our diagnostic test, which had a sensitivity of 97% and specificity of 90%, what is the probability that a single individual who has the HIV antibody in the general population will test positive with the new procedure? This would be the question of interest in evidence-based practice. Assuming only our sample of 500 volunteers the answer would be:

$$p(D \mid T) = \frac{p(D \cap T)}{p(T)} = \frac{.194}{.274} = .708$$

Sensitivity and specificity are evaluators for the test procedure. However, we are more interested in the ability to detect a disease or condition based on the test results; specifically, the probability of disease given a positive test result (called the **predicted value positive, *PVP***) and the probability of no disease given a negative test result (termed the **predicted value negative, *PVN***). In other words, we are interested in the general population and want to know the probability that a person having the HIV antibody will give a positive result on our test. In order to accomplish this we can expand upon Bayes' theorem.

$$p(A|B) = \frac{p(B|A) \cdot p(A)}{p(B)}$$

As discussed in Chapter 2, an event can be expressed as the sum of probabilities of the intersection of the event with all possible outcomes of a second event:

$$p(B) = \sum p(B \cap A_i)$$

With conditional probabilities the relationship can be expressed as

$$p(B) = \sum p(B|A_i)p(A_i)$$

Substituting our symbols for disease the result is:

$$p(T) = p(T|D)p(D) + p(T|\overline{D})p(\overline{D})$$

The result is used in the denominator of Bayes' theorem to produce what is termed the predicted value positive:

$$PVP = p(D|T) = \frac{p(T|D)p(D)}{p(T|D)p(D) + p(T|\overline{D})p(\overline{D})} \qquad \text{Eq. 19.8}$$

It is possible also to determine the probability of having HIV antibodies given a negative diagnostic result or a *PVN*:

$$PVN = p(\overline{D}|\overline{T}) = \frac{p(\overline{T}|\overline{D})p(\overline{D})}{p(\overline{T}|\overline{D})p(\overline{D}) + p(\overline{T}|D)p(D)} \qquad \text{Eq. 19.9}$$

These predictive values will help redefine probability in the patient's specific population and will provide information on the likelihood a disease is present or absent in a specific patient. If a disease or condition is either extremely rare, or conversely, very common, then only an extremely definitive test is likely to change the posttest probabilities. However, midrange probabilities (between .20 and .80) can change greatly on the basis of even a reasonably definitive test.

If we apply these equations to the results for our 500 volunteers we should expect to calculate the same result as seen in the first conditional probability in this section. Using the proportions in Figure 19.3; based on other gold standard tests, we know the prevalence of the disease specific to only our volunteers is:

$$p(D) = .200 \qquad and \qquad p(\overline{D}) = .800$$

Using conditional probabilities we were able to calculate the probabilities for true positives (sensitivity) and true negatives (specificity)

$$p(T|D) = .970 \qquad and \qquad p(\overline{T}|\overline{D}) = .900$$

and calculate the probabilities of false positive and false negative results:

$$p(\overline{T}|D) = .030 \qquad and \qquad p(T|\overline{D}) = .100$$

Applying this information the *PVP* and *PVN* for our sample can be calculated:

$$PVP = p(D\,|\,T) = \frac{p(T\,|\,D)p(D)}{p(T\,|\,D)p(D) + p(T\,|\,\overline{D})p(\overline{D})}$$

$$PVP = \frac{(.97)(.20)}{(.97)(.20)+(.10)(.80)} = .708$$

$$PVN = p(\overline{D}\,|\,\overline{T}) = \frac{p(\overline{T}\,|\,\overline{D})p(\overline{D})}{p(\overline{T}\,|\,\overline{D})p(\overline{D}) + p(\overline{T}\,|\,D)p(D)}$$

$$PVN = \frac{(.90)(.80)}{(.90)(.80)+(.03)(.20)} = 0.992$$

Similar to the previous equations using for a two-by-two contingency table (Figure 19.4), the equations for *PVP* and *PVN* can be simplified. The *PVP* is the proportion of patients with a positive test result who actually have the disease or condition:

$$PVP = \frac{TP}{TP+FP} = \frac{a}{a+b} \qquad \text{Eq. 19.10}$$

The *PVN* is the percent of patients with a negative result who do not truly have the condition or disease:

$$PVN = \frac{TN}{FN+TN} = \frac{d}{c+d} \qquad \text{Eq. 19.11}$$

Notice in these two equations we are dealing with horizontal information presented in the two-by-two contingency table. Using the information in Figure 19.2 we find the same results using either set of formulas:

$$PVP = \frac{a}{a+b} = \frac{97}{137} = .708$$

$$PVN = \frac{d}{c+d} = \frac{360}{363} = .992$$

If we define the proportion of patients with the disease (in this case 100 out of 500 volunteers) as a prevalence, we can further rewrite Eqs. 19.8 and 19.9 to be stated as follows:

$$PVP = \frac{(sensitivity)(prevalence)}{[(sensitivity)(prevalence)]+[(1-specificity)(1-prevalence)]}$$

Eq. 19.12

$$PVN = \frac{(specificity)(1-prevalance)}{[(specificity)(1-prevalence)]+[(1-sensitivity)(prevalence)]}$$

Eq. 19.13

Without going through the entire derivation of these two formulas, we will prove the equations using the data from Figure 19.4. With our knowledge of the associated sensitivity and specificity from these volunteers, we can calculate *PVP* and *PVN* where prevalence is .20 (100 out of 500 volunteers):

$$PVP = \frac{(sensitivity)(prevalence)}{[(sensitivity)(prevalence)]+[(1-specificity)(1-prevalence)]}$$

$$PVP = \frac{(.97)(.20)}{(.97)(.20)+(1-.90)(1-.20)} = 0.708$$

$$PVN = \frac{(specificity)(1-prevalance)}{[(specificity)(1-prevalence)]+[(1-sensitivity)(prevalence)]}$$

$$PVN = \frac{(.90)(.80)}{(.90)(.80)+(.03)(.20)} = \frac{(.90)(.80)}{(.90)(.80)+(.03)(.20)} = 0.992$$

Using Equations 19.12 and 19.13 we have simplified our equation to requiring only three pieces of information: sensitivity and specificity of the diagnostic test and the prevalence of the disease or condition. In the previous case our prevalence was based on our knowledge of only 500 volunteer in the study. To extend these equations for the general population or a subpopulation we will use an estimate of the prevalence of a given disease. Prevalence is the probability of persons in a defined population having a specific disease or characteristic of interest. For illustrative purposes, let us assume that a review of the literature revealed that the prevalence of HIV antibodies (*D*) in the general U.S. population is 5%. We would replace the previous $p(D)$ and $p(\overline{D})$ with the information for the U.S. population and recalculate the *PVP* to be:

$$PVP = \frac{(sensitivity)(prevalence)}{[(sensitivity)(prevalence)] + [(1 - specificity)(1 - prevalence)]}$$

$$PVP = \frac{(.970)(.050)}{(.970)(.050) + (.100)(.950)} = .338$$

Thus, based on initial trials with our diagnostic test, there is only a 33.8% chance that an individual with HIV antibodies will be identified using our test. The negative predictive value is:

$$PVN = \frac{(specificity)(1 - prevalance)}{[(specificity)(1 - prevalence)] + [(1 - sensitivity)(prevalence)]}$$

$$PVN = \frac{(.90)(.95)}{(.90)(.95) + (.03)(.05)} = 0.998$$

However, based on these same initial measures of sensitivity and specificity, there is a 99.8% chance that a patient with a negative test result actually does not have the disease. Therefore, selectivity and sensitivity of a procedure can be applied to a known prevalence to predict the ability to detect specific outcomes.

Notice in the previous examples we were dealing with dichotomous results (pass or fail, present or absent). Such dichotomies will be used for the following tests that are expansions of the chi square test of independence.

## Likelihood Ratios

An alternative, equivalent process for redefining pretest probability and create new posttest probability involves the likelihood ratio(s). Using this method we combine the likelihood ratio with information about the prevalence of the disease or condition to determine the posttest probability of disease. This is illustrated in Figure 19.6. Unfortunately, the direct relationship needs one final modification, namely, incorporating odds into the calculations.

As mentioned earlier, **pretest probability** or **prior probability** is a term used to describe the probability of an event occurring based on previous experience with that event. It is the probability of a given disease prior to performing any diagnostic procedure. Clinically this might be referred to as the practitioner's **index of suspicion**. For example, based on national data, the probability of a *certain disease* occurring in otherwise healthy individuals is .020. This prior probability is used with a likelihood ratio to calculate a **posttest probability** or **posterior probability**. This posttest result is the probability that a specific patient has the disease, given the result of the diagnostic procedure for that patient is positive. Calculating the likelihood ratio is based on the sensitivity and specificity of the diagnostic procedure used to determine the latter probability.

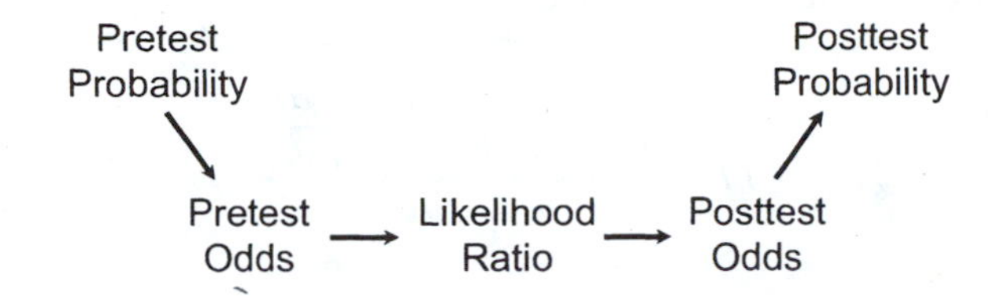


**Figure 19.6** Redefining probability using the likelihood ratio.

If an individual gives a positive test result, how many times more likely is this individual to actually have the disease present? As discussed previously, to evaluate the success or failure of a diagnostic procedure, the sensitivity is defined as the proportion of individuals with a given disease that are correctly identified as positive by the diagnostic test. Whereas, the specificity is that proportion of individuals without disease, that is correctly identified as negatives, by the diagnostic test. A diagnostic test may be very useful in one specific population, but could possibly be worthless for screening in a different population. This is determined by the **likelihood ratio,** which is dependent on both the sensitivity and specificity of the test:

$$LR^{+} = \frac{Sensitivity}{1 - Specificity} \qquad \text{Eq. 19.14}$$

The resultant value for the likelihood ratio can range from zero to infinity. The $LR^+$ is the likelihood of a particular test result in someone *with* disease divided by the likelihood of the same test results in someone *without* the disease. If a calculated likelihood ratio is 8.0, then the individual with a positive test result is eight times more likely to have the disease than someone with a negative test result. This is sometimes referred to as the **likelihood ratio for a positive result** and symbolized as $LR^+$.

It is also possible to calculate the **likelihood ratio for a negative result**:

$$LR^{-} = \frac{1 - Sensitivity}{Specificity} \qquad \text{Eq. 19.15}$$

Similar to the description above, the $LR^-$ is the likelihood of a negative test result in someone *with* disease divided by the likelihood of the same test results in someone *without* the disease. In this case an $LR^-$ of 8.0 would indicated that an individual patient with a negative test result is eight times more likely to not have the disease than another patient with a positive test result.

These two likelihood ratios do not require a 2 x 2 contingency table and are easy to calculate if information in the literature provides only sensitivity and specificity for a diagnostic test or procedure. But looking at Equations 19.14 and 19.15 we can see where they can be derived from such a table:

$$LR^{+} = \frac{sensitivity}{1-specificity} = \frac{\dfrac{a}{a+c}}{\dfrac{b}{b+d}} \qquad \text{Eq. 19.16}$$

$$LR^{-} = \frac{1-specificity}{sensitivity} = \frac{\dfrac{c}{a+c}}{\dfrac{d}{b+d}} \qquad \text{Eq. 19.17}$$

Using data from our previous example of the HIV diagnostic test, with a sensitivity of .970 and specificity of .900, the two likelihood ratios would be:

$$LR^{+} = \frac{Sensitivity}{1-Specificity} = \frac{.970}{.100} = 9.70$$

$$LR^{-} = \frac{1-Sensitivity}{Specificity} = \frac{.030}{.900} = .033$$

or taking the results directly from Figure 19.2:

$$LR^{+} = \frac{\dfrac{a}{a+c}}{\dfrac{b}{b+d}} = \frac{\dfrac{97}{100}}{\dfrac{40}{400}} = \frac{.970}{.100} = 9.70$$

$$LR^{-} = \frac{\dfrac{c}{a+c}}{\dfrac{d}{b+d}} = \frac{\dfrac{3}{100}}{\dfrac{360}{400}} = \frac{.030}{.900} = .033$$

In this case, if a patient has a positive test result, he or she is 9.7 time more likely to have the disease than a patient with a negative result.
How does one interpret the likelihood ratio with respect to the value of a diagnostic test? In general, the greater the $LR^{+}$, the better the test at diagnosing the disease or condition. Likelihood ratios equal to or greater than 10 are considered to be a useful test. In contrast, the smaller the negative $LR^{-}$, the better the test at excluding the disease or condition. Negative likelihood ratios equal to or less than 0.1 are considered a useful test.

**Table 19.2** Impact of Likelihood Ratios of the Posttest Probability

| Likelihood Ratio | Posttest Probability |
|---|---|
| 0 | No disease |
| 0.1 | Lower incidence |
| 1 | No change |
| 10 | Higher incidence |
| ∞ | Disease is certain |

Modified from: Go, A.S. (1998). "Refining Probability: An Introduction to the Use of Diagnostic Tests" (1998). *Evidence-based Medicine: A Framework for Clinical Practice*, Friedland, D.J., ed., Appleton and Lange, Stamford, CT, p.24

An advantage to using likelihood ratios is they can be derived from knowing only the test sensitivities and test specificities. The likelihood ratio can be used as a quick estimate of the posttest probability and the amount of certainty of the disease being present (Table 19.2). Another advantage is that only one number is required for the calculations (*LR*) whereas the *PVP* and *PVN* require that both sensitivity and specificity be involved in the formulas. A final advantage, as will be seen later, if independent tests are involved they can be multiplied together to calculate a single estimate of a specific patient outcome.

The likelihood ratio combines information about test sensitivity and specificity and provides an indication of how much the odds of the presence of a disease or condition change based on a positive or a negative diagnostic result. However, in order to apply the likelihood ratio, one needs to know the pretest odds (also a ratio). With this information in hand, one can multiply the pretest odds by the likelihood ratio to calculate the posttest odds.

As discussed in Chapter 18, an odds is the number of time a given outcome occurs, divided by the number of times that specific event does not occur, which differs from probability (the number of outcomes divided by the total number of events). The use of odds is another way of calculating the likelihood or probability of an event and are fairly easy to understand and can be useful in applying the likelihood ratio. Equation 18.1 could be modified to express odds as follows:

$$odds = \frac{p}{1-p} \qquad \text{Eq. 19.18}$$

By manipulating this equation, a probability can be calculated for any odds:

$$probability = \frac{odds}{odds+1} \qquad \text{Eq. 19.19}$$

**Table 19.3** Comparison of Probabilities to Odds

| Probability | Odds |
|---|---|
| 0.01 | 1 to 99 |
| 0.05 | 1 to 19 |
| 0.10 | 1 to 9 |
| 0.20 | 1 to 4 |
| 0.25 | 1 to 3 |
| 0.33 | 1 to 2 |
| 0.50 | 1 to 1 |
| 0.66 | 2 to 1 |
| 0.75 | 3 to 1 |
| 0.80 | 4 to 1 |
| 0.90 | 9 to 1 |
| 0.95 | 19 to 1 |
| 0.99 | 99 to 1 |

Some examples of the conversion from probability to odds are presented in Table 19.3.

With respect to the pretest odds involving the likelihood ratio, such a value is calculated by dividing the probability of the condition (prevalence, based on the literature), by the complementary probability of not having the condition:

$$Pretest\ odds = \frac{p(D^+)}{p(D^-)} \qquad \text{Eq. 19.20}$$

Thinking of these likelihood ratios in terms of odds ratios (Chapter 18), the $LR^+$ represents how much the odds of having a disease increases in the presence of a positive test results. The $LR^-$ indicates how much the odds of the disease decrease when the test result is negative.

Consider the administration of a diagnostic test; if the researcher has specific information about anticipated odds of an outcome before the test, it can be multiplied by the likelihood ratio to create the posttest odds for that outcome:

$$odds_{post} = (odds_{pre})(LR^+) \qquad \text{Eq. 19.21}$$

As seen in the equation, the magnitude of the likelihood ratio will have a direct effect on the magnitude of the posttest probability. These posttest odds represent the chance that a specific patient with a positive test result actually has a disease. Thus, if the researcher can combine the likelihood ratio with information about the prevalence of a specific disease, characteristics of the patient population, and information about the particular patient (represented as the pretest odds), it is possible to predict the odds of the disease being present. This forms the basis of evidence-based practice.

The calculation of the posttest probability is presented in Figure 19.6. The steps required to calculate the redefined probability are:

1. Estimate the pretest probability (prevalence)
2. Convert the pretest probability to pretest odds (Eq. 19.20)
3. Multiply the likelihood ratio by the pretest odds to create the posttest odds (Eq. 19.21)
4. Convert the posttest odds to a posttest probability (Eq. 19.19)

Using this process we can calculate the probability of a patient having an HIV if they test positive to our new diagnostic test. As defined in a previous section the prevalence of HIV infections is 5% or a pretest probability of .050. The pretest odds would be:

$$odds_{pre} = \frac{p}{1-p} = \frac{.050}{.950} = .0526$$

Multiplying the pretest odds by the likelihood ratio calculated in the previous section, the posttest odds would be:

$$odds_{post} = (odds_{pre})(LR^{+}) = (.0526)(9.70) = .5102$$

Finally, the conversion of the posttest odds to a posttest probability would be:

$$posttest\ probability = \frac{odds_{post}}{odds_{post}+1} = \frac{.5102}{1.5102} = .338$$

Therefore, a positive diagnostic result for our new test would mean the patient has a 34% chance of truly being infected. The result is identical to the value we calculated for the *PVP* using Bayes' theorem. Thus, either approach would give us the same answer.

The postprobability for not having the disease, given a negative test result can be calculated in a similar manner, substituting the *1 − prevalence* for the pretest probability. However, in this case the $LR^{-}$ is used as the likelihood ratio and become the denominator in the equation.

$$odds(-)_{post} = \frac{odds(-)_{pre}}{LR^{-}} \qquad \text{Eq. 19.22}$$

Using our HIV example once again:

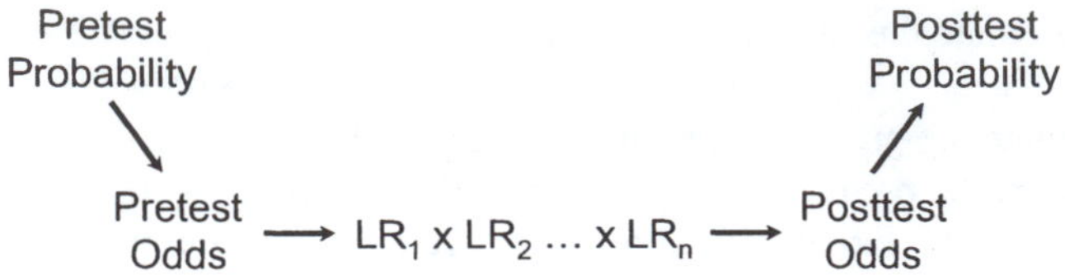

**Figure 19.7** Redefining probability for multiple independent tests.

$$odds(-)_{pre} = \frac{p}{1-p} = \frac{.950}{.050} = 19.0$$

$$odds(-)_{post} = \frac{odds(-)_{pre}}{LR^-} = \frac{19.0}{0.033} = 575.76$$

$$posttest\ probability(-) = \frac{odds(-)_{post}}{odds(-)_{post} + 1} = \frac{575.76}{576.76} = .998$$

In this case the posttest probability is equal to the PVN using Bayes' rule. The terms predicted value positive and posttest probability or posterior probability of having the disease are synonymous. Similarly, the predicted value negative and posttest probability of not having the disease or condition are also synonymous.

A third approach to determining posttest probability would be through the use of a visual graphic. Go (1998) provides a simple visual method for calculating posttest probability using a nomogram. It represents a simplification of Fagan's earlier nomogram in the *New England Journal of Medicine* (1975). On three vertical axes are pretest probability, likelihood ratio, and posttest probability. Using a ruler (or similar straightedge) to line up the pretest probability and the likelihood ratio, this straightedge crosses the third line at a value for the posttest probability (labeled as percents).

As mentioned previously, starting with the pretest odds, it is possible to combine the results from multiple tests to produce a final posttest odds. This process can be used if there are multiple diagnostic criteria, since one of the useful properties of likelihood ratios is that they may be used in sequence. Therefore, determination of the posttest probability can involve combining likelihood ratios, but only if the diagnostic tests are independent and not influenced by the outcomes of the other tests (Figure 19.7). Thus, we can keep modifying the posttest probability on the basis of a series of test results.

$$odds_{post} = (odds_{pre})(LR_1^+)(LR_2^+)...(LR_k^+) \qquad \text{Eq. 19.23}$$

One additional advantage of the likelihood ratio is that it can be used for continuous or ordinal data and measure the magnitude of these results.

**References**

Brian, H.R. (2001). "Of studies, syntheses, synopses and systems: the '4S' evolution of services for finding current best evidence," *American College of Physicians Journal Club* 134(2):A11-A13.

Fagan, T.J. (1975). "Nomogram for Bayes's Theorem," *New England Journal of Medicine* 293:257.

Go, A.S. (1998). "Refining Probability: An Introduction to the Use of Diagnostic Tests," *Evidence-Based Medicine: A Framework for Clinical Practice*, Friedland, D.J., ed., Appleton and Lange, Stamford, CT, p. 27

Pauker, S.G. and Kassirer, J.P. (1980). "The threshold approach to clinical decision making," *New England Journal of Medicine* 302:1109-1117.

Shlipak, M.G. (1998). "Decision Analysis," *Evidence-Based Medicine: A Framework for Clinical Practice*, Friedland, D.J., ed., Appleton and Lange, Stamford, CT, pp. 35-57.

**Suggested Supplemental Readings**

Bland M. and Peacock, J. (2000). *Statistical Questions in Evidence-Based Medicine*, Oxford University Press, Oxford, UK.

Friedland, D.J., ed. (1998). *Evidence-Based Medicine: A Framework for Clinical Practice*, Appleton and Lange, Stamford, CT.

Forthofer, R.N. and Lee, E.S. (1995). *Introduction to Biostatistics: A Guide to Design, Analysis and Discovery*, Academic Press, San Deigo, pp. 104-107.

Lee, P.M. (1997). *Bayesian Statistics: An Introduction*, Wiley and Sons, New York.

Mayer, D. (2004). *Essential Evidence-Based Medicine*, Cambridge University Press, Cambridge, UK.

Press, S.J. (1989). *Bayesian Statistics: Principles, Models, and Applications*, Wiley and Sons, New York.

Sackett, D.L. (2000). *Evidence-Based Medicine: How to Practice and Teach EBM*, Saunders, Philadelphia.

## Example Problems

1. Returning to the first example in the problem set for Chapter 2, we employed 150 healthy female volunteers to take part in a multicenter study of a new urine testing kit to determine pregnancy. One-half of the volunteers were pregnant, in their first trimester. Based on test results with our new agent we found the following:

| | | Study Volunteers | | |
|---|---|---|---|---|
| | | Pregnant | Not Pregnant | |
| Test Results for Pregnancy | Positive | 73 | 5 | 78 |
| | Negative | 2 | 70 | 72 |
| | | 75 | 75 | 150 |

What is the specificity and selectivity of our test?

2. One test for occult blood in the feces has a sensitivity of 52% and a specificity of 91% for colorectal cancer. At the same time the estimated incidence of colorectal cancer in the U.S. for 40-59 year-old males is 0.87%. What is the probability of colorectal cancer in a 52 year-old male with a positive result with this occult blood test? Use both a Bayesian and non-Bayesian approach.

3. Assume that we suspect 15% of the patients with a given risk factor will develop a particular disease. From the literature (or online databases) given the test has a sensitivity of 0.75 and specificity of 0.80. If a specific patient, with the given risk factor tests positive, what is the probability that she will develop the given disease? Alternatively, if the same patient has a negative response to the test, what is the probability that she will not develop the disease?

## Answers to Problems

1. Sensitivity, specificity, and probability of a false negative result for a trial urine pregnancy test.

| | | Study Volunteers | | |
|---|---|---|---|---|
| | | Pregnant | Not Pregnant | |
| Test Results for Pregnancy | Positive | 73 | 5 | 78 |
| | Negative | 2 | 70 | 72 |
| | | 75 | 75 | 150 |

$$Sensitivity = \frac{a}{a+c} = \frac{73}{75} = .973$$

$$Specificity = \frac{d}{b+d} = \frac{70}{75} = .933$$

2. Probability of colorectal cancer in a 52 year-old male having a positive result on a fecal occult blood test.

   a. Bayesian approach

   Based on the information provided we know the prevalence (preprobability) and the probability of not having the disease:

$$p(D) = .0087 \qquad and \qquad p(\overline{D}) = .9913$$

   Additional information is available about true positives (sensitivity) and true negatives (specificity)

$$Sensitivity = p(T|D) = .52$$

$$Specificity = p(\overline{T}|\overline{D}) = .91$$

   The probabilities of false positive and false negative results:

$$p(\overline{T}|D) = .48 \quad and \quad p(T|\overline{D}) = .09$$

   The postprobability of the disease given a positive test results is:

$$PVP = p(D \mid T) = \frac{p(T \mid D)p(D)}{p(T \mid D)p(D) + p(T \mid \overline{D})p(\overline{D})}$$

$$PVP = \frac{(.52)(.0087)}{(.52)(.0087) + (.09)(.9913)} = \frac{.004524}{.093741} = .0483$$

   The postprobability of not having the disease given a negative test result is:

$$PVN = p(\overline{D} \mid \overline{T}) = \frac{p(\overline{T} \mid \overline{D})p(\overline{D})}{p(\overline{T} \mid \overline{D})p(\overline{D}) + p(\overline{T} \mid D)p(D)}$$

$$PVN = \frac{(.91)(.9913)}{(.91)(.9913) + (.48)(.0087)} = \frac{.902083}{.906259} = .9954$$

b. Frequentist approach

$$prevalence = p(D) = .0087$$

$$LR^{+} = \frac{Sensitivity}{1-Specificity} = \frac{.52}{.09} = 5.7778$$

$$odds_{pre} = \frac{p}{1-p} = \frac{0.0087}{0.9913} = .00878$$

$$odds_{post} = (odds_{pre})(LR^{+}) = (.00878)(5.7778) = .0507$$

$$posttest\ probability = \frac{odds_{post}}{odds_{post}+1} = \frac{.0507}{1.0507} = 0.0483$$

$$LR^{-} = \frac{1-Sensitivity}{Specificity} = \frac{.48}{.91} = .5275$$

$$odds(-)_{pre} = \frac{p}{1-p} = \frac{.9913}{.0087} = 113.8425$$

$$odds(-)_{post} = \frac{odds(-)_{pre}}{LR^{-}} = \frac{113.8425}{0.5275} = 216.0047$$

$$posttest\ probability(-) = \frac{odds(-)_{post}}{odds(-)_{post}+1} = \frac{216.0047}{217.0047} = .9954$$

3. Based on the information provided we know the following:

$p(D)$ = prevalence = 0.15 ; the complement $p(\overline{D}) = 0.85$
$p(T|D)$ = sensitivity = 0.75; the complement $p(\overline{T}|D) = 0.25$
$p(\overline{T}|\overline{D})$ = specificity = 0.80; the complement $p(T|\overline{D}) = 0.20$

Using Bayes' theorem the probability of developing the disease given a positive test, or the predictive value positive, is:

$$PVP = \frac{(sensitivity)(prevalence)}{[(sensitivity)(prevalence)] + [(1 - specificity)(1 - prevalence)]}$$

$$PVP = \frac{(.75)(.15)}{(.75)(.15) + (.20)(.85)} = \frac{.1125}{.2825} = .3982$$

Alternatively, the probability of not developing the disease given a negative test, or the predictive value negative, is:

$$PVN = \frac{(specificity)(1 - prevalance)}{[(specificity)(1 - prevalence)] + [(1 - sensitivity)(prevalence)]}$$

$$PVN = \frac{(.80)(.85)}{(.80)(.85) + (.25)(.15)} = \frac{.6800}{.7175} = 0.9477$$

Using the pretest probability of having the disease (.15) and the $LR^+$ the posttest probability would be:

$$LR^+ = \frac{Sensitivity}{1 - Specificity} = \frac{.75}{.20} = 3.75$$

$$odds_{pre} = \frac{p}{1-p} = \frac{.15}{.85} = .1765$$

$$odds_{post} = (odds_{pre})(LR^+) = (.01765)(3.75) = .6619$$

$$posttest\ probability = \frac{odds_{post}}{odds_{post} + 1} = \frac{.6619}{1.6619} = .3982$$

Using the pretest probability of not having the disease (.85) and the $LR^-$ the posttest probability would be:

$$LR^- = \frac{1 - Sensitivity}{Specificity} = \frac{.25}{.80} = .3125$$

$$odds(-)_{pre} = \frac{p}{1-p} = \frac{.85}{.15} = 5.6667$$

$$odds(-)_{post} = \frac{odds(-)_{pre}}{LR^{-}} = \frac{5.6667}{.3125} = 18.1334$$

$$posttest\ probability(-) = \frac{odds(-)_{post}}{odds(-)_{post} + 1} = \frac{18.1334}{19.1334} = .9477$$

# 20

# Survival Statistics

In certain clinical studies, the researcher may wish to evaluate the progress of patients over a certain time period and observe their responses to a therapeutic intervention(s). Patients are monitored from the time they enter the study until some "well-defined" event. This event is often death, but may include other outcomes such as time to hospitalization, organ failure/rejection, or the next seizure. They could also be positive outcomes such as time to recovery, to discharge from the hospital, return to normal renal function, or cessation of symptoms.

At first glance it would seem possible to compare two or more survival rates using previously discussed statistics such as the t-test or analysis of variance to compare the mean survival times. Unfortunately these methods may not work for two reasons. First, up to this point in the book, all the statistical procedures have involved "complete" observations. There were measurable outcomes for all the people or items associated with the data. With survival data we may not know the ultimate outcome for all the potential measures because the study may end before all reach the well-defined event. The second reason is that the survival times usually do not follow a normal distribution. Nonparametric alternative (such as the Mann-Whitney U or Kruskal-Wallis tests to be discussed in Chapter 21) could be used if all the people in the study reach the well-defined endpoint. Unfortunately, in many cases, study result will be evaluated before all the patients have died or reached the outcome of interest. Therefore, a new set of statistical tests are needed to evaluate data that measure the amount of time elapsing between the two events. These types of evaluations are referred to as survival statistics.

**Survival statistics,** or survival analysis, is part of a larger group of test referred to generically as "time-to-event" models. For production or industrial data, the end date might be defined as "time-to-failure" for a particular application. The examples used in this chapter will focus on clinical events and primarily "time-to-death" analysis. However, time-to-failure data could be handled with similar methods.

Although these tests can be used to assess any well-defined event, by convention these are all referred to a survival statistics. Often survival data involves the creation of a graphic representation of the outcomes from the study, referred to as survival curves. This chapter will consider the two most commonly used methods for evaluating survival curves: 1) actuarial (life) tables and 2) the product limit method

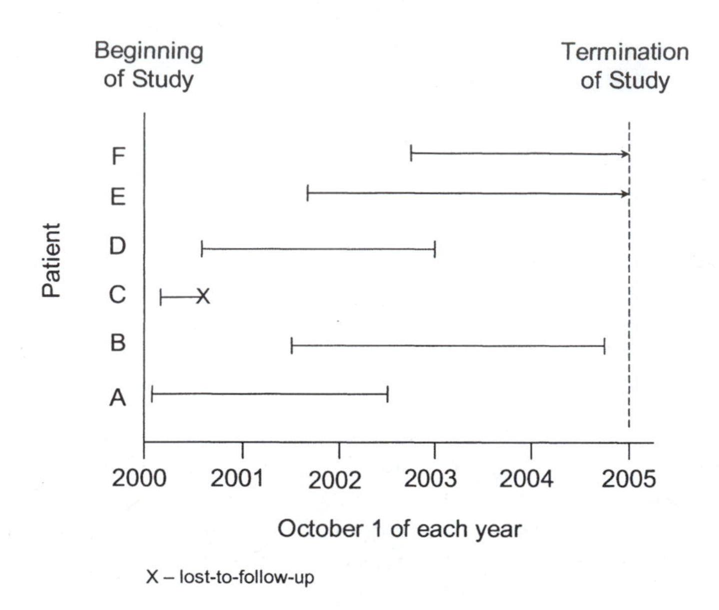


**Figure 20.1** Illustration of various survival times.

(illustrated by the Kaplan-Meier procedure). The tests are similar and can be used not only to create survival curves, but estimated confidence limits about the curves and median survival times.

Once survival curves are established, different conditions (i.e., treatment vs. active control) can be compared using statistical tests. The log rank and Cochran-Mantel-Haenszel test statistics will be presented for this type of comparison.

## Censored Survival Data

The amount of time that elapses between the point at which the subject entered the study and the time that the patient experiences the well-defined terminal event is the **survival time**. The collection of these survival times is referred to as the **survival data** and these data will be used to create survival curves and make decisions about the relative importance of the sample information and possible predictor variables. For survival data the outcomes are binary discrete results (i.e., survival or death, hospitalized or not hospitalized) and usually measured as an estimate of time with specific types of therapeutic interventions or under different conditions. However, as mentioned in the introduction, in most cases not all the patients will begin the study at exactly the same point in time and some patients may not have reached the terminal event before the study is concluded. This is one of the primary reasons why we need special methods to analyze survival data.

Using the definition above, the survival time cannot be calculated for patients who have not reached the terminal event by the closing date of the study. Also, for longer studies some patient may have been lost on follow-up and their health status may be unknown. These incomplete observations are called **censored data,** or censored survival times, and are divided into two types: 1) those alive at the end of the study (if death is the endpoint), these are labeled as "withdrawn alive"; and 2) those patients whose status could not be assessed label as "lost-to-follow-up" (this may be due to actual loss or noncompliance). For example, Figure 20.1 illustrated the data for the survival time of eight patients in a clinical trial. The *x*-axis represents the dates when patients entered the trial and left the trial. Note that patients A, B, and D provide complete survival information. Unfortunately, patient C was lost-to-follow-up during the second year he was enrolled. Also, for patients E and F, where the entry times are not simultaneous and the patients are still in the study when data analysis was performed, these patients are said to be **progressively censored**. With these progressively censored patients we know that they survived up to a certain time but we do not have any useful information about what happened after the time of data analysis. Patients C, E, and F represent censored data; their inclusion in the data analysis would artificially lower the average survival time because there is incomplete survival information. Even with censored data it is possible to analyze the survival times of these patients. Survival analysis is not restricted to only those who reach the definitive event, but incorporates data from all the patients enrolled in the study.

Patients who die from causes other than the disease being studied (i.e., sudden coronary or automobile accident) might be handled as either censored data or deaths. Both approaches have merit, and the investigator should determine how such data will be handled prior to starting the study.

### Life Table Analysis

**Life table analysis**, also referred to as **actuarial** analysis, is a type of survival analysis involving time lines that are divided into equally spaced intervals and number of outcomes are observed for each interval. For example, intervals may be every 60 days, in six-month intervals or as one-year periods. To illustrate the use of the various survival analyses, consider the fictional clinical trial where we followed 30 patients diagnosed with Stage IV melanoma over a five-year period. Beginning on October 1, 2000, as the newly diagnosed patients (meeting very specific inclusion and exclusion criteria) enter the study, they are randomly assigned to the current gold standard for treatment (control) or the gold standard plus a new RAF kinase inhibitor (experimental). The study was terminated on September 30, 2005 and data was analyzed for the five-year period (Table 20.1). Five patients represent censored data (patients 2, 19, 27, 29, and 30). For this and the following section we will ignore whether the patients were in the control or experimental group and first evaluate the congregate data.

This actuarial method is simpler to calculate than the product limit method discussed in the next session and at one time was the predominant method used in survival analysis. In some of the older literature it is referred to as the **Cutler-Ederer method** (Cutler and Ederer, 1958). The actual time intervals chosen for the analysis

**Table 20.1** Survival Data for Patients Enrolled in Study with Stage IV Melanoma

| Patient | Entered Study | Ended Study | Survival (months) | Result* | Group |
|---|---|---|---|---|---|
| 1 | 10/2/2000 | 5/28/2003 | 31.8 | DOD | Control |
| 2 | 10/7/2000 | 12/1/2001 | 13.8 | LTF | Control |
| 3 | 10/14/2000 | 12/12/2002 | 25.9 | DOD | Experimental |
| 4 | 11/15/2000 | 1/3/2004 | 37.6 | DOD | Control |
| 5 | 11/19/2000 | 9/19/2004 | 46.0 | DOD | Experimental |
| 6 | 12/12/2000 | 9/1/2002 | 20.6 | DOD | Control |
| 7 | 1/13/2001 | 4/26/2004 | 39.4 | DOD | Experimental |
| 8 | 2/1/2001 | 1/29/2004 | 35.9 | DOD | Experimental |
| 9 | 3/15/2001 | 9/23/2003 | 30.3 | DOD | Control |
| 10 | 3/21/2001 | 10/14/2004 | 42.8 | DOD | Experimental |
| 11 | 6/23/2001 | 7/16/2004 | 36.8 | DOD | Experimental |
| 12 | 7/14/2001 | 2/18/2003 | 19.2 | DOD | Experimental |
| 13 | 9/11/2001 | 6/2/2005 | 44.7 | DOD | Experimental |
| 14 | 11/11/2001 | 4/20/2002 | 5.3 | DOD | Control |
| 15 | 12/1/2001 | 10/17/2002 | 10.5 | DOD | Control |
| 16 | 3/4/2002 | 8/15/2004 | 29.4 | DOD | Control |
| 17 | 3/21/2002 | 4/15/2005 | 36.8 | DOD | Control |
| 18 | 4/30/2002 | 9/15/2005 | 40.5 | DOD | Experimental |
| 19 | 6/11/2002 | 9/30/2005 | 39.7 | WA | Experimental |
| 20 | 8/14/2002 | 10/23/2002 | 2.3 | DOD | Control |
| 21 | 9/21/2002 | 3/4/2005 | 29.4 | DOD | Control |
| 22 | 12/6/2002 | 7/2/2003 | 6.8 | DOD | Control |
| 23 | 3/14/2003 | 9/15/2005 | 30.1 | DOD | Experimental |
| 24 | 3/18/2003 | 8/2/2005 | 28.5 | DOD | Experimental |
| 25 | 5/11/2003 | 4/17/2005 | 23.2 | DOD | Control |
| 26 | 5/28/2003 | 7/26/2004 | 14.0 | DOD | Experimental |
| 27 | 7/13/2003 | 9/30/2005 | 26.6 | WA | Control |
| 28 | 7/15/2003 | 10/16/2004 | 15.1 | DOD | Experimental |
| 29 | 8/1/2003 | 9/30/2005 | 26.0 | WA | Control |
| 30 | 8/23/2003 | 9/30/2005 | 25.3 | WA | Experimental |

* Study results: DOD = dead of disease; WA = withdrawn alive; LTF = lost-to-follow-up.

are arbitrary, but should be selected so there are a reasonable number to evaluate and should not include a large number of censored observations in any one interval. Also, the interval widths should be equidistant. Since our example data includes five years, we will evaluate survivals using six-month intervals in our actuarial table. First, the data for all 30 patients is rank ordered by length of survival (Table 20.2). Note at this point the actual enrollment dates become irrelevant and only the length of time to the event is considered for analysis. Next a table is created indicating the results for each

**Table 20.2** Congregate Results for Survival Example

| Subject | Time (months) | Censored | Subject | Time (months) | Censored |
|---|---|---|---|---|---|
| 20 | 2.3 | N | 16 | 29.4 | N |
| 14 | 5.3 | N | 21 | 29.4 | N |
| 22 | 6.8 | N | 23 | 30.1 | N |
| 15 | 10.5 | N | 9 | 30.3 | N |
| 2 | 13.8 | Y | 1 | 31.8 | N |
| 26 | 14.0 | N | 8 | 35.9 | N |
| 28 | 15.1 | N | 11 | 36.8 | N |
| 12 | 19.2 | N | 17 | 36.8 | N |
| 6 | 20.6 | N | 4 | 37.6 | N |
| 25 | 23.2 | N | 7 | 39.4 | N |
| 30 | 25.3 | Y | 19 | 39.7 | Y |
| 3 | 25.9 | N | 18 | 40.5 | N |
| 29 | 26.0 | Y | 10 | 42.8 | N |
| 27 | 26.6 | Y | 13 | 44.7 | N |
| 24 | 28.5 | N | 5 | 46.0 | N |

**Table 20.3** Life Table for Congregate Results for Melanoma Patients

| Months | $n_i$ | $d_i$ | $w_i$ | $n_i'$ | $q_i$ | $p_i$ | $s_i$ | SE ($s_i$) |
|---|---|---|---|---|---|---|---|---|
| 0.0 - 6.0 | 30 | 2 | 0 | 30 | 0.0667 | 0.9333 | 0.9333 | 0.0455 |
| 6.1 - 12.0 | 28 | 2 | 0 | 28 | 0.0714 | 0.9286 | 0.8667 | 0.0621 |
| 12.1 - 18.0 | 26 | 2 | 1 | 25.5 | 0.0784 | 0.9216 | 0.7987 | 0.0735 |
| 18.1 - 24.0 | 23 | 3 | 0 | 23 | 0.1304 | 0.8696 | 0.6945 | 0.0850 |
| 24.1 - 30.0 | 20 | 4 | 3 | 18.5 | 0.2162 | 0.7838 | 0.5443 | 0.0941 |
| 30.1 - 36.0 | 13 | 4 | 0 | 13 | 0.3077 | 0.6923 | 0.3769 | 0.0954 |
| 36.1 - 42.0 | 9 | 5 | 1 | 8.5 | 0.5882 | 0.4118 | 0.1552 | 0.0748 |
| >42.0 | 3 | 3 | 0 | 3 | 1.0000 | 0.0000 | … | … |

interval in the study (Table 20.3). In this table $n_i$ is the number of patients in the study at the beginning of the interval, $d_i$ is the number of patients who reached the event during the interval (in this example death was the terminal event) and $w_i$ are the number of patient who were "withdrawn" from the study during the interval (either through lost to follow-up or were alive at the point of data analysis). The fifth column, $n_i'$, represent the number of observations correcting for the number of withdrawals during the interval:

$$n_i' = n_i - \frac{w_i}{2} \qquad \text{Eq. 20.1}$$

Using the information in the first five columns of Table 20.3 the proportion terminating in any *i*th interval is calculated using the following formula:

$$q_i = \frac{d_i}{n_i'} \qquad \text{Eq. 20.2}$$

and the proportion surviving would be the complement of those terminating the study during any given interval:

$$p_i = 1 - q_i \qquad \text{Eq. 20.3}$$

These results are expressed in the sixth and seventh columns of Table 20.3. The actuarial method evaluates the number of patients at the beginning of the interval but not at the end. It assumes that patients are randomly removed from the study throughout any one interval; therefore, withdrawal is measured halfway though the time represented by the interval. Patients ending the study are given credit for surviving half of the interval. Therefore, in the error term, the denominator (Eq. 20.2) is reduced by half of the number of patients who withdraw during the period. If the *i*th interval is conditional on a previous event (*i*th – 1), the probability of their joint occurrence is determined by multiplying the probabilities of the two conditional events. Thus, the cumulative probability of surviving interval *i* along with all the previous intervals is calculated by multiplying *i*th $p_i$, and all previous $p_i$s:

$$\hat{S}_i = p_i \cdot p_{i-1} \cdot p_{i-2} \cdot \ldots \cdot p_1 \qquad \text{Eq. 20.4}$$

which can be also written as:

$$\hat{S}_i = \Pi(p_i) \qquad \text{Eq. 20.5}$$

where $\Pi$ is the symbol for product, similar to $\Sigma$ for sum. The eighth column represents the cumulative proportions of survival ($\hat{S}_i$) for our sample data, which is the called the **survival function**. The survival function, (synonyms are survivor function or survivorship function) is our best estimate of the probability of surviving past a given time point:

$$S_i = p(T > t_i) \qquad \text{Eq. 20.6}$$

where $T$ is the time of death and $t_i$ is the time under consideration. In other words, survival function is the probability that the death or other well-defined event will occur later than some specific time interval.

An important point is that the event of interest can only happen once for each patient or object (in the case of time-to-failure studies). If an event can occur

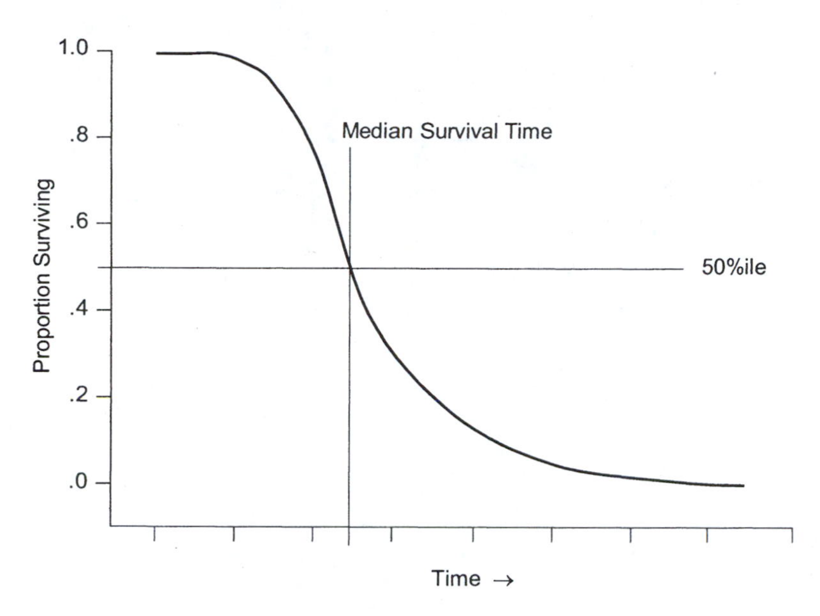


**Figure 20.2** Hypothetical survival curve.

multiple times, then the **recurring event model** (or **repeated event model**) can be employed and results are often relevant to system reliability. These measurements involve a reliability function and fall beyond the scope of this book.

## Survival Curve

Usually results are presented as a survival curve, rather than as a table (i.e., Table 20.3). The survival function ($S_i$) is the parameter for the population(s) we are studying. Figure 20.2 illustrates a hypothetical survival function where at time zero ($t_i$ = 0) 100% of the patients are alive ($p_i$ = 1.00). The proportion of patients surviving will gradually decrease over time and at some endpoint none of the patients will be alive ($p_i$ = 0). In survival analysis we estimate this curve by using sample data. The curve for the sample data is created plotting the cumulative proportions of survival on the *y*-axis and time on the *x*-axis (Figure 20.3). Instead of a smooth curve represented by population data and the curve for sample data is a series of steps downward at the end of each interval using our best estimate the sample survival functions ($\hat{S}_i$). Once again, we begin a $t_i$ = 0 with $p_i$ = 1.00 (all patients are alive or have not yet reached some other well-defined event), and the results from our example are illustrated in Figure 20.3. The beginning of the *y*-axis, time zero, does not refer to a particular month or year, it is the time at which each subject was entered into the study.

A common measure of survival is the **median survival time**, which is the point in time where 50% of the patients reach the well-defined endpoint in the study. Using the sample survival curve, it is relatively simple to determine the median survival time visually by drawing a horizontal line at the .50 point on the *y*-axis. Where it

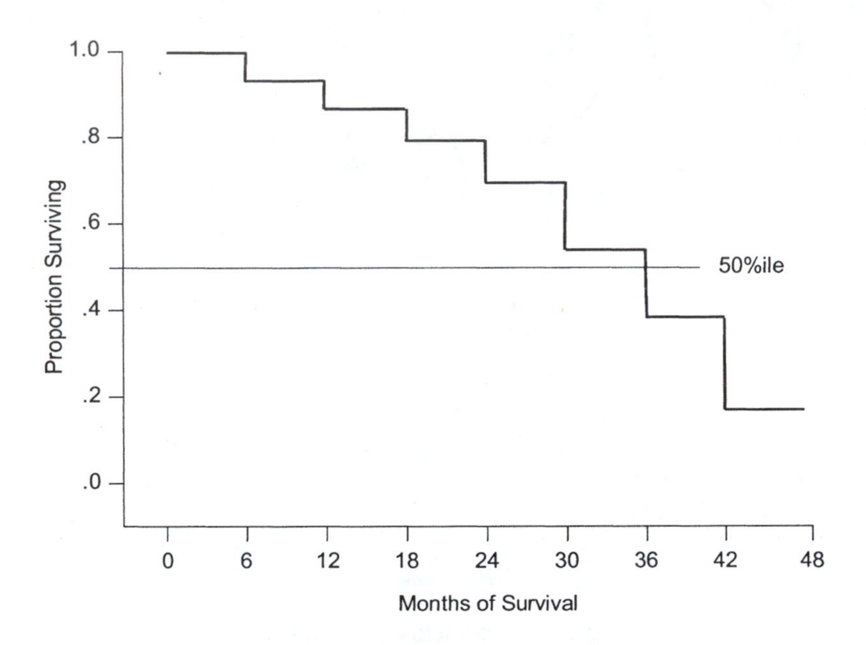


**Figure 20.3** Actuarial life table curve with median line.

meets the survival curve, moving vertically to the *x*-axis defines the median survival time. This is illustrated in our hypothetical model (Figure 20.2). In our example problem the horizontal line in Figure 20.3 meets the curve at 36 months, which is the median survival time for the congregate data. If the p=.50 line intercepts at a horizontal line, the average of the two extremes of that horizontal line is defined as the median survival time. It is possible to have no median survival if the survival curve fails to reach .50 by the end of the study.

Often these curves include dotted or dashed lines on either side of the survival curve that represent confidence bands. Normally these confidence intervals will become wider as time progresses, illustrating a decreased confidence in the estimate due to decreasing sample sizes. Applying the survival function defined above and data presented in Table 20.3, it is possible to calculate an estimated standard error term for each interval:

$$SE(\hat{S}_i) = \hat{S}_i \sqrt{\sum \frac{q_i}{n_i'(p_i)}} \qquad \text{Eq. 20.7}$$

For example the standard error for the 30.1- and 36.0-month interval would be:

$$SE(\hat{S}_i) = 0.3769\sqrt{\frac{0.0667}{30(.9333)} + \frac{0.0714}{28(.9286)} + \ldots \frac{.3077}{13(.6923)}}$$

$$SE(\hat{S}_i) = 0.3769(0.2532) = 0.0954$$

The results for all the intervals are presented in the last column of Table 20.3. This formula assumes a reasonably large sample size and only a relatively small number of censored observations. It is assumed that the proportion of survival at any interval is approximately normally distributed. Using this error term from Eq. 20.7 and a desired level of confidence represented by the $z_{1-\alpha/2}$ reliability coefficient (i.e., 1.96 for 95% confidence) it is possible to define the confidence bands:

$$S_i = \hat{S}_i \pm z_{1-\alpha/2} \cdot SE(\hat{S}_i) \qquad \text{Eq. 20.8}$$

For example, the 95% confidence interval for an interval of 30.1 to 36.0 months would be:

$$S_i = .3769 \pm 1.96(0.0954) = .3769 \pm .1870$$

$$.1899 < S_i < .5639$$

With 95% confidence the true $p_i$ for surviving 30.1 to 36.0 months, based on our sample on only 30 patients is somewhere between a probability of .1899 to .5639. The resulting confidence interval is very large because of the small sample size of patients still living after 36 months of therapy. Because the $p_i$-value cannot be greater than 1.0 or less than zero, some intervals may need to be truncated. For example, for the first interval (up to 6.0 months) the upper confidence bond would be greater than 1.0.

$$S_i = .9333 \pm 1.96(.0455) = .9333 \pm .0893$$

$$.8440 < S_i < 1.0226$$

Therefore, the ceiling for the probability would be truncated to 1.000.

$$.8440 < S_i < 1.000$$

Based on the study results, patients would have a .8440 or greater probability of surviving at least 6 months. The results for all the confidence intervals are listed in Table 20.4. These are graphically represented in Figure 20.4.

The 95% confidence bands can be used to estimate the median survival time by locating where the .50 line crosses the two vertical bands around the survival curve. For our example in Figure 20.4, the 95% confidence intervals for the median would be 24 and 48 months.

There are two major assumptions for using the actuarial time. First, that an individual withdrawal during a specific interval, on the average, occurs at the

**Table 20.4** Confidence Intervals for Life Table for Melanoma Patients

| Months | Lower Band | $s_i$ | Upper Band | Band Width |
|---|---|---|---|---|
| 0.0 - 6.0 | 0.8440 | 0.9333 | 1.0000 | ... |
| 6.1 - 12.0 | 0.7451 | 0.8667 | 0.9883 | 0.2433 |
| 12.1 - 18.0 | 0.6547 | 0.7987 | 0.9427 | 0.2881 |
| 18.1 - 24.0 | 0.5279 | 0.6945 | 0.8611 | 0.3333 |
| 24.1 - 30.0 | 0.3598 | 0.5443 | 0.7288 | 0.3690 |
| 30.1 - 36.0 | 0.1899 | 0.3769 | 0.5639 | 0.3740 |
| 36.1 - 42.0 | 0.0087 | 0.1552 | 0.3017 | 0.2931 |
| >42.0 | ... | ... | ... | ... |

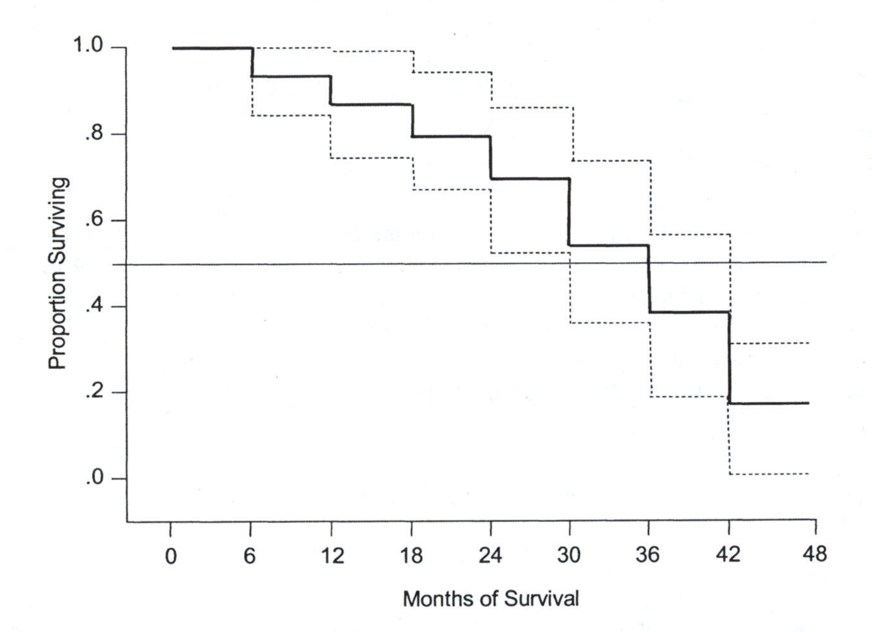


**Figure 20.4** Actuarial curve with 95% confidence bands.

midpoint of the interval. This is a problem with the censored patients in that we do not know their actual length of survival either within the interval or after that interval. The advantage of using the Kaplan-Meier method (discussed in the following section) is that it overcomes the problem of an averaged midpoint. The second assumption is that even though the survival in a specific interval ($i$) depends on survival in all previous periods, the probability of survival at one specific interval is independent of the probability of survival at any of the other periods.

### Kaplan-Meier Procedure

As will be discussed below, this procedure involves successive multiplications of individual estimated probabilities (the survival functions $\hat{S}_i$), for this reason the **Kaplan-Meier procedure** is sometimes referred to as the **product-limit method** of estimating survival probabilities. Similar to the actuarial table curve, the Kaplan-Meier survival curve plots the proportion of survival as a function of time. However, unlike the previous method, with the product limit method each death is a downward step in the curve, rather than considering the number of deaths within a specific interval. Each time one patient dies, there is subsequent decease in the $p_i$ and $\hat{S}_i$. Because the Kaplan-Meier procedure is based on the ranking of all the individual survival times, it may be mathematically tedious to apply large data sets (greater than 100 patients). However, with the aid of computer programs it would be the preferred method for determining survival curves and subsequent statistics.

Use of the Kaplan-Meier method is appropriate in studies involving a smaller number of patients and is the preferred procedure for survival analysis, unless there are a large number of patients in the study. Because withdrawals or censored patients are ignored, the procedure involves fewer calculations than the actuarial method. These calculations involve determining the proportions of patients in a sample who survive for various lengths of time ($p_i$s). However, at times when a patient is censored (withdrawn), the survival curve does not step down since no one has died. Step-downs in the curve only occur only with a death and the survival curve changes precisely at the time points when patients die. With the Kaplan-Meier method, censored observations have not been excluded from the analysis. They are used to determine the number of patients at risk for each time of relapse. If censored withdrawals were excluded from the survival analysis, the estimate of the survival probabilities ($p_i$) for the remaining observations would be different.

The first step in the Kaplan-Meier procedure is to list the times-to-event in rank order. For our example problem on melanoma patients, data has already been ranked and previously presented in Table 20.2. A new table is created to calculate various probabilities, similar to the actuarial table. In this table (Table 20.5) the first column are the times-to-event in rank order. The second column is the number of patients in the remaining previous period ($n_{i-1}$) who are beginning the new period (for the first period this would be the number of patients entering the study). The third column is the number of patients censored during the interval ($w_i$) and the fourth represents the number of patients at risk ($n_i$), which is the number of patients beginning the period less the number censored.

$$n_i = n_{i-1}' - w_i \quad \text{Eq. 20.9}$$

Note again, that the interval ends only with a death or other well-defined end-point. The fifth column are patients-who-died-events during the period (usually one, unless more died at the exact same duration of time in the study. The sixth column is the number of patients remaining at the end of the period:

**Table 20.5** Determination of Cumulative Survival for Kaplan-Meier Example

| Event (Months) | $n_{i-1}'$ | $w_i$ | $n_i$ | $d_i$ | $n_i'$ | $p_i$ | $S_i$ |
|---|---|---|---|---|---|---|---|
| 2.3 | 30 | 0 | 30 | 1 | 29 | 0.9667 | 0.9667 |
| 5.3 | 29 | 0 | 29 | 1 | 28 | 0.9655 | 0.9333 |
| 6.8 | 28 | 0 | 28 | 1 | 27 | 0.9643 | 0.9000 |
| 10.5 | 27 | 0 | 27 | 1 | 26 | 0.9630 | 0.8667 |
| 14.0 | 26 | 1 | 25 | 1 | 24 | 0.9600 | 0.8320 |
| 15.1 | 24 | 0 | 24 | 1 | 23 | 0.9583 | 0.7973 |
| 19.2 | 23 | 0 | 23 | 1 | 22 | 0.9565 | 0.7627 |
| 20.6 | 22 | 0 | 22 | 1 | 21 | 0.9545 | 0.7280 |
| 23.2 | 21 | 0 | 21 | 1 | 20 | 0.9524 | 0.6933 |
| 25.9 | 20 | 1 | 19 | 1 | 18 | 0.9474 | 0.6568 |
| 28.5 | 18 | 2 | 16 | 1 | 15 | 0.9375 | 0.6158 |
| 29.4 | 15 | 0 | 15 | 2 | 13 | 0.8667 | 0.5337 |
| 30.1 | 13 | 0 | 13 | 1 | 12 | 0.9231 | 0.4926 |
| 30.3 | 12 | 0 | 12 | 1 | 11 | 0.9167 | 0.4516 |
| 31.8 | 11 | 0 | 11 | 1 | 10 | 0.9091 | 0.4105 |
| 35.9 | 10 | 0 | 10 | 1 | 9 | 0.9000 | 0.3695 |
| 36.8 | 9 | 0 | 9 | 2 | 7 | 0.7778 | 0.2874 |
| 37.6 | 7 | 0 | 7 | 1 | 6 | 0.8571 | 0.2463 |
| 39.4 | 6 | 0 | 6 | 1 | 5 | 0.8333 | 0.2053 |
| 40.5 | 5 | 1 | 4 | 1 | 3 | 0.7500 | 0.1539 |
| 42.8 | 3 | 0 | 3 | 1 | 2 | 0.6667 | 0.1026 |
| 44.7 | 2 | 0 | 2 | 1 | 1 | 0.5000 | 0.0513 |
| 46.0 | 1 | 0 | 1 | 1 | 0 | 0.0000 | ... |

$$n_i' = n_i - d_i \qquad \text{Eq. 20.10}$$

The seventh column is the probability of survival at the end of the period with the number of patients at risk divided by the number surviving at the end of the period:

$$p_i = \frac{n_i'}{n_i} \qquad \text{Eq. 20.11}$$

The eighth column is the cumulative survival determined each time a patient dies (Eq. 20.4 or Eq. 20.5). Note the $n_i'$ used in the Kaplan-Meier method automatically accounts for censored patients by reducing the numerator. The survival curve is then created similar to the actuarial curve, plotting the cumulative probability on the *y*-axis and the time on the *x*-axis. Data from Table 20.5 is presented in Figure 20.5. Note that unlike the actuarial curve, the widths of the periods will vary and are dependent on the survival times of the individual patients in the study. Also, note that in both curves presented on Figures 20.3 and 20.5, the curve does not reach the value

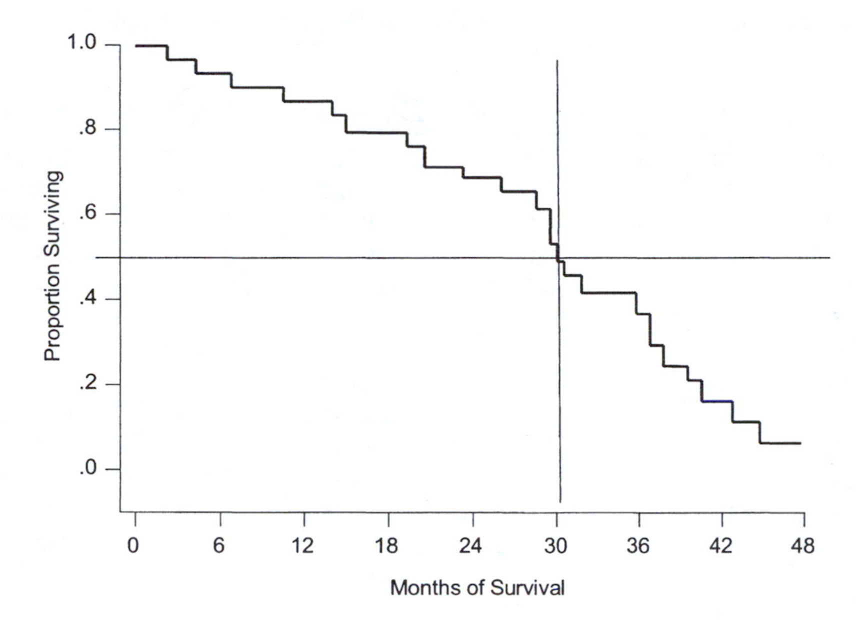


**Figure 20.5** Kaplan-Meier curve for patients with melanoma.

$p_i = 0$. Some textbooks and computer software packages may present a vertical line at the end of the survival curve extending to zero at the point of the last observation. This approach would be appropriate if there were no censored data. However, when there is censored data there are still individuals or objects that have not reached the well-defined end-point, therefore a better representation of the data to end with is a horizontal line at the smallest value greater than zero.

The standard error calculation for the cumulative survival estimate $S_i$ is similar to the error term for the actuarial:

$$SE(\hat{S}_i) = \hat{S}_i \sqrt{\sum \frac{d_i}{n_i(n_i - d_i)}} \qquad \text{Eq. 20.12}$$

Calculations for the standard error terms for the various periods for our example problem on stage IV melanoma patients are presented in Table 20.6. Similar to the actuarial life table, to extrapolate from our sample information to a population, a survival curve is more informative when it includes confidence intervals. The standard error term in the last column of Table 20.6 can be used in Eq. 20.8 to determine the bands for these intervals, the result of which are presented in Table 20.7. Once again, like the actuarial method, calculations may create bands that exceed 1.00 or are less than zero. The bands may need to be adjusted to 1.00 or zero to reflect the possible limits of statistical probability. If there are censored patients, the right side of a survival curve represents fewer patients than the left side, and the

**Table 20.6** Determination of Standard Errors for Kaplan-Meier Example

| Event (Months) | $n_i$ | $d_i$ | $d_i/n_i(n_i\text{-}_{di})$ | $\Sigma d_i/n_i(n_i\text{-}_{di})$ | $s_i$ | $SE(s_i)$ |
|---|---|---|---|---|---|---|
| 2.3 | 30 | 1 | 0.0011 | 0.0011 | 0.9667 | 0.0328 |
| 5.3 | 29 | 1 | 0.0012 | 0.0024 | 0.9333 | 0.0455 |
| 6.8 | 28 | 1 | 0.0013 | 0.0037 | 0.9000 | 0.0548 |
| 10.5 | 27 | 1 | 0.0014 | 0.0051 | 0.8667 | 0.0621 |
| 14.0 | 25 | 1 | 0.0017 | 0.0068 | 0.8320 | 0.0686 |
| 15.1 | 24 | 1 | 0.0018 | 0.0086 | 0.7973 | 0.0740 |
| 19.2 | 23 | 1 | 0.0020 | 0.0106 | 0.7627 | 0.0785 |
| 20.6 | 22 | 1 | 0.0022 | 0.0127 | 0.7280 | 0.0822 |
| 23.2 | 21 | 1 | 0.0024 | 0.0151 | 0.6933 | 0.0853 |
| 25.9 | 19 | 1 | 0.0029 | 0.0181 | 0.6568 | 0.0883 |
| 28.5 | 16 | 1 | 0.0042 | 0.0222 | 0.6158 | 0.0918 |
| 29.4 | 15 | 2 | 0.0103 | 0.0325 | 0.5337 | 0.0962 |
| 30.1 | 13 | 1 | 0.0064 | 0.0389 | 0.4926 | 0.0971 |
| 30.3 | 12 | 1 | 0.0076 | 0.0465 | 0.4516 | 0.0973 |
| 31.8 | 11 | 1 | 0.0091 | 0.0556 | 0.4105 | 0.0968 |
| 35.9 | 10 | 1 | 0.0111 | 0.0667 | 0.3695 | 0.0954 |
| 36.8 | 9 | 2 | 0.0317 | 0.0984 | 0.2874 | 0.0901 |
| 37.6 | 7 | 1 | 0.0238 | 0.1222 | 0.2463 | 0.0861 |
| 39.4 | 6 | 1 | 0.0333 | 0.1556 | 0.2053 | 0.0810 |
| 40.5 | 4 | 1 | 0.0833 | 0.2389 | 0.1539 | 0.0752 |
| 42.8 | 3 | 1 | 0.1667 | 0.4056 | 0.1026 | 0.0654 |
| 44.7 | 2 | 1 | 0.5000 | 0.9056 | 0.0513 | 0.0488 |
| 46.0 | 1 | 1 | 0.0011 | 0.0011 | ... | ... |

confidence interval will become wider as time progresses and eventually collapse at zero survival. The confidence bands for our example problem using the Kalpan-Meier procedure are presented in Table 20.7.

The median survival time can be determined by locating the time at which the cumulative survival proportion is equal to .50. Like the actuarial table curve, this can be visually estimated on a time plot by identifying the corresponding value on the *x*-axis for .50 on the *y*-axis. If this point occurs at a vertical line on the plot, the extreme values at the ends of the vertical line are averaged.

### Visual Comparison of Two Survival Curves

In most research situations, the investigator will be interested in comparing the survival curves for two or more groups of patients (i.e., a control vs. experimental group). Visually comparing the two curves is the simplest method. In our original example of stage IV melanoma, the patients received two therapies: 1) the gold standard (control) and 2) the gold standard plus new RAF kinase inhibitor. To

**Table 20.7** Confidence Bands for Kaplan-Meier Table for Melanoma Patients

| Months | Lower Band | $S_i$ | Upper Band |
|---|---|---|---|
| 2.3 | 0.9024 | 0.9667 | 1.0000 |
| 5.3 | 0.8441 | 0.9333 | 1.0000 |
| 6.8 | 0.7926 | 0.9000 | 1.0000 |
| 10.5 | 0.7450 | 0.8667 | 0.9883 |
| 14.0 | 0.6976 | 0.8320 | 0.9664 |
| 15.1 | 0.6524 | 0.7973 | 0.9423 |
| 19.2 | 0.6089 | 0.7627 | 0.9164 |
| 20.6 | 0.5669 | 0.7280 | 0.8891 |
| 23.2 | 0.5262 | 0.6933 | 0.8605 |
| 25.9 | 0.4839 | 0.6568 | 0.8298 |
| 28.5 | 0.4359 | 0.6158 | 0.7957 |
| 29.4 | 0.3452 | 0.5337 | 0.7222 |
| 30.1 | 0.3022 | 0.4926 | 0.6830 |
| 30.3 | 0.2608 | 0.4516 | 0.6424 |
| 31.8 | 0.2209 | 0.4105 | 0.6002 |
| 35.9 | 0.1825 | 0.3695 | 0.5564 |
| 36.8 | 0.1107 | 0.2874 | 0.4641 |
| 37.6 | 0.0775 | 0.2463 | 0.4151 |
| 39.4 | 0.0466 | 0.2053 | 0.3639 |
| 40.5 | 0.0065 | 0.1539 | 0.3014 |
| 42.8 | 0.0000 | 0.1026 | 0.2307 |
| 44.7 | 0.0000 | 0.0513 | 0.1470 |
| 46.0 | ... | ... | ... |

compare these two therapies, a Kaplan-Meier table for each therapy is prepared (Table 20.8) and plotted (Figure 20.6).

Visually we can see a difference between the two curves, with the experimental appearing to represent a better survival curve. If a line were drawn at $p_i$ = .50, it would indicate that the median survival for the experimental groups was 36.8 months, whereas the median for the control group was only 29.4 months. So, one quick comparison is to evaluate the median survival times. One then must question whether these differences are due simply to chance or whether the difference between the two groups is statistically significant? To answer this question one will need to employ hypothesis testing. In this example, the null hypotheses would be that there is no difference between the two survival functions:

$$H_0: \ S_i\,(\text{control}) = S_i\,(\text{experimental})$$
$$H_1: \ S_i\,(\text{control}) \neq S_i\,(\text{experimental})$$

In testing the hypotheses we are interested in three pieces of information about each patient: 1) which treatment they received (experimental or control); 2) the length of time was the patient was enrolled in the study; and 3) if the experience is the defined

**Table 20.8** Cumulative Survival for Experimental and Control Groups

| Event (Months) | $n_{i-1}'$ | $w_i$ | $n_i$ | $d_i$ | $n_i'$ | $p_i$ | $s_i$ | $SE(s_i)$ |
|---|---|---|---|---|---|---|---|---|
| Results for the Experimental Group: | | | | | | | | |
| 0-14.0 | 15 | 0 | 15 | 1 | 14 | 0.9333 | 0.9333 | 0.0644 |
| 14.1-15.1 | 14 | 0 | 14 | 1 | 13 | 0.9286 | 0.8667 | 0.0642 |
| 15.2-19.2 | 13 | 0 | 13 | 1 | 12 | 0.9231 | 0.8000 | 0.0641 |
| 19.3-25.9 | 12 | 1 | 11 | 1 | 10 | 0.9091 | 0.7273 | 0.0693 |
| 26.0-28.5 | 10 | 0 | 10 | 1 | 9 | 0.9000 | 0.6545 | 0.0690 |
| 28.6-30.1 | 9 | 0 | 9 | 1 | 8 | 0.8889 | 0.5818 | 0.0686 |
| 30.2-35.9 | 8 | 0 | 8 | 1 | 7 | 0.8750 | 0.5091 | 0.0680 |
| 36.0-36.8 | 7 | 0 | 7 | 1 | 6 | 0.8571 | 0.4364 | 0.0673 |
| 37.9-39.4 | 6 | 0 | 6 | 1 | 5 | 0.8333 | 0.3636 | 0.0664 |
| 39.5-40.5 | 5 | 1 | 4 | 1 | 3 | 0.7500 | 0.2727 | 0.0787 |
| 40.6-42.8 | 3 | 0 | 3 | 1 | 2 | 0.6667 | 0.1818 | 0.0742 |
| 42.9-44.7 | 2 | 0 | 2 | 1 | 1 | 0.5000 | 0.0909 | 0.0643 |
| 44.8-46.0 | 1 | 0 | 1 | 1 | 0 | 0.0000 | ... | ... |
| Results for the Control Group: | | | | | | | | |
| 0-2.3 | 15 | 0 | 15 | 1 | 14 | 0.9333 | 0.9333 | 0.0644 |
| 2.4-5.3 | 14 | 0 | 14 | 1 | 13 | 0.9286 | 0.8667 | 0.0878 |
| 5.4-6.8 | 13 | 0 | 13 | 1 | 12 | 0.9231 | 0.8000 | 0.1033 |
| 6.9-10.5 | 12 | 0 | 12 | 1 | 11 | 0.9167 | 0.7333 | 0.1142 |
| 10.6-20.6 | 11 | 1 | 10 | 1 | 9 | 0.9000 | 0.6600 | 0.1241 |
| 20.7-23.2 | 9 | 0 | 9 | 1 | 8 | 0.8889 | 0.5867 | 0.1302 |
| 23.3-29.4 | 8 | 2 | 6 | 2 | 4 | 0.6667 | 0.3911 | 0.1424 |
| 29.5-30.3 | 4 | 0 | 4 | 1 | 3 | 0.7500 | 0.2933 | 0.1363 |
| 30.4-31.8 | 3 | 0 | 3 | 1 | 2 | 0.6667 | 0.1956 | 0.1210 |
| 31.9-36.8 | 2 | 0 | 2 | 1 | 1 | 0.5000 | 0.0978 | 0.0919 |
| 36.9-37.6 | 1 | 0 | 1 | 1 | 0 | 0.0000 | ... | ... |

event of interest (in this case death) or had been withdrawn from the study (either lost to follow-up or alive at the end of the study).

With either the actuarial or product limit method it is assumed that patients were randomly assigned to the two treatment levels and the results represent independent observations. There must be consistent inclusion and exclusion criteria and consistent definition "survival."

### Tests to Compare Two Levels of an Independent Variable

One possible method for testing the hypotheses for comparing two survival curves is called the **log-rank test**. The log-rank test provides an objective comparison of the two survival curves to determine if they are statistically significantly different. We

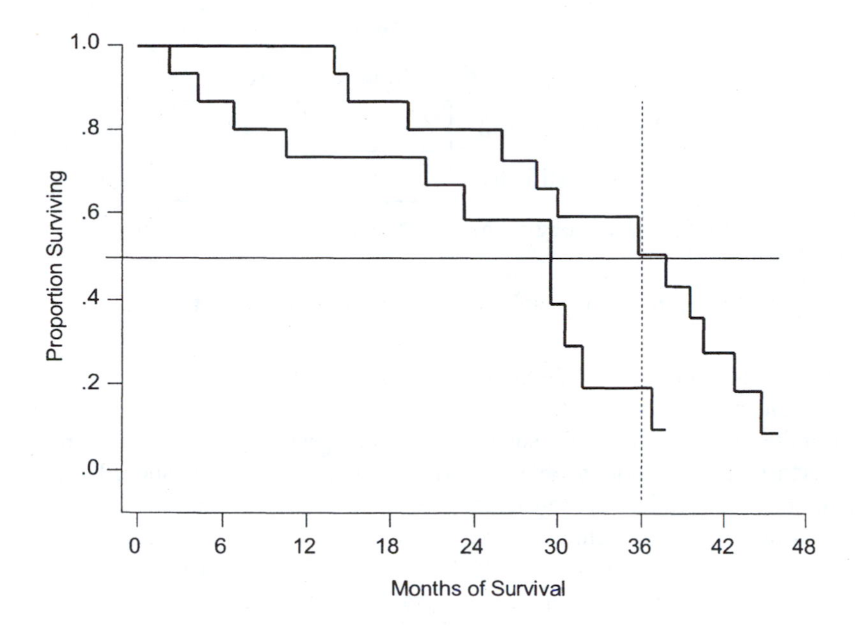


**Figure 20.6** Kaplan-Meier curve for experimental and control groups.

test the null hypothesis that there is no difference in survival experience between the two populations. The alternative hypothesis is that the difference between the two populations is significant and not due to chance variation.

$$H_0: \text{Survival (level 1)} = \text{Survival (level 2)}$$
$$H_1: \text{Survival (level 1)} \neq \text{Survival (level 2)}$$

Unfortunately, as seen in previous chapters, synonyms or multiple names for the same test are commonplace in statistics. This is true also with survival statistics and the log-rank test has been given numerous names in literature, including the **Mantel log-rank test**, the **Cox-Mantel log-rank test**, the **Cochran-Mantel-Haensel test**, or the **CMH test**. Technically the log-rank test and CMH-type tests are different but produce equivalent results. One is interpretable based on the chi square distribution and one by the standardized normal distribution. Both methods will produce the same *p*-value. In this section we will test the null hypothesis using both methods. CMH test will be discussed first because we are already familiar with this test.

In order to compare two survival curves it is assumed that: 1) patients are randomly assigned to the different groups; 2) the times are independent measures; 3) there are consistent criteria throughout the time of the study; 4) the baseline survival rate is not changing over time (inclusion and exclusion criteria remain constant); and 5) on the average, survival of censored patients would be the same patients reaching the endpoint of the study. At each time interval (actuarial or product-limit method) there is a comparison of the number of observed deaths for each group with the

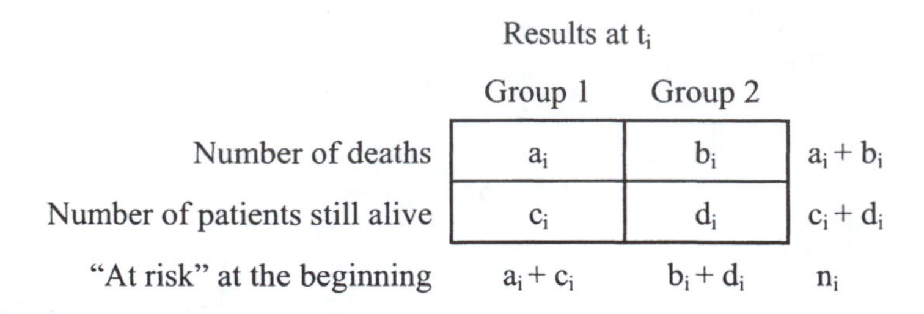

Results at $t_i$

| | Group 1 | Group 2 | |
|---|---|---|---|
| Number of deaths | $a_i$ | $b_i$ | $a_i + b_i$ |
| Number of patients still alive | $c_i$ | $d_i$ | $c_i + d_i$ |
| "At risk" at the beginning | $a_i + c_i$ | $b_i + d_i$ | $n_i$ |

**Figure 20.7** Contingency table for each stratum for the CMH test.

expected number of deaths if the null hypothesis were true.

In Chapter 16 we used the Mantel-Haensel test to evaluate a possible confounding variable for a chi square test of independence. To avoid confusion we will discuss the calculations for the CMH test and refer to it as such. However, the calculations are identical to the Mantel-Haensel test.The calculations of the Cochran-Mantel-Haensel test are cumbersome and use the same equations as the Mantel-Haenszel test (Eq. 16.16 to Eq. 16.19). For readability, we will renumber the equations and include them in this paragraph. First, order the survival times until death for both groups combined (omitting censored times) and each time will constitutes a stratum of our matrix. Each stratum represents time $t_i$ and we construct a 2 x 2 contingency table (Figure 20.7). In each table the first row contains the number of observed deaths, the second row contains the number of patients still living. The columns represent the results for the two groups. The CMH formula is:

$$\chi^2_{CMH} = \frac{\left[\sum \frac{a_i d_i - b_i c_i}{n_i}\right]^2}{\sum \frac{(a+b)_i (c+d)_i (a+c)_i (b+d)_i}{(n_i - 1)(n_i^2)}} \qquad \text{Eq. 20.13}$$

To simplify this equation, for each stratum compute the expected frequency for the upper left-hand cell (deaths in Group 1):

$$e_i = \frac{(a_i + b_i)(a_i + c_i)}{n_i} \qquad \text{Eq. 20.14}$$

Then for each stratum the $v_i$ intermediate is computed:

$$v_i = \frac{(a_i + b_i)(c_i + d_i)(a_i + c_i)(b_i + d_i)}{n_i^2 (n_i - 1)} \qquad \text{Eq. 20.15}$$

| | Interval ending 2.3 months | | | Interval ending 14.0 months | | |
|---|---|---|---|---|---|---|
| | Exper. | Control | | Exper. | Control | |
| Deaths | 0 | 1 | 1 | 1 | 0 | 1 |
| Remaining | 15 | 14 | 29 | 14 | 10 | 24 |
| At risk | 15 | 15 | 30 | 15 | 10 | 25 |

**Figure 20.8** Example of two strata for example CMH test.

Finally, the Cochran-Mantel-Haensel statistic is calculated by summing the results for each interval and creating a chi square statistic:

$$\chi^2_{CMH} = \frac{[\Sigma(a_i - e_i)]^2}{\Sigma v_i} \qquad \text{Eq. 20.16}$$

The results are compared to the chi square critical value (Table B15) with one degree of freedom ($\chi^2$=3.84). If the calculated Cochran-Mantel-Haensel statistic exceeds 3.84 there is a significant difference between the two curves. If 3.84 or less, one fails to identify a difference.

The test could be used for comparing two curves using either the actuarial or product-limit methods. For our previous example of patients with stage IV melanoma, we will use the Kaplan-Meier results. Each of the possible 23 intervals identified in the combined curves (Table 20.8 and Figure 20.6) are evaluated to determine their respective $e_i$ and $v_i$ values. For example, at the end of the first time period there would still be 29 patients alive, 15 in the experiment and 14 in the control group. These results appear on the left side of Figure 20.8. By the end of the fifth interval, 24 patients are still alive, 10 in the control group and 14 in the experimental group. The results for all 23 intervals are presented in Table 20.9. As mentioned censored data is not included in the calculations, with the exception of the appropriate reduction in the $n_i$ values (as seen by the drops in the total number of patients at risk in intervals 5, 10, 11, and 19). Using the sums for Table 20.9, the Cochran-Mantel-Haensel statistic is:

$$\chi^2_{CMH} = \frac{[\Sigma(a_i - e_i)]^2}{\Sigma v_i} = \frac{(-5.677)^2}{7.323} = 7.393$$

Since the results are greater than 3.84, we reject the null hypothesis and show that the two curves are statistically different. The exact $p$-value is 0.0065 and can be determined using Excel [CHIDIST(x,1)}.

Initial preparation for the log rank test is similar to the CMH test. The first step is to calculate the expected value ($e_i$) for cell $a_i$ in a two-by-two contingency table for each point on the Kaplan-Meier or actuarial curve (Eq. 20.14). These have already

**Table 20.9** Determination of Strata and CMH Test for Example Data

| Event (Months) | $a_i$ | $b_i$ | $c_i$ | $d_i$ | $n_i$ | $e_i$ | $a_i - e_i$ | $v_i$ | $e_i(b_i)$ |
|---|---|---|---|---|---|---|---|---|---|
| 2.3 | 0 | 1 | 15 | 14 | 30 | 0.500 | 0.500 | 0.250 | 0.500 |
| 5.3 | 0 | 1 | 15 | 13 | 29 | 0.517 | 0.483 | 0.250 | 0.483 |
| 6.8 | 0 | 1 | 15 | 12 | 28 | 0.536 | 0.464 | 0.249 | 0.464 |
| 10.5 | 0 | 1 | 15 | 11 | 27 | 0.556 | 0.444 | 0.247 | 0.444 |
| 14.0 | 1 | 0 | 14 | 10 | 25 | 0.600 | −0.600 | 0.240 | 0.400 |
| 15.1 | 1 | 0 | 13 | 10 | 24 | 0.583 | −0.583 | 0.243 | 0.417 |
| 19.2 | 1 | 0 | 12 | 10 | 23 | 0.565 | −0.565 | 0.246 | 0.435 |
| 20.6 | 0 | 1 | 12 | 9 | 22 | 0.545 | 0.455 | 0.248 | 0.455 |
| 23.2 | 0 | 1 | 12 | 8 | 21 | 0.571 | 0.429 | 0.245 | 0.429 |
| 25.9 | 1 | 0 | 10 | 8 | 19 | 0.579 | −0.579 | 0.244 | 0.421 |
| 28.5 | 1 | 0 | 9 | 6 | 16 | 0.625 | −0.625 | 0.234 | 0.375 |
| 29.4 | 0 | 2 | 9 | 4 | 15 | 1.200 | 0.800 | 0.446 | 0.800 |
| 30.1 | 1 | 0 | 8 | 4 | 13 | 0.692 | −0.692 | 0.213 | 0.308 |
| 30.3 | 0 | 1 | 8 | 3 | 12 | 0.667 | 0.333 | 0.222 | 0.333 |
| 31.8 | 0 | 1 | 8 | 2 | 11 | 0.727 | 0.273 | 0.198 | 0.273 |
| 35.9 | 1 | 0 | 7 | 2 | 10 | 0.800 | −0.800 | 0.160 | 0.200 |
| 36.8 | 1 | 1 | 6 | 1 | 9 | 1.556 | −0.556 | 0.302 | 0.444 |
| 37.6 | 0 | 1 | 6 | 0 | 7 | 0.857 | 0.143 | 0.122 | 0.143 |
| 39.4 | 1 | 0 | 5 | 0 | 6 | 1.000 | −1.000 | 0.000 | 0.000 |
| 40.5 | 1 | 0 | 3 | 0 | 4 | 1.000 | −1.000 | 0.000 | 0.000 |
| 42.8 | 1 | 0 | 2 | 0 | 3 | 1.000 | −1.000 | 0.000 | 0.000 |
| 44.7 | 1 | 0 | 1 | 0 | 2 | 1.000 | −1.000 | 0.000 | 0.000 |
| 46.0 | 1 | 0 | 0 | 0 | 1 | 1.000 | −1.000 | 0.000 | 0.000 |
| Sums | 13 | 12 | | | | 17.677 | −5.677 | 4.359 | 7.323 |

been calculated for our example problem and presented in the eighth column of Table 20.9). Next the sum of the differences between the observed and expected results is calculated for $a_i$:

$$U_L = \sum(a_i - e_i) \qquad \text{Eq. 20.17}$$

For our example problem this has already been reported by the summation reported at the bottom of the eighth column in Table 20.9. If the $U_L$ is relatively small there is probably no difference between the two levels of the independent variable. If the $U_L$ is large the null hypothesis will be rejected that the groups being compared will be deemed statistically different. But how large should the $U_L$ be to determine significance? To answer this question we need some measure of data variability. This is provided by calculating an error term. This measurement is determined using the following equation and assumes that the sampling distribution is approximately normal:

$$S_{U_L} = \sqrt{\sum \frac{(a_i + c_i)(b_i + d_i)(a_i + b_i)[n_i - (a_i + b_i)]}{n_i^2 (n_i - 1)}} \qquad \text{Eq. 20.18}$$

With an estimate of the differences between the observed and expected values and a measure of variability, we can calculate a ratio between the two measures:

$$z = \frac{U_L}{S_{U_L}} \qquad \text{Eq. 20.19}$$

The resultant value can be interpreted using the standardized normal distribution. As discussed in Chapter 16, since the data is based on a discrete sampling distribution, but evaluating the results are based on a continuous distribution, we may wish to be more conservative in our decision making process. Once again we have a Yates' correction to make this adjustment:

$$z_{Yates} = \frac{|U_L| - 0.5}{S_{U_L}} \qquad \text{Eq. 20.20}$$

With adjustment in the numerator of the equation the $z_{Yates}$ will always be smaller and more difficult to reject the null hypothesis.

Using this approach, let us once again look at the sample problem of the Stage IV melanoma. From Table 20.9 we know that

$$U_L = \sum (a_i - e_i) = -5.677$$

The error term is

$$S_{U_L} = \sqrt{\sum \frac{(a_i + c_i)(b_i + d_i)(a_i + b_i)[n_i - (a_i + b_i)]}{n_i^2 (n_i - 1)}}$$

$$S_{U_L} = \sqrt{\frac{15 \cdot 15 \cdot 1 \cdot (30 - 1)}{30^2 \cdot (30 - 1)} + \frac{15 \cdot 14 \cdot 1 \cdot (29 - 1)}{29^2 \cdot (29 - 1)} + \ldots \frac{1 \cdot 0 \cdot 1 \cdot (1) \cdot}{1^2 \cdot (1 - 1)}} = 2.088$$

and the ratio is

$$z = \frac{U_L}{S_{U_L}} = \frac{-5.677}{2.088} = -2.719$$

A z-value of -2.719 represents $p$ = 0.0065 [calculated using Excel code (1 –

(NORMSDIST(ABS(-2.719))))*2]. This $p$-value is exactly the same as the $p$-value from our earlier calculation of the CMH tests.

If we wish to apply Yates' correction the result would be

$$z_{Yates} = \frac{|U_L| - 0.5}{S_{U_L}} = \frac{|-5.677| - 0.5}{2.088} = 2.479$$

The $p$-value associated with this $z$-value is 0.0125. Thus, with the CMH test, the log rank test, and Yates' correction on the log rank test we would reject the hypothesis and conclude there is a significant difference, with the addition of the RAF kinase inhibitor to the regimen producing a significantly longer survival time..

Both the log rank and CMH tests involve a series of 2 x 2 contingency tables. From this information an odds ratio for survival could be calculated for each contingency table. It is recommended that the CMH test statistic be used only when the odds ratios are similar across the various 2 x 2 tables or intervals for the survival distributions (Frothofer, p. 341). Recall the odds ratio is experimental event odds divided by the control event odds (Chapter 18). If the plots of the two survival curves cross one another, then the odds ratios will not be similar across all the tables. The estimate of a pooled odds ratio can be used for descriptive purposes:

$$OR = \frac{\sum\left(\frac{a \cdot d}{n}\right)}{\sum\left(\frac{b \cdot c}{n}\right)} \qquad \text{Eq. 20.21}$$

For the example we have been using throughout this chapter and presented in Table 20.10, the odds ratio would be:

$$OR = \frac{\sum\left(\frac{a \cdot d}{n}\right)}{\sum\left(\frac{b \cdot c}{n}\right)} = \frac{7.343}{2.666} = 2.754$$

If one is interested in comparing more than two survival curves, multiple pair-wise comparisons can be performed. Also, since survival data does not follow any particular probability distribution it is appropriate to consider this test a nonparametric procedure (see Chapter 21).

**Hazard Ratios**

Another way to assess survival is to evaluate the hazard risk to the patients in a study. The **hazard function** is an estimate of the probability that a subject who has

**Table 20.10** Determination of Strata and Log Rank Test for Example Data

| Interval | $a_i$ | $b_i$ | $c_i$ | $d_i$ | $n_i$ | $(a_i \cdot d_i)/n_i$ | $(b_i \cdot c_i)/n_i$ |
|---|---|---|---|---|---|---|---|
| 0-2.3 | 1 | 0 | 14 | 15 | 30 | 0.5000 | 0.0000 |
| 2.4-5.3 | 1 | 0 | 13 | 15 | 29 | 0.5172 | 0.0000 |
| 5.4-6.8 | 1 | 0 | 12 | 15 | 28 | 0.5357 | 0.0000 |
| 6.9-10.5 | 1 | 0 | 11 | 15 | 27 | 0.5556 | 0.0000 |
| 10.6-14.0 | 0 | 1 | 10 | 14 | 25 | 0.0000 | 0.4000 |
| 14.1-15.1 | 0 | 1 | 10 | 13 | 24 | 0.0000 | 0.4167 |
| 15.2-19.2 | 0 | 1 | 10 | 12 | 23 | 0.0000 | 0.4348 |
| 19.3-20.6 | 1 | 0 | 9 | 12 | 22 | 0.5455 | 0.0000 |
| 20.7-23.2 | 1 | 0 | 8 | 12 | 21 | 0.5714 | 0.0000 |
| 23.3-25.9 | 0 | 1 | 8 | 10 | 19 | 0.0000 | 0.4211 |
| 25.6-28.5 | 0 | 1 | 6 | 9 | 16 | 0.0000 | 0.3750 |
| 29.2-29.4 | 2 | 0 | 4 | 9 | 15 | 1.2000 | 0.0000 |
| 29.5-30.1 | 0 | 1 | 4 | 8 | 13 | 0.0000 | 0.3077 |
| 30.2-30.3 | 1 | 0 | 3 | 8 | 12 | 0.6667 | 0.0000 |
| 30.4-31.8 | 1 | 0 | 2 | 8 | 11 | 0.7273 | 0.0000 |
| 31.9-35.9 | 0 | 1 | 2 | 7 | 10 | 0.0000 | 0.2000 |
| 36.3-36.8 | 1 | 1 | 1 | 6 | 9 | 0.6667 | 0.1111 |
| 36.9-37.6 | 1 | 0 | 0 | 6 | 7 | 0.8571 | 0.0000 |
| 37.7-39.4 | 0 | 1 | 0 | 5 | 6 | 0.0000 | 0.0000 |
| 39.5-40.5 | 0 | 1 | 0 | 3 | 4 | 0.0000 | 0.0000 |
| 40.6-42.8 | 0 | 1 | 0 | 2 | 3 | 0.0000 | 0.0000 |
| 42.9-44.7 | 0 | 1 | 0 | 1 | 2 | 0.0000 | 0.0000 |
| 44.8-46.0 | 0 | 1 | 0 | 0 | 1 | 0.0000 | 0.0000 |
| | | | | | Σ = | 7.3431 | 2.6663 |

survived to the beginning of a study interval (actuarial or product-limit methods) will experience the definable event during that particular period. It is calculated as the negative natural log of the survival function:

$$\hat{h}(t_i) = -ln(\hat{S}_i) \qquad \text{Eq. 20.22}$$

The hazard function is also referred to as the **hazard rate**, the **instantaneous failure rate**, the **force of morality**, or the **life-table mortality rate**. In the case where death is the endpoint, the hazard rate is the proportion of patients dying in an interval per unit of time. The hazard function must be greater than zero and can be any positive value. An error term and confidence intervals can be calculated using the following equations:

$$SE(\hat{h}_i) = \frac{SE(\hat{S}_i)}{\hat{S}_i} \qquad \text{Eq. 20.23}$$

**Table 20.11** Determination of Hazard Function from Table 20.6

| Event (Months) | $n_i$ | $d_i$ | $s_i$ | $SE(s_i)$ | $h_i$ | $SE(h_i)$ |
|---|---|---|---|---|---|---|
| 2.3 | 30 | 1 | 0.9667 | 0.0328 | 0.0339 | 0.0339 |
| 5.3 | 29 | 1 | 0.9333 | 0.0455 | 0.0690 | 0.0488 |
| 6.8 | 28 | 1 | 0.9000 | 0.0548 | 0.1054 | 0.0609 |
| 10.5 | 27 | 1 | 0.8667 | 0.0621 | 0.1431 | 0.0716 |
| 14.0 | 25 | 1 | 0.8320 | 0.0686 | 0.1839 | 0.0824 |
| 15.1 | 24 | 1 | 0.7973 | 0.0740 | 0.2265 | 0.0928 |
| 19.2 | 23 | 1 | 0.7627 | 0.0785 | 0.2709 | 0.1029 |
| 20.6 | 22 | 1 | 0.7280 | 0.0822 | 0.3175 | 0.1129 |
| 23.2 | 21 | 1 | 0.6933 | 0.0853 | 0.3662 | 0.1230 |
| 25.9 | 19 | 1 | 0.6568 | 0.0883 | 0.4203 | 0.1344 |
| 28.5 | 16 | 1 | 0.6158 | 0.0918 | 0.4849 | 0.1491 |
| 29.4 | 15 | 2 | 0.5337 | 0.0962 | 0.6280 | 0.1802 |
| 30.1 | 13 | 1 | 0.4926 | 0.0971 | 0.7080 | 0.1972 |
| 30.3 | 12 | 1 | 0.4516 | 0.0973 | 0.7950 | 0.2155 |
| 31.8 | 11 | 1 | 0.4105 | 0.0968 | 0.8903 | 0.2357 |
| 35.9 | 10 | 1 | 0.3695 | 0.0954 | 0.9957 | 0.2582 |
| 36.8 | 9 | 2 | 0.2874 | 0.0901 | 1.2470 | 0.3137 |
| 37.6 | 7 | 1 | 0.2463 | 0.0861 | 1.4011 | 0.3496 |
| 39.4 | 6 | 1 | 0.2053 | 0.0810 | 1.5835 | 0.3944 |
| 40.5 | 4 | 1 | 0.1539 | 0.0752 | 1.8711 | 0.4888 |
| 42.8 | 3 | 1 | 0.1026 | 0.0654 | 2.2766 | 0.6368 |
| 44.7 | 2 | 1 | 0.0513 | 0.0488 | 2.9698 | 0.9516 |
| 46.0 | 1 | 1 | ... | ... | ... | ... |

$$h_i = \hat{h}_i \pm z_{1-\alpha/2} \cdot SE(\hat{h}_i) \qquad \text{Eq. 20.24}$$

The hazard functions and error terms for all the intervals in our Kaplan-Meier example are presented in Table 20.11.

One can think of a hazard ratio the same as relative risk. If the ratio is 0.25, then the relative risk of event in one group is one-quarter the risk of that event in the second group. The **cumulative hazard function** is the difference between the observed death rate and the expected rate of death, for all time periods, if there was no significant difference between the two treatment groups.

$$h_i = \frac{\sum O_i}{\sum E_i} = \frac{\sum a_i}{\sum e_i} \qquad \text{Eq. 20.25}$$

These two values have already been reported or calculated for the first treatment level

($a_i$ and $e_i$ ) in order to determine the Cochran-Mantel-Haenszel chi square test. Using the same method it is possible to calculate the expected values for the second treatment level ($b_i$):

$$e_i(b_i) = \frac{(a_i + b_i)(b_i + d_i)}{n_i} \qquad \text{Eq. 20.26}$$

Using our example data in Table 20.9, we have already reported the reported the observed outcomes for both the experimental and control groups (the second and third columns, respectively). In the previous section we calculated the expected outcome for the experimental group ($e_i$ in column seven). Using Eq. 20.26 the expected values are reported in the tenth column. The sums are reported for the observed and expected results at the bottom of Table 20.9. The hazard function for the experimental group is:

$$h_E = \frac{\sum a_i}{\sum e_i} = \frac{13}{17.677} = 0.735$$

and the controlled group is:

$$h_C = \frac{\sum b_i}{\sum e_i(b_i)} = \frac{12}{7.323} = 1.639$$

The larger the hazard rate, the lower the chance of survival. Thus, it appears that chance of survival in the experimental group is greater than that of the control group. This is visually supported in Figure 20.6.

The **hazard ratio** is the relative risk of reaching the defined endpoint at any given time interval. The hazard ratio is a useful description statistic when used in the context of the log-rank statistic, for comparing two groups. Another way to think of hazard, with respect to the survival curves created in the previous sections, is that hazard represents the slopes of the survival curves. It measures how rapidly subjects are dying or reaching some other endpoint. In the comparison of two survival curves, the hazard ratio compares two treatment levels. The results are interpreted similar to the relative risk or the odds ratio described in the previous chapter. A hazard ratio of 1.0 indicates that the two groups being compared are identical. If the hazard ratio is 6.0, the group in the numerator has a six times greater risk compared to the group in the denominator. To compare two groups the hazard ratio can be estimated by

$$\text{Hazard ratio} = \frac{h_C}{h_E} \qquad \text{Eq. 20.27}$$

For illustration, using our example of treatment alternatives for stage IV melanoma, the hazard ratio of control group to the experimental groups would be:

$$Hazard\ ratio = \frac{1.639}{0.735} = 2.220$$

Based on our study of 30 patients, the risk of dying is more than twice as great for the control group compared to the experimental groups receiving the additional RAF kinase inhibitor. One limitation with the hazard ratio is that it is assumed that the risk of death or other endpoint is constant throughout the period of time studied.

**Multiple Regression with Survival Data: Proportional Hazards Regression**

Up to this point we have looked at survival analysis with only one independent variable, in our example, two treatment levels. However, we may wish to control for additional characteristics, or covariates, for patients volunteering for a study (i.e., age, gender, ethnicity). One of the most commonly used method is the Cox regression model, or **Cox proportional hazard regression** model, which accounts for the effects of predictor continuous and discrete variables on the dependent variable, which can include censored time-until-event data. The method is named after D.R. Cox who first proposed applying regression methodology to survival studies, involves a proportional hazard regression model (Daniel). This model is a multivariate analysis used to identify a combination of variables that best predicts the outcomes in the group of patients. It may also independently test the effect of individual variables. It is a hazards model commonly used for survival analyses. The detailed description of this regression goes beyond the scope of this book, but excellent discussions of this method can be found in Kleinbaum (1996, pp. 86-112) or Klein and Moeschnerger (2003, pp. 243-287). A brief overview is presented below.

As discussed in the previous section, the hazard function [$h(t_i)$] describes the conditional probability that an event will occur, given survival up to that point in time. Similar to the multiple linear regression model discussed in Chapter 14, the model to measure $k$ covariates can be described as:

$$h(t_i) = h_0(t_i)exp(\beta_1 x_1 + \beta_2 x_2 + .... + \beta_k x_k) \qquad \text{Eq. 20.28}$$

where $\beta_i$ represents the beta coefficients (or weights) for each $x_i$ covariate. Modifying the equation, the results can be interpreted as hazard ratios.

$$\frac{h(t_i)}{h_0(t_i)} = exp(\beta_1 x_1 + \beta_2 x_2 + .... + \beta_k x_k) \qquad \text{Eq. 20.29}$$

These regression coefficients represent the amount of change in the hazard resulting from the risk factors. This rearranged equation indicates that the exponentiated coefficient is the ratio of the conditional probabilities or the hazard ratio. It serves as an estimate of the odds ratio from the coefficient, similar to logistic regression from Chapter 18.

Using this method is it possible to compare survival in two or more levels of an independent variable adjusting for multiple covariables. Unfortunately the calculations for these tests are so cumbersome that they require computer programs to determine the best fit and calculate proportional hazards for each of the risk factors, or covariate) as hazard ratios. Most will also calculate 95% confidence intervals around each estimated proportional hazard. These are interpreted similarly to the ratios discussed in Chapter 19, the location of the value 1 with respect to the interval.

## Other Measures and Tests of Survival

Based on visual examination of survival curves, it is possible to estimate the **time of survival percentiles**. Most commonly this would be the 25th and 75th percentiles, in addition the previously identified 50th percentile (median survival time).

**Mortality rates** (i.e, three- or five-year survival rates) are popular ways to deal with survival data. These are commonly used in oncology, but unfortunately the mortality rate cannot be used for all patients the until end of the specific length of time.

Another measure of survival is **person-years of observation**. Sometime used in epidemiology it is the number of deaths per each 100 person-years of observations. It may be useful in comparing the results during one specific period of time compared to another period or compared to the results of another investigation. However, a problem with this measurement is that no statistical methods exist for comparing different intervals. A second problem is that the person-year of observation measure assumes that the risk of the definable event is constant though study.

The traditional comparison of two independent groups (i.e., t-test) is not appropriate, since survival times are usually not normally distributed and tend to be positively skewed. Also, censored data cannot be used if all the patients would need to reach the endpoint before the data can be analyzed. However, there are additional procedures for testing the null hypothesis that two survival curves are identical. The **Breslow test** (also referred to as the **Gehan test**, a generalized Wilcoxon test or a generalized Kruskal-Wallis test) and the **Tarone-Ware test** both involve weighted differences between actual and expected numbers of deaths at the observed time intervals. Another test called the **Peto log-rank test**, which gives more weight to the initial interval of the study where there are the largest numbers of patients at risk. If the rate of deaths is similar over time, the Peto log-rank test and the logrank test will produce similar results. Information about these tests can be found in the following references: Breslow test (Breslow; Gehan; Lee and Wang, pp. 107-109; Glantz, pp. 396,397); Tarone-Ware test (Tarone and Ware; Miller, pp. 104-118); and Peto (Lee and Wang, 116,117; Kleinbaum, pp. 65,66).

## References

Breslow, N.E. (1970). "A generalized Kruskal-Wallis test for comparing K samples subject to unequal patterns of censorship," *Biometrika* 57:579-594.

Cutler, S. and Ederer, F. (1958). "Maximum utilization of the lifetable method in analyzing survival," *Journal of Chronic Diseases* 8:699-712.

Daniel, W.W. (1999). *Biostatistics: A Foundation for Analysis in the Health Sciences*, Seventh edition, John Wiley and Sons, New York, p. 636.

Gehan, E.A. (1965). "A generalized Wilcoxon test for comparing arbitrarily singly censored samples," *Biometrika* 52:203-223.

Glantz, S.A. (2002). *Primer of Biostatistics*, McGraw-Hill, New York, pp. 396,397.

Kaplan, E.L. and Meier, P. (1958). "Nonparametric estimation from incomplete observations," *Journal of the American Statistical Association* 53:457-81.

Klein, J.P. and Moeschberger, M.L. (2003). *Survival Analysis: Techniques for Censored and Truncated Data*, Springer, New York.

Kleinbaum, D.G. (1996). *Survival Analysis: A Self-learning Text*, Springer, New York.

Lee, E.T. and Wang, J.W. (2003). *Statistical Methods for Survival Data Analysis*, John Wiley and Sons, Hoboken, NJ.

Miller, R.G., Jr. (1981). *Survival Analysis*, John Wiley and Sons, New York, pp.104-118.

Tarone, R.E. and Ware, J.H. (1977). "On distribution-free tests for equality for survivl distributions," *Biometrika* 64:156-160.

**Suggested Supplemental Readings**

Altman, D.G. (1991). *Practical Statistics for Medical Research*, Chapman and Hall, London, pp. 365-394.

Kleinbaum, D.G. (1996). *Survival Analysis: A Self-learning Text*, Springer, New York.

Lee, E.T. and Wang, J.W. (2003). *Statistical Methods for Survival Data Analysis*, John Wiley and Sons, Hoboken, NJ, pp. 116,117.

Peto R. and Peto, J. (1972). "Asymptotically efficient rank invariant test procedures," *Journal of the Royal Statistical Society A* 135:185-206.

**Table 20.12** Number of Closure Openings until Failure

| | | | | | |
|---|---|---|---|---|---|
| 36 | 150 | 174 | 186 | 195 | 200* |
| 65 | 154 | 175 | 187 | 195 | 200* |
| 81 | 154 | 178 | 187 | 196 | 200* |
| 97 | 156 | 179 | 189 | 197 | 200* |
| 107 | 157 | 180 | 190 | 198 | 200* |
| 115 | 159 | 180 | 190 | 198 | 200* |
| 121 | 159 | 181 | 190 | 198 | 200* |
| 128 | 162 | 182 | 191 | 200 | 200* |
| 132 | 162 | 182 | 191 | 200* | 200* |
| 134 | 163 | 182 | 192 | 200* | 200* |
| 136 | 165 | 184 | 193 | 200* | 200* |
| 139 | 166 | 185 | 193 | 200* | 200* |
| 142 | 169 | 185 | 194 | 200* | 200* |
| 146 | 172 | 185 | 194 | 200* | 200* |
| 148 | 172 | 186 | 194 | 200* | 200* |

* Censored data.

## Example Problems

1. A container manufacturer has developed a new safety closure system for prescription vials. The company tests these closures by asking 30 volunteers to open and close a vial 200 times or until there is a physical failure in the closure system. Each volunteer is asked to repeat this process with three vials. Failure is clearly defined in the study protocol and the number of repetitions assumes that a maximum requirement for such a vial would be 120 (four openings per day for a 30-day supply of medication). The results are presented in Table 20.12. Using both the actuarial and Kaplan-Meier methods for estimating survival, calculate the survival function (with confidence intervals) and median number of closures before failure.

2. Infection is a common problem associated with a specific surgical procedure. The P&T Committee, based on a review of the literature, wanted to evaluate new Antibiotic B compared to the current Antibiotic A that they were using to prevent infection following this procedure. Forty patients were randomly divided into two treatment groups, receiving either Antibiotic A or Antibiotic B. They were followed to determine the number of hours (following survey) before they were discharged, infection free, from the hospital. The results are presented below (* indicates censored data):

   Antibiotic A: 42, 57, 63, 98, 104* 105, 132, 132, 132, 133, 133, 133, 139, 140, 161, 180, 180, 195, 195, 233*

Antibiotic B: 43, 65, 88, 88, 90, 92, 106, 108, 112, 116, 116*, 120, 127, 130, 133, 135, 144*, 146, 165, 203

Was there a significant difference between the time-to-event (discharge) based on the type of antibiotic received?

**Answers to Problems**

1. Listed in Table 20.13 and Table 20.14 are the results from calculating the survival function and confidence interval using both the actuarial and Kaplan-Meier methods. Below are presented the actual calculations for test results 150 times-to-failure.

   Actuarial method:

$$n_i' = n_i - \frac{w_i}{2} = 83 - \frac{0}{2} = 83$$

$$q_i = \frac{d_i}{n_i'} = \frac{9}{83} = 0.108$$

$$p_i = 1 - q_i = 1 - 0.108 = 0.892$$

$$\hat{S}_i = \Pi(p_i) = (1.000 \cdot 0.989 \cdot \ldots \cdot 0.892) = 0.822$$

$$SE(\hat{S}_i) = \hat{S}_i \sqrt{\sum \frac{q_i}{n_i'(p_i)}}$$

**Table 20.13** Actuarial Method for Determining $\hat{S}_i$ for Container Failures

| Max. Times | $n_i$ | $d_i$ | $w_i$ | $q_i$ | $p_i$ | $s_i$ | SE ($s_i$) | Confidence Limits Lower | Upper |
|---|---|---|---|---|---|---|---|---|---|
| 25 | 90 | 0 | 0 | 0.000 | 1.000 | 1.000 | 0.000 | 1.000 | 1.000 |
| 50 | 90 | 1 | 0 | 0.011 | 0.989 | 0.989 | 0.011 | 0.967 | 1.000 |
| 75 | 89 | 1 | 0 | 0.011 | 0.989 | 0.978 | 0.016 | 0.947 | 1.000 |
| 100 | 88 | 2 | 0 | 0.023 | 0.977 | 0.956 | 0.022 | 0.913 | 0.998 |
| 125 | 86 | 3 | 0 | 0.035 | 0.965 | 0.922 | 0.028 | 0.867 | 0.978 |
| 150 | 83 | 9 | 0 | 0.108 | 0.892 | 0.822 | 0.040 | 0.744 | 0.900 |
| 175 | 74 | 16 | 0 | 0.216 | 0.784 | 0.644 | 0.051 | 0.546 | 0.743 |
| 200 | 58 | 36 | 22 | 0.766 | 0.234 | 0.151 | 0.042 | 0.070 | 0.232 |

**Table 20.14** Kaplan-Meier Method for Determining $\hat{S}_i$ for Container Failures

| Max. Time | $n_{i-1}'$ | $w_i$ | $n_i$ | $d_i$ | $n_i'$ | $p_i$ | $s_i$ | SE ($s_i$) | Confidence Limits Lower | Confidence Limits Upper |
|---|---|---|---|---|---|---|---|---|---|---|
| 36 | 90 | 0 | 90 | 1 | 89 | 0.989 | 0.989 | 0.011 | 0.967 | 1.000 |
| 65 | 89 | 0 | 89 | 1 | 88 | 0.989 | 0.978 | 0.016 | 0.947 | 1.000 |
| 81 | 88 | 0 | 88 | 1 | 87 | 0.989 | 0.967 | 0.019 | 0.930 | 1.000 |
| 97 | 87 | 0 | 87 | 1 | 86 | 0.989 | 0.956 | 0.022 | 0.913 | 0.998 |
| 107 | 86 | 0 | 86 | 1 | 85 | 0.988 | 0.944 | 0.024 | 0.897 | 0.992 |
| 115 | 85 | 0 | 85 | 1 | 84 | 0.988 | 0.933 | 0.026 | 0.882 | 0.985 |
| 121 | 84 | 0 | 84 | 1 | 83 | 0.988 | 0.922 | 0.028 | 0.867 | 0.978 |
| 128 | 83 | 0 | 83 | 1 | 82 | 0.988 | 0.911 | 0.030 | 0.852 | 0.970 |
| 132 | 82 | 0 | 82 | 1 | 81 | 0.988 | 0.900 | 0.032 | 0.838 | 0.962 |
| 134 | 81 | 0 | 81 | 1 | 80 | 0.988 | 0.889 | 0.033 | 0.824 | 0.954 |
| 136 | 80 | 0 | 80 | 1 | 79 | 0.988 | 0.878 | 0.035 | 0.810 | 0.945 |
| 139 | 79 | 0 | 79 | 1 | 78 | 0.987 | 0.867 | 0.036 | 0.796 | 0.937 |
| 142 | 78 | 0 | 78 | 1 | 77 | 0.987 | 0.856 | 0.037 | 0.783 | 0.928 |
| 146 | 77 | 0 | 77 | 1 | 76 | 0.987 | 0.844 | 0.038 | 0.770 | 0.919 |
| 148 | 76 | 0 | 76 | 1 | 75 | 0.987 | 0.833 | 0.039 | 0.756 | 0.910 |
| 150 | 75 | 0 | 75 | 1 | 74 | 0.987 | 0.822 | 0.040 | 0.744 | 0.900 |
| 154 | 74 | 0 | 74 | 2 | 72 | 0.973 | 0.800 | 0.042 | 0.717 | 0.883 |
| 156 | 72 | 0 | 72 | 1 | 71 | 0.986 | 0.789 | 0.043 | 0.705 | 0.873 |
| 157 | 71 | 0 | 71 | 1 | 70 | 0.985 | 0.778 | 0.044 | 0.692 | 0.864 |
| 159 | 70 | 0 | 70 | 2 | 68 | 0.971 | 0.756 | 0.045 | 0.667 | 0.844 |
| 162 | 68 | 0 | 68 | 2 | 66 | 0.971 | 0.733 | 0.047 | 0.642 | 0.825 |
| 163 | 66 | 0 | 66 | 1 | 65 | 0.985 | 0.722 | 0.047 | 0.628 | 0.815 |
| 165 | 65 | 0 | 65 | 1 | 64 | 0.985 | 0.711 | 0.048 | 0.618 | 0.805 |
| 166 | 64 | 0 | 64 | 1 | 63 | 0.984 | 0.700 | 0.048 | 0.605 | 0.795 |
| 169 | 63 | 0 | 63 | 1 | 62 | 0.984 | 0.689 | 0.049 | 0.593 | 0.785 |
| 172 | 62 | 0 | 62 | 2 | 60 | 0.968 | 0.667 | 0.050 | 0.569 | 0.764 |
| 174 | 60 | 0 | 60 | 1 | 59 | 0.983 | 0.656 | 0.050 | 0.557 | 0.754 |
| 175 | 59 | 0 | 59 | 1 | 58 | 0.983 | 0.644 | 0.051 | 0.546 | 0.743 |
| 178 | 58 | 0 | 58 | 1 | 57 | 0.983 | 0.633 | 0.051 | 0.534 | 0.733 |
| 179 | 57 | 0 | 57 | 1 | 56 | 0.983 | 0.622 | 0.051 | 0.522 | 0.722 |
| 180 | 56 | 0 | 56 | 2 | 54 | 0.964 | 0.600 | 0.052 | 0.499 | 0.701 |
| 181 | 54 | 0 | 54 | 1 | 53 | 0.982 | 0.589 | 0.052 | 0.487 | 0.691 |
| 182 | 53 | 0 | 53 | 3 | 50 | 0.943 | 0.556 | 0.052 | 0.453 | 0.658 |
| 184 | 50 | 0 | 50 | 1 | 49 | 0.980 | 0.544 | 0.053 | 0.442 | 0.647 |
| 185 | 49 | 0 | 49 | 3 | 46 | 0.939 | 0.511 | 0.053 | 0.408 | 0.614 |
| 186 | 46 | 0 | 46 | 2 | 44 | 0.957 | 0.489 | 0.053 | 0.386 | 0.592 |
| 187 | 44 | 0 | 44 | 2 | 42 | 0.955 | 0.467 | 0.053 | 0.364 | 0.570 |

continued

**Table 20.14** Kaplan-Meier Method for Determining $\hat{S}_i$ for Container Failures (continued)

| Max. Time | $n_{i-1}'$ | $w_i$ | $n_i$ | $d_i$ | $n_i'$ | $p_i$ | $s_i$ | SE ($s_i$) | Confidence Limits Lower | Upper |
|---|---|---|---|---|---|---|---|---|---|---|
| 189 | 42 | 0 | 42 | 1 | 41 | 0.976 | 0.456 | 0.053 | 0.353 | 0.558 |
| 190 | 41 | 0 | 41 | 3 | 38 | 0.927 | 0.422 | 0.052 | 0.321 | 0.524 |
| 191 | 38 | 0 | 38 | 2 | 36 | 0.947 | 0.400 | 0.052 | 0.299 | 0.501 |
| 192 | 36 | 0 | 36 | 1 | 35 | 0.972 | 0.389 | 0.051 | 0.288 | 0.490 |
| 193 | 35 | 0 | 35 | 2 | 33 | 0.943 | 0.367 | 0.051 | 0.267 | 0.466 |
| 194 | 33 | 0 | 33 | 3 | 30 | 0.909 | 0.333 | 0.050 | 0.236 | 0.431 |
| 195 | 30 | 0 | 30 | 2 | 28 | 0.933 | 0.311 | 0.049 | 0.216 | 0.407 |
| 196 | 28 | 0 | 28 | 1 | 27 | 0.964 | 0.300 | 0.048 | 0.205 | 0.395 |
| 197 | 27 | 0 | 27 | 1 | 26 | 0.963 | 0.289 | 0.048 | 0.195 | 0.383 |
| 198 | 26 | 0 | 26 | 3 | 23 | 0.885 | 0.256 | 0.046 | 0.165 | 0.346 |
| 200 | 23 | 22 | 1 | 1 | 0 | 0.000 | 0.000 | … | … | … |

$$SE(\hat{S}_i) = 0.822\sqrt{\frac{0}{90(1.000)} + \frac{0.011}{90(0.989)} + \ldots + \frac{0.108}{83(0.892)}} = 0.040$$

$$S_i = \hat{S}_i \pm z_{1-\alpha/2} \cdot SE(\hat{S}_i) = 0.822 \pm 1.96(0.040)$$

$$0.744 < S_i < 0.900$$

Kaplan-Meier:

$$n_i = n_{i-1}' - w_i = 75 - 0 = 75$$

$$n_i' = n_i - d_i = 75 - 1 = 74$$

$$p_i = \frac{n_i'}{n_i} = \frac{74}{75} = 0.987$$

$$\hat{S}_i = \Pi(p_i) = (0.989 \cdot 0.989 \cdot \ldots \cdot 0.987) = 0.822$$

$$SE(\hat{S}_i) = \hat{S}_i\sqrt{\sum \frac{d_i}{n_i(n_i - d_i)}}$$

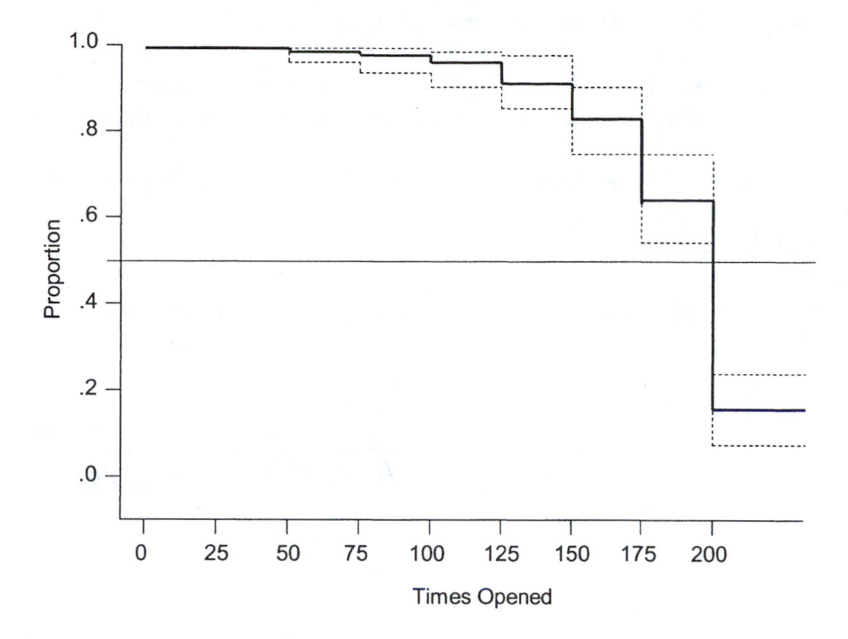


**Figure 20.9** Actuarial curve with 95% confidence bands for example problem.

$$SE(\hat{S}_i) = \sqrt{\frac{1}{90(90-1)} + \frac{1}{89(89-1)} + \ldots + \frac{1}{75(75-1)}} = 0.040$$

$$S_i = \hat{S}_i \pm z_{1-\alpha/2} \cdot SE(\hat{S}_i) = 0.822 \pm 1.96(0.040)$$

$$0.744 < S_i < 0.900$$

The median survival function would be the point on the curve it crosses 0.5. Looking at Tables 20.13 and 20.14, the first times point below 0.5 would be:

Actuarial method median survival = 200 times

Kaplan-Meier median survival = 186 times

Figure 20.9 presents a graphic representation of the survival curve for the actuarial method. The Kaplan-Meier method would produce a similar curve, but with 48 intervals instead of just eight from the actuarial method.

2. Comparison on time-to-event comparing two antibiotics.

Hypotheses: $H_0$: Time-to-event(antibiotic A) = Time-to-event(antibiotic B)
$H_1$: Time-to-event(antibiotic A) ≠ Time-to-event(antibiotic B)

Decision rule: With $\alpha = 0.05$, reject $H_0$, if $z > z_{(1-\alpha/2)} = 1.96$ or $z < -1.96$ or if $\chi^2_{CMH} > \chi_1^2 = 3.84$.

Calculations (log rank test):

Table 20.15 contains the calculations for each $U_L$ and $S_{U_L}$:

$$U_L = \sum(a_i - e_i) = -3.555$$

$$S_{U_L} = \sqrt{\sum \frac{(a_i + c_i)(b_i + d_i)(a_i + b_i)[n_i - (a_i + b_i)]}{n_i^2(n_i - 1)}}$$

$$S_{U_L} = \sqrt{7.904} = 2.811$$

$$z = \frac{U_L}{S_{U_L}} = \frac{-3.555}{2.811} = -1.265$$

Decision: With $z$ greater than −1.96, fail to reject the null hypothesis and assume there is no difference in the time to discharge between antibiotics A and B.

Calculations (Cochran-Mantel-Haensel test):

Table 20.15 contains the calculations for each $e_i$ and $v_i$:

$$e_i = \frac{(a_i + b_i)(a_i + c_i)}{n_i}$$

$$\sum(a_i - e_i) = -3.555$$

$$v_i = \frac{(a_i + b_i)(c_i + d_i)(a_i + c_i)(b_i + d_i)}{n_i^2(n_i - 1)}$$

$$\sum v_i = 7.935$$

**Table 20.15** Comparison of Two Antibiotics and Time-to-Event (Discharge)

| Event (Hours) | $a_i$ | $b_i$ | $c_i$ | $d_i$ | $n_i$ | $e_i$ | $a_i - e_i$ | $v_i$ | SLU Int* |
|---|---|---|---|---|---|---|---|---|---|
| 42 | 1 | 0 | 19 | 20 | 40 | 0.500 | −0.500 | 0.250 | 0.250 |
| 43 | 0 | 1 | 19 | 19 | 39 | 0.487 | 0.513 | 0.250 | 0.250 |
| 57 | 1 | 0 | 18 | 19 | 38 | 0.500 | −0.500 | 0.250 | 0.250 |
| 63 | 1 | 0 | 17 | 19 | 37 | 0.486 | −0.486 | 0.250 | 0.250 |
| 65 | 0 | 1 | 17 | 18 | 36 | 0.472 | 0.528 | 0.249 | 0.249 |
| 88 | 0 | 2 | 17 | 16 | 35 | 0.971 | 1.029 | 0.485 | 0.485 |
| 90 | 0 | 1 | 17 | 15 | 33 | 0.515 | 0.485 | 0.250 | 0.250 |
| 92 | 0 | 1 | 17 | 14 | 32 | 0.531 | 0.469 | 0.249 | 0.249 |
| 98 | 1 | 0 | 16 | 14 | 31 | 0.548 | −0.548 | 0.248 | 0.248 |
| 105 | 1 | 0 | 14 | 14 | 29 | 0.517 | −0.517 | 0.250 | 0.250 |
| 106 | 0 | 1 | 14 | 13 | 28 | 0.500 | 0.500 | 0.250 | 0.250 |
| 108 | 0 | 1 | 14 | 12 | 27 | 0.519 | 0.481 | 0.250 | 0.250 |
| 112 | 0 | 1 | 14 | 11 | 26 | 0.538 | 0.462 | 0.249 | 0.249 |
| 116 | 0 | 1 | 14 | 9 | 24 | 0.583 | 0.417 | 0.243 | 0.243 |
| 120 | 0 | 1 | 14 | 8 | 23 | 0.609 | 0.391 | 0.238 | 0.238 |
| 127 | 0 | 1 | 13 | 8 | 22 | 0.591 | 0.409 | 0.242 | 0.242 |
| 130 | 0 | 1 | 13 | 7 | 21 | 0.619 | 0.381 | 0.236 | 0.236 |
| 132 | 3 | 0 | 10 | 7 | 20 | 1.950 | −1.950 | 0.611 | 0.611 |
| 133 | 3 | 1 | 7 | 6 | 17 | 2.353 | −1.353 | 0.787 | 0.787 |
| 135 | 0 | 1 | 7 | 5 | 13 | 0.538 | 0.462 | 0.249 | 0.249 |
| 139 | 1 | 0 | 7 | 4 | 12 | 0.667 | −0.667 | 0.222 | 0.222 |
| 140 | 1 | 0 | 6 | 4 | 11 | 0.636 | −0.636 | 0.231 | 0.231 |
| 146 | 0 | 1 | 6 | 2 | 9 | 0.667 | 0.333 | 0.222 | 0.222 |
| 161 | 1 | 0 | 6 | 2 | 8 | 0.875 | −0.875 | 0.250 | 0.219 |
| 165 | 0 | 1 | 5 | 1 | 7 | 0.714 | 0.286 | 0.204 | 0.204 |
| 180 | 2 | 0 | 3 | 1 | 6 | 1.667 | −1.667 | 0.222 | 0.222 |
| 195 | 2 | 0 | 1 | 1 | 4 | 1.500 | −1.500 | 0.250 | 0.250 |
| 203 | 0 | 1 | 1 | 0 | 2 | 0.500 | 0.500 | 0.250 | 0.250 |
| | | | | | Σ = | 21.555 | −3.555 | 7.935 | 7.904 |

* SLU Intermediate = $((a_i + c_i)(b_i + d_i)(a_i + b_i)(n_i - (a_i + b_i)))/(n_i^2(n_i - 1))$.

The calculation of the Cochran-Mantel-Haensel chi square is as follows:

$$\chi^2_{CMH} = \frac{[\Sigma(a_i - e_i)]^2}{\Sigma v_i}$$

$$\chi^2_{CMH} = \frac{(-3.555)^2}{7.935} = 1.593$$

Decision: With $\chi^2_{CMH}$ less than 3.84, fail to reject the null hypothesis and assume there is no difference in the time to discharge between antibiotics A and B.

# 21

# Nonparametric Tests

Nonparametric statistical tests can be useful when dealing with extremely small sample sizes or when the requirements of normality and homoscedasticity cannot be met or assumed. These tests are simple to calculate, but are traditionally less powerful and the researcher needs to evaluate the risk of a Type II error. Often referred to as **distribution-free statistics**, nonparametric statistical tests do not make any assumptions about the population distribution. One does not need to meet the requirements of normality or homogeneity of variance associated with the parametric procedures (z-test, t-tests, F-tests, correlation and regression). Chi square tests are often cited as distribution-free tests and have been covered in a previous chapter.

These distribution-free tests have been slow to gain favor in the pharmaceutical community, but are currently being seen with greater frequency, often in parallel with the parametric counterparts. This is seen in the following example of a 1989 clinical trial protocol:

> If the variables to be analyzed are normally distributed and homogenous with respect to variance, a parametric analysis of variance that models the cross-over design will be applied. If these criteria are not fulfilled, suitable nonparametric tests will be used.

Nonparametric tests are relatively simple to calculate. Their speed and convenience offers a distinct advantage over the parametric alternatives discussed in the previous chapters. Therefore, as investigators we can use these procedures as a quick method for evaluating data.

### Use of Nonparametric Tests

Nonparametric tests usually involve ranking or categorizing the data and by doing so we decrease the accuracy of our information (changing from the raw data to a relative ranking). We may obscure the true differences and make it difficult to identify differences that are significant. In other words, nonparametric tests require differences to be larger if they are to be found significant. We increase the risk that we will accept a false null hypothesis (Type II error). It may be to the researcher's advantage to tolerate minor doubts about normality and homogeneity associated with a given parametric test, rather than to risk the greater error possible with a nonparametric procedure.

A **robust statistic** refers to test-based populations with assumed normality distributions and similar variances even when the underlying population may not be normal. Some of the parametric tests discussed previously (notably the t-tests are known to be robust against the assumption of normality, especially if there are large sample sizes. However, other authors (i.e., Conover, 1999) would argue that nonparametric tests are preferable and even more powerful than parametric tests if the assumptions (normality and homogeneity) are false. Thus, results showing extremely different variances should be tested using the appropriate nonparametric procedure.

When dealing with ordinal dependent variable results, the nonparametric tests become the tests of choice. As discussed in Chapter 1, units on an ordinal scale may not be equidistant and violate assumption required for parametric procedures. For example, consider the following commonly used scale for investigators to assess the cognitive functioning of Alzheimer's patients:

Cognitive Performance Scale Description

| Score | Assessment |
|---|---|
| 0 | Intact |
| 1 | Borderline intact |
| 2 | Mild Impairment |
| 3 | Moderate Impairment |
| 4 | Moderate to Severe Impairment |
| 5 | Severe Impairment |
| 6 | Very Severe Impairment |

Is the difference between mild and moderate to severe impairment twice the difference between mild and moderate impairment? The answer is probably not. Therefore the conversion from the initial ordinal scale to the relative positioning of a rank order scale would be the more appropriate statistical test.

Nonparametric tests are particularly useful when there are potential outliers (to be discussed in Chapter 23). Because of the ranking involved, extremely large or small observation will receive the ranks on 1 or *N*. For example, assume the following numbers: 2, 3, 3, 4, 4, 5, 6, 7, and 15. In this case 15 would seem to different from the other eight observations. However, when ranking the data the number 15 would be converted to rank 9 and its difference from the other observations would be minimized. What if the last value was 150 or even 15,000? The same rank of 9 would be assigned. Thus, nonparametric statistics are generally not affected by outliers.

This chapter will explore a few of the most commonly used nonparametric tests that can be used in place of the previously discussed methods (i.e., t-tests, F-tests, correlation) Nonparametric tests that analyze differences between two discrete levels of the independent variable include the: 1) Mann-Whitney U test and 2) median test.

For comparing how paired groups of data relate to each other, appropriate tests include: 1) Wilcoxon's signed-rank test and 2) sign test. The analyses of variance models can be evaluated using: 1) the Kruskal-Wallis test or 2) Friedman two-way analysis of variance. These nonparametric procedures are extremely valuable and in many cases more appropriate when testing small sample sizes. Lastly, for correlations, the Spearman rho test may be substituted.

## Ranking of Information

Most nonparametric tests require that the data be ranked on an ordinal scale. Ranking involves assigning the value 1 to the smallest observation, 2 to the second smallest, and continuing this process until $N$ is assigned to the largest observation. For example:

| Data | Rank | |
|---|---|---|
| 12 | 1 | |
| 18 | 5 | |
| 16 | 3 | $N = 5$ |
| 15 | 2 | |
| 17 | 4 | |

In the case of ties, the average of the rank values is assigned to each tied observation.

| Data | Rank | |
|---|---|---|
| 12 | 1 | |
| 18 | 9 | |
| 16 | 6 | |
| 15 | 4 | |
| 17 | 7.5 | $N = 10$ |
| 14 | 2 | |
| 15 | 4 | |
| 15 | 4 | |
| 17 | 7.5 | |
| 20 | 10 | |

In this example there were three 15s (ranks 3,4, and 5) with an average rank of 4 and two 17s (ranks 7 and 8) with an average rank of 7.5.

When comparing sets of data from different groups or different treatment levels (levels of the independent variable), ranking involves all of the observations regardless of the discrete level in which the observation occurs:

| Group A (n = 5) | | Group B (n = 7) | | Group C (n = 8) | | Total (N = 20) |
|---|---|---|---|---|---|---|
| Data | Rank | Data | Rank | Data | Rank | |
| 12 | 3 | 11 | 2 | 15 | 8.5 | |
| 18 | 17.5 | 13 | 4.5 | 15 | 8.5 | |
| 16 | 12 | 19 | 19.5 | 17 | 15 | |
| 15 | 8.5 | 17 | 15 | 19 | 19.5 | |
| 17 | 15 | 16 | 12 | 18 | 17.5 | |
| | | 15 | 8.5 | 16 | 12 | |
| | | 14 | 6 | 13 | 4.5 | |
| | | | | 10 | 1 | |
| $\Sigma =$ | 56.0 | $\Sigma =$ | 67.5 | $\Sigma =$ | 86.5 | $\Sigma\Sigma = 210$ |

Accuracy of the ranking process may be checked in two ways. First, the last rank assigned should be equal to the total *N* (in this example the largest rank was a tie between two observations (ranks 19 and 20), the average of which was 19.5. The second way to check the accuracy of the ranking procedure is the fact that the sum of all the summed ranks should equal $N(N + 1)/2$, where *N* equals the total number of observations:

$$Sum\ of\ Summed\ Ranks = \Sigma\Sigma R_i = \frac{N(N+1)}{2} \qquad \text{Eq. 21.1}$$

For the above example this check for accuracy in the ranking would be:

$$56.0 + 67.5 + 86.5 = 210 = \frac{20(21)}{2} = \frac{N(N+1)}{2}$$

**Mann-Whitney U Test**

The Mann-Whitney U test is a procedure for the situation where the independent variable has two discrete levels and there is a continuous dependent variable (similar to the two-sample t-test). Data are ranked and a formula is applied. Note that the hypotheses are not concerned with the means of the populations. The parameters of normality and homogeneity of variance are not considered, where the t-test evaluated the null hypothesis the $\mu_1 = \mu_2$, the hypotheses for this nonparametric procedure are:

$H_0$: Samples are from the same population
$H_1$: Samples are drawn from different populations

For this test the data are ranked and the sums of the ranks of the dependent variables is calculated for one level of the independent variable.

| Data Level 1 | Rank | Data Level 2 | Rank |
|---|---|---|---|
| $d_{11}$ | $R_{11}$ | $d_{21}$ | $R_{21}$ |
| $d_{12}$ | $R_{12}$ | $d_{22}$ | $R_{22}$ |
| $d_{13}$ | $R_{13}$ | $d_{23}$ | $R_{23}$ |
| ... | ... | ... | ... |
| $d_{1j}$ | $R_{1j}$ | $d_{2j}$ | $R_{2j}$ |
| | $\Sigma R_{1j}$ | | |

Either the first or second ranking could be used for the statistical sum of the ranks. The statistical values are calculated using the following two formulas where $\Sigma R_{1j}$ is associated with $n_1$:

$$U = n_1 n_2 + \frac{n_1(n_1+1)}{2} - \sum_{i=1}^{I} R_{1j} \qquad \text{Eq. 21.2}$$

Here $n_2$ is the number of observation in the level of independent variable not summed. This $U$-value is converted to a $z$-value by applying a second formula:

$$z = \frac{U - \frac{n_1 n_2}{2}}{\sqrt{\frac{n_1 n_2 \cdot [n_1 + (n_2 + 1)]}{12}}} \qquad \text{Eq. 21.3}$$

The calculated $z$-value is then compared to values in the normalized standard distribution (Table B2, Appendix B). If the calculated $z$-value is to the extreme of the critical $z$-value (positive or negative) then $H_0$ is rejected. In the case of 95% confidence, the critical $z$-values would be either a –1.96 or +1.96. The numerator of the equation is similar to the $z$-test of proportions; we are comparing an observed $U$-value to an expected value that is the average of the ranks ($n_1 n_2/2$).

As an example of the Mann-Whitney U test, a pharmacology experiment was conducted to determine the effect of atropine on the release of acetylcholine (ACh) from rat neostriata brain slices. The measure of ACh release through stimulation was measured twice. Half of the sample received atropine before the second measurement. The ratios (stimulation 2 divided by stimulation 1) are presented in the first and third columns of Table 21.1. Is there a difference in the ratios between the control group and those administered the atropine? The hypotheses are:

$H_0$: Samples are from the same population
(i.e., no difference in response)
$H_1$: Samples are drawn from different populations
(i.e., difference in response)

**Table 21.1** Sample Data for the Mann-Whitney U Test

| Control | Rank | Received Atropine | Rank |
|---|---|---|---|
| 0.7974 | 3 | 1.7695 | 13 |
| 0.8762 | 4 | 1.6022 | 12 |
| 0.6067 | 1 | 1.0632 | 7 |
| 1.1268 | 9 | 2.7831 | 14 |
| 0.7184 | 2 | 1.0475 | 6 |
| 1.0422 | 5 | 1.4411 | 11 |
| 1.3590 | 10 | 1.0990 | 8 |
| Σ = | 34 | Σ = | 71 |

The decision rule is, with $\alpha$ = .05, reject $H_0$, if $|z|$ > critical $z_{(.975)}$ = 1.96. The rankings of the data are presented in the second and fourth columns of Table 21.1. A quick computational check for accuracy of the ranking shows that the ranking was done correctly:

$$\frac{N(N+1)}{2} = \frac{14(15)}{2} = 105 = 34 + 71$$

The calculation of the Mann-Whitney test statistics would be:

$$U = n_1 n_2 + \frac{n_1(n_1+1)}{2} - \Sigma R_{1j}$$

$$U = (7)(7) + \frac{(7)(8)}{2} - 34 = 43$$

$$z = \frac{U - \frac{n_1 n_2}{2}}{\sqrt{\frac{n_1 n_2 \cdot [n_1 + (n_2+1)]}{12}}}$$

$$z = \frac{43 - \frac{(7)(7)}{2}}{\sqrt{\frac{(7)(7)\cdot[7+8)]}{12}}} = \frac{43 - 24.5}{7.83} = 2.36$$

Note that reversing Level 1 and Level 2 would produce identical results. In the above case the $\Sigma R_{ij}$ is 71 and $n_1$ is 7:

$$U = (7)(7) + \frac{(7)(8)}{2} - 71 = 6$$

$$z = \frac{6 - \frac{(7)(7)}{2}}{\sqrt{\frac{(7)(7) \cdot [7 + 8)]}{12}}} = \frac{6 - 24.5}{7.83} = -2.36$$

The decision, either way, would be with $z > z_{critical} = 1.96$, reject $H_0$ and conclude that the samples are drawn from different populations and the response of the rat's neostriata release of ACh is affected by atropine.

## Median Test

The median test may also be used for an independent variable with two discrete levels. This test utilizes the median for all of the data points observed. In many nonparametric statistics, the median is used instead of the mean as a measure of central tendency. The hypotheses are the same as the Mann-Whitney test.

$H_0$: Samples are from the same population
$H_1$: Samples are drawn from different populations

The first step is to create a 2 x 2 table using the *grand median* for all of the observations in both levels of the independent variable. As discussed previously, one valuable property of the median is that it is not affected by an outlier (extreme values).

| | Group 1 | Group 2 |
|---|---|---|
| Above the median | a | b |
| Below the median | c | d |

n = total observations

The calculated $p$-value is determined using a formula that incorporates a numerator of all the margin values ($a + b$, $c + d$, $a + c$ and $b + d$) and a denominator involving each cell:

$$p = \frac{(a+b)!\,(c+d)!\,(a+c)!\,(b+d)!}{n!\,a!\,b!\,c!\,d!} \qquad \text{Eq. 21.4}$$

The decision rule is to reject $H_0$, if the calculated $p$-value is less than the critical $p(\alpha)$ in a normal standardized distribution, for example, $\alpha = 0.05$. Note that this formula is exactly the same as the Fisher Exact test presented in Chapter 16. The difference between the two tests is that the median is created based on an ordinal or higher scaled data and the results are based solely on the observed results and not any more extreme scenarios as seen with the Fisher Exact test.

As an example of the median test, the same data used for the Mann-Whitney U test will be considered. In this case the grand median is between data points 1.0632 and 1.0990 (ranks 7 and 8). The data for each level of the independent variable is classified as above or below the median and the results are presented in the following table:

| | Control | Atropine | |
|---|---|---|---|
| Above the median | 2 | 5 | N = 14 |
| Below the median | 5 | 2 | |

In this example, all of the margin values (i.e., $a+b$) are seven and the computation of the probability of the occurrence is:

$$p = \frac{(2+5)!\,(2+5)!\,(5+2)!\,(2+5)!}{14!\,2!\,5!\,5!\,2!}$$

$$p = \frac{6.45 \times 10^{14}}{5.02 \times 10^{15}} = 0.128$$

With the calculated $p = 0.128$, there is a probability of this occurring 12.8% of the time by chance alone. We cannot reject $H_0$. The researcher cannot find a significant difference and must assume that the animals are drawn from the same population and there is no treatment effect.

Note that when using the Mann-Whitney test $H_0$ at the 0.05 level of significance, $H_0$ was rejected, but could not be rejected with the median test. If the same data is run using a t-test, the results are identical to the Mann-Whitney test:

| Significance level: | 0.1 | 0.05 | 0.01 |
|---|---|---|---|
| Mann-Whitney U test | Reject $H_0$ | Reject $H_0$ | Accept $H_0$ |
| Median test | Reject $H_0$ | Accept $H_0$ | Accept $H_0$ |
| t-test | Reject $H_0$ | Reject $H_0$ | Accept $H_0$ |

It appears that the median test is a slightly more conservative test than either the Mann-Whitney or t-tests, and more likely to result in a Type II error. This is due in part to the small amount of information available from the median test, results are dichotomized into above and below the median, and only two outcomes are possible.

### Wilcoxon Matched-Pairs Test

The Wilcoxon matched-pairs test offers a parallel to the matched-pair t-test discussed in Chapter 9. To accomplish this test, a traditional pre-posttest (before-after) table is constructed and the differences are calculated similar to the matched-pair t-test. For example:

| Subject | Before | After | d |
|---|---|---|---|
| 1 | 67 | 71 | +4 |
| 2 | 70 | 73 | +3 |
| 3 | 85 | 81 | –4 |
| 4 | 80 | 82 | +2 |
| 5 | 72 | 75 | +3 |
| 6 | 78 | 76 | –2 |

The *absolute* differences (regardless of sign, positive or negative) are then ranked from smallest to largest.

| Subject | Before | After | d | Rank \|d\| |
|---|---|---|---|---|
| 1 | 67 | 71 | +4 | 5.5 |
| 2 | 70 | 73 | +3 | 3.5 |
| 3 | 85 | 81 | –4 | 5.5 |
| 4 | 80 | 82 | +2 | 1.5 |
| 5 | 72 | 75 | +3 | 3.5 |
| 6 | 78 | 76 | –2 | 1.5 |

Notice that the fourth and sixth subjects have identical differences (even though the signs are different): therefore, they share the average rank of 1.5 (ranks 1 and 2). Thus, the ranking process measures the magnitude of the difference regardless of the direction (positive or negative). A *T*-value is calculated for the sum of the ranks associated with the *least frequent* sign (+ or –).

| Sub. | Before | After | d | Rank \|d\| | Rank associated with the least frequent sign |
|---|---|---|---|---|---|
| 1 | 67 | 71 | +4 | 5.5 | |
| 2 | 70 | 73 | +3 | 3.5 | |
| 3 | 85 | 81 | –4 | 5.5 | 5.5 |
| 4 | 80 | 82 | +2 | 1.5 | |
| 5 | 72 | 75 | +3 | 3.5 | |
| 6 | 78 | 76 | –2 | 1.5 | 1.5 |
| | | | | T = Σ = | 7.0 |

Note in the above example that the third and sixth subjects were the only two with negative differences (the least frequent sign); therefore, their associated ranks were

**Table 21.2** Example of Data for a Wilcoxon Matched-Pairs Test

| Before | After | d | Rank \|d\| | Rank associated with least frequent sign |
|---|---|---|---|---|
| 81 | 86 | +5 | 6.5 | |
| 81 | 93 | +12 | 8 | |
| 79 | 74 | −4 | 4.5 | 4.5 |
| 80 | 80 | 0 | - | |
| 74 | 76 | +2 | 3 | |
| 78 | 83 | +5 | 6.5 | |
| 90 | 91 | +1 | 1.5 | |
| 95 | 95 | 0 | - | |
| 68 | 72 | +4 | 4.5 | |
| 75 | 74 | −1 | 1.5 | 1.5 |
| n = 8 | Σ = | 0 | | T = Σ = 6 |

the only ones carried over to the last column and summed to produce the *T*-value. If all the signs are positive or negative then the *T*-value would be zero and no ranks would be associated with the least frequent sign and $T = 0$.

A unique aspect of this test is that a certain amount of data may be ignored. If a difference is zero, there is no measurable difference in either the positive or negative direction; therefore, a sign cannot be assigned. Thus, data associated with no differences are eliminated and the number of pairs (*n*) is reduced appropriately. To illustrate this point, note the example in Table 21.2. In this case *n* is reduced from 10 pairs to $n = 8$ pairs, because two of the results have zero differences. Also note that the least frequent sign was a negative, thus the *T*-value is calculated by summing only those rank scores with negative differences. The hypotheses for the Wilcoxon matched-pairs test are not concerned with mean differences, as seen with the t-test (where the null hypothesis was $\mu_d = 0$) and stated as follows:

$H_0$: No difference between pre- and post-measurements
$H_1$: Difference between pre- and post-measurements

One simple calculation is to determine, under a zero change, the expected *T*-value or *E(T)* if there was no difference between the pre- and post-measurements. The expected total for the ranks is $E(Total) = n(n + 1)/2$. If $H_0$ is true then the total for each sign rank (+ or −) should be equal to half the total ranks (Eq. 21.1). Thus:

$$E(T) = \frac{n(n+1)}{2} \cdot \frac{1}{2} \quad or \quad E(T) = \frac{n(n+1)}{4} \qquad \text{Eq. 21.5}$$

The test statistic once again involves a numerator that compares the difference between an expected value and an observed result, in this case the *T*-value:

$$z = \frac{T - E(T)}{\sqrt{\frac{n(n+1)(2n+1)}{24}}} \qquad \text{Eq. 21.6}$$

As with previous equations, if the observed and expected values are identical the numerator would be zero and the $z$-value would be zero. As the difference increases the $z$-value increases until it reaches a point of statistical significance with a given Type I error rate. In this procedure the decision rule is with a predetermined $\alpha$, to reject $H_0$ if $z$ is greater than $z(\alpha/2)$ from the normal standardized distribution (Table B2, Appendix B). For the example presented in Table 21.2 the decision rule would be, with $\alpha = .05$, reject $H_0$ if $z > 1.96$ and the computations would be as follows:

$$E(T) = \frac{(8)(9)}{4} = 18$$

$$z = \frac{6 - 18}{\sqrt{\frac{8(9)(2(8)+1)}{24}}} = \frac{-12}{\sqrt{51}} = -1.68$$

The decision is with $z < 1.96$, we cannot reject $H_0$ and we are unable to find a significant difference between pre- and post-measurements.

## Sign Test

The sign test is a second method for determining significant differences between paired observations and is based on the binomial distribution. It is among the simplest of all nonparametric procedures. Similar to the Wilcoxon test, differences are considered and any pairs with zero differences are dropped, and the $n$ of the sample is reduced. A table for the pairs is constructed and only the sign (+ or –) is considered. Using the same example presented for the Wilcoxon test we find signs listed in Table 21.3. If there are no significant differences between the before and after measurements we would expect half the numbers to be positive (+) and half to be negative (–). Thus $p(+) = 0.50$ and $p(-) = 0.50$. If there was no significant difference between the before-and-after measurements, the null hypotheses would be that the proportion of positive and negative signs would be equal.

$H_0$: No difference between measurement or $H_0$: $p(+) = 0.50$
$H_1$: Difference between measurements exists $H_1$: $p(+) \neq 0.50$

The more the proportion of (+)s or (–)s differ from 0.50, the more likely that there is a significant difference and that the difference is not due to random error alone.

For sample sizes less than 10 the binomial distribution can be used and Eq. 2.12 would be used to define the probabilities associated with the distribution.

**Table 21.3** Sample Data for a Sign Test

| Before | After | d | Sign |
|---|---|---|---|
| 81 | 86 | +5 | + |
| 81 | 93 | +12 | + |
| 79 | 74 | −4 | - |
| 80 | 80 | 0 | 0 |
| 74 | 76 | +2 | + |
| 78 | 83 | +5 | + |
| 90 | 91 | +1 | + |
| 95 | 95 | 0 | 0 |
| 68 | 72 | +4 | + |
| 75 | 74 | −1 | - |

$$p(x) = \binom{n}{x} p^x q^{n-x}$$

Dropping the two zero differences the final number of paired observations is eight. What is the probability of six or more positive values out of eight differences, given that the probability of a positive value equals 0.50?

$$p(6\ positives) = \binom{8}{6}(.50)^6(.50)^2 = 0.1092$$

$$p(7\ positives) = \binom{8}{7}(.50)^7(.50)^1 = 0.0313$$

$$p(8\ positives) = \binom{8}{8}(.50)^8(.50)^0 = 0.0039$$

$$p(>5\ positives) = \Sigma = 0.1444$$

Thus, there is almost a 15% chance that there will be six or more positive differences out of the 8 pairs by chance alone. Thus, we cannot reject $H_0$.

For 10 or more pairs of observations, we can employ Yates' correction for continuity for the one-sample z-test for proportions (modified from Eq. 15.2):

$$z = \frac{|p - P_0| - \frac{1}{n}}{\sqrt{\frac{(P_0)(1 - P_0)}{n}}} \qquad \text{Eq. 21.7}$$

where $p$ is the number of positive outcomes divided by the total number of pairs. In this particular case:

$$p = \frac{6}{8} = .75$$

$$z = \frac{|.75 - .50| - \frac{1}{8}}{\sqrt{\frac{(.50)(.50)}{8}}} = \frac{.25 - .125}{\sqrt{.0313}} = 0.71$$

In a normal standardized distribution table (Table B2, Appendix B) the area below the point where $z = 0.71$ is .7611 (.5000 + .2611). Thus, the probability of being above $z = 0.71$ is .2389 and therefore not significant.

**Kruskal-Wallis Test**

Much as the F-test is an extension of the t-test, Kruskal-Wallis is an equivalent nonparametric extension of the Mann-Whitney U test for more than two levels of an independent discrete variable. The hypotheses are:

$H_0$: Samples are from the same population
$H_1$: Samples are drawn from different populations

Like the Mann-Whitney test, data are ranked and rank sums calculated, then a new statistical formula is applied to the summed ranks.

| Level 1 | Rank | Level 2 | Rank | ... | Level k | Rank |
|---|---|---|---|---|---|---|
| $d_{11}$ | $R_{11}$ | $d_{21}$ | $R_{21}$ | ... | $d_{k1}$ | $R_{k1}$ |
| $d_{12}$ | $R_{12}$ | $d_{22}$ | $R_{22}$ | ... | $d_{k2}$ | $R_{k2}$ |
| $d_{13}$ | $R_{13}$ | $d_{23}$ | $R_{22}$ | ... | $d_{k3}$ | $R_{k3}$ |
| ... | ... | ... | ... | ... | ... | ... |
| $d_{1j}$ | $R_{1j}$ | $d_{2j}$ | $R_{2j}$ | ... | $d_{kj}$ | $R_{kj}$ |
| | $\Sigma R_{1j}$ | | $\Sigma R_{2j}$ | | | $\Sigma R_{kj}$ |

For the Kruskal-Wallis test the formula for the test statistic is:

$$H = \frac{12}{N(N+1)}\left[\Sigma \frac{(\Sigma R_{ij})^2}{n_j}\right] - 3(N+1) \qquad \text{Eq. 21.8}$$

The middle section of the equation involves the squaring of the individual sum of

**Table 21.4** Data for a Kruskal-Wallis Example

| Instrument A | | Instrument B | | Instrument C | |
|---|---|---|---|---|---|
| Assay | Rank | Assay | Rank | Assay | Rank |
| 12.12 | 8 | 12.47 | 14 | 12.20 | 10 |
| 13.03 | 18 | 13.95 | 21 | 11.23 | 1 |
| 11.97 | 7 | 12.75 | 16 | 11.28 | 2 |
| 11.53 | 3 | 12.21 | 11 | 12.89 | 17 |
| 11.82 | 6 | 13.32 | 19 | 12.46 | 13 |
| 11.75 | 5 | 13.60 | 20 | 12.56 | 15 |
| 12.25 | 12 | | | 11.69 | 4 |
| 12.16 | 9 | | | | |
| Σ = | 68 | | 101 | | 62 |

ranks for each of the $k$ levels of the independent variable, dividing those by their respective number of observations and then summing these $k$ results. The decision rule in this test is to compare the calculated Kruskal-Wallis H-statistic with a $\chi^2$-critical value from Table B15 in Appendix B. The degrees of freedom is based on the number of levels of the discrete independent variable minus one for bias ($K - 1$).

For an example of the Kruskal-Wallis test, assume that three instruments located in different laboratories were compared to determine if all three instruments could be used for the same assay (Table 21.4). Is there a significant difference based on the results (mg/tablet) seen in Table 21.4? The hypotheses are:

$H_0$: Samples are from the same population
(no difference between instruments)
$H_1$: Samples are drawn from different populations

The decision rule is: with $\alpha = .05$, reject $H_0$, if $H > \chi^2_{k-1}(.95)$. With three discrete levels in our independent variable, the number of degrees of freedom is two and $\chi^2_2$ equals 5.99. The calculations are as follows:

$$H = \frac{12}{N(N+1)}\left[\Sigma\frac{(\Sigma R_{ij})^2}{n_j}\right] - 3(N+1)$$

$$H = \frac{12}{21(22)}\left[\frac{(68)^2}{8} + \frac{(101)^2}{6} + \frac{(62)^2}{7}\right] - 3(22)$$

$$H = 0.026(578.5 + 1700.2 + 549.1) - 66 = 7.52$$

The decision in this case, with $H > 5.99$, is to reject $H_0$ and conclude that there is a significant difference among the three pieces of equipment and they are not equal in their assay results.

Some statisticians (i.e., Zar, p. 198) recommend a correction for ties (sharing of the same ranks) in the data, especially when there are a large number of such ties. This correction factor is:

$$C = 1 - \left[ \frac{\Sigma(t^3 - t)}{N^3 - N} \right] \quad \text{Eq. 21.9}$$

For example four sets of pair ties, and three sets of triplicate ties are:

$$4\left|(2)^3 - 2\right| + 3\left|(3)^3 - 3\right|$$

$N$ equals the total number of observations. In this particular example, the correction would be as follows:

$$C = 1 - \left[ \frac{4[(2)^3 - 2] + 3[(3)^3 - 3]}{(21)^3 - 21} \right]$$

$$C = 1 - \frac{96}{9240} = 1 - 0.0104 = 0.9896$$

The corrected $H$ statistic ($H'$) is:

$$H' = \frac{H}{C} \quad \text{Eq. 21.10}$$

since the denominator will be less than 1, this correction will give a slightly higher value than the original $H$ statistic. The decision rule is to reject $H_0$, if $H'$ is greater than $\chi^2_{K-1}(1 - \alpha)$, which is the chi square value from Table B15. In the example above, $H'$ is:

$$H' = \frac{7.52}{0.9896} = 7.60$$

In most cases the adjustment is negligible. Unlike Yates corrections, which produce a more conservative test statistic, the correction for ties produced a number more likely to find a significant difference, thus a more conservative approach would be to use the original $H$-statistic.

### *Post hoc* Comparisons Using Kruskal-Wallis

The Kruskal-Wallis *post hoc* comparison is a parallel to the Tukey test (Chapter 11) and uses the $q$-statistic for pair-wise differences between ranked sums. In this test, the numerator is the difference between the two sums of ranks ($\Sigma R_{ij}$) and the denominator represents is a new standard error term. For equal numbers of observations per $k$-levels of the independent variable, the formula is as follows:

$$q = \frac{R_A - R_B}{\sqrt{\dfrac{n(nk)(nk+1)}{12}}} \qquad \text{Eq. 21.11}$$

Since only pair-wise comparisons can be performed, $R_A$ is the sum of the ranks for the first level and $R_B$ is the sum of the ranks for the second level of the independent variable. If the cell sizes are not equal the formula is adjusted as follows:

$$q = \frac{R_A - R_B}{\sqrt{\dfrac{N(N+1)}{12}\left(\dfrac{1}{n_A} + \dfrac{1}{n_B}\right)}} \qquad \text{Eq. 21.12}$$

It can be further modified to correct for ties

$$q = \frac{R_A - R_B}{\sqrt{\dfrac{N(N+1)}{12} - \dfrac{\sum T}{12(N-1)}\left(\dfrac{1}{n_A} + \dfrac{1}{n_B}\right)}} \qquad \text{Eq. 21.13}$$

where:

$$\sum T = \sum_{i=1}^{m}(t_i^3 - t_i) \qquad \text{Eq. 21.14}$$

To illustrate this test, consider the significant results identified with the previous Kruskal-Wallis test evaluating the results produced by three analytical instruments, where the sum of ranks and $n$'s were as follows:

| Instrument | ΣR | n |
|---|---|---|
| A | 68 | 8 |
| B | 101 | 6 |
| C | 62 | 7 |
| | N = | 21 |

**Table 21.5** Results of Kruskal-Wallis *post hoc* Comparisons

| Pairing | q-statistic | Critical Value | Results |
|---|---|---|---|
| $R_A - R_B$ | −9.85 | 3.61 | Significant |
| $R_A - R_C$ | 1.87 | 3.61 | |
| $R_B - R_C$ | 11.30 | 3.61 | Significant |

Since the sample sizes differ per instrument and there were no tied ranks, Eq. 21.12 will be used for the three possible pair-wise comparisons. Comparing Instrument A and B, the result for this *post hoc* procedure is:

$$q = \frac{68-101}{\sqrt{\frac{21(21+1)}{12}\left(\frac{1}{8}+\frac{1}{6}\right)}} = \frac{-33}{3.351} = -9.85$$

The interpretation of significance uses the same procedure discussed for the *q*-statistic in Chapter 11. If $q > q_{\alpha,k,N-k}$ of $q < -q_{\alpha,k,N-k}$ from Table B10 (Appendix B), reject the hypothesis of no difference between the two levels being compared. The results of all three pair-wise comparisons are presented in Table 21.5.

**Friedman Two-Way Analysis of Variance**

The Friedman procedure can be employed for data meeting the design for the complete randomized block design (Chapter 10), but that fail to conform to the criteria for parametric procedures. The hypotheses test for differences in the various treatment levels, controlling for the effects of blocking, is.

$H_0$: No difference in the treatment levels
$H_1$: A difference exists in the treatment levels

The summed ranks are used in the following test statistic:

$$\chi_r^2 = \frac{12}{nk(k+1)}\Sigma(R_j)^2 - 3n(k+1) \qquad \text{Eq. 21.15}$$

Where *k* represents the number of levels of the independent variable (treatments) and *n* is the total number of rows (blocks). Critical values for small sample sizes (i.e., less than five blocks or rows) are available (Daniel, 1999). Larger sample sizes can be approximated from the standard chi square table for *k* – 1 degrees of freedom. If the calculated $\chi_r^2$ is greater than the critical $\chi^2$ value (Table B15, Appendix B), $H_0$ is rejected.

**Table 21.6** Results of Three Formulations Administered at Random to Twelve Volunteers

| Subject | Formula A | Formula B | Formula C |
|---|---|---|---|
| 1 | 125 | 149 | 126 |
| 2 | 128 | 132 | 126 |
| 3 | 131 | 142 | 117 |
| 4 | 119 | 136 | 119 |
| 5 | 130 | 151 | 140 |
| 6 | 121 | 141 | 121 |
| 7 | 129 | 130 | 126 |
| 8 | 133 | 138 | 136 |
| 9 | 135 | 130 | 135 |
| 10 | 123 | 129 | 127 |
| 11 | 120 | 122 | 122 |
| 12 | 125 | 140 | 141 |

First, the treatment effect for the blocking variables is calculated by ranking each level of the column variable per row. For example if the column variable consisted of four levels, each row for the blocking variable would be ranked and assigned values 1, 2, 3, and 4 per row. Ties would be averages, similar to previous tests. The data is ranked separately for each row. Then the ranks associated with each column are summed ($R_j$) and applied to Eq. 21.15.

To illustrate this process, assume we are attempting to determine if there is any significant difference between the three formulas. To reduce intersubject variability we administer all three formulations to the same subjects (in a randomized order). The results are presented in Table 21.6. The hypothesis would be as follows:

$H_0$: No difference exists between the two formulations
$H_1$: A difference exists between the two formulations

In this case the decision rule is to reject $H_0$ if the calculated $\chi_r^2$ is greater than $\chi_2^2(.95)$, which equals 5.99 (note that $n$ equals 12, which is large enough to use the critical value from the chi square table). The degrees of freedom for the chi square value is based on $k - 1$ treatment levels. The ranking of the data is presented in Table 21.7 where the responses for each subject (block) is ranked independently of all other subjects. Finally the ranks are summed for each of the treatment levels (columns) and presented at the bottom of Table 21.7. The computation of the $\chi_r^2$ is:

$$\chi_r^2 = \frac{12}{12(3)(4)}[(17.5)^2 + (32.5)^2 + (22)^2] - 3(12)(4)$$

$$\chi_r^2 = (0.0833)(1846.5) - 144 = 9.81$$

**Table 21.7** Example of the Freidman ANOVA for Data in Table 21.6

| | Formula A | | Formula B | | Formula C | |
|---|---|---|---|---|---|---|
| Subject | Data | Rank | Data | Rank | Data | Rank |
| 1 | 125 | 1 | 149 | 3 | 126 | 2 |
| 2 | 128 | 2 | 132 | 3 | 126 | 1 |
| 3 | 131 | 2 | 142 | 3 | 117 | 1 |
| 4 | 119 | 1.5 | 136 | 3 | 119 | 1.5 |
| 5 | 130 | 1 | 151 | 3 | 140 | 2 |
| 6 | 121 | 1.5 | 141 | 3 | 121 | 1.5 |
| 7 | 129 | 2 | 130 | 3 | 126 | 1 |
| 8 | 133 | 1 | 138 | 3 | 136 | 2 |
| 9 | 135 | 2.5 | 130 | 1 | 135 | 2.5 |
| 10 | 123 | 1 | 129 | 3 | 127 | 2 |
| 11 | 120 | 1 | 122 | 2.5 | 122 | 2.5 |
| 12 | 125 | 1 | 140 | 2 | 141 | 3 |
| $\Sigma =$ | | 17.5 | | 32.5 | | 22 |

Therefore, with the calculated $\chi_r^2$ greater than 5.99 we would reject $H_0$ and assume that there is a significant difference between formulations A, B, and C.

## Spearman Rank-Order Correlation

A **rank correlation coefficient** is a special type of bivariate correlation coefficient for relating two ordinal scaled variables. The Spearman rank-order correlation (also referred to as **Spearman rho**) is an example of a rank correlation coefficient. Similar to other nonparametric tests, this procedure ranks the observations, but each variable ($x$ and $y$) is ranked individually and then the difference between the two ranks becomes part of the test statistic. As seen in the following example, a table (similar to Table 21.8) is created and the sum of the differences squared is inserted into the following formula:

$$\rho = 1 - \frac{6(\sum d^2)}{n^3 - n} \qquad \text{Eq. 21.16}$$

Unlike the correlation coefficient, which is concerned with the means for both the $x$ and $y$ variables, here the investigator is interested in the correlation between the rankings.

To illustrate this process the previous data regarding volunteer heights and weights (Table 13.2) will once again be used. The results of the ranking process for each continuous variable are presented in Table 21.8. The computation for the Spearman rho is:

**Table 21.8** Sample Data for Spearman Correlation

| | Observed | | Ranked | | | |
|---|---|---|---|---|---|---|
| Subject | Wgt. | Hgt. | Wgt. | Hgt. | D | $D^2$ |
| 1 | 96.0 | 1.88 | 5 | 6 | −1 | 1 |
| 2 | 77.7 | 1.80 | 2 | 3 | −1 | 1 |
| 3 | 100.9 | 1.85 | 6 | 5 | 1 | 1 |
| 4 | 79.0 | 1.77 | 3 | 2 | 1 | 1 |
| 5 | 73.0 | 1.73 | 1 | 1 | 0 | 0 |
| 6 | 84.5 | 1.83 | 4 | 4 | 0 | 0 |
| | | | | | $\sum d^2 =$ | 4 |

$$\rho = 1 - \frac{6(\sum d^2)}{n^3 - n} = 1 - \frac{6(4)}{6^3 - 6} = 1 - \frac{24}{210} = 0.886$$

A perfect positive or a perfect negative correlation will both produce a $\sum d^2 = 0$; therefore, the result will always be a positive number. Thus, this procedure does not indicate the direction of the relationship. However, because the Spearman rho is used for small data sets, information can be quickly plotted on graph paper and the resulting scatter plot will indicate if the correlation is positive or negative. If the two continuous variables are normally distributed, the Pearson's correlation coefficient is more powerful than the test for Spearman's rank correlation. Spearman's statistic is useful when one of the variables is not normally distributed, if ordinal scales are involved or if the sample sizes are very small.

**Kendall's coefficient of concordance** is another nonparametric procedure for comparing two or more ordinal variables. Data is ranked for each variable and the strength of the agreement between variables is assessed based on a chi square distribution. The test statistic is:

$$W = \frac{\sum R_i^2 - \frac{(\sum R_i)^2}{n}}{\frac{M^2(n^3 - n)}{12}}$$

where $M$ in the number of ranked variables and $n$ is the number of observations for each variable. This coefficient can also be used to evaluation the agreement among two or more evaluators or raters (see interrated reliability in Chapter 17). **Kendall's tau** tests (Chapter 17) could also be used for rank-order correlations. However, it is felt that the Spearman correlation is a better procedure (Zar, p .395) and for a larger $n$, Spearman is easier to calculate. More information about these latter tests can be found in Bradley (1968).

**Theil's Incomplete Method**

As discussed in Chapter 14, linear regression models assume that the dependent variable is normally distributed. If the $y$-variable is not normally distributed, several nonparametric approaches can be used to fit a straight line through the set of data points. Possibly the simplest method is Theil's "incomplete" method.

As with most nonparametric procedures, the first step is to rank the points in ascending order for the values of $x$. If the number of points is odd, the middle point (the median) is deleted, thus creating an even number of data points that is required for the test. Data points are then paired based on their order (the smallest with the smallest above the median, the second smallest with second smallest above the median) until the last pairing represents the largest $x$-value below the median with the overall largest $x$-value.

For any pair of points, where $x_j > x_i$, the slope, $b_{ij}$, of a straight line joining the two points can be calculated as follows:

$$b_{ij} = \frac{(y_j - y_i)}{(x_j - x_i)} \qquad \text{Eq. 21.17}$$

These paired slope estimates are themselves ranked in ascending order and the median value becomes the estimated slope of the straight line that best fits all the data points. This estimated value of $b$ is inserted into the straight line equation ($y = a + bx$) for each data point and each corresponding intercept is calculated ($a = y - bx$) for each line. These intercepts are then arranged in ascending order and the median value is used as the best estimate of the intercept.

As an example, consider the following. During an early Phase I clinical trial of a new therapeutic agent the following AUCs (area under the curve) were observed at different dosages of the formulation. The data is already rank ordered by the $x$-variable.

| Dosage (mg) | AUC (hr·μg/ml) |
|---|---|
| 100 | 1.07 |
| 300 | 5.82 |
| 600 | 15.85 |
| 900 | 25.18 |
| 1200 | 33.12 |

Because there are an odd number of measurements ($n = 5$) the median value is removed from the data base:

| Point | Dosage | AUC |
|---|---|---|
| 1 | 100 | 1.07 |
| 2 | 300 | 5.82 |
| | ~~600~~ | ~~15.85~~ |
| 3 | 900 | 25.18 |
| 4 | 1200 | 33.12 |

The slopes of the two lines are then calculated by the pairings of points 1 and 3, and 2 and 4. These slopes are:

$$b_{13} = \frac{25.18 - 1.07}{900 - 100} = \frac{24.11}{800} = 0.0301$$

$$b_{24} = \frac{33.12 - 5.82}{1200 - 300} = \frac{27.3}{900} = 0.0303$$

The median slope ($b$) is the average of the two slopes (0.0302). This measure is then placed in the formula for a straight line and the intercept is calculated for all three pairings.

$$a = y - bx$$

$$a_1 = 1.07 - (0.0302)(100) = -1.95$$

$$a_2 = 5.82 - (0.0302)(300) = -3.24$$

$$a_3 = 25.18 - (0.0302)(900) = -2.00$$

$$a_4 = 33.12 - (0.0302)(1200) = -3.12$$

The new intercept is the median for these four calculations, which is the average of the third and fourth ranked values:

$$Median\ \ intercept\,(a) = \frac{(-2.00) + (-3.12)}{2} = -2.56$$

These results are slightly different than the slope (0.0299) and intercept (–2.33) if calculated using a traditional linear regression model.

Theil's method offers three advantages over traditional regression analysis: 1) it does not assume that errors are solely in the $y$-direction; 2) it does not assume that the populations for either the $x$- or $y$-variables are normally distributed; and 3) it is not affected by extreme values (outliers). With respect to the last point, in the traditional least-squares calculation, an outlier might carry more weight than the other points and this is avoided with Theil's incomplete method.

**Kolmogorov-Smirnov Goodness-of-Fit Test**

The Kolmogorov-Smirnov test (**K-S test**) is a nonparametric alternative to the chi square goodness-of-fit (Chapter 16) test when smaller sample sizes are involved. The test is named for two Russian mathematicians (Andrei Nikolaevich Kolmogorov and N.V. Smirnov) who created two similar tests during the 1930s. Smirnov's work focused on the two-sample case to determine if the distributions for two samples were taken from the same population. This is sometimes referred to as the **Kolmogorov-Smirnov two-sample test.** A.N. Kolmogorov's work addressed the one-sample case and the determination if the sample data was distributed according to the expectations of the population distribution. The test is referred to as the **Kolmogorov-Smirnov one-sample test** or **Kolmogorov goodness-of-fit test.**

The one-sample K-S test can be used to decide if the distribution of sample data comes from a population with a specific distribution (i.e., normal or skewed distribution). Two cumulative distribution functions are compared to determine if there is a significant difference between them. Distribution functions are compared for given values of *x*, on both distributions. The first is the distribution of interest where the probability of a random value being equal to or less than x is defined as $F_0(x)$. Sample data are collected and this second observed or **empirical distribution function**, *S(x)*, is the best estimate of the distribution *F(x)* from which the sample was taken. The magnitude of the difference between these two functions is used to determine where $H_0$ should be rejected. The hypotheses for these would be:

$H_0$: $F(x) = F_0(x)$ for all values of x
The data follow a specified distribution

$H_1$: $F(x) \neq F_0(x)$ for at least one value of x
The data do not follow the specified distribution

The sample distribution function *S(x)*, being the best estimate of *F(x)*, is used to determine the cumulative probability function for any given value of *x*:

$$S(x) = \frac{number\ of\ sample\ observations \leq x}{n} \qquad \text{Eq. 21.18}$$

Similarly, the probabilities $F_0(x)$ are calculated for the same points (*x*) of the proposed distribution to which the sample is being compared. For a two-sided test, the test statistic is:

$$D = sup\left|S(x) - F_0(x)\right| \qquad \text{Eq. 21.19}$$

Where *sup* is the supremum value or that point where the absolute difference is greatest. If the two distributions are presented graphically, *D* is the greatest vertical

**Table 21.9** Comparison of Sample Data to Expected Population Distribution

| % LC | z-value | $F_0(x)$ $p \leq$ %LC | S(x) $P \leq$ %LC | $\lvert S(x) - F_0(x)\rvert$ |
|---|---|---|---|---|
| 90 | −1.667 | 0.048 | | |
| 91 | −1.500 | 0.067 | 0.100 | 0.033 |
| 92 | −1.333 | 0.091 | | |
| 93 | −1.167 | 0.122 | 0.200 | 0.078 |
| 94 | −1.000 | 0.159 | | |
| 95 | −0.833 | 0.202 | | |
| 96 | −0.667 | 0.252 | | |
| 97 | −0.500 | 0.309 | 0.300 | 0.009 |
| 98 | −0.333 | 0.369 | | |
| 99 | −0.167 | 0.434 | 0.400 | 0.034 |
| 100 | 0.000 | 0.500 | 0.600 | 0.100 |
| 101 | 0.167 | 0.566 | 0.700 | 0.134 |
| 102 | 0.333 | 0.631 | 0.800 | 0.169 |
| 103 | 0.500 | 0.691 | | |
| 104 | 0.667 | 0.748 | | |
| 105 | 0.833 | 0.798 | 0.900 | 0.102 |
| 106 | 1.000 | 0.841 | | |
| 107 | 1.167 | 0.878 | | |
| 108 | 1.333 | 0.909 | | |
| 109 | 1.500 | 0.933 | 1.000 | 0.067 |
| 110 | 1.667 | 0.952 | | |

difference between $S(x)$ and $F_0(x)$. The $D$-value is compared to the critical values presented in Table B16 in Appendix B. If $D$ exceeds the critical value based on the number of sample observations, there is a significant difference between the two distributions and $H_0$ is rejected.

As an example, ten samples are taken from the batch or a particular pharmaceutical and assayed. The results, reported as percent label claim, are 101, 93, 97, 100, 109,102, 100, 99, 91, and 105 percent. Based on historical data it is assumed that a batch of this product is normally distributed with a mean of 100% label claim and a standard deviation of 6%. Does the sample come from our expected population (have distribution characteristics of a batch of this drug)? If both the population batch and sample are expected to be normally distributed we can use Eq. 6.3 to estimate the $z$-value for any percent label claim and use Table B2 in Appendix to determine the proportion of the results that should be below or equal to that point on the curve. The $S(x)$ is calculated using Eq. 21.18 for the results of the ten samples. These results are presented in Table 21.9. In this example the largest difference (the supremum) is:

$$D = sup\lvert 0.800 - 0.631\rvert = 0.169$$

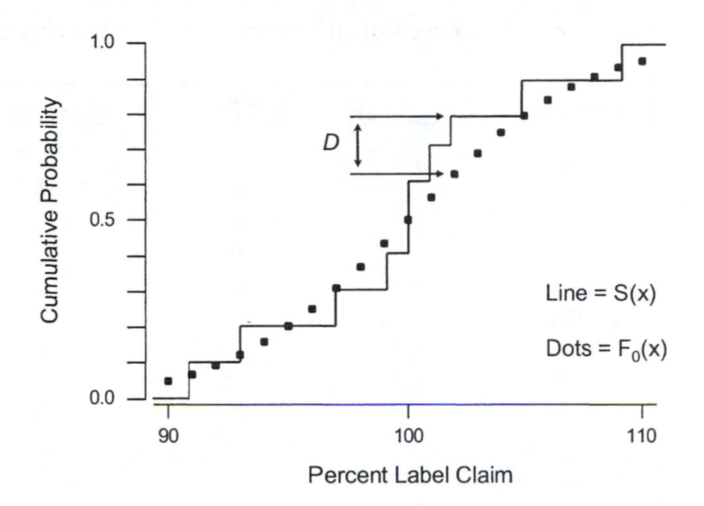


**Figure 21.1** Illustration of a comparison between sample and predicted population distributions.

Using Table B16, *D* is less than the critical value of 0.409; therefore, we fail to reject the null hypothesis and assume our sample data comes from the same distribution we would expect for our batch of drug. This result can be graphically represented as seen in Figure 21.1.

The previous example assumed a normal distribution. One advantage of the K-S test is that it does not depend on the underlying cumulative distribution function being tested. Also, it is an exact test (the chi square goodness-of-fit test depends on an adequate sample size for the approximations to be valid). Often the K-S test is preferred to the chi square for interval data and may be more powerful. However, despite these advantages, the test has limitations: 1) it applies to continuous distributions only, including ordinal scales; 2) it appears to be more sensitive near the center of the distribution and not at the tails; and 4) the entire distribution must be specified. The last limitation is the most serious and if the location, scale, and shape of the distribution are estimated based on the data, the critical region of the K-S test may no longer be valid. Due to this and the less sensitivity at the tails of the distribution, some statisticians prefer using the Anderson-Darling test, which is discussed below.

As mentioned, the **Kolmogorov-Smirnov two-sample test** is available to test if two sample sets or two levels of a discrete independent variable come from the same distribution (same population). This test is based on the previously mentioned work of Smirnov. In this test we have two independent samples from ordinal or higher scales and we compare two empirical distributions, $F_1(x)$ and $F_2(x)$ and the hypotheses are:

$$H_0: \quad F_1(x) = F_2(x) \text{ for all values of x}$$

$$H_1: \quad F_1(x) \neq F_2(x) \text{ for at least one value of x}$$

**Table 21.10** Comparison of Two Levels of an Independent Variable Using the K-S Test

| Control | Experimental | $p \le F_1(x)$ | $P \le F_2(x)$ | $\lvert F_1(x) - F_2(x) \rvert$ |
|---|---|---|---|---|
| 0.6067 | | 1/7 | 0 | 1/7 |
| 0.7184 | | 2/7 | 0 | 2/7 |
| 0.7974 | | 3/7 | 0 | 3/7 |
| 0.8762 | | 4/7 | 0 | 4/7 |
| 1.0422 | | 5/7 | 0 | 5/7 |
| | 1.0475 | 5/7 | 1/7 | 4/7 |
| | 1.0632 | 5/7 | 2/7 | 3/7 |
| | 1.0990 | 5/7 | 3/7 | 2/7 |
| 1.1268 | | 6/7 | 3/7 | 3/7 |
| 1.3590 | | 7/7 | 3/7 | 4/7 |
| | 1.4411 | 7/7 | 4/7 | 3/7 |
| | 1.6022 | 7/7 | 5/7 | 2/7 |
| | 1.7695 | 7/7 | 6/7 | 1/7 |
| | 2.7831 | 7/7 | 7/7 | 0 |

The best estimates for the population distributions are the sample results, $S_1(x)$ and $S_2(x)$. Calculated similarly to the one-sample, case each $S(x)$ is based on the number of observation at given point and the probability of being equal to or less than that value.

As an example, consider the Mann-Whitney U example previously presented comparing control group to animals receiving atropine and the amount of ACH being released (Table 21.1). In this particular example there are seven observations in each level for a total of 14 results. The data are presented in Table 21.10 where the fractions of results being equal to or below each given point are expressed for each level of the independent variable and the differences between these fractions are presented in the last column. Once again, the supremum (or largest difference) is identified and compared to the critical values on Table B17.

$$D = sup\lvert F_1(x) - F_2(x)\rvert \qquad \text{Eq. 21.20}$$

In this case the $D$ is 5/7 and equals the critical value of 5/7 on Table B17. Since it does not exceed the critical value, we would fail to reject the null hypotheses and, unlike the Mann-Whitney results, assume the two distributions are the same.

## Anderson-Darling Test

The Anderson-Darling test is a modification of the Kolmogorov-Smirnov test to determine if sample data came from a population with a specific distribution. Where Kolmogorov-Smirnov is distribution-free, the Anderson-Darling test makes use of the specific distribution in calculating critical values and is a more sensitive test. The

Anderson-Darling test can be used as an alternative to the either the chi square or Kolmogorov-Smirnov goodness-of-fit tests. The critical values for the Anderson-Darling test are dependent on the specific distribution that is being tested (i.e., normal, lognormal, or logistic distributions). The statistic for the Anderson-Darling is:

$$A_n^2 = -n - n^{-1}\sum(2i-1)[ln(P_i) + ln(1-P_{n+1-i})] \qquad \text{Eq. 21.21}$$

where, in the case of a normal distribution, $P_i$ is the probability that the standard normal distribution is less than $(x_i - \overline{X}/s)$. Even though it is possible to calculate the Anderson-Darling statistic, it is more convenient to use computer software designed to do the calculation. To interpretation of the results, the larger the $A_n^2$, the less likely the data comes from a normally distributed population.

## Runs Tests

A runs test can be used to evaluate the randomness of sample data. As indicated in Chapter 8 random sampling is a requirement for all inferential statistics. If a sample fails the runs test, it indicates that there are unusual, non-random periods in the order with which the sample was collected. It is used in studies where measurements are made according to some well defined sequence (either in time or space). A **run** is defined as a sequence of identical events that is preceded and followed by an event of a different type, or by nothing at all (in a sequence of events this latter condition would apply to the first and last event). There are two different types of runs: 1) for continuous data it refers to the values in a consecutively increasing or decreasing order; or 2) in the case of dichotomous results if refers to consecutive data points with the same value. In the former case the test addresses the question of whether the average value of the measurement is different at different points in the sequence and a run is defined dichotomously as a series of increasing values or decreasing values. The number of increasing values or decreasing values is defined as the length of the run. If the data set is random, the probability that the $(n + 1)$th value is larger or smaller than the $n$th value will follows a binomial distribution. The runs test is usually not as powerful as the Kolmogorov test or chi square test.

As an example of a dichotomous outcome and to illustrate defining a run as the number of consecutive identical results, we could record the results for a series of coin tosses. A run would be consecutive heads or consecutive tails. Assume the result of 20 tosses is as follows:

HHTTTHTHHHHTTHTTTHTH

In this case, the first run is two heads, followed by a second run of three tails, followed by a run of one head, etc. Using spacing we can see that our 20 tosses represent 11 runs:

HH TTT H T HHHH TT H TTT H T H

The statistical test will be a determination if the outcome of 11 runs is acceptable for a random set of data or if 11 runs too few or too many runs for a random process. For example, assume ten volunteers in a clinical trial are assigned to either a control or experimental group. We would hope that the assignment is at random; however, if there are only two runs based on the sequence within which the volunteers were enrolled (CCCCCEEEEE) one must question the randomization process since the number of runs is so small. Similarly randomization would be questionable if there were 10 runs (CECECECECE). Both scenarios appear to involve systematic assignment patterns, not random assignment.

Such runs tests could be used in quality control procedures (Chapter 7) where the sequential results are recorded as above or below the target value or in regression analysis (Chapter 14) where the residuals about the regression live would be expected to be above or below the line-of-best fit at random. In the later case if there were too few or too many runs, it might indicate that the relationship is not linear.

A **one-sample runs** test is illustrated by the previous coin-tossing experiment. Where we are considering whether a sequence of events are the result of a random process. In the case the hypotheses are:

$H_0$: The pattern of occurrence is determined by a random process
$H_1$: The pattern of occurrences is not random

To test the null hypothesis, observation are recorded for two mutually exclusive outcomes, $N$ is the total sample size, $n_1$ is the number of observations for the first type, and $n_2$ is the number of observations for the second type. The test statistic is $r$, the total number of runs. Using our previous example of coin tosses the results would be: $N = 20$, $n_1 = 10$ (heads), $n_2 = 10$ (tails) and $r = 11$. There are several formulas for runs test in the literature; we will use the simple approach of referring to a table of critical values for the number of runs, based on the sample size. This table developed by Swed and Eisenbar at the University of Wisconsin is presented as Table B18 in Appendix B. Using this table, if the number of runs exceeds the number in the fourth column in each section or is less than the number in the third column in each section, the $H_0$ is rejected. Note that this is a two-tailed test, modifications can be made to test for one-tailed tests (Daniel, 1978, pp. 54,55).

When either $n_1$ or $n_2$ exceed 20 observations the following formula can be used for large samples:

$$z = \frac{r - \left( \frac{2n_1 n_2}{n_1 + n_2} + 1 \right)}{\sqrt{\frac{2n_1 n_2 (2n_1 n_2 - n_1 - n_2)}{(n_1 + n_2)^2 (n_1 + n_2 - 1)}}} \qquad \text{Eq. 21.22}$$

The distribution approximates the standard normal distribution in Table B2 in Appendix B, and interpretation can be made by rejecting the $H_0$ if the absolute $z$-value exceeds he critical value of $z_{1-\alpha/2}$.

The **Wald-Wolfowitz runs test** is a nonparametric procedure to test that two samples come from the same population (similar to the Mann-Whitney U test) with the same distribution. The test evaluated the number of runs to determine if the samples come from identical populations:

$H_0$: The two samples come from identically distributed populations
$H_1$: The two samples are not from identically distributed populations

If these are too few runs (runs in this case being consecutive observations from the same level) it suggests that the two samples come from different populations. It is assumed that the samples are independent and the dependent variable is measured on a continuous scale.

Once again the test statistic is $r$ for the number of runs presented in both levels of the independent variable. The observations from the two samples (or levels of an independent variable) are ranked from smallest to largest regardless of level. However, it is important to keep track which level the sample represents. For this particular test we will use $A$ to denote the first level and $B$ for the second. As an example, let us use the data already used for the Mann-Whitney test and presented in Table 21.1. In this table the ranking has already been preformed, but here we will count the runs associated with the control ($A$) and atropine ($B$) groups:

| 0.6067 | 0.7184 | 0.7974 | 0.8762 | 1.0422 | 1.0475 | 1.0632 |
|---|---|---|---|---|---|---|
| A | A | A | A | A | B | B |
| 1.0990 | 1.1268 | 1.3590 | 1.4411 | 1.6022 | 1.7695 | 2.7831 |
| B | A | A | B | B | B | B |

In this case the $r = 4$ runs (AAAAA BBB AA BBBB) and $n_1 = 7$ and $n_2 = 7$. Using Table B18 in Appendix B. It would require less than four or more than 12 runs to reject the null hypothesis that the two samples came from identical populations. Once again the values in Table B18 represent a two-tailed test.

Unfortunately, runs tests have very little power (Conover, 1999) and in both one-sample and two-sample cases can be replaced by more powerful nonparametric procedures, the K-S goodness-of-fit and Mann-Whitney U test, respectively.

**Range Tests**

Although not really considered nonparametric tests, there are several quick and useful tests that can be performed using the range(s) for experimental data. In previous chapters, the standard deviation has been used as the most common measure of dispersion. For these procedures the **whole range** ($w$) of the sample is used (the difference between the largest and smallest observation). They are not considered nonparametric, because the sample means are involved in the calculations; therefore, the populations from which the samples are taken are assumed to be normally distributed.

The first test is a simple **range test**, which can be used instead of a one-sample t-test. In this case the results of a sample are evaluated to determine if it comes from a given population.

$$H_0: \ \overline{X} = \mu_0$$
$$H_1: \ \overline{X} \neq \mu_0$$

As with previous tests, a ratio is established with the numerator representing the difference between the observed (sample mean, $\overline{X}$) and the expected (population mean, $\mu_0$). The denominator represents a measure of dispersion (the range, $w$).

$$T_I = \frac{|\overline{X} - \mu_0|}{w} \qquad \text{Eq. 21.23}$$

The calculated $T_I$ is then compared to a critical value presented in Table B19 in Appendix B. If the calculated $T_I$ is greater than the critical table value, $H_O$ is rejected and a significant difference is assumed to exist between the sample and proposed population. As an example, assume that a dissolution test for a specific drug, under specific conditions (media, equipment, and paddle speed) is expected to be 75% at ten minutes. During one test the following values were observed: 73, 69, 73, 73, 67, and 76%. With the resultant sample mean of 71.8 and range of 9 (76 – 67). Do these results vary significantly from the expected dissolution result ($\mu_0$) of 75%?

$$T_I = \frac{|71.8 - 75|}{9} = \frac{3.2}{9} = 0.356$$

The calculated $T_I$ of 0.356 does not exceed the critical $T_I$-value of 0.399, therefore the null hypothesis cannot be rejected.

Similar to the one-sample t-test, a confidence interval can also be constructed using the same information and the critical value from Table B19, Appendix B.

$$\mu_0 = \overline{X} \pm T_{cv,n}(w) \qquad \text{Eq. 21.24}$$

This interval is equivalent to that previously described as Eq. 7.4:

$$\begin{matrix}\textit{Population} \\ \textit{mean}\end{matrix} = \begin{matrix}\textit{Estimated} \\ \textit{Sample mean}\end{matrix} \pm \begin{matrix}\textit{Reliability} \\ \textit{Coefficient}\end{matrix} \ x \ \begin{matrix}\textit{Standard} \\ \textit{Error}\end{matrix}$$

Using the same dissolution sample data, we can create a confidence interval for the population from which our six tablets were sampled at 10 minutes:

$$\mu_0 = 71.8 \pm 0.399(9) = 71.8 \pm 3.59$$

$$68.21 < \mu_0 < 75.39$$

The expected population value of 75% falls within the interval and produces the same result: failure to reject the null hypothesis.

A second range test, the **Lord's range test**, can be used as a parallel to the two-sample t-test. Here two sample means are compared to determine if they are equal:

$$H_0: \ \mu_A = \mu_B$$
$$H_1: \ \mu_A \neq \mu_B$$

Similar to the two-sample t-test a ratio is established with the difference between the means in the numerator and the degree of dispersion controlled in the denominator. In this case we substitute $w_1$ and $w_2$ for $S_1$ and $S_2$:

$$L = \frac{|\overline{X}_1 - \overline{X}_2|}{\frac{(w_1 + w_2)}{2}} \qquad \text{Eq. 21.25}$$

Here the calculated $L$-value is compared to the critical $T_I$-value in Table B19 in Appendix B. If the resultant value is greater than the critical value the null hypothesis is rejected. In this case it is also assumed that the dispersions are similar for the two samples.

To illustrate this, consider problem 4 at the end of Chapter 9. Samples are taken from a specific batch of drug and randomly divided into two groups of tablets. One group is assayed by the manufacturer's own quality control laboratories. The second group of tablets is sent to a contract laboratory for identical analysis. Is there a significant difference between the results generated by the two labs? The means for manufacturer's lab and contact lab were 99.83 and 98.95, respectively. The range of observations for the manufacturer's data is 2.4 (101.1 – 98.7) and the contract lab range is 3.6 (101.1 – 97.5). Note first that the dispersions are fairly similar: 2.4 versus 3.6 and the sample sizes are equal $n_m = n_{cl}$. The critical value from Table B19 for $n$ = 6 at $\alpha = 0.05$ is 0.399. The calculation of Lord's range test is as follows:

$$L = \frac{|99.83 - 98.95|}{(2.4 + 3.6)} = \frac{0.88}{6} = 0.15$$

The resultant 0.15 does not exceed the critical value of 0.399; therefore, we fail to reject $H_O$ of equality and assume that the results are similar for both laboratories. These are the same results found in the answer to this problem at the end of Chapter 9.

Another quick test using ranges is associated with a test for the homogeneity of variance. This can be used to replace the $F_{max}$ or Cochran C test, discussed in Chapter 10, for comparisons of the spreads of two sets of data. For the range test $F_R$ is computed using the following formula:

$$F_R = \frac{w_1}{w_2} \text{ or } \frac{w_2}{w_1} \qquad \text{Equ. 21.26}$$

whichever ratio is greater than 1 is compared to the critical value in Table B20, Appendix B. The sample size should be equal for both samples and if the computer $F_R$-value is greater than the critical table value then the hypothesis of equal dispersions is rejected. Using the previous example of the contract laboratory, we can test to see if ranges 2.4 and 3.6 represent similar dispersions.

$$F_R = \frac{w_2}{w_1} = \frac{3.6}{2.4} = 1.5$$

With $n$ = 6 associated with both the numerator and denominator ranges, the critical value from Table B20 is 2.8 for a two-tailed test. Because the $F_R$ is less than 2.8 we fail to reject the hypothesis of equal dispersion.

The last use of a range test is involved with outlier tests. This is discussed under the Dixon Q test in Chapter 23.

**References**

Conover, W.J. (1999). *Practical Nonparametric Statistics*, Third edition, John Wiley and Sons, New York, p. 3.

Daniel, W.W. (1999). *Biostatistics: A Foundation for Analysis in the Health Sciences*, Seventh edition, John Wiley and Sons, New York, pp. 701-706.

Zar, J.H. (1999). *Biostatistical Analysis*, Fourth edition, Prentice-Hall, Englewood Cliffs, NJ.

Bradley, J.V. (1968). *Distribution-free Statistical Tests*, Prentice-Hall, Englewood Cliffs, NJ, pp. 284-287.

**Suggested Supplemental Readings**

Conover, W.J. (1999). *Practical Nonparametric Statistics*, Third edition, John Wiley and Sons, New York.

Daniel, W.W. (1999). *Biostatistics: A Foundation for Analysis in the Health Sciences*, Seventh edition, John Wiley and Sons, New York, pp. 658-719.

Daniel, W.W. (1978). *Applied Nonparametric Statistics*, Houghton Mifflin Company, Boston.

Gibbs, J.D. and Chakraborti, S. (1992). *Nonparametric Statistical Inference*, Marcel Dekker, Inc., New York.

**Example Problems**

Use the appropriate nonparametric test to answer all of the following questions.

1. Two groups of physical therapy patients were subjected to two different treatment regimens. At the end of the study period, patients were evaluated on specific criteria to measure percent of desired range of motion. Do the results listed below indicate a significant difference between the two therapies at the 95% confidence level?

| Group 1 | | | Group 2 | | |
|---|---|---|---|---|---|
| 78 | 88 | 87 | 75 | 84 | 81 |
| 87 | 91 | 65 | 88 | 71 | 86 |
| 75 | 82 | 80 | 93 | 91 | 89 |
| | | | 86 | 79 | |

2. Following training on content uniformity testing, comparisons were made between the analytical result of the newly trained chemist with those of a senior chemist. Samples of four different drugs (compressed tablets) were selected from different batches and assayed by both individuals. The results are presented in Table 21.11.

**Table 21.11** Results of Content Uniformity Testing

| Sample Drug, Batch | New Chemist | Senior Chemist |
|---|---|---|
| A,42 | 99.8 | 99.9 |
| A,43 | 99.6 | 99.8 |
| A,44 | 101.5 | 100.7 |
| B,96 | 99.5 | 100.1 |
| B,97 | 99.2 | 98.9 |
| C,112 | 100.8 | 101.0 |
| C,113 | 98.7 | 97.9 |
| D,21 | 100.1 | 99.9 |
| D,22 | 99.0 | 99.3 |
| D,23 | 99.1 | 99.2 |

3. The absorption of ultraviolet light is compared among three samples. Are there any significant differences between Samples A, B, and C?

| Sample A | Sample B | Sample C |
|---|---|---|
| 7.256 | 7.227 | 7.287 |
| 7.237 | 7.240 | 7.288 |
| 7.229 | 7.257 | 7.271 |
| 7.245 | 7.241 | 7.269 |
| 7.223 | 7.267 | 7.282 |

4. Two scales are used to measure certain analytical outcome. Method A is an established test instrument, while Method B (which has been developed by the researchers) is quicker and easier to complete. Using Spearman's rho, is there a correlation between the two measures?

| Sample | Method A | Method B |
|---|---|---|
| 1 | 66 | 67 |
| 2 | 77 | 75 |
| 3 | 57 | 57 |
| 4 | 59 | 59 |
| 5 | 70 | 69 |
| 6 | 57 | 59 |
| 7 | 55 | 56 |
| 8 | 53 | 51 |
| 9 | 67 | 68 |
| 10 | 72 | 74 |

5. Six healthy male volunteers are randomly assigned to receive a single dose of an experimental anticoagulant at various dosages. Using Theil's incomplete method, define the line that best fits these six data points.

| Subject | Dose (mg) | Prothrombin Time (seconds) |
|---|---|---|
| 1 | 200 | 20 |
| 2 | 180 | 18 |
| 3 | 190 | 19 |
| 4 | 220 | 21 |
| 5 | 210 | 19 |
| 6 | 230 | 20 |

6. Thirty volunteers for a clinical trial are to be randomly divided into two groups of 15 subjects each. Using a random number table the assignments are presented in Table 21.12. Using the runs test, was the process successful?

**Table 21.12** Results of a Randomization Process

| Experimental Group | | | Control Group | | |
|---|---|---|---|---|---|
| 02 | 15 | 23 | 01 | 10 | 20 |
| 05 | 16 | 24 | 03 | 11 | 21 |
| 06 | 18 | 25 | 04 | 13 | 28 |
| 09 | 19 | 26 | 07 | 14 | 29 |
| 12 | 22 | 27 | 08 | 17 | 30 |

Numbers assigned in order of enrollment, 01 to the first volunteer and 30 to the last volunteer.

## Answers to Problems

1. Comparison of two physical therapy regimens.
   Independent variable: two physical therapy regimens (discrete)
   Dependent variable: percent range of motion (ranked to ordinal scale)
   Statistical test: Mann-Whitney U test and Median Test

   a. Mann-Whitney U

   Hypotheses: $H_0$: Samples are from the same population
   $H_1$: Samples are drawn from different populations

   Decision rule: With $\alpha = 0.05$, reject $H_0$, if $|z| >$ critical $z_{(.975)} = 1.96$

   Data: Table 21.13

   Calculations:

$$U = n_1 n_2 + \frac{n_1(n_1+1)}{2} - \sum R_{ij}$$

$$U = (9)(11) + \frac{(9)(10)}{2} - 86.5 = 57.5$$

$$Z = \frac{U - \frac{n_1 n_2}{2}}{\sqrt{\frac{n_1 n_2 \cdot [n_1 + (n_2+1)]}{12}}}$$

**Table 21.13** Data and Ranking Associated with Comparison of Two Groups of Physical Therapy Patients

| Group 1 | Ranks | Group 2 | Ranks |
|---|---|---|---|
| 78 | 5 | 75 | 3.5 |
| 87 | 13.5 | 88 | 15.5 |
| 75 | 3.5 | 93 | 20 |
| 88 | 15.5 | 86 | 11.5 |
| 91 | 18.5 | 84 | 10 |
| 82 | 9 | 71 | 2 |
| 87 | 13.5 | 91 | 18.5 |
| 65 | 1 | 79 | 6 |
| 80 | 7 | 81 | 8 |
| | | 86 | 11.5 |
| | | 89 | 17 |
| ΣR = | 86.5 | ΣR = | 123.5 |

$$Z = \frac{57.5 - \frac{(9)(11)}{2}}{\sqrt{\frac{(9)(11) \cdot [9+12)]}{12}}} = \frac{57.5 - 49.5}{13.16} = 0.61$$

Decision: With z < 1.96, fail to reject $H_0$ and fail to show a significant difference between the two types of physical therapy.

b. Median Test

Median for all the values in both groups:

$$Median = \frac{84+86}{2} = 85$$

| | Group 1 | Group 2 |
|---|---|---|
| Above the median | 4 | 6 |
| Below the median | 5 | 5 |

$$p = \frac{(a+b)!\,(c+d)!\,(a+c)!\,(b+d)!}{n!\,a!\,b!\,c!\,d!}$$

$$p = \frac{10!\,10!\,9!\,11!}{20!\,4!\,6!\,5!\,5!} = \frac{3969}{12597} = 0.315$$

Decision: With $p > 0.05$, fail to reject $H_0$ and fail to show a significant difference between the two types of physical therapy.

2. Comparisons between the analytical results of the newly trained chemist and senior chemist.
   Independent variable: two time periods (each sample serves as own control)
   Dependent variable: assay results (ranked to ordinal scale)
   Test statistic: Wilcoxon matched-pairs test, sign test, or Friedman two-way analysis of variance

   Hypotheses: $H_0$: No difference between the two chemists
   $H_1$: Difference exists between the two chemists

   a. Wilcoxon matched-pairs test

      Decision rule: With $\alpha = 0.05$, reject $H_0$ if $|z| > 1.96$.

      Data: Table 21.14

      Calculations:

$$E(T) = \frac{n(n+1)}{4} = \frac{(10)(11)}{4} = 27.5$$

**Table 21.14** Data and Ranking Associated with Comparison of Two Chemists for the Wilcoxon Matched-Pairs Test

| Sample batch | New chemist | Senior chemist | d | Rank d | Rank associated with least frequent sign |
|---|---|---|---|---|---|
| A,42 | 99.8 | 99.9 | 0.1 | 1.5 | |
| A,43 | 99.6 | 99.8 | 0.2 | 4 | |
| A,44 | 101.5 | 100.7 | −0.8 | 9.5 | 9.5 |
| B,96 | 99.5 | 100.1 | 0.6 | 8 | |
| B,97 | 99.2 | 98.9 | −0.3 | 6.5 | 6.5 |
| C,112 | 100.8 | 101.0 | 0.2 | 4 | |
| C,113 | 98.7 | 97.9 | −0.8 | 9.5 | 9.5 |
| D,21 | 100.1 | 99.9 | −0.2 | 4 | 4 |
| D,22 | 99.0 | 99.3 | 0.3 | 6.5 | |
| D,23 | 99.1 | 99.2 | 0.1 | 1.5 | |
| | | | | | $T = \sum = 29.5$ |

$$Z = \frac{T - E(T)}{\sqrt{\frac{n(n+1)(2n+1)}{24}}}$$

$$Z = \frac{29.5 - 27.5}{\sqrt{\frac{10(11)(21)}{24}}} = \frac{2}{\sqrt{96.25}} = 0.20$$

Decision: Using the Wilcoxon matched-pairs test, the result is a z < 1.96. Thus we fail to reject $H_0$ and fail to show a significant difference in the assay results for the two scientists.

b. Sign test

$H_0$: $p(+) = 0.50$
$H_1$: $p(+) \neq 0.50$

Using the data presented in Table 21.14
Number of negative results = 6
Total number of events = 10

$$p(x) = \binom{n}{x} p^x q^{n-x}$$

$$p(6\ positives) = \binom{10}{6}(.50)^6(.50)^4 = 0.205$$

$$p(7\ positives) = \binom{10}{7}(.50)^7(.50)^3 = 0.117$$

$$p(8\ positives) = \binom{10}{8}(.50)^8(.50)^2 = 0.044$$

$$p(9\ positives) = \binom{10}{9}(.50)^9(.50)^1 = 0.0098$$

$$p(10\ positives) = \binom{10}{10}(.50)^{10}(.50)^0 = 0.00098$$

$$p(\geq 6\ positives) = \Sigma = 0.377$$

**Table 21.15** Data and Ranking Associated with Comparison of Two Chemists for the Friedman Two-Way Analysis of Variance

| | New Chemist | | Senior Chemist | |
|---|---|---|---|---|
| Sample, Batch | Data | Rank | Data | Rank |
| A,42 | 99.8 | 1 | 99.9 | 2 |
| A,43 | 99.6 | 1 | 99.8 | 2 |
| A,44 | 101.5 | 2 | 100.7 | 1 |
| B,96 | 99.5 | 1 | 100.1 | 2 |
| B,97 | 99.2 | 2 | 98.9 | 1 |
| C,112 | 100.8 | 1 | 101.0 | 2 |
| C,113 | 98.7 | 2 | 97.9 | 1 |
| D,21 | 100.1 | 2 | 99.9 | 1 |
| D,22 | 99.0 | 1 | 99.3 | 2 |
| D,23 | 99.1 | 1 | 99.2 | 2 |
| $\Sigma =$ | | 14 | | 16 |

Fail to reject $H_0$ because $p > 0.05$.

c. Friedman two-way analysis of variance - data (Table 21.15)

Decision rule: With $\alpha = 0.05$, reject $\chi_r^2 > \chi_1^2 = 3.84$.

Calculations:

$$\chi_r^2 = \frac{12}{nk(k+1)} \Sigma (R_j)^2 - 3n(k+1)$$

$$\chi_r^2 = \frac{12}{10(2)(3)} [(14)^2 + (16)^2] - 3(10)(3)$$

$$\chi_r^2 = (0.02)(452) - 90 = 0.40$$

Decision: Using the Friedman two-way analysis of variance, the result is a $\chi_1^2 < 3.84$. Thus we fail to reject $H_0$ and fail to show a significant difference in the assay results for the two scientists.

3. Comparison of ultraviolet data for three different samples
   Independent variable: samples (discrete, 3 levels)
   Dependent variable: ultraviolet data (based on continuous scale)
   Statistical test: Kruskal-Wallis

**Table 21.6** Results of Three Formulations Administered at Random to Twelve Volunteers

| Subject | Formula A | Formula B | Formula C |
|---|---|---|---|
| 1 | 125 | 149 | 126 |
| 2 | 128 | 132 | 126 |
| 3 | 131 | 142 | 117 |
| 4 | 119 | 136 | 119 |
| 5 | 130 | 151 | 140 |
| 6 | 121 | 141 | 121 |
| 7 | 129 | 130 | 126 |
| 8 | 133 | 138 | 136 |
| 9 | 135 | 130 | 135 |
| 10 | 123 | 129 | 127 |
| 11 | 120 | 122 | 122 |
| 12 | 125 | 140 | 141 |

Hypothesis:

$H_0$: All three samples are from the same population
$H_1$: All three samples are not from the same population

Decision rule: With $\alpha = 0.05$, reject $H_0$ if $H > \chi^2_2(.95) = 5.99$.

Data: Table 21.16

Calculations:

$$H = \frac{12}{N(N+1)}\left[\Sigma\frac{(\Sigma R_{ij})^2}{n_j}\right] - 3(N+1)$$

$$H = \frac{15}{15(16)}\left[\frac{(23)^2}{5} + \frac{(33)^2}{5} + \frac{(64)^2}{5}\right] - 3(16)$$

$$H = 0.0625(105.8 + 217.8 + 819.2) - 48 = 23.425$$

Decision: With $H > 5.99$, reject $H_0$,conclude that there is a significant difference between the three samples and that they are not from the same population.

*Post hoc* comparison for location(s) of significant difference(s):

Comparison of Sample A and B:

$$q = \frac{R_A - R_B}{\sqrt{\frac{n(nk)(nk+1)}{12}}}$$

$$q = \frac{23 - 33}{\sqrt{\frac{5(5\cdot 3)[(5\cdot 3)+1]}{12}}} = \frac{-10}{10} = -1.0$$

Results for all three Kruskal-Wallis *post hoc* comparisons:

| Pairing | q-statistic | Critical Value | Results |
|---|---|---|---|
| $R_A - R_B$ | −1.0 | 3.73 | |
| $R_A - R_C$ | −4.1 | 3.73 | Significant |
| $R_B - R_C$ | −3.1 | 3.73 | |

Decision: The only significant difference was between Samples A and C.

4. Comparison of results from two analytical methods.
   Independent variable: Continuous (Method A)
   Dependent variable: Continuous (Method B)
   Statistical test: Spearman rho correlation

   Data: Table 21.17

   Computation:

$$\rho = 1 - \frac{6(\Sigma d^2)}{n^3 - n}$$

$$\rho = 1 - \frac{6(9)}{10^3 - 10} = 1 - \frac{54}{990} = .945$$

   Decision: There is a very strong correlation between the two analytical methods. Plotting the data we would see that the correlation is positive.

5. Comparison of various doses of an anticoagulant and prothrombin times.
   Independent variable: dosages (continuous)
   Dependent variable: prothrombin times (continuous)

**Table 21.17** Data and Ranking Associated with Comparison of Two Methods Using the Spearman Rho Test

| | Method A | | Method B | | | |
|---|---|---|---|---|---|---|
| Sample | x | Rank | y | Rank | d | $d^2$ |
| 1 | 66 | 6 | 67 | 6 | 0 | 0 |
| 2 | 77 | 10 | 75 | 10 | 0 | 0 |
| 3 | 57 | 3.5 | 57 | 3 | −0.5 | 0.25 |
| 4 | 59 | 5 | 59 | 4.5 | −0.5 | 0.25 |
| 5 | 70 | 8 | 69 | 8 | 0 | 0 |
| 6 | 57 | 3.5 | 59 | 4.5 | +1 | 1.00 |
| 7 | 55 | 2 | 56 | 2 | 0 | 0 |
| 8 | 53 | 1 | 51 | 1 | 0 | 0 |
| 9 | 67 | 7 | 68 | 7 | 0 | 0 |
| 10 | 72 | 9 | 74 | 9 | 0 | 0 |
| | | | | | Σ = | 1.50 |

Statistical test: Theil's incomplete method

| Subject | Dose (mg) | Prothrombin Time (seconds) |
|---|---|---|
| 2(1) | 180 | 18 |
| 3(2) | 190 | 19 |
| 1(3) | 200 | 20 |
| 5(4) | 210 | 19 |
| 4(5) | 220 | 21 |
| 6(6) | 230 | 20 |

Calculate the median slope:

$$b_{ij} = \frac{(y_j - y_i)}{(x_j - x_i)}$$

$$b_{14} = \frac{19-18}{210-180} = \frac{1}{30} = 0.033$$

$$b_{25} = \frac{21-19}{220-190} = \frac{2}{30} = 0.067$$

$$b_{36} = \frac{20-20}{230-200} = \frac{0}{30} = 0$$

$$Median\ b = 0.033$$

Calculation of the median intercept:

$$a = y - bx$$

$$a_1 = 18 - (0.033)(180) = 12.06$$

$$a_2 = 19 - (0.033)(190) = 12.73$$

$$a_3 = 20 - (0.033)(200) = 13.40$$

$$a_4 = 19 - (0.033)(210) = 12.07$$

$$a_5 = 21 - (0.033)(220) = 13.47$$

$$a_6 = 20 - (0.033)(230) = 12.41$$

$$Median\ \ intercept\ (a) = \frac{(12.41) + (12.73)}{2} = 12.57$$

Line of best fit:

$$y = a + bx = 12.57 + 0.033x$$

6. Runs test to determine if random sampling of volunteers was successful (Table 21.12). The volunteer will be recoded as E (experimental) and C (control) base on the sequence in which they volunteered for the study.

CECCEECCECCECCEECEECCEEEEEECCC

Hypotheses: $H_0$: The pattern of occurrence is determined by a random process
$H_1$: The pattern of occurrences is not random

Decision rule: Table B18, with $n_1$ = 15 and $n_2$ = 15, reject $H_0$ if $r$ is < 11 or > 21.

Spacing the sequence in to runs, there are 15 runs.

C E CC EE CC E CC E CC EE C EE CC EEEEEE CCC

Therefore, we fail to reject $H_0$ and assume that the randomization process was successful.

# 22

# Statistical Tests for Equivalence

Up to this point, most of the statistical tests we have discussed are concerned with null hypotheses stating equality (i.e., $H_0$: $\mu_1 = \mu_2$). These tests were designed to identify significant differences and by rejecting the null hypothesis, prove inequality. As discussed in Chapter 8, when finding a result that is not statistically significant we do not accept the null hypothesis, we simply fail to reject it. The analogy was presented of jurisprudence where the jury will render a verdict of "not guilty," but never "innocent." They failed to prove the client guilty beyond a reasonable doubt. Similarly, if our data fails to show a statistically significant difference exists, we do not prove equivalency. But what if we do want to show equality or at least similarity with a certain degree of confidence?

To address this topic several tests will be presented that are commonly used for bioequivalence testing in pharmacy and a relatively recent approach in clinical trials referred to as noninferiority studies. In the former case, if we produce a new generic product, is it the same as the originator's product? Are we producing the same product from batch to batch, or are there significant variations between batches of our drug product? In the latter case, the FDA and other agencies are asking manufacturers to prove that their new therapeutic agents are at least as good as existing agents and not inferior. The tests presented in this chapter will help answer these questions.

### Bioequivalence Testing

In order for an oral or injectable product to be effective it must reach the site of action in a concentration large enough to exert its effect. Bioavailability indicates the rate and/or amount of active drug ingredient that is absorbed from the product and available at the site of action. *Remington: The Science and Practice of Pharmacy* (Malinowski, p. 995) defines bioequivalence as an indication "that a drug in two or more similar dosage forms reaches the general circulation at the same relative rate and the same relative extent." Thus, two drug products are bioequivalent if their bioavailabilities are the same and may be used interchangeably for the same therapeutic effect. In contrast to previous tests that attempted to prove differences, the objective of most of these bioequivalence statistics is to prove that two dosage forms are the same or at least close enough to be considered equal, beyond a reasonable doubt.

The measures of bioavailability are based upon measures of the concentration of the drug in the blood and we must assume that there is a direct relationship between the concentration of drug we detect in the blood and the concentration of the drug at the site of action. These usually involve the evaluation of the peak plasma concentration ($C_{max}$), the time to reach the peak concentration ($T_{max}$) and/or the area under plasma concentration-time curve (AUC). The AUC measures the extent of absorption and the amount of drug that is absorbed by the body, and the parameter most commonly evaluated in bioequivalence studies. Many excellent text books deal with the issues associated with measuring pharmacokinetic parameters: the extent of bioavailability and bioequivalence (Welling and Tse, 1995; Evans, Schentag, and Jusko, 1992; Winter, 1994). The purpose of this discussion is to focus solely on the statistical manipulation of bioequivalence data.

There are three situations requiring bioequivalence testing: a) when a proposed marketed dosage form differs significantly from that used in the major clinical trials for the product; b) when there are major changes in the manufacturing process for a marketed product; and c) when a new generic product is compared to the innovator's marketed product (Benet and Goyan, 1995). Regulatory agencies allow the assumption of safety and effectiveness if the pharmaceutical manufacturers can demonstrate bioequivalence with their product formulations.

**Experimental Designs for Bioequivalence Studies**

Before volunteers are recruited and the actual clinical trial is conducted, an insightful and organized study is developed by the principle investigator. As discussed in Chapter 1, the first two steps in the statistical process is to identify the questions to be answered and the hypotheses to be tested (defined in the study objectives). Then the appropriate research design is selected (to be discussed below) and the appropriate statistical tests are selected. For *in vivo* bioavailability study, the FDA requires that the research design identify the scientific questions to be answered, the drugs(s) and dosage form(s) to be tested, the analytical methods used to assess the outcomes of treatment, and benefit-risk considerations involving human testing (21 *Code of Federal Regulations*, 320.25(b)).

Study protocols should not only include the objectives of the study, the patient inclusion and exclusion criteria, the study design, dosing schedules, and physiological measures; but also a statistics section describing the sample size, power determinations, and the specific analyses that will be performed. These protocols are then reviewed by an Institutional Review Board to evaluate the benefit-risk considerations regarding the volunteers. Two types of study designs are generally used for comparing the bioavailability parameters for drugs. Each of these designs employ statistics or modifications of statistics presented in previous chapters.

The first design is a **parallel group design**, which is illustrated in Figure 22.1. In this design, volunteers are assigned to one of two "similar" groups and each group

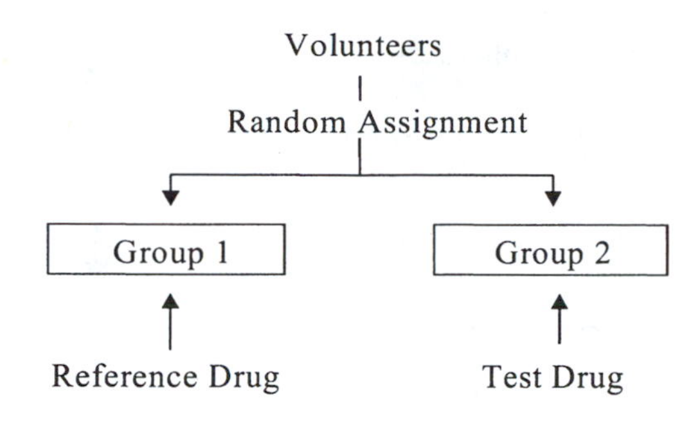


**Figure 22.1** Parallel design involving two groups.

receives only one treatment (either the test drug or the reference standard). In order to establish similar groups, volunteers are randomly assigned to one of the two groups using a random numbers table as discussed in Chapter 2. For example, assume that 30 healthy volunteers (15 per group) are required to compare two formulations of a particular product. Using a random numbers table, the volunteers (numbered 01 to 30) are assigned to one of the two groups (Table 22.1). Because of random assignment to the two treatment levels (groups), it is assumed that each set of volunteers is identical to the other (i.e., same average weight, average lean body mass, average physiological parameters). Therefore, any differences in the bioavailability measures are attributable to the drug formulation received. Results from this parallel design can be simply evaluated using a two sample t- test (Chapter 9). Also, if more that two formulations are involved, the volunteers can be randomly assigned to *k* treatment levels and the one-way analysis of variance can be employed (Chapter 10).

In the parallel group design each volunteer receives only one of the formulations of a drug. This design can be extremely useful for Phase II and Phase III clinical trials. It is easy to conduct and exposes volunteers to risk only once, but cannot control for intersubject variability. The design is appropriate when there is an anticipated small intersubject variability in response to the drug. To minimize

**Table 22.1** Results of a Random Sample of 30 Volunteers for a Clinical Trial

| Group 1 | | | Group 2 | | |
|---|---|---|---|---|---|
| 02 | 15 | 23 | 01 | 10 | 20 |
| 05 | 16 | 24 | 03 | 11 | 21 |
| 06 | 18 | 25 | 04 | 13 | 28 |
| 09 | 19 | 26 | 07 | 14 | 29 |
| 12 | 22 | 27 | 08 | 17 | 30 |

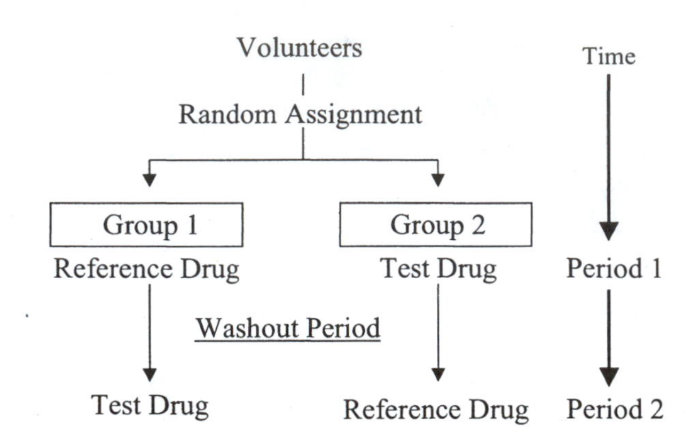


**Figure 22.2** Two period crossover design for two groups.

patient risk, the parallel group design can be used for studies involving drugs with long elimination half-life and potential toxicity. Also, the design can be employed with ill patients or those involving long periods to determine therapeutic response. However, the parallel group design is not appropriate for most bioavailability or bioequivalence studies. With intersubject variability, unaccounted for in this design, it provides a less precise method for determining bioavailability differences.

To overcome some of the disadvantages of the parallel design, a second more rigorous approach is the **crossover study design**. In this design, volunteers are once again randomly assigned to two groups, but each group receives all the treatments in the study. In the case of the two formulations described above, each volunteer would receive both treatments. The order in which the volunteers received the formulations would depend on the group to which they were assigned (Figure 22.2). Using the same volunteers from our example in Table 22.1, if we employee a crossover study design, those subjects randomly assigned to Group 1 (volunteers 02, 05, 06, etc.) will first receive the reference drug (*R*). After an appropriate "washout" period, the same volunteers will receive the test drug (*T*). For those volunteers assigned to Group 2 the order of the drug will be reversed; with the test drug first, followed by the reference standard. In this simple two-period crossover study design (referred to as a standard 2 x 2 crossover design). The subjects in Group 1 receive an *RT* sequence and those in Group 2 a *TR* sequence. Note that every volunteer will receive both the test and reference drug.

The washout mentioned above is a predetermined period of time between the two treatment periods. It is intended to prevent any carryover of effects from the first treatment to the second treatment period. In this type of design, the washout period should be long enough for the first treatment to wear off. This washout period could be based on the half-life of the drug being evaluated. In five half-lives the drug can be considered removed from the body, with approximately 96.9% of the drug eliminated. Obviously, if the washout period is not sufficiently long there is a

**carryover effect** and the second bioavailability measures will not be independent of the first measurements and would violate statistical criteria. Using well designed studies it is assumed that the washout period is sufficiently long enough to prevent any carryover effects.

In clinical trials, individual volunteers can contribute a large amount of variability to pharmacokinetic measures. Thus the crossover design provides a method for removing intersubject variability by having individuals serve as their own controls. The FDA recommend the crossover design when evaluating pharmacokinetic parameters (21 *Code of Federal Regulations* 320.26(b) and 320.27(b)). In addition to having volunteers serving as their own controls and reduce intersubject variability, these study designs also require fewer subjects to provide the same statistical power because the same volunteers are assessed for each treatment level.

Results from the crossover design presented on Figure 22.2 could be evaluated using either the paired t-test (Chapter 9), a complete randomized block design (Chapter 10) or Latin square design (Chapter 12). If more than two formulations are involved the volunteers can be randomly assigned to *k* treatment levels and the complete randomized block or Latin square design can be used.

A third possible research design is a **balanced incomplete block design**. This last method overcomes several disadvantages associated with the complete randomized block design used in crossover studies. When there are more than two treatment levels, the "complete" crossover design may not be practical since such a design would involve an extended period of time, with several washout periods and an increased likelihood of volunteers withdrawing from the study. Also, such designs would involve a larger number of blood draws, which increases the risk to the volunteers. An incomplete block design is similar to a complete block design, except not all formulations are administered to each block. The design is incomplete if the number of treatments for each block is less than the total number of treatments being evaluated in the study. Each block, or volunteer, is randomly assigned to a treatment sequence and the design is "balanced" if the resulting number of subjects receiving each treatment is equal. A complete discussion of this design is presented by Kirk (1968).

Selection of the most appropriate study design (parallel, crossover or balanced incomplete block design) depends on several factors. These include: 1) the objectives of the study; 2) the number of treatment levels being compared; 3) characteristics of the drug being evaluated; 4) availability of volunteers and anticipated withdrawals; 5) inter- and intrasubject variability; 6) duration of the study; and 7) financial resources (Chow and Liu, 2000).

### Two-Sample t-Test Example

When pharmaceutical manufacturers and regulatory agencies began studying the bioequivalence of drug products, the general approach was to use a simple two-sample t-test or analysis of variance to evaluate plasma concentration-time curve (i.e., $C_{max}$, $T_{max}$, AUC). Since these traditional statistical tests were designed to

**Table 22.2** Data from Two Randomly Assigned Groups (AUC in ng·hr/ml)

| Acme Chemical (New Product) | | Innovator (Reference Standard) | |
|---|---|---|---|
| 61.3 | 91.2 | 80.9 | 70.8 |
| 71.4 | 80.1 | 91.4 | 87.1 |
| 48.3 | 54.4 | 59.8 | 99.7 |
| 76.8 | 68.7 | 70.5 | 62.6 |
| 60.4 | 84.9 | 75.7 | 85.0 |
| Mean = | 69.75 | Mean = | 78.35 |
| S = | 13.76 | S = | 12.79 |

demonstrate differences rather than similarities, they were incorrectly used to interpret the early bioequivalence studies. In the 1970s researchers began to note that traditional hypothesis tests were not appropriate for evaluating bioequivalence (Metzler, 1974).

Most of the statistical procedures involved with bioequivalence testing require that the data approximate a normality distribution. However, most of the bioavailability measures (AUC, $t_{max}$, and $C_{max}$) have a tendency to be positively skewed. Therefore, a transformation of the data may be required before analysis. The log transformation (Chapter 6) on AUC is usually performed to remove the skew to the distribution. This log-transformed data is then analyzed using the procedures discussed below.

To illustrate the problems that exist when using some of our previous statistical tests, let us take an example of a clinical trial comparing Acme Chemical's new generic antihypertensive agent to the innovators original product. This would portray the third situation cited previously by Benet. We design a very simple study to compare the two formulations of the same chemical entity, by administering them to two groups of randomly assigned volunteers. Only ten volunteers are assigned to each group. Our primary pharmacokinetic parameter of interest is the AUC (ng·hr/ml). The results of our *in vivo* tests are presented in Table 22.2.

If we use our traditional two-sample t-test as discussed in Chapter 9, the hypotheses would be:

$$H_0: \mu_1 = \mu_2$$
$$H_1: \mu_1 \neq \mu_2$$

The decision rule, base on $\alpha$ of 0.05 is to reject $H_0$ if $t > t_{18}(.025) = +2.104$ or $t < -t_{18}(.025) = -2.104$. The statistical analysis using Eq. 9.3 and Eq. 9.6 would be as follows:

$$S_p^2 = \frac{(n_1-1)S_1^2+(n_2-1)S_2^2}{n_1+n_2-2} = \frac{9(13.76)^2+9(12.79)^2}{18} = 176.46$$

$$t = \frac{\overline{X}_1 - \overline{X}_2}{\sqrt{\frac{S_P^2}{n_1} + \frac{S_P^2}{n_2}}} = \frac{69.75 - 78.35}{\sqrt{\frac{176.46}{10} + \frac{176.46}{10}}} = \frac{-8.60}{5.94} = -1.45$$

The result is that we fail to reject $H_0$ because the $t$-value is less than our critical value of –2.104. Therefore, with 95% confidence, we failed to prove a difference between the two formulations. However, at the same time we *did not* prove that the formulations were equal.

Since in most cases the sample sizes are the same, we can make the following substitution for the denominator in Eq. 9.6. However, if we do run into unequal sample sizes ($n_1 \neq n_2$) we can substitute the left side of equation for the standard error portion in any of the formulas discussed in this chapter.

$$\sqrt{\frac{S_P^2}{n_1} + \frac{S_P^2}{n_2}} = \sqrt{\frac{2S_p^2}{n}} \qquad \text{Eq. 22.1}$$

A potential problem exists with the Type II error in our statistical analysis. As discussed in Chapter 8, $\beta$ is the error of failing to reject $H_0$ (equality) when there is a true difference between the formulations we are testing. As shown in Figure 8.5, with smaller sample sizes there is a greater likelihood of creating a Type II error. If an unethical entrepreneur wished to prove his product was equal to an innovator's drug, the easiest way to accomplish this would be to use very small sample sizes, apply traditional statistical methods, fail to reject $H_0$, and conclude that the two products were equivalent. To avoid such deceptions the FDA has developed guidelines to ensure adequate power in bioequivalence tests (i.e., the 80/20 rule discussed below).

## Power in Bioequivalence Tests

For most bioequivalence studies, the same size is usually 18-24 healthy normal volunteers. To detect a clinically important difference (20%), a power calculation is often performed prior to the study to determine the number of subjects needed to have the desired power (80%). For example, the following is a typical statement associated with a proposed protocol: "A sample size of 28 healthy males will be enrolled in this study to ensure study completion by at least 24 patients. Based on (a previous study cited) a sample size of 20 patients can provide at least 80% probability to show that the 90% confidence interval of the mean AUC value for the clinical lot of (test drug name) is within ±20% of the reference mean AUC value." Note that the investigators increased the sample size to ensure that there would be sufficient power once the data was collected. Also, more than the required number of subjects are recruited to anticipate possible replacements for dropouts.

In the previous example we were unable to reject the null hypothesis that $\mu_1 = \mu_2$ based on 10 volunteers for each product. However, we might ask ourselves, if there was a difference between the two formulations, was our sample size large enough to detect a difference? In other words, was our statistical test powerful enough to detect a desired difference? Let us assume that we want to be able to detect a 10% difference from our reference standard (78.35 x 0.10 = 7.84 = $\delta$). Using a formula extracted from Zar (1999), the power determination formula would be:

$$t_{\beta} \geq \frac{\delta}{\sqrt{\frac{2S_p^2}{n}}} - t_{\alpha/2} \qquad \text{Eq. 22.2}$$

where $t_{\alpha/2}$ is the critical $t$-value for $\alpha = 0.05$, $n$ is our sample size per level of our discrete independent variable and the resultant $t_{\beta}$ is the $t$-value associated with our Type II error. To determine the power we will need to find the complement $(1 - \beta)$ of Type II error. Using our data we find the following:

$$t_{\beta} \geq \frac{7.84}{\sqrt{\frac{2(176.46)}{10}}} - 1.96$$

$$t_{\beta} \geq \frac{7.84}{5.89} - 1.96 = 1.32 - 1.96 = -0.64$$

If we used a full table of critical t-values (for example, *Geigy Scientific Tables*, Seventh, Ciba-Geigy Corp., Ardsley, NY, 1974, pp. 32-35) or used Excel function [TDIST($t_{\beta}$,df,1*tailed*)], unlike the abbreviated version presented as Table B3 in Appendix B, we would find the table probability associated with t-values with 18 degrees of freedom at $p = 0.25$ for $t = -0.6884$ and $p = 0.30$ for $t = -0.5338$. Through interpolation, a calculated $t$-value of –0.64 has a probability of 0.27. Using Excel software the $p$-value would be 0.2651, or approximately 0.27. This represents the Type II error. The complement 0.73 (1 – 0.27), is the power associated with rejecting $H_0$ (bioequivalence) when in truth $H_0$ is false.

Let us further assume that we want to have at least 80% power to be able to detect a 10% difference between our two sets of tablets. We can modify the above formula to identify the appropriate sample size:

$$n \geq \frac{2S_p^2}{\delta^2}(t_{\beta} + t_{\alpha/2})^2 \qquad \text{Eq. 22.3}$$

If we look at the first column of Table B3 in Appendix B, the values listed for the various degrees of freedom represent our $t$-value for a one-tailed test with $\beta = 0.20$. In this case we would interpolate the $t$-value to be 0.862 for 18 degrees of freedom. The $t(1 - \alpha/2)$ for 18 degrees of freedom is 2.10. Applied to our example:

$$n \geq \frac{2(173.46)}{(7.84)^2}(0.862 + 2.10)^2 \geq (5.64)(8.77) \geq 49.48$$

In this case, the sample size we should have used to ensure a power of at least 80%, to detect a difference as small as 10%, would have been a minimum of 50 volunteers per group.

## Rules for Bioequivalence

To control the quality of bioequivalence studies the FDA has considered three possible standards: 1) the 75/75 rule; 2) the 80/20 rule; and 3) the ± 20 rule. The **75/75 rule** for bioequivalence requires that bioavailability measures for the test product be within 25% of those for the reference product (greater than 75% and less than 125%) in at least 75% of the subjects involved in the clinical trials (*Federal Register*, 1978). This rule was easy to apply and compared the relative bioavailability by individual subject, removing intersubject variability. The rule was very sensitive when the size of the sample was relatively small, but was not valuable as a scientifically based decision rule. This 1977 rule was criticized for its poor statistical nature, was never finalized, and was finally abandoned in 1980.

A more acceptable FDA criterion has focused on preventing too much Type II error and requires that manufacturers perform a retrospective assessment of the power associated with their bioequivalence studies. In any study, there must be at least an 80% power to detect a 20% difference. In other words, this **80/20 rule** states that if the null hypothesis cannot be rejected at the 95% confidence level ($1 - \alpha$), the sample size must be sufficiently large to have a power of at least 80% for a 20% difference to be detected between the test product and reference standard. (*Federal Register*, 1977). This 20% difference appears to have been an arbitrary selection to represent the minimum difference that can be regarded as clinically significant. Once again using the previous example, based on a pooled variance of 173.46, a desired difference of 20% (in this case 15.67 ng·hr/ml, 78.35 x 0.20 = $\delta$), a Type I error rate of 0.05, and a Type II error rate of 0.20, the required sample size would be at least 12 volunteers per group.

$$n \geq \frac{2(173.46)}{(15.67)^2}(0.862 + 2.10)^2 \geq (1.41)(8.77) \geq 12.37$$

This seems like a dramatic drop in the amount of subjects required (at least 50 for a 10% difference and only 13 for a 20% difference), but it demonstrates how important it is to define the difference the researcher considers to be important (Table 22.3).

But even if we have enough power to detect a significant difference we still have failed to prove that the null hypothesis is true. Alternative tests are needed to work with the data presented. Similar to the approach used in Chapter 9 presenting the t-test, we will first use a confidence interval approach and then a hypothesis testing format to prove that even if there are differences between the new product and the

**Table 22.3** Sample Size Required to Detect Various Differences with 80% Power Where the Reference Standard Mean is 78.35 (Table 21.2)

| Difference (%) | Minimum Sample Size |
|---|---|
| 5 | 180 |
| 10 | 45 |
| 15 | 20 |
| 20 | 12 |
| 25 | 8 |
| 30 | 5 |

reference standard, that difference falls within acceptable limits.

The last measure of bioequivalence, the **±20 rule**, concerns the average bioavailability and states that the test product must be within 20% of the reference drug (between 80% and 120%). The ±20 rule appears to be most acceptable to the FDA. As will be seen in the following sections the ±20 rule can be tested by use of either a confidence interval or two one-tailed t-tests. These two methods are briefly introduced for comparisons for one test product to a reference standard. For a more in-depth discussion of these tests and more complex bioequivalence tests, readers are referred to the excellent text by Chow and Liu (2000).

## Creating Confidence Intervals

Considering our earlier discussion of the comparison of our new generic product to the innovator's product, we could write our hypotheses as follows, where the innovator's drug is referred to as the reference standard:

$$H_0: \mu_T = \mu_R$$
$$H_1: \mu_T \neq \mu_R$$

Where $\mu_T$ represents our new or "test" product and $\mu_R$ the "reference" or innovator's product. An alternative method for writing these hypotheses was seen in Chapter 9 when we discussed confidence intervals:

$$H_0: \mu_T - \mu_R = 0$$
$$H_1: \mu_T - \mu_R \neq 0$$

But, as discussed, we cannot prove true equality ($\delta = 0$). Rather we will establish an acceptable range and if a confidence interval falls within those limits we can conclude that any difference is not therapeutically significant. Using this method for testing bioequivalence we create a confidence interval for the population difference, $\mu_T - \mu_R$, based on our sample results, $\overline{X}_T - \overline{X}_R$. Currently the FDA recommendations use a 90% confidence interval ($\alpha = 0.10$). If the 90% confidence interval falls completely between 0.80 and 1.20, the two products are considered bioequivalence (an absolute difference less than 20%). With respect to a comparison of a test product to a reference standard, we want the test product to fall between 0.80 and 1.20:

$$0.80 < \mu_T - \mu_R < 1.20$$

As noted earlier in this chapter, pharmacokinetic parameters, such as $C_{max}$ and AUC often involve log transformations before the data is analyzed to ensure a normal distribution. The general formula for such a confidence interval would be:

$$\mu_T - \mu_R = (\overline{X}_T - \overline{X}_R) \pm t_{\upsilon(1-\alpha)} \sqrt{\frac{2S_p^2}{n}} \qquad \text{Eq. 22.4}$$

This is almost identical to Eq. 9.4 for the two-sample t-test. Because of formulas discussed later in this chapter, we will simplify the formula to replacing the sample difference with $d$ and our standard error term with $SE$:

$$d = \overline{X}_T - \overline{X}_R \qquad \text{Eq. 22.5}$$

$$SE = t_\upsilon(1-\alpha) \sqrt{\frac{2S_p^2}{n}} \qquad \text{Eq. 22.6}$$

If one thinks of this problem as an ANOVA with $v_1 = 1$ in Chapter 10, the $MS_W$ (mean square within) from the ANOVA table can be substituted for the $S_p^2$ term. Also, note that we are performing two one-tailed tests with 5% error loaded on each tail $(1 - \alpha)$. Also, if the sample sizes are not equal the standard error portion of the equation can be rewritten as:

$$SE = t_\upsilon(1-\alpha) \sqrt{\frac{S_p^2}{n_1} + \frac{S_p^2}{n_2}} \qquad \text{Eq. 22.7}$$

Using Eqs. 22.4 through 22.7 we can create a confidence interval based on the same units of measure as the original data (i.e., AUC in ng·hr/ml). A better approach would be to calculate confidence intervals about the observed relative bioavailability between the test product and the reference standard; converting the information into percentages of the reference standard. With the FDA's recommendation of at least 80% bioavailability in order to claim bioequivalence, the ratio of the two products are more often statistically evaluated than the differences between the AUCs.

$$80\% < \frac{\mu_T}{\mu_R} < 120\%$$

This ratio of bioavailabilities between 80 and 120% is an acceptable standard by the FDA and pharmaceutical regulatory agencies in most countries. The last step is to create a ratio between the change and the reference standard so outcomes can be expressed as percent of the reference standard:

$$Lower\ Limit = \frac{(d - SE) + \overline{X}_R}{\overline{X}_R} x\ 100\% \qquad \text{Eq. 22.8}$$

$$Upper\ Limit = \frac{(d + SE) + \overline{X}_R}{\overline{X}_R} x\ 100\% \qquad \text{Eq. 22.9}$$

Finally the resultant confidence interval is expressed as:

$$Lower\ Limit < \frac{\mu_T}{\mu_R} < Upper\ Limit \qquad \text{Eq. 22.10}$$

What we create is a confidence interval within which we can state with 95% confidence where the true population ratio falls based on our sample.

Applying these formulas to our previous example (Table 22.2) for Acme Chemical's generic and the Innovator's product, we find the following results:

$$SE = t_v(1-\alpha)\sqrt{\frac{2S_p^2}{n}} = (1.734)\sqrt{\frac{2(176.46)}{10}} = 10.30$$

$$d = \overline{X}_T - \overline{X}_R = 69.75 - 78.35 = -8.6$$

$$Upper\ Limit = \frac{(-8.6 + 10.3) + 78.35}{78.35} x100\% = 102.17\%$$

$$Lower\ Limit = \frac{(-8.6 - 10.3) + 78.35}{78.35} x100\% = 75.88\%$$

Thus, in this case, with 95% confidence, the true population ratio is between:

$$75.88\% < \frac{\mu_T}{\mu_R} < 102.17\%$$

This fails to meet the FDA requirement of falling within the 80% to 120% range. Therefore, we would conclude that the two products are not equivalent.

**Comparison Using Two One-Sided t-Tests**

The last method we will explore is to involve hypothesis testing to determine if we can satisfy the requirements for bioequivalence. As discussed previously, the absolute difference between the two products should be less than 20% of the reference standard:

$$\left|\mu_T - \mu_R\right| < 20\%\ \mu_R$$

This method, proposed by Hauck and Anderson (1984), overcomes some of the negative aspects of the previous approaches by using two one-sided t-tests to evaluate bioequivalence. In this case we deal with two null hypotheses, which indicate outcomes outside of the acceptable differences for bioequivalency:

$$H_{01}: \mu_T - \mu_R \leq -20\%$$
$$H_{02}: \mu_T - \mu_R \geq +20\%$$

The two alternate hypotheses represent outcomes that fall short of the extremes:

$$H_{11}: \mu_T - \mu_R > -20\%$$
$$H_{12}: \mu_T - \mu_R < +20\%$$

Obviously, both of the null hypothesis must be rejected in order to prove:

$$80\% < \mu_T - \mu_R < 120\%$$

The equations for these two one-tailed tests involves two *thetas* that define the "equivalence interval" where $\theta_1 < \theta_2$. In other words, $\theta_2$ is always the upper equivalence limit and $\theta_1$ the lower limit. In the case of equivalency being less than 20%, each theta represents a 20% difference in the units from which the data was collected: $\theta_2 = +20\%$ value and $\theta_1 = -20\%$ value. Schuirmann's (1987) formulas for calculating the two one-sided t-tests are:

$$t_1 = \frac{(\overline{X}_T - \overline{X}_R) - \theta_1}{\sqrt{MS_E}\ \sqrt{2/n}} \qquad \text{Eq. 22.11}$$

$$t_2 = \frac{\theta_2 - (\overline{X}_T - \overline{X}_R)}{\sqrt{MS_E}\ \sqrt{2/n}} \qquad \text{Eq. 22.12}$$

These tests are $H_{01}$ and $H_{02}$, respectively. As with past tests of hypotheses, we establish a decision rule based on the sample size and a 95% confidence in our decision. Our decision rule is with $\alpha = 0.05$, reject $H_{01}$ or $H_{02}$ if $t > t_{df}(1 - \alpha)$. Each hypothesis is tested with a Type I error of 0.05 ($\alpha$). Traditionally we have tested out the hypothesis with a total $\alpha = .05$; in the procedure we actually use $1 - 2\alpha$ rather than $1 - \alpha$

(Westlake, 1988). This would correspond to the 90% confidence intervals discussed in the previous section.

In this case theta represents our desired detectable difference (δ) and, as discussed previous, the $MS_E$ or $MS_W$ for only two levels of the discrete independent variable ($\nu_1 = 1$) is the same as $S_p^2$. Therefore, the equations can be rewritten as follows:

$$t_1 = \frac{(\overline{X}_T - \overline{X}_R) - \delta_1}{\sqrt{\frac{2S_p^2}{n}}} \qquad \text{Eq. 22.13}$$

$$t_2 = \frac{\delta_2 - (\overline{X}_T - \overline{X}_R)}{\sqrt{\frac{2S_p^2}{n}}} \qquad \text{Eq. 22.14}$$

Using our previous example (Table 22.2) and once again assuming we wish to be able to detect a 20% difference for an innovator's product:

$$\delta = 78.35 \ x \ 0.20 = 15.67$$

Therefore, $\delta_1 = -15.67$; $\delta_2 = +15.67$, $S_p^2 = 173.46$ and our critical value through interpolation for $t_{18}(1-\alpha)$ is 1.73. The decision rule, with $\alpha = 0.05$, is to reject $H_{01}$ or $H_{02}$ if $t > 1.73$.

$$t_1 = \frac{(-8.6) - (-15.67)}{\sqrt{\frac{2(176.46)}{10}}} = \frac{7.07}{5.94} = 1.20$$

$$t_2 = \frac{15.67 - (-8.6)}{\sqrt{\frac{2(176.46)}{10}}} = \frac{24.27}{5.94} = 4.09$$

In this case we were able to reject $H_{02}$ and prove that the difference was less than 120% ($\mu_{Test} - \mu_{Reference} < +20\%$), but failed to reject $H_{01}$. We were not able to prove that $\mu_{Test} - \mu_{Reference}$ was greater than 80%. Therefore, similar to our confidence interval in the previous section, we are unable to show bioequivalency between Acme's generic and the Innovator's reference standard.

**Clinical Equivalence and Noninferiority studies:**

Noninferiority studies are similar to equivalence studies. Based on the researcher's objectives clinical trials used to compare a new product to an already approved agent could be designed to: 1) test the equivalence of the two products (previously discussed); 2) establish the superiority of the new product; or 3) show noninferiority of the new product. This section will focus primarily on the last type of assessment.

For completeness, a **superiority trial** is designed to evaluate the response to an investigational agent and determine if it is superior to that of a comparative product. Superiority studies are the most effective way to established efficacy, either by showing: 1) superiority to a placebo (placebo-controlled trial); 2) superiority to an active control; or 3) a dose-response relationship. Thus, the comparator could be either an active or placebo control. However, using a placebo control raises serious ethical questions, especially if there is an alternative effective therapy available: "In cases where an available treatment is known to prevent serious harm, such as death or irreversible morbidity in the study population, it is generally inappropriate to use a placebo control" (ICH, 1999). In most cases superiority studies could be handled as a one-tailed two-sample t-test (Chapter 9) with the hypotheses:

$$H_0:\ \mu_T \leq \mu_C$$
$$H_1:\ \mu_T > \mu_C$$

where $\mu_T$ is the response to the new (test) product and $\mu_C$ is the active control (or comparator agent). If there is sufficient data to reject the null hypothesis with a certain degree of confidence (i.e., $1 - \alpha = 0.95$), than the new agent is proven to be superior to the comparator. The hypotheses also can be written as a one-tailed confidence interval:

$$H_0:\ \mu_T - \mu_C \leq 0$$
$$H_1:\ \mu_T - \mu_C > 0$$

If a confidence interval is created using Eq. 9.4 and all the results are positive (zero does not fall within the confidence interval), we can reject the null hypothesis and with 95% confidence conclude that the test product is superior to the control. This is illustrated in Figure 22.3 as confidence interval *A*.

Noninferiority is a relatively new term, dating back to the late 1970s. For a while in the 1990s the terms equivalence and noninferiority were sometimes used interchangeably and both referred to an equivalency test (Wang, 2003). As discussed in the first part of this chapter an **equivalence trial** (or bioequivalence test) is intended to show that the difference in the amount of response to two or more treatments is clinically unimportant. This difference (previously defined as the difference between sample means, Eqs. 22.9 and 22.10) represent equivalence if the results fell between the established upper and lower limits :

$$H_{01}:\ \mu_T - \mu_C \leq -\delta$$
$$H_{02}:\ \mu_T - \mu_C \geq +\delta$$

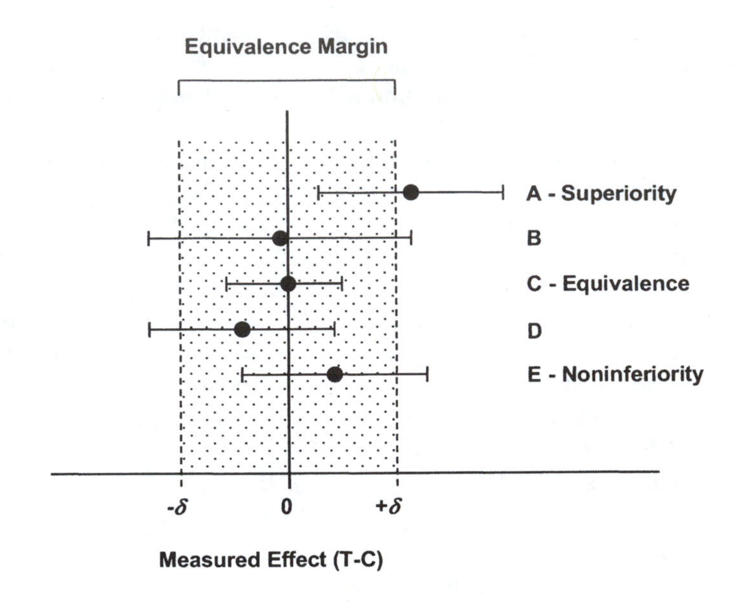


**Figure 22.3** Illustrations of various confidence intervals.

$$H_{11}: \mu_T - \mu_C > -\delta$$
$$H_{12}: \mu_T - \mu_C < +\delta$$

If both null hypotheses are rejected then the following would be proven using this approach:

$$-\delta < \mu_T - \mu_C < +\delta$$

It is virtually impossible to prove that the results form two treatments are exactly equivalent ($\delta = 0$). Therefore, as seen in the previous hypotheses, the goal was to show that the results differ by no more than a certain amount (i.e., $\delta < 10\%$). This acceptable difference is termed the **equivalence margin**. For equivalence testing, if the results from the two treatments differ by more than the equivalence margin in either direction, then the assumption of equivalence cannot be proven. The *deltas* can be thought of as the boundaries for an equivalence margin or as clinically acceptable differences. So equivalency trials are designed to show that two treatments do not differ by more than some predetermined equivalency margin (illustrated as confidence interval C in Figure 22.3). Note with confidence interval B in this same figure, both the lower and upper limits of the confidence interval extend beyond the boundaries of the equivalence margin. Another name for the area between the two boundaries is the **zone of indifference**. For equivalence testing the statistical analysis of the difference is based on the two-sided confidence interval. However, as seen previously, operationally this testing involves two simultaneous one-sided tests to test two null hypothesis that the treatment difference is outside an acceptable limit. In most cases, each hypothesis being tested with 5% Type I error rate, with a resulting 90% confidence interval. Failure to reject either of the null hypotheses would be visually represented by one of the ends of the interval extending beyond its respective boundary.

In contrast to equivalence testing, a **noninferiority trial** is concerned only with the lower limits of the equivalency margin. A simple way to think of noninferiority trials is to view them as one-sided equivalency tests.

$$H_{01}: \mu_T - \mu_C \leq -\delta$$
$$H_{11}: \mu_T - \mu_C > -\delta$$

With a noninferiority trial the primary goal is to prove the alternative hypothesis that the investigational agent is not clinically inferior to the comparative agent. These studies are intended to show that the effect of a new treatment is not worse than that of an active control by more than a specified margin. A confidence interval approach can be used to test the outcome for a noninferiority trial. Similar to the previous bioequivalence studies, a single one-sided 95% confidence interval is created and if the estimated population differences between the two agents (test drug and comparator) fall entirely within the positive side of the noninferiority margin ($>-\delta$) the null hypothesis is rejected. Any improvement (a positive $\delta$) meets the criteria of noninferiority. In Figure 22.3, confidence intervals D would represent an unsuccessful test, where as E would be a successful test of noninferiority. In many cases the established evidence of effectiveness for an experimental treatment through noninferiority studies will be a regulatory requirement for drug approval. So an important question is how large is the margin to be clinically insignificant?

Choosing the $\delta$ value is crucial. One possible approach to determine the equivalence margin is to base it on a clinical determination of what is considered a minimally important effect (Snapinn, 2000). According to the ICH, "this margin is the largest difference that can be judged as being clinically acceptable and should be smaller than differences observed in superiority trials of the active comparator" (ICH, 1998). The choice of $\delta$ will be based on the purpose for conduction the clinical trial and should be clearly stated in the protocol. The selection of $\delta$ should provide, at the minimum, assurance that difference ($\mu_T - \mu_C$) has a clinical effect greater than zero. Also, the choice of the margin should be independent of any power considerations. The sample sizes for these types of studies are very sensitive to the assumed effect of the new drug relative to the control. For a discussion of power and sample size see Chan (2002). The ICH provides some guidance (E-9 and E-10) on the design and analysis of such trials, but do not set specific limits for $\delta$. These require decisions by the primary investigator base on sound clinical judgments. The decision on $\delta$ should always be made on both realistic clinical judgments and sound statistical grounds. The decision is made on a study-by-study basis and no rule of thumb that applies to all clinical situations.

A potential problem is the choice of active comparator in these noninferiority studies. As mentioned previously the use of a placebo control raises ethical concerns. Thus, an active control is usually used. However, the assumption is made that the active control is effective. For that reason the comparator should be chosen with care. If the comparator is not effective, proving noninferiority will not result in the conclusion that the new treatment drug is effective. The ability to distinguish between an active and placebo control is **assay sensitivity**. If the assay sensitivity cannot be assumed, a noninferiority study cannot demonstrate the effectiveness of a new agent, because assay sensitivity is not measured in a noninferiority trial. Assay sensitivity is dependent on the size of the effect one is interested in detecting. Either a noninferiority or equivalence trial may have assay sensitivity for an effect of 20% but not an effect of 10%. Therefore, it is essential to know the effect of the control drug. Assay sensitivity can be accomplished by using concurrent placebo control or through historical evidence. Therefore, sensitivity must be assumed based on historical experience with the comparator agent and requires evidence external to the study. The ICH guidelines list several factors that can reduce assay sensitivity, including: poor patient compliance; poor diagnostic criteria; concomitant medications; excessive variability in the measurements; and a biased end-point assessment (ICH 1999). For that reason, some studies involve three arms in the study: new test drug, active control, and placebo control. Such a study would be optimal because it: 1) assesses assay sensitivity; 2) measures the effect of the new drug; and 3) compares the effects of the two active treatments (Temple and Ellenberg, 2000). A discussion of the evaluation of these three-way studies is presented by Pigeot et al. (2003).

As an example, consider the following fictitious clinical trial. One hundred and twenty newly diagnosed hyperlipidemic patients are randomly assigned to one of two legs in a clinical trial; the first group receives StatinA which is on the hospital formulary (the comparator agent). The second group receives a newly marked agent (StatinB), which reportedly has a better safety profile. Patients are followed for six months. At the end of the study period the change in total cholesterol levels are recorded for each group. The two possible scenarios and their summary statistics are presented in Table 22.4. As seen in the Table, the average decrease in total cholesterol for the comparator product was –40 mg/dl. Prior to the study it is determined that the noninferiority for the new product will be based on a less than 10% difference compared to the comparator product. Since a negative result is desired, we would not want to see a positive, increase in total cholesterol. Thus, the upper bounds of equivalency margin would be a change equal to +4 mg/dl.

$$H_0: \mu_{StatinB} - \mu_{StatinA} \geq +4 \text{ mg/dl}$$
$$H_1: \mu_{StatinB} - \mu_{StatinA} < +4 \text{ mg/dl}$$

To evaluate the null hypothesis we will use a one-tailed, two-sample confidence interval created by a Student t-test with $\alpha = 0.05$ (modified from Eq. 9.4).

$$\mu_B - \mu_A = (\overline{X}_B - \overline{X}_A) + t_{n_B+n_A-2}(1-\alpha)\sqrt{\frac{S_p^2}{n_B} + \frac{S_p^2}{n_A}} \qquad \text{Eq. 22.15}$$

**Table 22.4** Two Potential Results Involving a Noninferiority Trial

| | StatinA (C) | StatinB (T) | Difference (T – C) |
|---|---|---|---|
| Scenario A | | | |
| $\overline{X}_d =$ | –40.0 | –41.1 | 1.1 mg/dl lower |
| $S_d =$ | 15.4 | 20.3 | |
| $n =$ | 60 | 60 | |
| Scenario B | | | |
| $\overline{X}_d =$ | –40.0 | –39.8 | 0.2 mg/dl higher |
| $S_d =$ | 15.4 | 7.7 | |
| $n =$ | 60 | 60 | |

In scenario A, even though the new StatinB performs slightly better than StatinA, it fails the test for noninferiority (where $S_p^2 = 324.63$) because the upper limit is greater than +4.

$$\mu_B - \mu_A = [-41.1 - (-40.0)] + 1.66\sqrt{\frac{324.63}{60} + \frac{3.24.63}{60}}$$

$$\mu_B - \mu_A = -1.1 + 1.66(3.29) = -1.1 + 5.46 = +4.36$$

However, in scenario B, StatinB on the average did not perform quite as well as the comparator StatinA, but it does pass the test for noninferiority (where $S_p^2 = 148.23$) because the upper limit is less than +4:

$$\mu_B - \mu_A = [(-39.8 - (-40.0)] + 1.66\sqrt{\frac{148.23}{60} + \frac{148.23}{60}}$$

$$\mu_B - \mu_A = +0.2 + 1.66(2.22) = +0.2 + 3.69 = +3.89$$

As seen in Figure 22.4 the primary contributing cause for these different results is the width of the interval caused by the much greater variance in the StatinB in scenario A. This greater variance results in an overall wider interval and failure to have an interval less than +4 mg/dl. Displayed in Figure 22.4 are the entire 90% confidence intervals for both scenarios.

There are a number of other statistical tests involving rate ratios that can be used for the evaluation of differences between treatments (i.e., odds ratio, relative risk, hazard ratio). In these cases the same principles apply, except the assessment of "no difference" is represented by the value one, not zero. For example, using hazard ratio (Chapter 19), if the new treatment is evaluated to be non-inferior compared to an active control, the object of the trial is to demonstrate the effectiveness of this new

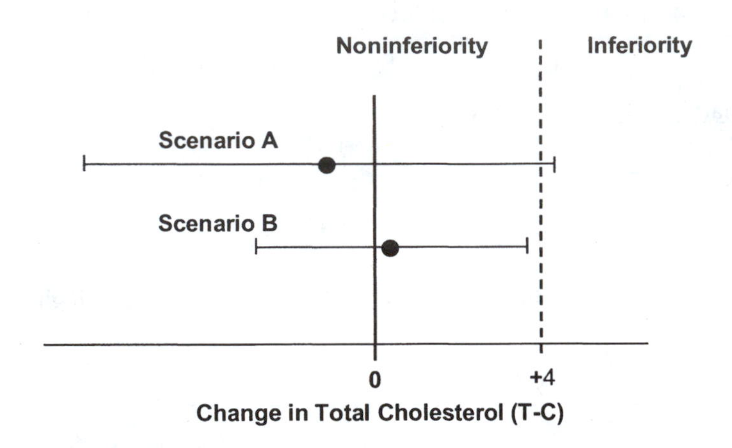


**Figure 22.4** Confidence intervals created by data in Table 22.4.

treatment by demonstrating noninferiority. In this case the hypotheses are:

$$H_0: HR(T/C) \geq 1 + \delta$$
$$H_1: HR(T/C) < 1 + \delta$$

where $\delta > 0$ is the noninferiority margin. The null hypothesis is rejected if $\tau_0(\delta)$ less than −1.96 or −2.58 for 95% or 99% confidence, respectively. If the log of the hazard ratio is used the hypotheses would be:

$$H_0: \log HR(T/C) \geq 1 + \delta$$
$$H_1: \log HR(T/C) < 1 + \delta$$

and the null hypotheses rejected if $log\ HR(T/C) + 1.96SE[log\ hr(T/C)] < \delta$. Both these hypotheses are tested at the one-sided 2.5% significance level. In both cases, if $H_0$ is rejected, it is possible to conclude that the new treatment is non-inferior and no worse than the active control within this fixed margin $\delta$.

## Dissolution Testing

Dissolution tests provide an *in vitro* method to determine if products produced by various manufacturers or various batches from the same manufacturer are in compliance with compendia or regulatory requirements. For example, the *United States Pharmacopeia* (2005) states that aspirin tablets ($C_9H_8O_4$) must have "not less than 90% and not more than 110% of labeled amount of $C_9H_8O_4$." In addition, the tolerance level for dissolution testing is that "not less than 80% of the labeled amount of $C_9H_8O_4$ is dissolved in 30 minutes."

Dissolution profiles can be used to compare multiple batches, different manufacturers, or different production sites to determine if the products are similar with respect to percent of drug dissolved over given periods of time. The assumption made is that the rate of dissolution and availability will correlate to absorption in the gut and eventually similar effects at the site of action. This assumption can be significantly enhanced if manufacturers can establish an *in vivo-in vitro* correlation between their dissolution measures and bioavailability outcomes (FDA, 1997, p. 7).

Using aspirin tablets as an example, consider the two sets of profiles seen in Figure 22.4. All batches meet the dissolution criteria of 80% in 30 minutes, but the profiles vary. Are they the same or different enough to consider the batches as not equivalent?

## SUPAC-IR Guidance

To answer the question of equivalency in dissolution profiles the FDA has proposed a guidance for manufacturers issued as "Scale-up and Post-Approval Changes for Immediate Release Solid Oral Dosage Forms" (SUPAC-IR). This guidance is designed to provide recommendations for manufacturers submitting new drug applications, abbreviated new drug applications and abbreviated antibiotic applications who wish to change the process, equipment or production sites following approval of their previous drug submission (*Federal Register*, 1995). Previous evaluations involved single-point dissolution tests (i.e., the previous aspirin monograph). The SUPAC-IR guidance can assist manufacturers with changes associated with: 1) scale-up procedures; 2) site changes in the manufacturing facilities; 3) equipment or process changes; and 4) changes in component or composition of the finished dosage form.

Under SUPAC-IR there are two factors that can be calculated: 1) a difference factor ($f_1$), and 2) a similarity factor ($f_2$). The published formulas are as follows:

$$f_1 = \{[\sum|R_t - T_t|] \;/\; [\sum R_t]\} \cdot 100 \qquad \text{Eq. 22.16}$$

$$f_2 = 50\, Log\,\{\, [1 + \frac{1}{n}\Sigma(R_t - T_t)^2\,]^{-0.5} \cdot 100\,\} \qquad \text{Eq. 22.17}$$

where $n$ is the number of time points in the dissolution profile, $R_t$ is the percent dissolved for the reference standard at each time period, $\mathbf{T_t}$ is percent dissolved for the test product at the same time period, and *log* is the logarithm base 10. We will slightly rewrite these formulas to remove the negative, fractional root terminology:

$$f_1 = \frac{\sum|R_t - T_t|}{\sum R_t} x\,100 \qquad \text{Eq. 22.18}$$

**Table 22.5** Example of Data From Dissolution Tests on Two Drug Batches

| Time (minutes): | 15 | 30 | 45 | 60 |
|---|---|---|---|---|
| | Batch Produced Using Original Equipment | | | |
| | 63.9 | 85.9 | 85.4 | 93.6 |
| | 42.9 | 75.8 | 74.5 | 87.4 |
| | 58.1 | 77.3 | 83.2 | 86.4 |
| | 62.4 | 79.3 | 76.2 | 79.2 |
| | 52.5 | 74.5 | 90.3 | 94.5 |
| | 59.1 | 65.1 | 87.5 | 86.1 |
| Mean: | 56.48 | 76.32 | 82.85 | 87.87 |
| SD: | 7.74 | 6.79 | 6.29 | 5.61 |
| RSD: | 13.71 | 8.91 | 7.59 | 6.38 |
| | Batch Produced Using Newer Equipment | | | |
| | 78.5 | 85.6 | 88.4 | 92.9 |
| | 67.2 | 72.1 | 80.2 | 86.8 |
| | 56.5 | 80.4 | 83.1 | 85.4 |
| | 78.9 | 85.2 | 89.8 | 91.4 |
| | 72.3 | 84.1 | 85.4 | 94.1 |
| | 84.9 | 72.1 | 79.0 | 85.9 |
| Mean: | 73.05 | 79.92 | 84.32 | 89.42 |
| SD: | 10.13 | 6.33 | 4.35 | 3.83 |
| RSD: | 13.87 | 7.91 | 5.16 | 4.28 |

$$f_2 = 50\, \text{Log}\left[\frac{1}{\sqrt{1+\frac{1}{n}\Sigma(R_t - T_t)^2}} \times 100\right] \qquad \text{Eq. 22.19}$$

The guidance for equivalency is that the $f_1$-value should be close to 0 (generally values less than 15) and the $f_2$-value should be close to 100, with values greater than 50 ensuring equivalency.

If the two dissolution profiles are exactly the same (one laying exactly over the second) the $f_2$ value will be 100. As the $f_2$-value gets smaller there is a greater difference between the two profiles. An $f_2$ of 50 represents a 10% difference, thus the SUPAC-IR guidance requires a calculated $f_2$-value between 50 and 100 for equivalency. As an example, consider the data presented in Table 22.5 and Figure 22.5, which show the results of dissolution tests performed on two batches of the same drug, one produced with the original equipment used for products NDA application, and the second with newer equipment. Are the following two profiles the same (less than a 10% difference) based on the $f_1$ and $f_2$ formulas proposed under SUPAC-IR?

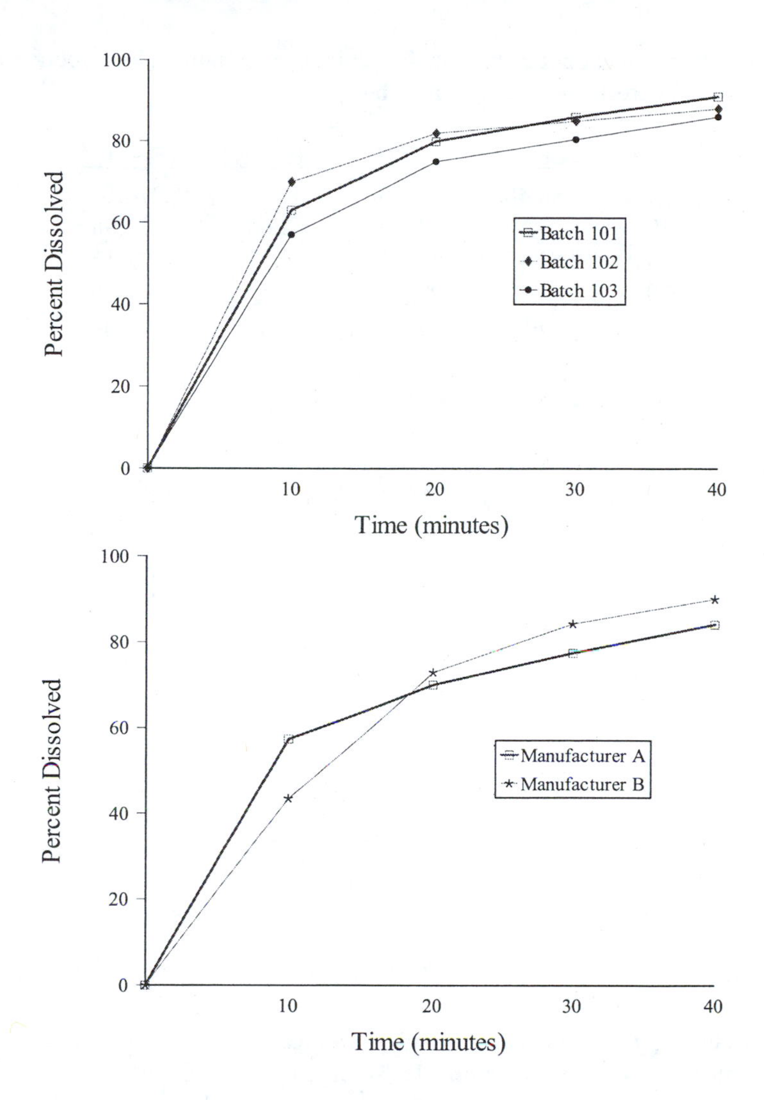


**Figure 22.5** Examples of dissolution profiles.

Several criteria must be met in order to apply the $f_1$ and $f_2$ calculations (FDA, 1997). These include: 1) test and reference batches should be tested under exactly the same conditions, including the same time points; 2) only one time point should be considered after 85% dissolution for both batches; and 3) the "percent coefficient of variation" (what we have called the relative standard deviation in Chapter 5) at the earlier time points should be no more than 20% and at other time points should be no more than 10%. The rationale for these criteria is discussed by Shah and colleagues (1998).

Looking at the data presented in Table 22.5, our data fulfills all three criteria. Therefore, both the $f_1$ and $f_2$ statistics can be used to evaluate the equivalency of these two types of production equipment. To calculate certain values required by the statistics, we can create an intermediate table:

| Time | $R_t$ | $T_t$ | $\lvert R_t - T_t \rvert$ | $(R_t - T_t)^2$ |
|---|---|---|---|---|
| 15 | 56.48 | 73.05 | 16.57 | 274.56 |
| 30 | 76.32 | 79.92 | 3.60 | 12.96 |
| 45 | 82.85 | 84.32 | 1.47 | 2.16 |
| 60 | 87.87 | 89.42 | 1.55 | 2.40 |
| Σ= | 303.52 | 326.71 | 23.19 | 292.08 |

Using these numbers produces the following results:

$$f_1 = \frac{\sum \lvert R_t - T_t \rvert}{\sum R_t} x\,100 = \frac{23.19}{303.52} x100 = 7.64$$

$$f_2 = 50 \cdot \log \left[ \frac{1}{\sqrt{1 + \frac{1}{n} \Sigma (R_t - T_t)^2}} x\,100 \right]$$

$$f_2 = 50 \cdot \log \left[ \frac{1}{\sqrt{1 + \frac{1}{4} (292.08)}} x\,100 \right]$$

$$f_2 = 50 \cdot \log (11.62) = 50(1.06) = 53.3$$

In this example, $f_1$ is less than 15 and $f_2$ is greater than 50; therefore, we would conclude that the two dissolution profiles are not significantly different.

Although the tests presented in this chapter have focused strictly on bioequivalence, they provide us means for showing equivalency between levels of any discrete independent variables.

## References

*Federal Register* (1977). 42: 1648.

*Federal Register* (1978). 43: 6965-6969.

*Federal Register* (1995). 60: 61638-61643.

FDA (1997). “Guidance for industry: dissolution testing of immediate release solid oral dosage forms,” (BP1), Center for Drug Evaluation and Research, Food and Drug Administration, Rockville, MD, p. 9.

ICH Steering Committee (1998). “ICH E9 – Statistical principles for clinical trials,” International Conference on Harmonization of Technical Requirements for Registration of Pharmaceuticals for Human Use. *Federal Register* 63:49583-49598.

ICH Steering Committee (1999). “E10 – Choice of control group and related issues in clinical trials,” International Conference on Harmonization of Technical Requirements for Registration of Pharmaceuticals for Human Use. *Federal Register* 64:51767-51780.

*United States Pharmacopeia* (2005). 28th revision, United States Pharmacopeial Convention, Rockville, MD, p. 183.

Benet, L.Z. and Goyan, J.E. (1995). “Bioequivalence and narrow therapeutic index drugs,” *Pharmacotherapy* 15:433-440.

Chan, I.S. (2002). “Power and sample size determination for noninferiority trials using an exact method,*” Journal of Biopharmaceutical Statistics* 12: 457-469.

Chow, S.C. and Liu, J.P. (2000). *Design and Analysis of Bioavailability and Bioequivalence Studies*, Second edition, Marcel Dekker, Inc., New York.

Evans, W.E., Schentag, J.J., and Jusko, W.J. (eds), (1992). *Applied Pharmacokinetics: Principles of Therapeutic Drug Monitoring*, Third edition, Applied Therapeutics, Vancouver, WA.

Hauck, W.W. and Anderson, S. (1984). “A New Statistical Procedure for Testing Equivalence in Two-Group Comparative Bioavailability Trials,” *Journal of Pharmacokinetics and Biopharmaceutics* 12:83-91.

Kirk, R.E. (1968). *Experimental Design: Procedures for the Behavioral Sciences*, Brooks/Cole Publishing, Belmont, CA, pp. 424-440.

Malinowski, H.J. (2000). “Bioavailability and Bioequivalency Testing,” Chapter 53 in *Remington: The Science and Practice of Pharmacy*, Twentieth edition, Gennaro, A.R. (ed.), Lippincott, Williams and Wilkins, Baltimore, MD, pp. 995-1004.

Metzler, C.M. (1974). “Bioavailability: A problem in equivalence,” *Biometrics* 30:309-317.

Pigeot, I., Schäfer, J., Röhmel, J., and Hauschke, D. (2003). “Assessing noninferiority of a new treatment in a three-arm clinical trial including a placebo,” *Statistics in*

*Medicine* 22:883-899.

Schuirmann, D.J. (1987). "Comparison of the two one-sided tests procedure and the power approach for assessing the equivalence of average bioavailability," *Journal of Pharmacokinetics and Biopharmaceutics* 15:660.

Shah, V.P., et al. (1998). "*In Vitro* dissolution profile comparison – statistics and analysis of the similarity factor, $f_2$," *Pharmaceutical Research* 15:891-898.

Snapinn, S.M. (2000). "Noninferiority trials," *Current Controlled Trials in Cardiovascular Medicine* 1:19-21.

Temple, R. and Ellenberg, S.S. (2000). "Placebo-controlled trials and active-control trials in the evaluation of new treatments," *Annals of Internal Medicine* 133:455-463.

Wang, S.J., Hung, H.M.J., and Tsong, Y. (2003). "Noninferiority analysis in active controlled clinical trials," *Encyclopedia of Biopharmaceutical Statistics*, Chow, S.C. (ed.), Marcel Dekker, New York, p. 674.

Westlake, W.J. (1988). "Bioavailability and bioequivalence of pharmaceutical formulations," *Biopharmaceutical Statistics for Drug Development*. Peace, K.E., (ed.), Marcel Dekker, New York, p. 342.

Welling, P.G. and Tse, F.L.S. (1995). *Pharmacokinetics*, Second edition, Marcel Dekker, Inc., New York.

Winter, M.E. (1994). *Basic Clinical Pharmacokinetics*, Third edition, Mary Anne Koda-Kimble, M.A. and Young, L.Y. (eds), Applied Therapeutics, Vancouver, WA.

Zar, J.H. (1999). *Biostatistical Analysis*, Fourth edition., Prentice-Hall, Englewood Cliffs, NJ, pp. 134.

**Suggested Supplemental readings:**

Chan, I.S.F. (2004). "Noninferiority and equivalency trials," *Journal of Biopharmaceutical Statistics* 14: 261,262.

Chan, I.S.F. (2003). "Statistical analysis of noninferiority trials with a rate ratio in small-sample match-pair designs," *Biometrics* 59:1170-1177.

Hauck, W.W. and Anderson, S. (1984). "A New Statistical Procedure for Testing Equivalence in Two-Group Comparative Bioavailability Trials," *Journal of Pharmacokinetics and Biopharmaceutics* 12:83-91.

Rodda, B.E. (1990). "Bioavailability: design and analysis," *Statistical Methodology in the Pharmaceutical Sciences*. Berry, D.A., (ed.), Marcel Dekker, New York, pp. 57-82.

Schuirmann, D.J. (1987). "Comparison of the two one-sided tests procedure and the power approach for assessing the equivalence of average bioavailability," *Journal of Pharmacokinetics and Biopharmaceutics* 15:657-680.

Schuirmann, D.J. (1990). "Design of bioavailability/bioequivalence studies," Drug Information Journal 15:315-323.

Shah, V.P., et al. (1998). "*In Vitro* dissolution profile comparison – statistics and analysis of the similarity factor, $f_2$," *Pharmeutical Research* 15:891-898.

Westlake, W.J. (1988). "Bioavailability and bioequivalence of pharmaceutical formulations," *Biopharmaceutical Statistics for Drug Development.* Peace, K.E. (ed.), Marcel Dekker, New York, p.329-352.

**Example Problems**

1. In a clinical trial, data comparing Gigantic Drugs a new generic product was compared with the Innovator's branded antipsychotic; both products contain the exact same chemical entity. One subject did not complete the study. The results were as follows:

| | Innovator | Generic |
|---|---|---|
| Mean = | 289.7 | 271.6 |
| Standard Deviation = | 18.1 | 20.4 |
| n = | 24 | 23 |

   Use the confidence interval approach and the two one-tailed t-tests to check for bioequivalence, assuming there should be less than a 10% difference between the two products.

2. Production of a certain product in two different countries (A and B) were compared to the manufacturer's original production site (standard). Dissolution data is presented in Table 22.6 and Figure 22.6. Visually it appears that site B has a profile closer to the reference standard, but do both of the foreign facilities meet the SUPAC-IR guidelines for similarity?

**Answers to Problems**

1. Clinical trial data comparing a new generic product to an Innovator's branded drug. Is there less than a 10% difference between the products?

**Table 22.6** Dissolution Data (percent)

| Time (minutes) | Country A | Country B | Standard |
|---|---|---|---|
| 15 | 57.3 | 54.1 | 49.8 |
| 30 | 66.4 | 67.7 | 70.8 |
| 45 | 71.9 | 75.4 | 80.9 |
| 60 | 76.4 | 81.4 | 86.7 |
| 75 | 80.4 | 85.6 | 90.9 |
| 90 | 84.6 | 88.8 | 93.6 |

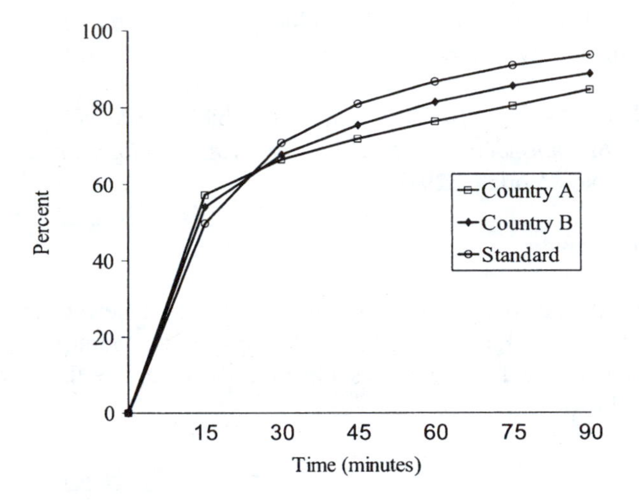


**Figure 22.6** Dissolution profiles for two foreign countries.

| | Innovator | Generic |
|---|---|---|
| Mean = | 289.7 | 271.6 |
| Standard Deviation = | 18.1 | 20.4 |
| n = | 24 | 23 |

10% difference = 28.97 ($\delta$=289.7 x 0.10)

Difference observed = 18.1 (289.7 – 271.6)

Pooled variance:

$$S_p^2 = \frac{(n_1 - 1)S_1^2 + (n_2 - 1)S_2^2}{n_1 + n_2 - 2} = \frac{23(18.1)^2 + 22(20.4)^2}{24 + 23 - 2} = 370.9$$

Standard error portion of the equations:

$$\sqrt{\frac{S_P^2}{n_1}+\frac{S_P^2}{n_2}}=\sqrt{\frac{370.9}{24}+\frac{370.9}{23}}=5.62$$

a. Confidence interval

$$Lower\ Limit=\frac{(d\text{ - }SE)+\overline{X}_R}{\overline{X}_R}\ x\ 100\%$$

$$Lower\ Limit=\frac{(18.1\text{ - }5.62)+289.7}{289.7}\ x\ 100\%=104.3\%$$

$$Upper\ Limit=\frac{(d+SE)+\overline{X}_R}{\overline{X}_R}\ x\ 100\%$$

$$Lower\ Limit=\frac{(18.1+5.62)+289.7}{289.7}\ x\ 100\%=108.2\%$$

The limits of our estimated interval are:

$$Lower\ Limit<\frac{\mu_T}{\mu_R}<Upper\ Limit$$

$$104.3\%<\frac{\mu_T}{\mu_R}<108.2\%$$

Therefore, we are 95% confident that we have equivalence because the difference is well within our criteria of ±10% and the true population ratio is somewhere between 104.3 and 108.2%.

b. Two one-tailed t-tests

Hypotheses: $H_{01}$: $\mu_T - \mu_R \leq 10\%$
$H_{11}$: $\mu_T - \mu_R > 10\%$

$H_{02}$: $\mu_T - \mu_R \geq 10\%$
$H_{12}$: $\mu_T - \mu_R < 10\%$

Decision rule: With $\alpha = 0.05$, reject $H_{01}$ or $H_{02}$ if $|t| > t_{45}(.95) \approx 1.679$

$$t_1 = \frac{(\overline{X}_T - \overline{X}_R) - \delta_1}{\sqrt{\frac{2S_p^2}{n}}} = \frac{18.1-(-28.97)}{5.62} = 8.38$$

$$t_2 = \frac{\delta_2 - (\overline{X}_T - \overline{X}_R)}{\sqrt{\frac{2S_p^2}{n}}} = \frac{28.97 - 18.1}{5.62} = 1.93$$

Decision: Reject $H_{01}$ and $H_{02}$, and conclude that there is a difference between the two populations are less than 10%.

2. To compare Country A and the "standard" original facility, the first step is to calculate the difference term in the denominator:

$$\Sigma(R_t - T_t)^2 = (49.8 - 57.3)^2 \;...\; + (93.6 - 84.6) = 453.95$$

The calculation of the remainder of the $f_2$ formula is as follows:

$$f_2 = 50 \cdot \log \left[ \frac{1}{\sqrt{1 + \frac{1}{n}\Sigma(R_t - T_t)^2}} x\,100 \right]$$

$$f_2 = 50 \cdot \log \left[ \frac{1}{\sqrt{1 + \frac{1}{6}(453.95)}} x\,100 \right]$$

$$f_2 = 50 \cdot \log(11.421) = 50 \cdot (1.058) = 52.9$$

Decision: With $f_2 > 50$ conclude that the two dissolution profiles are the same and that there is no significant difference between the product produced in Country A and the manufacturer's original production site.

To compare Country B and the "standard" original facility, the same process is used:

$$\Sigma(R_t - T_t)^2 = (49.8 - 54.1)^2 \;...\; + (93.6 - 88.8) = 137.56$$

$$f_2 = 50 \cdot \log \left[ \frac{1}{\sqrt{1 + \frac{1}{6}(137.56)}} x\,100 \right]$$

$$f_2 = 50 \cdot \log(20.444) = 50 \cdot (1.311) = 65.55$$

Decision: With $f_2 > 50$ conclude that the two dissolution profiles are the same and that there is no significant difference between the product produced in Country A and the manufacturer's original production site.

Note that Country B produced a higher $f_2$ and that confirms the visual assessment that the dissolution profile for Country B was closer to that of the original product.

# 23

# Outlier Tests

An outlier is an extreme data point that is significantly different from the remaining values in a set of observations. Based on information, either investigational or statistical,, an outlier value may be removed from the data set before performing an inferential test. However, removal of an outlier is discouraged unless the data point can be clearly demonstrated to be erroneous. Rodda (1990) provided an excellent description of outliers when he portrayed them as "... much like weeds; they are very difficult to define and are only called outliers because they are inconsistent with the environment in which they are observed." Outliers can dramatically affect the outcome of a statistical analysis. This is especially true if the sample size is small. However, we need to use care in our decision-making process to ensure that we remove the weed and not a budding piece of data.

**Regulatory Considerations**

Outliers are often referred to as **aberrant results** and have been the source of regulatory discussions and guidances. Prior to the introduction of USP Chapter <1010> in 2005, there were no compendia guidances on the treatment of outliers, except with respect to biological assays presented in USP <111>. This lack of guidance or "silence" on the part of USP, was noted in the 1993 litigation United States vs. Barr Laboratories, Inc. (Wolin, 1993). Judge Wolin's ruling in the Barr case pointed out the need for compendia guidance in this area of outliers, as well as other analytical measures. USP <1010> attempts to address many of these issues (USP, 2005). This chapter lists a litany of other synonyms for outlying results, including "anomalous, contaminated, discordant, spurious, suspicious or wild observations; and flyers, rogues, and mavericks."

In 1998 the FDA focused attention on a similar problem, out-of-specification (OOS) test results, and issued a draft guidance (FDA, 1998). In addition to outlier tests, the guidance attempts to address retesting, resampling, and averaging of test results.

Similar to other laboratory results, potential outliers must be documented and interpreted. Both USP <1010> and the FDA guidance propose a two-phase approach to identifying and dealing with outliers. When an outlier is suspected, the first phase is a thorough and systematic laboratory investigation to determine if there is a possible assignable cause for the aberrant result. Potential assignable causes include "human error, instrumentation error, calculation error, and product or component deficiency" (USP, 2005). If one can identify an assignable cause in the first phase, then the outlier can be removed and retesting of the same sample or a new sample is permissible. However, if no assignable cause can be identified, then the second phase is to evaluate the potential aberrant value using statistical outlier tests as part of the overall outlier investigation. When used correctly, the outlier tests described below are valuable statistical tools; however, any judgment about the acceptability of data in which outliers are observed requires careful interpretation.

The term "outlier labeling" refers to an informal recognition of a potential aberrant value (often performed visually using graphing procedures discussed in Chapter 4). Use of statistical procedures to determine if any value is truly aberrant is termed "outlier identification." Determining the most appropriate outlier test will depend on the assumed population distribution and the sample size.

If, as the result of either thorough investigation or outlier test, a value is removed as an outlier, this is termed an "outlier rejection." Both the FDA and USP note that using an outlier test cannot be the sole means for outlier rejection. Even though the outlier tests can be useful as part of the determination of the aberrant nature of a data point, the outlier test can never replace the value of a thorough laboratory investigation. All data, especially outliers, should be kept for future reference. Outliers are not used to calculate the final reportable values, but should be footnoted in tables or reports.

One simple way to address the issue of an aberrant value is to perform the intended statistical analysis both with and without the potential outlier(s). If the results of the analysis are the same (rejecting or failing to reject the null hypothesis), the question of whether a value is an outlier becomes a moot issue.

## Outliers on a Single Continuum

With both descriptive and inferential statistics it is common to report the center and distribution for the sample data. An uncharacteristic observation could be either a valid data point that falls to one of the extreme tailing ends of our continuum or due to some error in data collection. In the latter case, this would be considered an outlier. Many detectable and undetectable effects could cause such an extreme measurement, including: 1) a temporary equipment malfunction; 2) a technician or observer misreading the result; 3) errors in data entry; 4) calculation errors; 5) contamination; or 6) a very large or small measurement within the extremes of the distribution. With respect to the last point, an outlier does not necessarily imply that an error has occurred with the experiment, only that an extreme value has occurred. Vigilance is important with any data manipulation and an inspection of data for recording or transcribing errors is always warranted before the statistical analysis.

Another consideration is that a potential outlier could be a legitimate observation in a strongly skewed distribution and represent a value at the extreme end of the longer tail. Transforming data may be first required to create a normally distributed

**Table 23.1** Impact of a Potential Outlier on Measures of Central Tendency

| | 88% Included | 88% Not Included |
|---|---|---|
| Mean | 95.8 | 97.4 |
| Standard Deviation | 4.1 | 1.5 |
| Range | 11 | 4 |
| Median | 97.5 | 98 |

sample before performing some of the outlier tests. Even an extremely high value in a strong positively skewed distribution may be a true value and not necessarily an outlier. As discussed in Chapter 6, common transformations include using the logarithms or square roots of the individual data points. Alternatively, for non-normally distributed populations, there are robust measures for central tendency and spread (the median and median absolute deviation) and exploratory data analysis (EDA) methods. Use of a nonparametric procedure or other robust technique, is termed "outlier accommodation" and usually involve rank ordering the data that minimized the influence of outliers. Various transformations or ranking of the data can be used to minimize the effect of an outlier. This was pointed out in Chapter 21, when nonparametric statistics were described as being influenced less by outliers than are traditional parametric tests, whose calculations are affected by measures of dispersion (variance and standard deviation). In addition outliers could represent data points accidentally sampled from a population that is different from the intended population. Also, care should be taken that computer programs do not handle missing data as real values (in most cases assigning a value of zero).

Extreme values can greatly influence the most common measures of central tendency; they can distort the mean and greatly inflate the variance. This is especially true with small sample sizes. In contrast, the median and quartile measures are relatively insulated from the effects of outliers. For example consider the following assay results (in percents):

97, 98, 98, 95, 88, 99

Whether or not 88% is a true outlier, it has an important effect on the mean and spread (range and variance) of the sample and can be termed an **influential observation**, which will be discussed later in this chapter. Table 23.1 shows the impact this one observation can have on various measures of central tendency. As seen in the table, this extreme value pulls the mean in the direction of that value, increases the standard deviation by a factor of two, and the range is increased almost threefold. However, the median (97.5) is relatively unaffected. This would also be true even if the lowest value was 78 or even 68%. As mentioned, nonparametric tests rely on ranking of observations, in many cases the use the median as the center of the distribution, and are less affected by outliers. In fact, using the various statistical tests listed below, the value 88% would not be rejected as an outlier. It would be considered only an influential observation.

A second example of assay results is presented below. In this case the more

**Table 23.2** Impact of a Potential Outlier on Measures of Central Tendency with Two Sample Sizes

| | Case 1 | | |
|---|---|---|---|
| | 86% Not Included | 86% Included | Case 2 |
| n | 5 | 6 | 12 |
| Mean | 97.4 | 95.5 | 96.5 |
| S.D. | 1.5 | 4.8 | 3.5 |
| Range | 4 | 11 | 11 |
| Median | 98 | 97.5 | 98 |

extreme value (86%) would be defined as an outlier, with 95% confidence using the test procedures discussed below. In this particular sample there are only six tablets:

97, 98, 98, 95, 86, 99

For illustrative purposes, assume in this second case that these results were part of a larger sample of twelve tablets.

97, 98, 98, 95, 86, 99
98, 98, 97, 99, 98, 95

Without the outlier, both the first case and second case have approximately the same mean and standard deviation. Notice in Table 23.2, that the greater sample size "softens" the effect of the outlier. In the second case, 86% would not be identified as an outlier using the tests described in this chapter. If possible, additional measurements should be made when a suspect outlier occurs, particularly if the sample size is very small.

To test for outliers we need at least three observations. Naturally the more information we have (the larger the sample size), the more obvious an outlier will become, either visually or statistically. For a sample size as small as three observations, there would need to be a wide discrepancy for one data point to be deemed an outlier. If an outlier is identified, it is important to try and identify a possible cause for this extreme value (i.e., miscalculation, data entry error, contamination). The identification of an outlier can lead to future corrective action in the process or research being conducted, but it can also serve as a potential source of new information about the population.

A simple technique to "soften" the influence of possible outliers is called **winsorizing** (Dixon and Masey, 1969). Using this process the two most extreme observations (the largest value and the smallest value) are changed to the value of their next closest neighbor ($x_1 \rightarrow x_2$; $x_n \rightarrow x_{n-1}$). For example, consider the following rank ordered set of observations, where 11 might be an outlier:

11,21,24,25,26,26,27,28,29,31

Our suspected outlier would be replaced with the second lowest number. Also we would replace the largest value with the second largest value:

<u>21</u>,21,24,25,26,26,27,28,29,<u>29</u>

For the first set of data the mean and standard deviation are 24.8 ± 5.6 and for the winsorized data they are 25.6 ± 2.9. For this set of data the potential outlier has little impact (+3% change) on our sample mean, but a dramatic chance in the standard deviation (48% decrease). Although not a statistical test for outliers, winsorizing might provide a quick measure of the impact of extreme values on the measures of central tendency for our sample.

**Plotting and the Number of Standard Deviations from the Center**

By using various plotting methods to display the data, outliers may become readily visible. For example, box-and-whisker plots are specifically designed to identify possible outliers (Figure 23.1). As discussed in Chapter 4, each of the "whiskers" or t-bars extending from the box three semi-interquartile ranges (SIQR) above and below the median (the SIQR being the distance between the upper or lower quartile and the median, Eq. 4.1). Observations that fall above or below the whiskers can be identified as potential outliers. Potential outliers can also be observed using other graphic techniques including stem-and-leaf plots, histograms, line charts, or point plots. In addition, scatter plots can be useful in identifying potential outliers involving two or more continuous variables.

An example of the box-and-whisker plots will be presented later when discussing residuals under the bivariate outliers section.

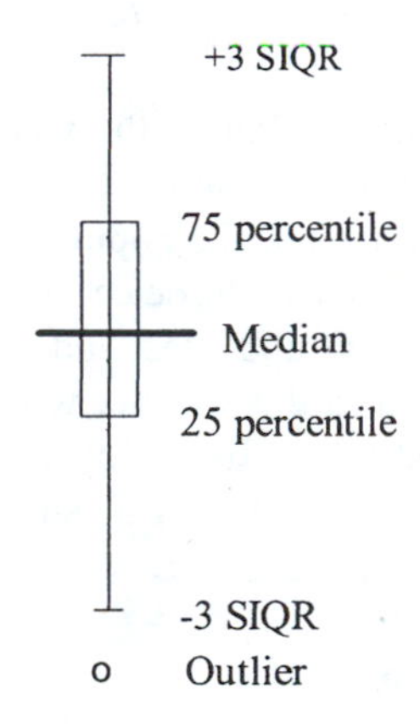


**Figure 23.1** Box-and-whisker plot.

### The "Huge" Rule

One method for detecting an aberrant value is to compare the potential outlier to the sample mean and standard deviation with the potential outlier removed from the calculations. This general rule of thumb is to consider the data point as an outlier if that point is located more than four standard deviations from the mean as calculated without the suspected outlier (Marascuilo, 1971). The rationale for this rule is that it is extremely unlikely ($p < 0.00005$) to find values more than four standard deviations from the expected center of a distribution. The distance, in standard deviations, is measured between the mean and the potential outliers:

$$M = \frac{|x_i - \overline{X}|}{S} \qquad \text{Eq. 23.1}$$

where $\overline{X}$ and $S$ are calculated from the sample data, ignoring the outlier value ($x_i$). If $M$ is greater than four, then the data point is considered to be an outlier.

To illustrate this rule of thumb test, consider the following observations:

99.3, 99.7, 98.6, 99.0, 99.1, 99.3, 99.5, 98.0,
98.9, 99.4, 99.0, 99.4, 99.2, 98.8, 99.2

Using this set of 15 observations, is data point 98.0 an outlier? For the huge rule, the mean and standard deviation are calculated without 98.0 and the number of standard deviations is calculated between this mean and 98.0. These sample results are $\overline{X}$ = 99.17 and $S$ = 0.29 without 98.0. The calculation of the number of standard deviations from the mean for our potential outlier is:

$$M = \frac{|x_i - \overline{X}|}{S} = \frac{|99.17 - 98.0|}{0.29} = \frac{1.17}{0.29} = 4.03$$

Since the data point 98.0 is more than 4.00 below the mean it is disregarded as an outlier. Several other procedures are available to statistically determine if observations are outliers or simply extremes of the population from which the sample is selected. The most commonly used statistics to detect univariate outliers (involving one discrete independent variable) are the Grubbs' test and the Dixon Q test and these will be discussed below. Also discussed in this chapter will be Hampel's rule. Other possible tests include: 1) Youden's test for outliers (Taylor, 1987); 2) Cochran's test for extreme values of variance (Taylor, 1987); and 3) studentized deleted residuals (Mason, 1989).

### Grubbs' Test for Outlying Observations

Grubbs' procedure involves ranking the observations from smallest to largest ($x_1 < x_2 < x_3 < \ldots x_n$) and calculating the mean and standard deviation for all of the observations in the data set (Grubbs, 1969). This test is also referred to as **Extreme Studentized Deviate test** or **ESD test**. One of the following two formulas is used, depending upon whether $x_1$ (the smallest value) or $x_n$ (the largest value), is suspected of being a possible outlier.

$$T = \frac{\overline{X} - x_1}{S} \quad or \quad T = \frac{x_n - \overline{X}}{S} \qquad \text{Eq. 23.2}$$

These formulas are occasionally referred to as the **T procedure** or **T method**. This resultant $T$ is compared to a critical value on Table B21 (Appendix B), based on the sample size ($n$) for a given allowable error ($\alpha$). The error level for interpreting the result of the Grubbs' test is the same as our previous discussion of hypothesis testing. Once again $\alpha$ will represent the researcher-controlled error rate. Assuming we want to be 95% confident in our decision and use the 5% level (right column in Table B21), we may incorrectly reject an outlier one in 20 times. If $T$ is greater than the critical value, the data point can be rejected as an outlier. Using the previous example, the information is first ranked in ascending order (Table 23.3). The mean and standard deviations are then calculated with the proposed outlier included. The results are: $\overline{X}$ = 99.09 and $S$ = 0.41. Using Grubbs' test we first identify the critical value on Table B21; in this case it is 2.409 for $n$ = 15 and $\alpha$ = .05. The calculation of the Grubbs' test is

$$T = \frac{\overline{X} - x_1}{S} = \frac{99.09 - 98.0}{0.41} = \frac{1.09}{0.41} = 2.66$$

**Table 23.3** Sample Rank Ordered Data for Outlier Tests

| | Value |
|---|---|
| $x_1$ | 98.0 |
| $x_2$ | 98.6 |
| $x_3$ | 98.8 |
| ... | 98.9 |
| | 99.0 |
| | 99.0 |
| | 99.1 |
| | 99.2 |
| | 99.2 |
| | 99.3 |
| | 99.3 |
| ... | 99.4 |
| $x_{n-2}$ | 99.4 |
| $x_{n-1}$ | 99.5 |
| $x_n$ | 99.7 |

Since our calculated value of 2.66 exceeds the critical value of 2.409, once again 98.0 is rejected as an outlier.

**Dixon Q Test**

A third method to determine if a suspected value is an outlier is to measure the difference between that data point with the next closest value and compare that difference to the total range of observations (Dixon, 1953). Various ratios of this type (absolute ratios without regard to sign) make up the **Dixon test** for outlying observations, also referred to as the **Dixon Q test**. Both the Grubbs' test and Dixon Q test assume that the population from which the sample is taken is normally distributed. The advantage of this test is that it is not required to estimate the standard deviation. First the observations are rank ordered similar to the Grubbs' test (Table 23.3):

$$x_1 < x_2 < x_3 < \ldots x_{n-2} < x_{n-1} < x_n$$

Formulas for the Dixon test use ratios of ranges and subranges within the data. The ratios are listed in Table 23.4 and the choice of ratio is dependent on the sample size and whether $x_1$ or $x_n$ is suspected to be an outlier. If the smallest observation is suspected of being an outlier, use the ratios are presented on the upper half of Table 23.4. However, if the largest value is evaluated as the outlier, use the ratios in the lower half of Table 23.4. The resultant ratio is compared to the critical values in Table B22 (Appendix B). If the calculated ratio is greater than the value in the table, the data point can be rejected as an outlier. Using the Dixon test for the data presented in Table 23.3, the critical value from Table B22 is $\tau = 0.525$, based on $n = 15$ and $\alpha = .05$. The calculated Dixon ratio would be:

$$\frac{(x_3 - x_1)}{(x_{n-2} - x_1)} = \frac{98.8 - 98.0}{99.4 - 98.0} = \frac{0.8}{1.4} = 0.57$$

Because this calculated value of 0.57 exceeds the critical value of 0.525, we reject 98.0 as an outlier.

The Grubbs' and Dixon's tests may not always agree regarding the rejection of the possible outlier, especially when the test statistic results are very close to the allowable error (i.e., 5% level). The simplicity of Dixon's test is of most benefit when small samples are involved and only one observation is suspected as an outlier. Grubbs' test requires more calculations (i.e., determining the sample mean and standard deviation), but is considered to be the more powerful of the two tests. Also, Grubbs' test can be used when there is more than one suspected outlier (Mason, p.512). As with any statistical test that measures the same type of outcomes, the researcher should select the outlier test he or she is most comfortable with before looking at the data.

As mentioned previously, both Grubbs' and Dixon's tests assume that the population from which the sample was taken is normal distributed. In the case of the

**Table 23.4** Ratios for Dixon's Test for Outliers

| Sample Size | Ratio | If $x_1$ is suspected | |
|---|---|---|---|
| $3 \leq n \leq 7$ | $\tau_{10}$ | $\frac{x_2 - x_1}{x_n - x_1}$ | Eq. 23.3 |
| $8 \leq n \leq 10$ | $\tau_{11}$ | $\frac{x_2 - x_1}{x_{n-1} - x_1}$ | Eq. 23.4 |
| $11 \leq n \leq 13$ | $\tau_{21}$ | $\frac{x_3 - x_1}{x_{n-1} - x_1}$ | Eq. 23.5 |
| $14 \leq n \leq 25$ | $\tau_{22}$ | $\frac{x_3 - x_1}{x_{n-2} - x_1}$ | Eq. 23.6 |
| Sample Size | Ratio | If $x_n$ is suspected | |
| $3 \leq n \leq 7$ | $\tau_{10}$ | $\frac{x_n - x_{n-1}}{x_n - x_1}$ | Eq. 23.7 |
| $8 \leq n \leq 10$ | $\tau_{11}$ | $\frac{x_n - x_{n-1}}{x_n - x_2}$ | Eq. 23.8 |
| $11 \leq n \leq 13$ | $\tau_{21}$ | $\frac{x_n - x_{n-2}}{x_n - x_2}$ | Eq. 23.9 |
| $14 \leq n \leq 25$ | $\tau_{22}$ | $\frac{x_n - x_{n-2}}{x_n - x_3}$ | Eq. 23.10 |

Grubbs' test with more than one outlier, the most extreme measurement will tend to be masked by the presence of other possible outliers. **Masking** occurs when two or more outliers have similar values. In a data set, if the two smallest (or largest) values are almost equal, an outlier test for the more extreme of the two values will not be statistically significant. This is especially true for sample sizes less than ten, where the numerator of the ratio for the Dixon Q test is the difference between the two most extreme values. Only a test for both of these two smallest observations will be statistically significant. Plotting the data can sometimes avoid the masking problem. **Swamping** is another problem and is seen when several good data points, that may be close to the suspected outlier, disguise its effect. Using graphing techniques, it is possible to identify a cluster of data points and these might influence tests for outliers.

### Hampel's Rule

The underlying assumption with both the Grubbs' and Dixon's tests is that the sample being evaluated comes from population with a normal distribution. Hampel's rule for testing outliers is based on the median and can be used for samples that have either normally or nonnormally distributed populations.

**Table 23.5** Example Using Hampel's Rule

| | Data | Absolute Deviations ($AD_i$) | Absolute Normalized Deviations ($NAD_i$) |
|---|---|---|---|
| | 99.7 | 0.5 | 1.686 |
| | 99.5 | 0.3 | 1.011 |
| | 99.4 | 0.2 | 0.674 |
| | 99.4 | 0.2 | 0.674 |
| | 99.3 | 0.1 | 0.337 |
| | 99.3 | 0.1 | 0.337 |
| | 99.2 | 0 | 0.000 |
| | 99.2 | 0 | 0.000 |
| | 99.1 | 0.1 | 0.337 |
| | 99.0 | 0.2 | 0.674 |
| | 99.0 | 0.2 | 0.674 |
| | 98.9 | 0.3 | 1.011 |
| | 98.8 | 0.4 | 1.349 |
| | 98.6 | 0.6 | 2.023 |
| | 98.0 | 1.2 | 4.046 |
| Median = | 99.2 | 0.2 | |
| MAD = | | 0.2966 | |

The first step in determining an outlier using Hampel's rule is to calculate an *MAD* value (which is the median for the absolute deviations from the median times a constant). To calculate the *MAD* the median is subtracted from each data point and expressed in absolute terms (called the **absolute deviations**).

$$AD_i = |x_i - Md| \qquad \text{Eq. 23.11}$$

For example, using our previous data set, the $AD_i$ for 98.0 is:

$$AD_i = |98.0 - 99.2| = |-1.2| = 1.2$$

These absolute derivations are presented in the second column of Table 23.5. The next step is to multiply the median for the absolute deviations by a constant 1.483[1] to produce the $MAD_i$.

$$MAD_i = Median(AD_i) \cdot 1.483 \qquad \text{Eq. 23.12}$$

[1] The constant 1.483 is the reciprocal of the range of values for a normal standardized distribution between the first and third quartiles. The area between -0.674 and +0.674 is 0.500 (1.483 = 1/0.674).

The third step is to normalize the $MAD_i$ data. However instead of subtracting each value from the mean and dividing the results by the standard deviation (similar to Grubbs' calculations), each value is subtracted from the median and divided by the *MAD*.

$$NAD_i = \frac{|Md - x_i|}{MAD_i} \qquad \text{Eq. 23.13}$$

These results are presented in the third column of Table 23.5. In the case of an assumed underlying normal distribution, if the most extreme value is greater than 3.5 it can be rejected as an outlier (more than 3.5 standard deviations based on the normalized median). In this example, 98.0 is once again removed as an outlier. Hampel provides other constants and critical values for non-normal situations (Hampel, 1985).

**Multiple Outliers**

Once an initial extreme outlier value has been determined and removed from the data, the researcher can determine if there is a possible second outlier using the same procedures with $n - 1$ data points. Using our data from the previous example (now with only 14 data points) is 98.6 a possible outlier? In this case the mean and standard deviation for the data would be:

| | With 98.6 | Without 98.6 |
|---|---|---|
| Mean | 99.17 | 99.22 |
| SD | 0.29 | 0.25 |
| n | 14 | 14 |

Using the Huge rule, the value 98.6 is less than four standard deviations below the mean and not an outlier:

$$M = \frac{|x_i - \overline{X}|}{S} = \frac{|99.22 - 98.6|}{0.25} = \frac{1.17}{0.29} = 2.14$$

Using the Grubbs' test we fail to reject 98.6 as an outlier because it does not exceed the critical value of 2.371.

$$T = \frac{\overline{X} - x_1}{S} = \frac{99.17 - 98.6}{0.29} = \frac{0.57}{0.29} = 1.97$$

Dixon's test shows similar results, with the calculated ratio not exceeding the critical value of 0.546.

**Table 23.6** Example Using Hampel's Rule without 98.0

| | Data | Absolute Deviations ($AD_i$) | Absolute Normalized Deviations ($NAD_i$) |
|---|---|---|---|
| | 99.7 | 0.5 | 1.686 |
| | 99.5 | 0.3 | 1.011 |
| | 99.4 | 0.2 | 0.674 |
| | 99.4 | 0.2 | 0.674 |
| | 99.3 | 0.1 | 0.337 |
| | 99.3 | 0.1 | 0.337 |
| | 99.2 | 0 | 0.000 |
| | 99.2 | 0 | 0.000 |
| | 99.1 | 0.1 | 0.337 |
| | 99.0 | 0.2 | 0.674 |
| | 99.0 | 0.2 | 0.674 |
| | 98.9 | 0.3 | 1.011 |
| | 98.8 | 0.4 | 1.349 |
| | 98.6 | 0.6 | 2.023 |
| Median = | 99.2 | 0.2 | |
| MAD = | | 0.2966 | |

$$\frac{(x_3 - x_1)}{(x_{n-2} - x_1)} = \frac{98.9 - 98.6}{99.4 - 98.6} = \frac{0.3}{0.8} = 0.375$$

Finally, the same results are found with Hampel's rule as seen in Table 23.6 where the absolute normalized deviation for 98.6 is less than 3.5. Note the values in Tables 23.5 and 23.6 are similar because the median value is the same in both cases.

## Bivariate Outliers in Correlation and Regression Analysis

In the case of correlation or regression, where each data point represents values on different axes, an outlier is a point clearly outside the range of the other data points on the respective axis. Outliers may greatly affect the results of correlation regression models. Outliers in regression analysis are data points that fall outside the linear pattern of the regression line. One rule of thumb is to consider any point on an outlier if its standardized residual value is greater than 3.3. This would correspond to an $\alpha = 0.001$. At the same time, many statistical tests for identifying multivariate outliers are prone to problems of masking, swamping, or both; and no single method is adequate for all given situations. For our discussion we will focus only on the simplest situations where we are analyzing just two continuous variables. Obviously problems will compound as additional variables enter into the analysis.

In linear regression-type models, outliers generally do not occur in the independent variable, because the levels for that variable are selected by the researcher and can usually be controlled. Potential problems then exist only with the dependent or response variable.

In contrast, with a correlation model, both variables can vary greatly, outliers may occur in either variable. As mentioned previously, variables are sometime referred to as the **predictor variable** and the **response variable** depending on the focus of our investigation. For example, as the dose of a medication changes (predictor variable), what type of response do we see in the physiological response in laboratory animals (response variable)?

Let us first look at the regression model where we can control the independent variable and are interested in possible outliers in the dependent (response) variable. Outlier detecting techniques are based on an evaluation of the residuals. The **residual** is the difference between the observed outcome ($y_i$) and the predicted outcome ($y_c$) based on the least square line that best fits the data ($r = y_i - y_c$). In Chapter 14, when evaluating if a linear relationship existed between our independent and dependent variable, we used residuals to explain the error with respect to the deviations about the regression line (Eqs. 14.4 and 14.5):

$$\Sigma(y_i - \overline{X}_y)^2 = \Sigma(y_c - \overline{X}_y)^2 + \Sigma(y_i - y_c)^2$$

$$SS_{total} = SS_{explained} + SS_{unexplained}$$

An outlier in linear regression is a data point that lies a great distance from the regression line. It can be defined as an observation with an extremely large residual.

To illustrate a potential outlier, consider the following example, where during one step in the synthesis of a biological product there is a brief fermentation period. The concentration (in percent) of one component is evaluated to determine if changes will influence the yield in units produced. The results of the experiment are presented in Table 23.7. If we perform a regression analysis (Table 23.8), as described in Chapter 14, we would reject the null hypothesis and conclude that there is a straight line relationship between our two variables. Therefore, we can draw a straight line through our data and graphically present it (Figure 23.2). Is the data point at the 4.5%

**Table 23.7** Data and Residuals Presented in Figure 23.2

| $x_i$ concentration | $y_i$ units | $y_c$ | r |
|---|---|---|---|
| 2.0 | 87.1 | 89.980 | −2.840 |
| 2.5 | 95.2 | 93.165 | +2.035 |
| 3.0 | 98.3 | 96.350 | +1.950 |
| 3.5 | 96.7 | 99.535 | −2.835 |
| 4.0 | 100.4 | 102.720 | −2.320 |
| 4.5 | 112.9 | 105.905 | +6.985 |
| 5.0 | 110.7 | 109.090 | +1.610 |
| 5.5 | 108.5 | 112.275 | −3.735 |
| 6.0 | 114.7 | 115.460 | −0.760 |
| | | Σ = | 0.000 |

**Table 23.8** Regression Analysis for Figure 23.2

| Source | SS | df | MS | F |
|---|---|---|---|---|
| Linear Regression | 608.65 | 1 | 608.65 | 43.79 |
| Residual | 97.29 | 7 | 13.90 | |
| Total | 705.94 | 8 | | |

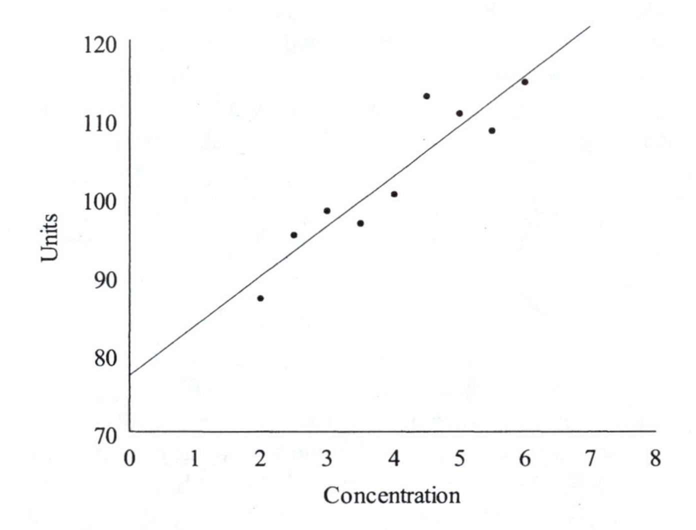


**Figure 23.2** Data and best-fit line for yield vs. various concentrations.

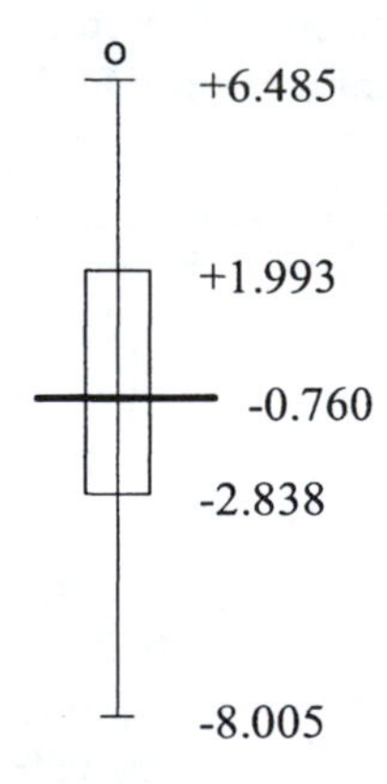


**Figure 23.3** Box-and-whisker plot of residuals.

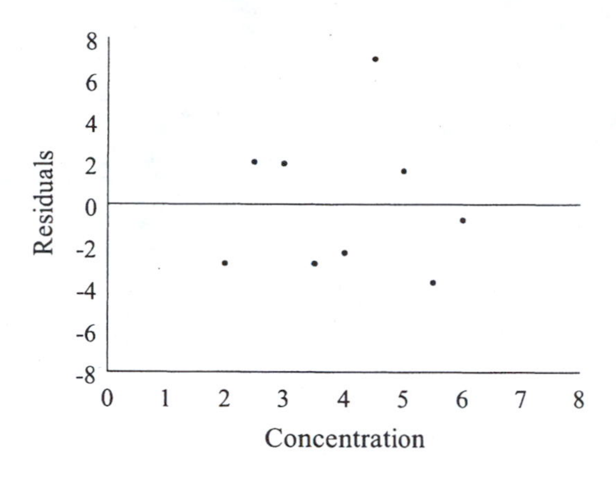


**Figure 23.4** Scatter diagram showing residuals.

concentration an outlier or simply an extreme measurement?

Graphing techniques involving residuals can be useful in identifying potential outliers in one variable. For example if the box-and-whisker plot method were applied (Figure 23.3) to the residuals in Table 23.7 we would see that the residual of +6.985 seems to be an outlier. Note that the second largest residual (3.735) does not fall outside the lower whisker and would not be considered an outlier using the visual method.

A second method would be to create **residuals plot**, which is a scatter plot of the residuals against their corresponding outcomes (dependent variable), where the independent variable is on the *x*-axis and the residuals plotted on the *y*-axis. The residuals seen in Table 23.7 are used and plotted in Figure 23.4. Once again the residual +6.985 visually appears to be an outlier. Similar to univariate outliers, the plotting of residuals can help with subjective decisions about the possibility that a data point is an outlier.

Residual plots, like the one seen in Figure 23.4 should be a random scattering of points and there should be no systematic pattern. There should be approximately as many positive points as negative ones. Note in Table 23.7 that the sum of the residuals equals zero. Outliers are identified as points far above or below the center line. Instead of plotting the residuals (Figure 23.4), we can plot the **studentized residuals** that are calculated:

$$t = \frac{y_i - y_c}{\sqrt{MS_E}} \qquad \text{Eq. 23.14}$$

where $MS_E$ is the $MS_{residual}$ taken off the ANOVA table used to test for linearity. These studentized values are scaled by the estimate of the standard error so their values follow a student *t*-distribution (Tables B5 and B6 in Appendix B). Use of the studentized residuals makes systematic trends and potential outliers more obvious. Figure 23.5 shows the studentized residual plot of the same data seen in Figure 23.4. Note that the studentized value at 4.5% concentration does not exceed the critical *t*-value of $t_8(.975) = 2.306$;

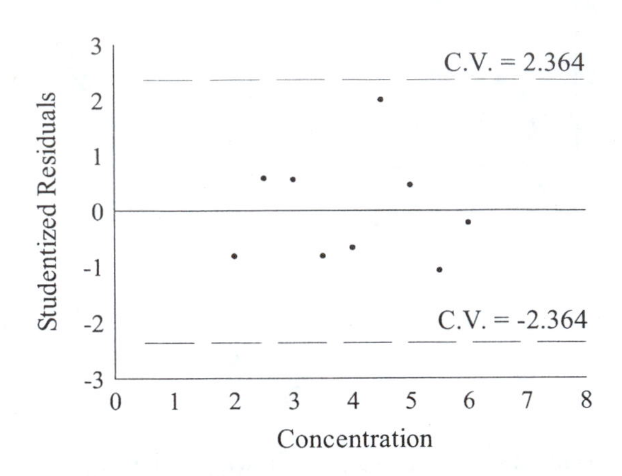


**Figure 23.5** Scatter diagram studentized residuals.

therefore, we cannot statistically reject this value as an outlier.

There are more objective statistical procedures available to evaluate such extreme points based on the residuals. One process known as **studentized deleted residuals** is a popular method for identifying outliers when there are multiple continuous variables. It involves deleting the outling observation and refitting the regression model with the remaining $n - 1$ observations. By refitting the model, it is possible to predict if the observation that was deleted from the data set was an outlier if the deleted residual was large. It requires calculations involving the standard error estimated for each deleted residual and are best handled through computer manipulation of the data. A detailed explanation of the studentized deleted residual method is found in Mason (1989, pp. 518-521).

For correlation problems, an outlier (represented by a pair of observations that are clearly out of the range of the other pairs) can have a marked effect on the correlation coefficient and often lead to misleading results. Such a paired data point may be extremely large or small compared to the bulk of the other sample data. This does not mean that there should not be a data point that is greatly different from the other data points on one axis as long as there is an equal difference on the second axis, which is consistent with the remainder of the data. For example, look at the two dispersions in Figure 23.6. It appears that the single lone data point (*A*) on the left scatter diagram is consistent with the remainder of the distribution (as x increases, y also appears to increase). In contrast, point (*B*) on the right scatter diagram is going in the opposite direction from the other sample points.

The problem occurs when one data point distorts the correlation coefficient or significantly changes the line of best-fit through the data points. The best check for a potential outlier is to remove the single observation and recalculate the correlation coefficient and determine its influence on the outcome of the sample. For example consider the data in Figure 23.7, where the data point at the extreme left side might be

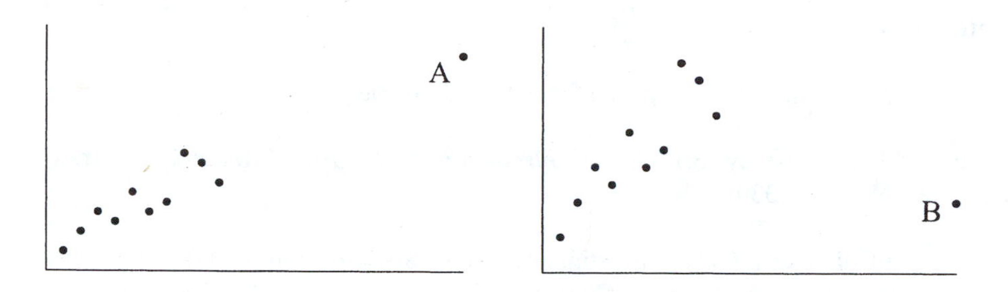


**Figure 23.6** Examples of two correlation distributions.

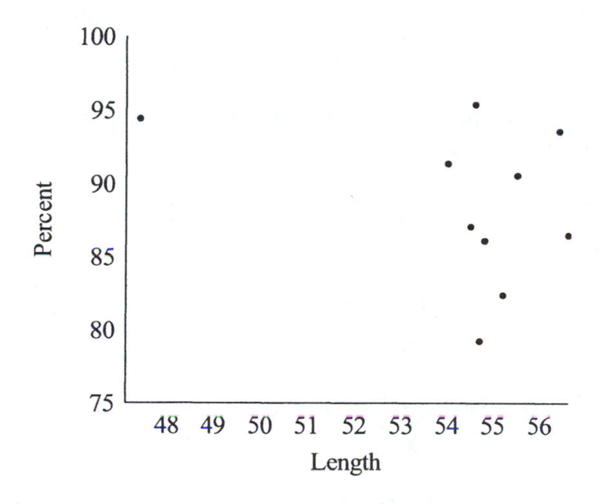


**Figure 23.7** Possible outlier with a correlation example.

an outlier. Without this one point there is virtually no correlation ($r$ = .07) and a best-fit line drawn between these points has slight positive slope ($b$ = +0.426). However, if this point is added into our calculations, there is a "low" negative correlation ($r$ = –.34) and our best-fit line changes to a negative slope ($b$ = –0.686). One method for deciding to classify a data point as an outlier might be to collect more data to determine if the number is a true outlier or just an extreme value of a trend that was not noted in the original data.

Two additional problems may be seen with bivariate outliers. The first is swamping, which was previously described as several good data points that may be close to the suspected outlier and mask its effect. Using graphing techniques, it is possible to identify a cluster of data points and these might influence tests for outliers. The second involves influential observations, which are data points that have a pronounced influence on the position of the regression line. If removed, the remaining data can be refitted and the position of the regression line may shift by a significant amount. An outlier and an influential observation are not necessarily the same. Studentized deleted residuals may be helpful in identifying influential observations.

**References**

Dixon, W.J. (1953). "Processing data for outliers," *Biometrics* 1:74-89.

Dixon, W.J. and Massey, F.J. (1969). *Introduction to Statistical Analysis*, McGraw-Hill, New York, pp. 330-332.

FDA Draft Guidance (1998). "Investigating Out of Specification (OOS) Test Results for Pharmaceutical Production, Guidance for Industry," FDA, Rockville, MD (www.fda.gov/cder/guidance/1212dft.pdf).

Grubbs, F.E. (1969). "Procedures for detecting outlying observations in samples," *Technometrics* 11:1-21.

Hampel, F.R. (1985). "The breakdown points of the mean combined with some rejection rules," *Technometrics* 27:95–107.

Marascuilo, L.A. (1971). *Statistical Methods for Behavioral Science Research*, McGraw Hill, New York, 1971, p. 199.

Mason, R.L., Gunst, R.F., Hess, J.L. (1989). *Statistical Design and Analysis of Experiments*, John Wiley and Sons, New York, pp. 518, 526.

Rodda, B.E. (1990). "Bioavailability: design and analysis," *Statistical Methodology in the Pharmaceutical Sciences*. Berry, D.A., ed., Marcel Dekker, New York, p. 78.

Taylor, J.K. (1987). *Quality Assurance of Chemical Measures*, Lewis Publishers, Chelsea, MI, pp. 37,38.

*USP* (2005). <1010> Analytical Data—Interpretation and Treatment, United States Pharmacopeia/National Formulary, Rockville, MD, pp. 2516-2526.

Wolin, A.M. (1993). "United States v. Barr Laboratories, Inc.," 812 F. Supp. 458, Newark District Federal Court, February.

**Suggested Supplemental Readings**

Barnett V., Lewis, T. (1994). *Outliers in Statistical Data*, Third edition, John Wiley and Sons, New York.

Bolton, S. (1997). *Pharmaceutical Statistics: Practical and Clinical Applications,* Third edition, Marcel Dekker, Inc., New York, pp. 355-382, 675-684.

Mason, R.L., Gunst, R.F., and Hess, J.L. (1989). *Statistical Design and Analysis of Experiments*, John Wiley and Sons, New York, pp. 510-527.

## Example Problems

1. Is the data point 12.9 an outlier from the following set of observations?

   12.3, 12.0, 12.9, 12.5, 12.4

2. The analytical laboratory at Acme Chemical assayed a solution that was assumed to be homogenous, but found the following assay results (in percent). Is 94.673 a possible outlier?

   89.470, 94.673, 89.578, 89.096, 88.975, 89.204
   87.765, 91.993, 89.954, 90.738, 90.122, 89.711

3. An experiment was designed to evaluate different theoretical concentrations of a particular agent. Based on HPLC analysis, the following recoveries were observed. Is the observation at 50% a possible outlier?

| Theoretical % | % Recovered | Theoretical % | % Recovered |
|---|---|---|---|
| 30 | 30.4 | 80 | 81.6 |
| 40 | 39.7 | 90 | 89.3 |
| 50 | 42.0 | 100 | 100.1 |
| 60 | 59.1 | 110 | 109.7 |
| 70 | 70.8 | 120 | 119.4 |

## Answers to Problems

1. Outlier tests to evaluate 12.9:

   a. Rank order of data: 12.0, 12.3, 12.4, 12.5, 12.9

   b. Mean and standard deviation:

   Without 12.9: $\overline{X} = 12.3$ $S = 0.22$
   With 12.9 included: $\overline{X} = 12.42$ $S = 0.33$

   c. Rule for huge error

$$M = \frac{|x_i - \overline{X}|}{S} = \frac{|12.3 - 12.9|}{0.22} = \frac{0.6}{0.22} = 2.73$$

   Decision with $2.73 < 4.00$, do not reject 12.9 as an outlier.

**Table 23.9** Hampel's Rule Applied to First Example Problem

| | Data | Absolute Deviations ($AD_i$) | Absolute Normalized Deviations ($NAD_i$) |
|---|---|---|---|
| | 12.0 | 0.4 | 2.697 |
| | 12.3 | 0.1 | 0.674 |
| | 12.4 | 0.0 | 0.000 |
| | 12.5 | 0.1 | –0.674 |
| | 12.9 | 0.5 | –3.372 |
| | 12.0 | 0.4 | 2.697 |
| Median = | 12.4 | 0.1 | |
| MAD = | | 0.1483 | |

d. Grubbs' test – critical value with n = 5 and $\alpha$ = .05 is 1.672.

$$T = \frac{X_n - \overline{X}}{S} = \frac{12.9 - 12.42}{0.33} = \frac{0.48}{0.33} = 1.45$$

Decision with 1.45 < 1.672, do not reject 12.9 as an outlier.

e. Dixon test – with n = 5 and $\alpha$ = .05, critical $\tau$ = 0.642.

$$\frac{(x_n - x_{n-1})}{(x_n - x_1)} = \frac{12.9 - 12.5}{12.9 - 12.0} = \frac{0.4}{0.9} = 0.44$$

Decision with 0.44 < 0.642, do not reject 12.9 as an outlier.

f. Hampel's rule

The results for the calculations appear in Table 23.9. The median for the five values is 12.4. For 12.9 the $AD_i$ is:

$$AD_i = |x_i - Md| = |12.9 - 12.4| = 0.5$$

The median $AD_i$ is 0.1 and the $MAD$ is 0.1(1.483) = 0.1483. For 12.9 the $NAD_i$ is:

$$NAD_i = \frac{|Md - x_i|}{MAD_i} = \frac{|12.4 - 12.9|}{0.1483} = 3.37$$

With the $NAD_i$ less than 3.5, do not reject 12.9 as an outlier.

2. Outlier tests to determine if 94.673% is an outlier.

   a. Rank order of data:

      87.765, 88.975, 89.096, 89.204, 89.470, 89.578
      89.711, 89.954, 90.122, 91.738, 91.993, 94.673

   b. Mean/standard deviation:

| | | |
|---|---|---|
| Without 94.673: | $\overline{X} = 89.69$ | S = 1.07 |
| With 94.673 included: | $\overline{X} = 90.11$ | S = 1.77 |

   c. Rule for huge error

$$M = \frac{|x_i - \overline{X}|}{S} = \frac{|89.69 - 94.673|}{1.07} = \frac{4.983}{1.07} = 4.66$$

Decision with 4.66 < 4.00, reject 94.673 as an outlier.

   d. Grubbs' test – critical value with n = 12 and α = .05 is 2.27.

$$T = \frac{x_n - \overline{X}}{S} = \frac{94.673 - 90.11}{1.77} = \frac{4.563}{1.77} = 2.58$$

Decision with 2.58 < 2.27, reject 94.673 as an outlier.

   e. Dixon test – with n = 12 and α = .05, critical τ = 0.546.

$$\frac{(x_n - x_{n-2})}{(x_n - x_2)} = \frac{94.673 - 90.738}{94.673 - 89.096} = \frac{3.935}{5.577} = 0.705$$

Decision with 0.705 < 0.546, reject 94.673 as an outlier.

   f. Hampel's rule

The results for the calculations appear in Table 23.10. The median for the twelve values is 89.645%. For 94.673 the $AD_i$ is:

$$AD_i = |x_i - Md| = |94.673 - 89.645| = 5.028$$

The median $AD_i$ is 0.513 and the *MAD* is 0.513(1.483) = 0.761. For 94.673 the $NAD_i$ is:

**Table 23.10.** Hampel's Rule Applied to Second Example Problem

| | Data | Absolute Deviations ($AD_i$) | Absolute Normalized Deviations ($NAD_i$) |
|---|---|---|---|
| | 89.470 | 0.175 | 0.229 |
| | 94.673 | 5.028 | 6.610 |
| | 89.578 | 0.067 | 0.087 |
| | 89.096 | 0.549 | 0.721 |
| | 88.975 | 0.670 | 0.880 |
| | 89.204 | 0.441 | 0.579 |
| | 87.765 | 1.880 | 2.470 |
| | 91.993 | 2.348 | 3.087 |
| | 89.954 | 0.309 | 0.407 |
| | 90.738 | 1.093 | 1.437 |
| | 90.122 | 0.477 | 0.628 |
| | 89.711 | 0.066 | 0.087 |
| Median = | 89.645 | 0.513 | |
| MAD = | | 0.761 | |

$$NAD_i = \frac{|Md - x_i|}{MAD_i} = \frac{|89.645 - 94.673|}{0.761} = 6.610$$

With the $NAD_i$ greater than 3.5, reject 94.673 as an outlier.

3. Evaluation of HPLC analysis to determine if 50% is a possible outlier. Listed below are the results of the typical regression analysis table and the calculated slope and *y*-intercept for all the data, and the data excluding the potential outlier.

| Outcomes: | With the potential outlier included | With the potential outlier excluded |
|---|---|---|
| n = | 10 | 9 |
| $\Sigma x$ = | 750 | 700 |
| $\Sigma y$ = | 742.1 | 700.1 |
| $\Sigma x^2$ = | 64,500 | 62,000 |
| $\Sigma y^2$ = | 63,713.21 | 61,949.21 |
| $\Sigma xy$ = | 64,072 | 61,972 |
| b = | +1.02 | +0.99 |
| a = | –2.29 | +0.79 |

As can be seen, the proposed outlier does affect the slope and intercept point, but is this effect significant and should the 50% response be considered an outlier?

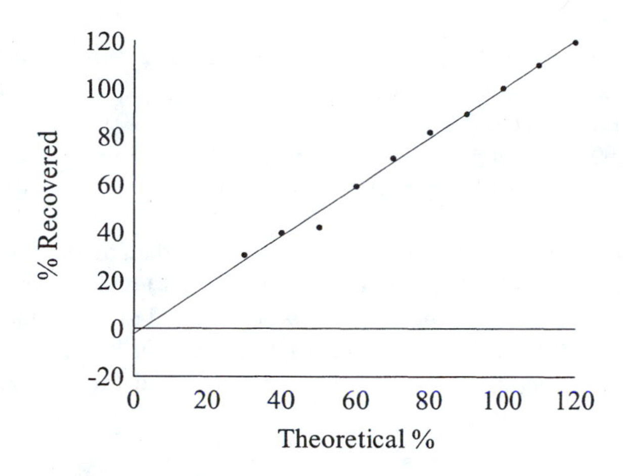


**Figure 23.8** Scatter plot of HPLC outcomes.

**Table 23.11** Residuals Presented in Figure 23.7

| x | $y_i$ | $y_c$ | r |
|---|---|---|---|
| 30 | 30.4 | 28.31 | +2.09 |
| 40 | 39.7 | 38.51 | +1.19 |
| 50 | 42.0 | 48.71 | –6.71 |
| 60 | 59.1 | 58.91 | +0.19 |
| 70 | 70.8 | 69.11 | +1.69 |
| 80 | 81.6 | 79.31 | +2.29 |
| 90 | 89.3 | 89.51 | –0.21 |
| 100 | 100.1 | 99.71 | +0.39 |
| 110 | 109.7 | 109.91 | –0.21 |
| 120 | 119.4 | 120.11 | –0.71 |
| | | | $\Sigma = 0.000$ |

Figure 23.8 shows a scatter plot for the HPLC data and the line of best fit. The results of the linear regression analysis would be as follows:

| Source | SS | df | MS | F |
|---|---|---|---|---|
| Linear Regression | 8583.30 | 1 | 8583.30 | 1170.98 |
| Residual | 58.67 | 8 | 7.33 | |
| Total | 8641.97 | 9 | | |

The values on the line of best fit can be calculated using the formula $y_c=a+bx$. These values and the residuals associated with the difference between the data ($y$) and $y_c$ is presented in Table 23.11. If the residuals are ranked from the lowest to the highest we find the following:

| x | $y_i$ | r | x | $y_i$ | r |
|---|---|---|---|---|---|
| 50 | 42.0 | −6.71 | 100 | 100.1 | +0.39 |
| 120 | 119.4 | −0.71 | 40 | 39.7 | +1.19 |
| 110 | 109.7 | −0.21 | 70 | 70.8 | +1.69 |
| 90 | 89.3 | −0.21 | 30 | 30.4 | +2.09 |
| 60 | 59.1 | +0.19 | 80 | 81.6 | +2.29 |

A box-and-whisker plot can be created with the median of +0.29 (average of fifth and sixth ranks), 25 percentile of −0.21 (third rank) and 75 percentile of +1.69 (eighth rank). In this case the whiskers would extend to −2.56 and +3.14. Clearly the value of −6.71 would be an outlier because it is located beyond the lower whisker. A studentized residuals plot can be created for each HPLC outcome. For example the value at 100% would be:

$$t = \frac{y_i - y_c}{\sqrt{MS_E}} = \frac{100.1 - 99.71}{\sqrt{7.33}} = 0.144$$

Each of the studentized residuals are plotted and the critical t-value is $t_{n-1}(1 - \alpha/2)$, which is $t_9(.975)$ or 2.26.

# 24

# Statistical Errors in the Literature

In the preface to this book, we discussed the need for a better understanding of statistics in order to avoid research mistakes and to be better able to identify possible errors in published documents. It only seems fitting to conclude this book by reviewing the prevalence of these mathematical misadventures and identifying some of the most common types of statistical errors.

The purpose of this chapter is to point out errors that can occur, not to criticize individual authors. It is doubtful that any of the errors described below were the result of intentional manipulation of findings or overt attempts to mislead the reader. More than likely, they are errors committed due to a misunderstanding or misinterpretation of the statistics involved with the evaluating the findings. Therefore, examples will be presented without reference to the specific author(s), article or journal of publication. However, the reader should appreciate that these are all actual errors that have occurred in refereed journals of medicine or pharmacy.

## Errors and the Peer Review Process

In recent years the use of statistical analysis in published works has increased greatly, due in no small part to the ease, accessibility, and power of modern desktop and laptop computers. This has also lead to an increase in the complexity of the procedures performed and reported in the literature. As noted by Altman (1991) there is an increasing trend to use statistics in the medical literature, which are usually not taught to medical students during their education and may not even be taught in postgraduate programs. He found a dramatic decrease between 1978 and 1990 in the percentage of papers that contained no statistics or only descriptive statistics (Table 24.1). The number of simple inferential statistics (i.e., t-test, chi square) remained the same, but more complex statistics increased greatly during that time period. Earlier work by Felson and colleagues (1984), showed an even more dramatic increase in

**Table 24.1** Changes in the Use of Statistics in the Literature

| | 1978 | 1990 |
|---|---|---|
| No statistics or descriptive only | 27% | 11% |
| t-tests | 44% | 39% |
| Chi square | 27% | 30% |
| Linear regression | 8% | 18% |
| Analysis of variance | 8% | 14% |
| Multiple regression | 5% | 6% |
| Nonparametric tests | 11% | 25% |

From: Altman, D.G. (1991). "Statistics in medical journals: developments in the 1980s," *Statistics in Medicine* 10:1899.

the use of statistics in Arthritis and Rheumatism, between the years 1967-1968 and 1982 (Table 24.2)

As pointed out by Glantz (1980), few researchers have had formal training in biostatistics and "assume that when an article appears in a journal, the reviewers and editors have scrutinized every aspect of the manuscript, including the statistical methods." As he noted this assumption was usually not correct. Have things changed that much in the past 25 years? Are today's researchers any more knowledgeable of statistics, even though they now have the power of very sophisticated software packages in their desktop computers? Most journals do not employ a statistician or involve a statistician in their review process. McGuigan (1995) noted that only a small portion of the articles he reviewed (24% to 30%) employed a statistician as coauthors or acknowledged their help in papers. In fact, in the peer review process, colleagues reviewing articles submitted to journals probably have about the same statistical expertise as the authors submitting the manuscript.

Over the last several decades there have been several articles presented in the medical literature that report the incidence and types of error seen in publications (Table 24.3). In these papers statisticians review either all the articles published during a given time period (usually one year) in a specific periodical or a random sample of articles from a publication over a longer period. These errors are related to mistakes in the medical literature, because this is an area where most of the research

**Table 24.2** Changes in the Use of Common Statistics

| | 1967-1968 | 1982 |
|---|---|---|
| t-tests | 17% | 50% |
| Chi square | 19% | 22% |
| Linear regression | 1% | 18% |

From: Felson, D.T. et al. (1994). "Misuse of statistical methods in *Arthritis and Rheumatism*," *Arthritis and Rheumatism* 27:1020.

**Table 24.3** Prevalence of Statistical Errors in the Literature (percent of articles with at least one statistical error)

| Percent | Journal(s) | Reference |
|---|---|---|
| 57 | *Canadian Medical Association Journal* and *Canadian Journal of Public Health*, 1960 | Badgley, 1961 |
| 60 | *Arthritis and Rheumatism*, 1967-1968 | Felson, 1984 |
| 42 | *British Medical Journal*, 1976 | Gore, 1976 |
| 44 | *Circulation*, 1977 | Glantz, 1980 |
| 45 | *British Journal of Psychiatry*, 1977-1978 | White, 1979 |
| 66 | *Arthritis and Rheumatism*, 1982 | Felson, 1984 |
| 65 | *British Journal of Anaesthesia*, 1990 | Goodman and Hughes, 1992 |
| 74 | *American Journal of Tropical Medicine and Hygiene*, 1988 | Cruess, 1989 |
| 54 | *Clinical Orthopaedics and Related Research*, *Spine*, *Journal of Pediatric Orthopaedics*, *Journal of Orthopaedic Research, Journal of Bone and Joint Surgery* and *Orthopedics*, 1970-1990 | Vrbos, 1993 |
| 75 | *Transfusion*, 1992-1993 | Kanter and Taylor, 1994 |
| 40 | *British Journal of Psychiatry*, 1993 | McGuigan, 1995 |

has been conducted. However, it is doubtful that the incidence of these errors is any less frequent in the pharmacy literature.

A problem to consider with the results presented in Table 24.3 was that most of these evaluations used different methods of assessing mistakes and there were no standardized criteria for defining statistical errors. Therefore, the same error may be defined differently or the researchers may have been focusing their attentions on different parameters for establishing such errors. As errors are discussed, citations will be made to the articles presented in Table 24.3 and the proportion of such errors identified by the various authors in their research of the medical literature.

### Problems with Experimental Design

Many of the problems reported in the literature relate to the design of the studies. Ultimately such experimental design problems will show flawed statistical results. For example, many studies have inadequate or no control groups as part of the design. These types of incidences were reported to be as high as 41% (McGuigan, 1995) and 58% (Glantz, 1980). Outcomes from various medical interventions are extremely difficult to evaluate without a control set of subjects to determine if the outcome would occur without the intervention.

As discussed in Chapter 3, there are two requirements for any statistical procedure, that 1) samples are selected or volunteers assigned by some random process and 2) each measurement is independent of all others (except in certain repeat measurement designs). Unfortunately McGuigan (1995) and Cruess (1989) found errors related to randomization in 43% and 12%, respectively, of the articles they evaluated. Also there was a disregard for statistical independence in 10% of the articles reviewed by Gore and colleagues (1977) and 5% of those reviewed by Kanter and Taylor (1994).

In one research project it was found that 5% of studies fail to state a null hypotheses (McGuigan, 1995) and in a second study, questionable conclusions were drawn from the results in 47.5% of the articles evaluated (Vrbos, 1993). Excellent books exist on research design studies, especially Friedman and colleagues (1998), that are more effective in evaluating the desired outcomes.

Another problem, commonly seen in the methodology section of papers, is a failure to state and/or reference statistics used in the article. Failure to cite the specific statistics used were found in 41.5% of the articles reviewed by McGuigan (1995) and 13% of those by Kanter and Taylor (1994). In addition, studies of the medical literature found that many times conclusions were stated without any indication which statistical tests were performed (49% for Kanter and Taylor, 1994; and 35.7% for Vrbos, 1993).

Another common problem is a failure of authors to cite references for lesser known statistical procedures employed in their data analysis. Commonly used procedures (t-tests, ANOVA, correlation, linear regression, and even some of the popular nonparametric tests) need not be referenced. But lesser used procedures should be referenced so readers can understand the inferential statistic(s) involved. Nothing is more frustrating than to have a colleague or student ask about A-B-C statistical procedure, then; 1) to search Medline for references to that test and find 10 to 15 articles mentioning the A-B-C test in the online abstract; 2) to retrieve all the articles from the library; and 3) to find that not one of the authors cite a source for the A-B-C test in the methodology sections. More than likely the A-B-C test was part of a printout involved with a sophisticated software package and referenced somewhere in that software's reference manual. Even referencing the software would help readers seeking more information about a specific test.

## Standard Deviations versus Standard Error of the Mean

When reporting continuous data, it is important to describe the centers of the distribution and provide information about the dispersion of observations around the center(s). Unfortunately, studies by Gore and colleagues (1977) and White (1979) reported inadequate description of basic data, including centers and dispersions in 16.1% and 12.9% of the articles they reviewed, respectively.

As discussed in Chapter 5, the standard deviation ($S$) measures dispersion of the sample and provides an estimate of the dispersion of the population from which the sample was taken. In contrast the standard error of the mean ($SEM$), or standard error ($SE$), is a measure of how all possible sample means might vary around the population mean. As seen in the following equation (Eq. 7.3), the $SEM$ will always be smaller than $S$.

**Table 24.4** Example of Failure to Identify S or SEM (n = 45)

| Parameter | Mean Baseline Value | Mean Value at 4-8 years (mean, 5.3 yrs) |
|---|---|---|
| Total cholesterol (nmol/L) | 7.17 ± 0.83 | 7.01 ± 0.92 |
| HDL cholesterol (nmol/L) | 1.17 ± 0.41 | 1.39 ± 0.36* |
| Triglycerides (nmol/L) | 1.38 ± 0.63 | 1.35 ± 0.61 |

*Statistically significant increase (p < 0.05).
HDL = high-density lipoprotein.

$$SEM = \frac{S}{\sqrt{n}}$$

Because *SEM* is smaller, investigators will often report that value because it gives the perception of greater precision.

Often authors fail to state the measurement to the right of the ± symbol (7.1% from White's research, 1979; 13% for Felson et al., 1984; and 24% for Kanter and Taylor, 1994). Is it the *S* or the *SE*, or even relative standard deviation (*RSD*)? If not stated, the reader cannot adequately interpret the results. Even if the authors state in the methodology what is represented by the value to the right of the ± symbol, tables should still be self-explanatory, so readers can evaluate the results. For example, in an article evaluating serum lipid levels after long-term therapy with a calcium channel blocking agent, the author made the following statement: "After a mean treatment period of 5.3 years, total cholesterol and triglyceride levels were not significantly different from baseline, whereas the mean high-density lipoprotein cholesterol value increased significantly from 1.17 ± 0.41 nmol/L at the initiation of treatment to 1.39 ± 0.36 nmol/l at 5.3 years ($p < 0.05$)." The findings were presented in a table and an abbreviated version of this table is presented in Table 24.4. Unfortunately, nowhere in the article did the author state whether the values to the right of the ± symbol in the table or the text represent the standard deviation or the standard error of the mean. Only after recalculating the statistics is it possible to determine that the values reflect the standard deviation. Looking solely at the HDL cholesterol data in Table 24.4, if the measure of dispersion was the standard deviation, a two-sample t-test produces a *t*-value of 2.705, $p < 0.003$. In contrast, if the figure to the right of the ± symbol was the SEM, the two-sample t-test result would be $t = 0.40$, $p > 0.35$. Thus, data in the original table represents the mean ± standard deviation. However, the only way to determine this is to actually recalculate the statistical outcome.

Another potential problem is using the standard deviation for nonnormal data. As discussed in Chapter 6, the standard deviation reflects certain mathematical characteristics associated with normally distributed data. The median and quartiles are more appropriate measures for skewed distributions. However, McGuigan (1995)

**Table 24.5** Examples of Skewed Data Evaluated Using ANOVA

| Original information cited in article (mean ± SE): | | | |
|---|---|---|---|
| Nasal EDN (ng/ml) | Drug A (n = 16) | Drug B (n = 14) | Placebo (n = 15) |
| Treatment day 1 | 245 ± 66 | 147 ± 49 | 275 ± 133 |
| Treatment day 15 | 78 ± 34* | 557 ± 200 | 400 ± 159 |
| Data modified to reflect dispersion of the sample (mean ± SD) | | | |
| Treatment day 1 | 245 ± 264 | 147 ± 183 | 275 ± 515 |
| Treatment day 1 | 78 ± 136* | 557 ± 748 | 400 ± 615 |

* p < 0.05 versus Drug B or placebo based on change from day 1 to day 15.

reported that 39 of the 164 papers he reviewed (24%) used the mean and standard deviation for describing skewed or ordinal data. This occurred with less frequency (19%) in the work by Kanter and Taylor (1994). An example of skewed data can be seen in a recent article comparing two drugs and their effects on the amount of eosinophile-derived neurotoxin (EDN). Part of the results are presented in the upper half of Table 24.5 and the authors report that they "compared between treatment groups using t-tests." Also, "values of $p < 0.05$ were considered statistically significant." Note that the outcomes are reported as mean ± standard error. Converting the dispersion to standard deviations ($S = SEM \cdot \sqrt{n}$) we find the results presented in the lower portion of Table 24.5. Note in all cases that the standard deviation is larger than the mean, indicating data that is positively skewed. A nonparametric procedure or log transformation of the original data would have been the preferred method for analyzing the data.

Another problem with data dispersion is the evaluation of ordinal data by calculating a mean and standard deviation. This was identified in 25% of articles reviewed by Avram and colleagues (1985). An example of the use of parametric procedures to evaluate ordinal data is presented in a publication from the 1980s, where women who received a lumpectomy or mastectomy for breast cancer were asked to rate their feelings of femininity. The authors used a simple three level ordinal scale (0 = no change, 1 = a little less feminine, and 2 = moderately less feminine). Unfortunately, the authors took the responses, calculated means and standard deviations for women with lumpectomies versus those with mastectomies, and evaluated the data using a two-sample t-test ("$t = 4.35$, $p < 0.01$" after 14 months). The more appropriate assessment would have been a chi square test of independence with frequencies of responses in each of the following cells:

| | No Change | A Little Less Feminine | Moderately Less Feminine |
|---|---|---|---|
| Lumpectomy | | | |
| Mastectomy | | | |

**Problems with Hypothesis Testing**

We know from our previous discussions in Chapter 8 that the Type I error rate can be expressed as either $\alpha$ or $p$ and provides the researcher with a certain degree of confidence $(1 - \alpha)$ in their statistics. Unfortunately in Vrbos' (1993) review of the literature there was confusion over the level of significance or meaning of "$p$" in 46% of the articles.

A second problem, which appears less frequently, is assuming the null hypothesis is true simply because the researcher fails to reject the null hypothesis. As discussed in Chapter 8 that the null hypothesis is never proven, we only fail to reject it.

A third problem related to hypothesis testing is the failure to perform a prestudy power calculation or the failure to have an adequate sample size. This was observed in 50% of the articles reviewed by McGuigan (1995). For example, in a recent study comparing two routes of administration of a hematopoetic growth factor the authors reported the data in Table 24.6. Note the small sample size, n = 4. If there was a significant difference (i.e., 20%) at the <100 U/Kg/wk dosage, how many subjects would be required to detect such a difference? The authors used an ANOVA to evaluate the results. Since there are only two levels of the independent variable, we can use the formula presented in Chapter 8 (Eq. 8.2) as a quick estimate of the number of subjects required to detect a 20% difference with 80% power. Performing the calculations found that the required number of subjects would be 188 per delivery system. This large number is due primarily to the large variance in the sample data.

The following is an example of a 1998 clinical trial protocol where the researchers have clearly attempted to control the Type II error rate. "A sample size of 28 healthy males will be enrolled in this study to ensure study completion by at least 24 patients. Based on *(a previous study)* a sample size of 24 patients can provide at least 80% probability to show that the 90% confidence interval of the mean AUC value for the clinical lot of *Drug B* is within ±20% of the reference (commercial lot) mean AUC value."

Readers should be cautious of papers that report unnecessarily small and overly exact probabilities. For example, in a 1988 publication the authors were reporting the difference in parasitic infection rates in children in a developing country and the change in the frequencies of infections before and after their particular intervention. The change reported "for prevalence in 1984 vs. 1985, $\chi^2 = 624$, $df = 1$, $p < 10^{-11}$)." In other words, the Type I error rate was less than 0.00000000001! This paper clearly overstates the obvious. A second example, illustrating probabilities that are too exact, comes from a 1993 article presenting volunteer demographics (Table 24.7). Good luck finding a statistical table that provides a column for p = 0.0539! Also, note that the authors failed to indicate what the values were to the right of the ± symbol. In both cases, it appears that the authors were simply reporting results directly from the computer printout, without any attempt to apply a reasonable explanation to their results. This type of presentation of statistical results should warn the reader to read the article with extreme caution to ensure that the appropriate analysis was performed and correct interpretation stated.

**Table 24.6** Comparison of Mean Posologies at the End (Day 120) of Study

| Dosage | Time | IV Group (n = 4) | SC Group (n = 4) | Statistical Difference |
|---|---|---|---|---|
| >150 U/Kg/wk | Day 120 | 255 ± 131 | 138 ± 105 | P < 0.01 |
| <100 U/Kg/wk | Day 120 | 69 ± 45 | 58 ± 43 | ns |

**Table 24.7** Volunteer Demographics

| | Group A | Group B |
|---|---|---|
| Age (yr) | 67.4 ± 5.8 | 61.4 ± 8.6 * |

* $p = 0.0539$

**Problems with Parametric Statistics**

As discussed in Chapter 9, the two additional underlying requirements for performing a parametric statistic (t-tests, F-tests, correlation, and regression) are that the data: 1) come from populations that are normally distributed and 2) that sample variances (which are reflective of the population variances) be approximately equal (homogeneity of variance).

One common error is to perform a parametric test on data that is obviously skewed. The incidence of such mistakes range from 8% (Kanter and Taylor, 1994) and 17.7% (Gore, 1977) to as large as 54% (McGuigan, 1995). Note in the data cited in Table 24.5 that the standard deviations are greater than the means that would indicate that the data is positively skewed.

One method for correcting this problem is to transform the data so the resultant distribution is approximately normal (Chapter 6); for example, the log transformation of data from a positively skewed distribution. This is illustrated in the statistical analysis section of a paper by Cohn and colleagues (1993), where they evaluate cardiac function: "Because values were extremely skewed to the right, the Holter monitor results were transformed using the logarithmic transformation…." An alternative approach would be to perform one of the nonparametric procedures.

A second type of error related to parametric and nonparametric procedures is confusing paired vs. unpaired data and performing an inappropriate statistical test (i.e., an ANOVA instead of a randomized block design or a paired t-test for unpaired data). Paired data obviously has advantages in that a person serves as their own control and it provides a more rigorous test, because we are evaluating changes within individual subjects. Kanter and Taylor (1994) noted that in 15% of the articles they studied that the wrong t-test (paired/unpaired) was used and McGuigan (1995) found that in 26% of the papers he studied that the type of t-test (paired/unpaired) was not mentioned. For example, in a recent article comparing the pharmacokinetic results between two time periods are presented in Table 24.8. As indicated in the

**Table 24.8** Comparison of Eight Subjects Following a Single Oral Dose of a Drug at 10 and 22 Hours

| | $C_{max}$ ng/ml$^{-1}$ | |
|---|---|---|
| Subject | 10.00 h | 22.00h |
| 1 | 59.5 | 18.6 |
| 2 | 75.2 | 7.5 |
| 3 | 33.6 | 18.9 |
| 4 | 37.6 | 33.9 |
| 5 | 27.8 | 20.8 |
| 6 | 28.4 | 14.9 |
| 7 | 76.8 | 29.7 |
| 8 | 37.5 | 15.0 |
| Mean (SD) | 47.1 (20.4) | 19.9 (8.4)* |

* $p < 0.05$ compared to 10.00 h (analysis of variance).

table and the methodology section of the original paper, "the statistical analysis employed analysis of variance." As seen in Table 24.8 this clearly represents paired data (each subject serves as his own control, being measured at two separate time periods). The authors obviously established a decision rule and rejected the results for any $p < 0.05$. Recalculating the statistics we find the results to be even more significant than reported in the article: $F = 12.09$, $df = 1,14$, $p < 0.005$. Obviously a two-sample t-test would produce the identical results: $t = 3.48$, $df = 14$, $p < 0.005$. However, a more rigorous paired t-test shows that there is even less type I error when such a design is employed: paired-$t = 3.41$, $df = 7$, $p < 0.0025$. Unfortunately, in this particular example the author failed to observe the requirement of homogeneity of variance in order to perform an ANOVA. Note that $S^2_{10h} = 416.16$ and $S^2_{22h} = 70.60$ are not close to being equal. Therefore the most appropriate statistic would have been a paired t-test looking at the difference for each subject or a nonparametric Wilcoxon matched-pairs test, the results of such a procedure would be $Z = 2.52$, $p < 0.02$.

Another common error, discussed in Chapter 11, is the use of multiple t-tests to address a significant ANOVA where $H_0$: $\mu_1 = \mu_2 = \mu_3 \ldots = \mu_k$ is false. The compounding of the error using multiple t-tests was defined as experimentwise error rate (Eq. 11.2):

$$a_{ew} = 1-(1-\alpha)^C$$

To correct this problem, multiple comparison procedures were presented in Chapter 11. The incidence of this type of error has been fairly consistent at around one out of every four articles reviewed (27% for Glantz, 1980; 24% for Altman, 1991; and 22% for Kanter and Taylor, 1994). An example of the misinterpretation of data due to experimentwise error is illustrated in an article evaluating different athletic mouth guards and their effect on air flow in young adults (ages 20-36). The authors'

**Table 24.9** Effects of Three Different Mouth Guards on Air Flow (n = 17)

| | $FEV_1$ (liters) | PEF (l/min) |
|---|---|---|
| No mouth guard | 3.46 (0.70) | 508.65 (70.25) |
| Mouth guard 1 | 3.17 (0.16)† | 472.88 (68.44) † |
| Mouth guard 2 | 2.97 (0.19) † | 432.31 (78.99) † |
| Mouth guard 3 | 3.04 (0.86) † | 428.38 (65.02) † |

* Values represent means (s.d.); † values are significantly different ($p < 0.05$; ANOVA) from the values recorded with no mouth guard.

findings are presented in Table 24.9. They concluded, based on this table, "that each of the three athletic mouth guards used in this study significantly reduced air flow ($p < 0.05$) .... Similarly, peak expiratory flow rates were significantly reduced by the different mouth guards ($p < 0.05$)." The authors clearly state in their table that the measure of dispersion is the standard deviation. Therefore, it is a relatively easy process to re-evaluate their data using the ANOVA formula presented in Chapter 10 and the multiple comparison procedures in Chapter 11. This re-evaluation finds that there was in fact a significant difference with respect to the mouth guards tested and the outcome measures for only the PEF. The calculated *F*-value was 4.85 where the critical F-value for 95% confidence is 2.53. In fact the outcome was significant with a $p < 0.005$. Assume the original hypothesis of equality was tested ($\alpha = 0.05$) the Scheffé *post hoc* pair-wise comparisons with the same error rate find that there were only two significant differences: no mouth guard > mouth guard 2 and no mouth guard > mouth guard 3. Unlike the authors' findings, there was no significant difference between the PEF for mouth guard 1 and no mouth guard. How could the authors have found a significant difference for all three mouth guards? If one calculates three separate two-sample t-tests comparing each mouth guard to no mouth guard, there is still no significant difference ($t = 1.05$). It appears that, finding a significant ANOVA, the authors simply assumed that all the mouth guards provided significantly less air flow. Without a statement in the methodology section on how significant ANOVAs were evaluated, the question must remain unanswered.

## Errors with the Chi Square Test of Independence

As discussed in Chapter 16 the chi square test of independence is used to evaluate the independence or relationship (lack of independence) between two discrete variables. Overall problems with chi square analysis were identified in 15% of the articles reviewed by McGuigan (1995).

Two criteria are required in order to perform this test: 1) there cannot be any empty cells (a cell within the matrix where the observed frequency equal to zero); and 2) the expected value for each cell must be equal to or greater than five. A common mistake in the literature is to proceed with the statistical analysis even though one or both of these criteria are violated. An excellent example of this type of error appears in an article evaluating the practice of breast self-examination (BSE) in relationship

**Table 24.10** Original Table Reporting Susceptibility Scores and Annual Frequency of BSE

| | Perceived Susceptibility Scores | | | |
|---|---|---|---|---|
| | High (15-19) | Moderate (9-14) | Low (9) | Total |
| More than monthly | 9 | 1 | 0 | 10 |
| Monthly | 31 | 5 | 0 | 36 |
| 6-11 times | 11 | 3 | 0 | 14 |
| 1-15 times | 19 | 3 | 0 | 22 |
| Less than yearly | 5 | 1 | 0 | 6 |
| Never | 13 | 10 | 1 | 24 |
| Total | 88 | 23 | 1 | 112 |

to "susceptibility" scores (risk factors) for developing breast cancer. The authors concluded the following: "Forty-one (36%) participants with high susceptibility scores practiced BSE monthly or more frequently (Table 24.10). However, chi square analysis showed no statistically significant difference in the level of perceived susceptibility of students and the frequency of BSE, $\chi^2(10) = 13.1925$, $p = .2131$, $\alpha = .05$". Note that 24% (5/21) of the cells are empty. If we calculated the expected values for each cell under complete independence we would determine that 67% of the cells fail to meet the criteria of expected values greater or equal to five. Clearly the use of the chi square test of independence was inappropriate for this contingency table. If we modify the data by collapsing the cells in a logical order, we can create a matrix which fulfills the criteria required (Table 24.11). However, in doing this, we arrive at a decision exactly the opposite that of the authors ($\chi^2(2) = 7.24$, $p < 0.05$). With $\alpha = 0.05$ there is a significant relationship between risk factors and the volunteers practice of BSE. Also, note in the original table that the frequency of the BSE variable did not represent mutually exclusive and exhaustive categories. It is assumed that this was a typographical error and the mid-range values should have been 1-5 times and 6-11 times, but it was presented in the article that the two categories overlapped.

If the sample size is too small or data fails to meet the required criteria, a Fisher's exact test should be utilized. The percent of articles with this type of error is approximately 5% (5% by Kanter and Taylor, 1994; and 6% by Felson, 1984). For example, Cruess (1989) discussed an article reporting a significant relationship between reactivity with parasite isolates based on primary or multiple attacks of malaria in subjects studied and presented the following results:

| | Reactivity | | |
|---|---|---|---|
| | Positive | Negative | |
| Primary Attack | 1 | 2 | 3 |
| Multiple Attacks | 5 | 0 | 5 |
| | 6 | 2 | 8 |

**Table 24.11** Data Modified from Table 24.10 to Meet Criteria for the Chi Square Test of Independence

| | High (15-19) | Low and Moderate (less than 15) | Total |
|---|---|---|---|
| 12 or more times per year | 40 | 6 | 46 |
| 1-11 times per year | 30 | 6 | 36 |
| Less than yearly or never | 18 | 11 | 30 |
| Total | 88 | 23 | 112 |

The authors used a chi square test and reported a significant relationship ($p = 0.03$). However, if the more appropriate Fisher's exact test is performed (since there is one empty cell and all expected values are less than five), the result is no significant relationship exists ($p = 0.107$). An example of the appropriate use of Fisher's exact test is described in the methodology section of an article in *Gastroenterology*: "The responses to interferon were compared between the cirrhotic and noncirrhotic patients at various times of treatment and follow up, using $\chi^2$ method or Fisher's exact test when appropriate" (Jouet, 1994).

Another type of problem with the chi square test of independence is the correction for continuity when there is only one degree of freedom. This type of error was identified with a frequency of occurring between 2.8% (McGuigan, 1995) and 4.8% (Gore, 1977). The following is a simple clarification in the methodology section by Parsch et al. (1997), which assists the reader in understanding the statistics involved in the manuscript: "Categorical demographic data and differences in clinical outcome were analyzed by $\chi^2$ with Yates correction factor … Statistical significance was established at a $p$-value of less than 0.05."

## Summary

The purpose of this chapter has been to identify the most frequent statistical errors seen in the literature to help you better identify these mistakes in your own readings and assist you in avoiding them as you prepare written reports or publishable manuscripts.

One should always view with caution articles published in the literature. Make sure that the drug design and statistical tests are clearly described in the methodology section of the article. Altman (1991), George (1985), and McGuigan (1995) have indicated methods for improving the peer review process. These include requiring authors to indicate who performed the statistical analysis on submissions. Journals should clearly state minimum requirements for submission, even provide a standardized format regarding the nature of the research, the research design and the statistical analyses used in preparing the manuscript. Lastly, papers should be more extensively reviewed by statisticians and possibly include a statistician among the reviewers for any papers submitted for publication. An incorrect or inappropriate statistical analysis can lead to the wrong conclusions and can eventually lead to a false credibility to naive readers (White, 1979).

Additional information on the type of statistical errors can be found in the classic publication by Huff (1954) or a more recent publication by Jaffee and Spirer (1987), which are listed in the suggested supplemental readings. For specific information on designing and evaluation of clinical trails, the reader is referred to the book by Friedman and colleagues (1998), also listed in the suggested readings.

**References**

Altman, D.G. (1991). "Statistics in medical journals: developments in the 1980s," Statistics in Medicine 10:1897-1913.

Avram, M.J., Shanks, C.A., Dykes, M.H., Ronai, A.K., and Stiers, W.M. (1985). "Statistical methods in anesthesia articles: an evaluation of two American journals during two six-month periods," *Anesth Analg* 64:607-611.

Badgley, R.F. (1961). "An assessment of research methods reported in 103 scientific articles in two Canadian medical journals," *Canadian Medical Association Journal*, 85, 246-250.

Cohn, J.B., Wilcox, C.S., and Goodman, L.I. (1993). "Antidepressant efficacy and cardiac safety of trimipramine in patients with mild heart disease," *Clinical Therapeutics* 15:114-122.

Cruess, D.F. (1989). "Review of use of statistics in the American Journal of Tropical Medicine and Hygiene for January-December 1988," *American Journal of Tropical Medicine and Hygiene* 41:619-626.

Felson, D.T., Cupples, L.A., and Meenan R.F. (1984). "Misuse of statistical methods in *Arthritis and Rheumatism* 1882 versus 1967-68," *Arthritis and Rheumatism* 27:1018-1022.

Glantz, S.A. (1980). "Biostatistics: how to detect, correct and prevent errors in the medical literature," Circulation 61:1-7.

Goodman, N.W. and Hughes, A.O. (1992). "Statistical awareness of research workers in British anaesthesia," *British Journal of Anaesthesia* 68:321-324.

Gore, S.M., Jones, I.G., and Rytter, E.C. (1977). "Misuse of statistical methods: critical assessment of articles in BMJ from January to March 1976," British Medical Journal 1:85-87.

Jouet, P. et al. (1994). "Comparative efficacy of interferon alfa in cirrhotic and noncirrhotic patients with non-A, non-B, C hepatitis," *Gastroenterology* 106:686-690.

Kanter, M.H. and Taylor, J.R. (1994). "Accuracy of statistical methods in *Transfusion*: a review of articles from July/August 1992 through June 1993," *Transfusion* 34:687-701.

McGuigan, S.M. (1995). "The use of statistics in the *British Journal of Psychiatry*," *British Journal of Psychiatry* 167:683-688.

Parsch, D.J. and Paladino, J.A. (1997) "Economics of sequential ofloxacin versus switch therapy," *Annals of Pharmacotherapy* 31:1137-1145

Vrbos, L.A., Lorenz, M.A., Peabody, E.H., et al. (1993). "Clinical methodologies and incidence of appropriate statistic testing in orthopaedic spine literature: are statistics misleading?" *Spine* 18:1021-1029.

White, S.J. (1979). "Statistical errors in papers in the *British Journal of Psychiatry*," *British Journal of Psychiatry* 135:336-342.

**Supplemental Suggested Readings**

Friedman, L.M., Furberg, C.D. and DeMets, D.L. (1998). *Fundamentals of Clinical Trials*, Third edition, Springer, New York.

Huff, D. (1954). *How to Lie with Statistics*, W.W. Norton and Company, New York.

Jaffee, A.J. and Spirer, H.F. (1987). *Misused Statistics: Straight Talk for Twisted Numbers*, Marcel Dekker, Inc., New York.

# Appendix A

# Flow Charts for Selection of Appropriate Inferential Tests

On the following pages are a series of panels that give direction on selecting the most appropriate inferential statistical test to use, based on the type of variables involved in the outcomes measurement.

For any given hypothesis being tested, the researcher must first identify the independent variable(s) and/or dependent variable(s). This begins the process seen in Panel A. Next the researcher must consider if the data presented by the respective variables involves discrete or continuous data (D/C?). Lastly, at various points in the decision making process the researcher must determine if the sample data comes from populations that are normally distributed and, if more than one level of a discrete independent variable, does there appear to be homogeneity of variance (ND/H?).

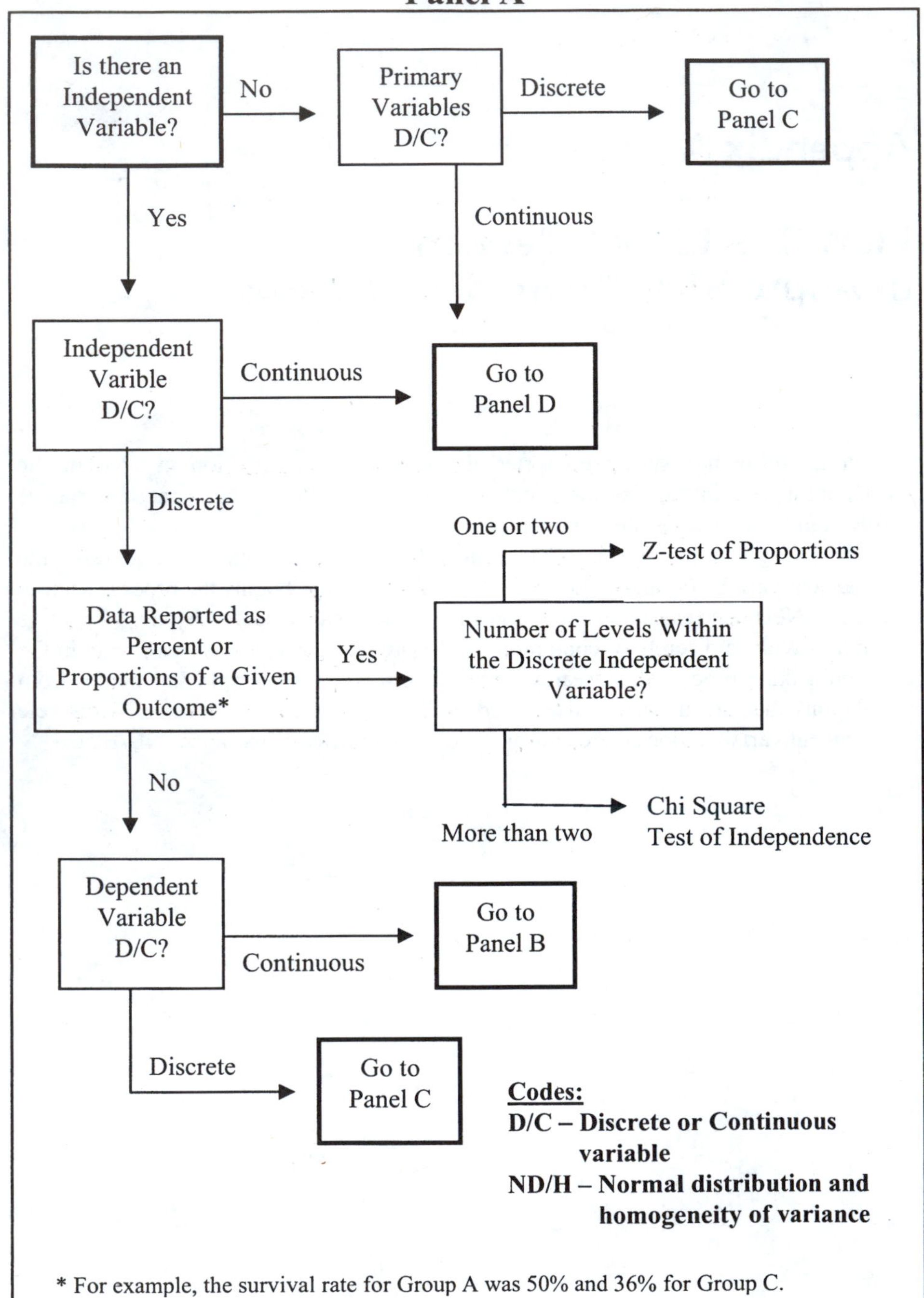
Panel A
Is there an Independent Variable?
No
Primary Variables D/C?
Discrete
Go to Panel C
Yes
Continuous
Independent Varible D/C?
Continuous
Go to Panel D
Discrete
One or two
Z-test of Proportions
Data Reported as Percent or Proportions of a Given Outcome*
Yes
Number of Levels Within the Discrete Independent Variable?
No
Chi Square Test of Independence
More than two
Dependent Variable D/C?
Go to Panel B
Continuous
Discrete
Go to Panel C
Codes:
D/C – Discrete or Continuous variable
ND/H – Normal distribution and homogeneity of variance
* For example, the survival rate for Group A was 50% and 36% for Group C.

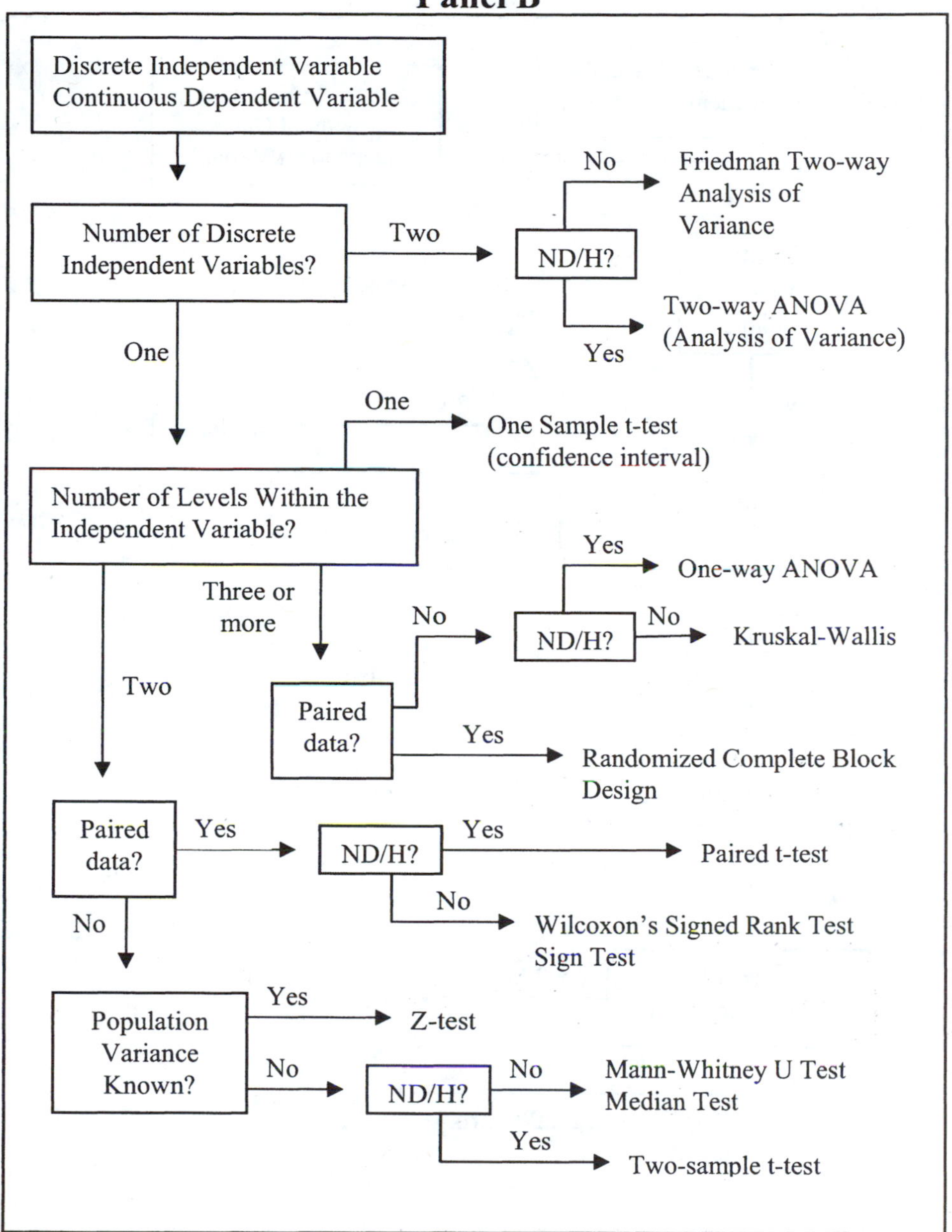
Panel B
Discrete Independent Variable
Continuous Dependent Variable
Number of Discrete Independent Variables?
Two
ND/H?
No
Friedman Two-way Analysis of Variance
Yes
Two-way ANOVA (Analysis of Variance)
One
Number of Levels Within the Independent Variable?
One
One Sample t-test (confidence interval)
Three or more
Paired data?
No
ND/H?
Yes
One-way ANOVA
No
Kruskal-Wallis
Yes
Randomized Complete Block Design
Two
Paired data?
Yes
ND/H?
Yes
Paired t-test
No
Wilcoxon's Signed Rank Test
Sign Test
No
Population Variance Known?
Yes
Z-test
No
ND/H?
No
Mann-Whitney U Test
Median Test
Yes
Two-sample t-test

## Panel C

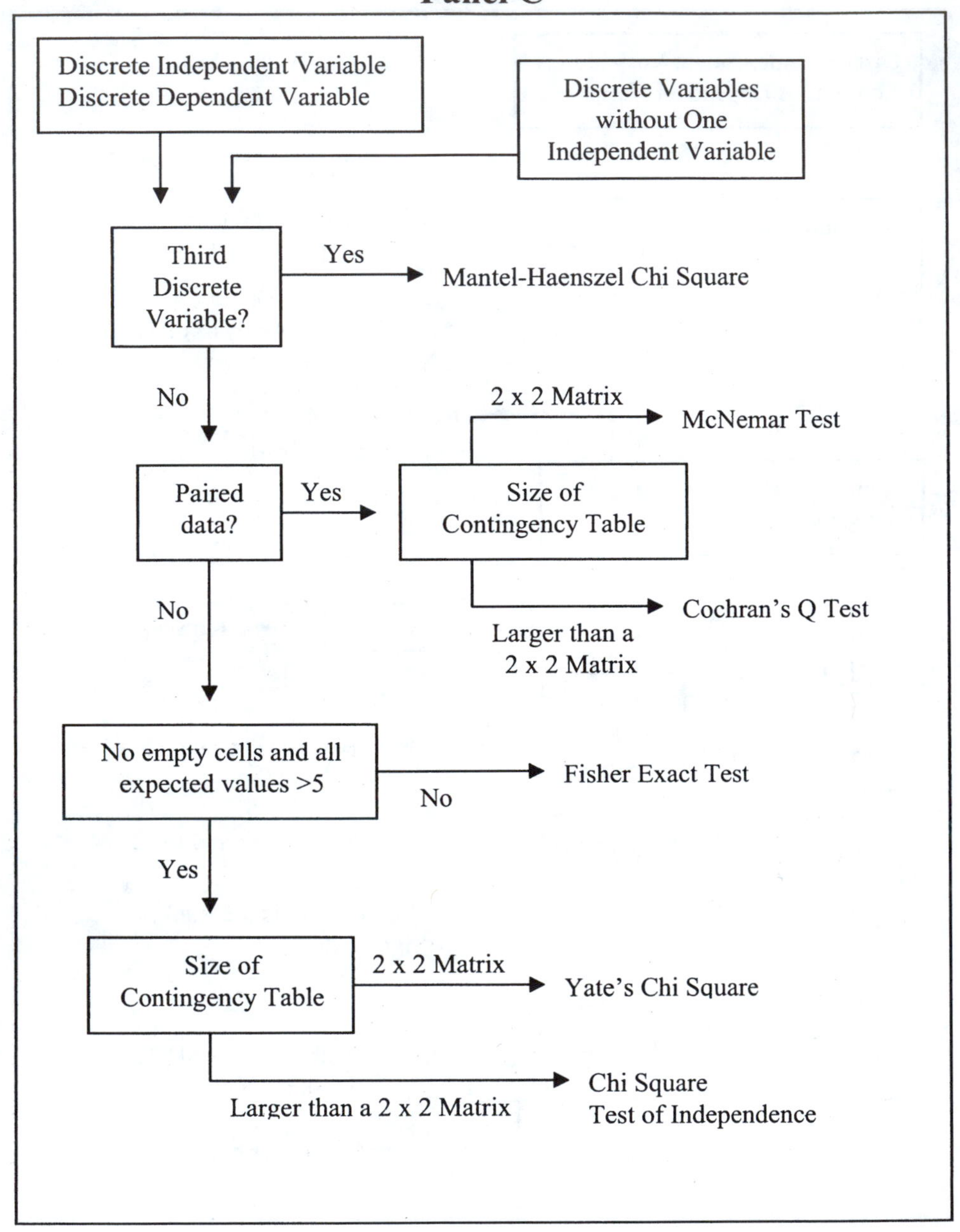
Discrete Independent Variable
Discrete Dependent Variable
Discrete Variables without One Independent Variable
Third Discrete Variable?
Yes
Mantel-Haenszel Chi Square
No
2 x 2 Matrix
McNemar Test
Paired data?
Yes
Size of Contingency Table
No
Cochran's Q Test
Larger than a 2 x 2 Matrix
No empty cells and all expected values >5
Fisher Exact Test
No
Yes
Size of Contingency Table
2 x 2 Matrix
Yate's Chi Square
Chi Square Test of Independence
Larger than a 2 x 2 Matrix

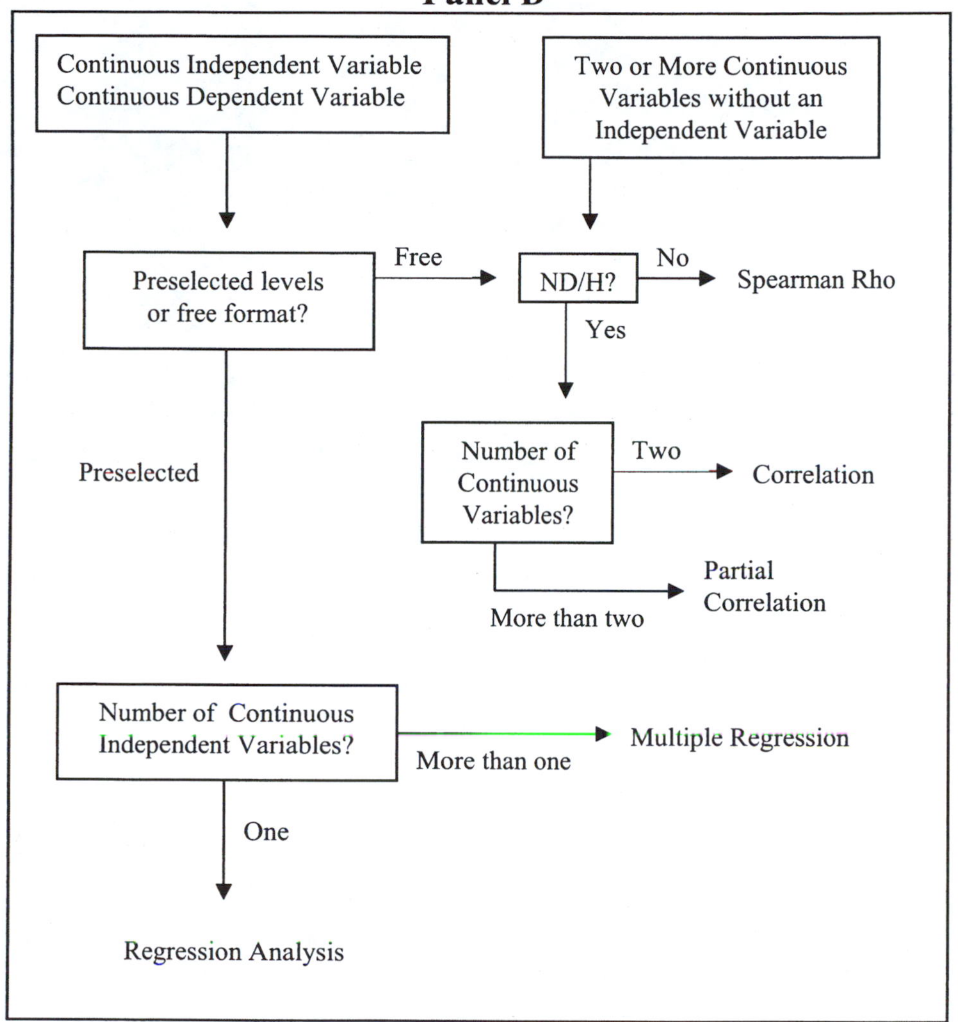
Panel D
Continuous Independent Variable
Continuous Dependent Variable
Two or More Continuous Variables without an Independent Variable
Preselected levels or free format?
Free
ND/H?
No
Spearman Rho
Yes
Preselected
Number of Continuous Variables?
Two
Correlation
Partial Correlation
More than two
Number of Continuous Independent Variables?
More than one
Multiple Regression
One
Regression Analysis

# Appendix B
# Statistical Tables

**Table B1** Random Numbers Table

| | | | | | | | | | |
|---|---|---|---|---|---|---|---|---|---|
| 42505 | 29928 | 18850 | 17263 | 70236 | 35432 | 61247 | 38337 | 87214 | 68897 |
| 32654 | 33712 | 97303 | 74982 | 30341 | 17824 | 38448 | 96101 | 58318 | 84892 |
| 09241 | 92732 | 66397 | 91735 | 20477 | 88736 | 14252 | 65579 | 71724 | 41661 |
| 60481 | 36875 | 52880 | 38061 | 76675 | 97108 | 70738 | 13808 | 86470 | 81613 |
| 00548 | 99401 | 29620 | 77382 | 62582 | 90279 | 51053 | 55882 | 23689 | 42138 |
| 14935 | 30864 | 23867 | 91238 | 43732 | 41176 | 27818 | 99720 | 82276 | 58577 |
| 01517 | 25915 | 86821 | 20550 | 13767 | 19657 | 39114 | 88111 | 62768 | 42600 |
| 85448 | 28625 | 27677 | 13522 | 00733 | 23616 | 45170 | 78646 | 77552 | 01582 |
| 11004 | 06949 | 40228 | 95804 | 06583 | 10471 | 83884 | 27164 | 50516 | 89635 |
| 38507 | 11952 | 75182 | 03552 | 58010 | 94680 | 28292 | 65340 | 34292 | 05896 |
| 99452 | 62431 | 36306 | 44997 | 71725 | 01887 | 74115 | 88038 | 98193 | 80710 |
| 87961 | 20548 | 03520 | 81159 | 62323 | 95340 | 10516 | 91057 | 64979 | 15326 |
| 91695 | 49105 | 11072 | 41328 | 45844 | 15199 | 52172 | 24889 | 99580 | 65735 |
| 90335 | 66089 | 33914 | 13927 | 17168 | 96354 | 35817 | 55119 | 77894 | 86274 |
| 74775 | 37096 | 60407 | 78405 | 04361 | 55394 | 09344 | 45095 | 88789 | 73620 |
| 65141 | 71286 | 54481 | 68757 | 28095 | 62329 | 66628 | 01479 | 47433 | 76801 |
| 30755 | 11466 | 35367 | 84313 | 19280 | 37714 | 06161 | 48322 | 23077 | 63845 |
| 40192 | 33948 | 28043 | 88427 | 73014 | 40780 | 16652 | 20279 | 09418 | 60695 |
| 94528 | 98786 | 62495 | 60668 | 41998 | 39213 | 17701 | 91582 | 91659 | 03018 |
| 21917 | 16043 | 24943 | 93160 | 97513 | 76195 | 08674 | 74415 | 81408 | 66525 |
| 36632 | 18689 | 89137 | 46685 | 11119 | 75330 | 03907 | 73296 | 43519 | 66437 |
| 90668 | 57765 | 80858 | 07179 | 35167 | 49098 | 57371 | 51101 | 08015 | 41710 |
| 71063 | 60441 | 53750 | 08240 | 85269 | 01440 | 04898 | 57359 | 55221 | 64656 |
| 21036 | 16589 | 79605 | 10277 | 52852 | 40111 | 77130 | 38429 | 31212 | 41578 |
| 88085 | 84496 | 81220 | 51929 | 00903 | 39425 | 61281 | 02201 | 03726 | 95044 |
| 27162 | 31340 | 60963 | 14372 | 21057 | 19015 | 14858 | 26932 | 85648 | 43430 |
| 12046 | 49063 | 03168 | 64138 | 55123 | 29232 | 59462 | 29850 | 79201 | 18349 |
| 33052 | 11252 | 53477 | 65078 | 09199 | 58814 | 07790 | 36148 | 18962 | 85602 |
| 84187 | 61668 | 03267 | 75095 | 13486 | 05438 | 01962 | 13994 | 16834 | 60262 |
| 67887 | 50033 | 32275 | 68259 | 05930 | 74797 | 66309 | 66181 | 37093 | 31528 |
| 70457 | 55716 | 87554 | 47943 | 42819 | 98810 | 02729 | 94043 | 54642 | 37974 |
| 86336 | 64926 | 01880 | 41598 | 64455 | 88602 | 81755 | 74262 | 74591 | 58802 |
| 94323 | 92053 | 79740 | 92794 | 69032 | 62871 | 07447 | 14192 | 16290 | 11747 |
| 13869 | 60770 | 04022 | 91154 | 72841 | 17275 | 52936 | 76317 | 89963 | 73241 |
| 94585 | 85528 | 41527 | 05795 | 59929 | 25458 | 38851 | 87484 | 18897 | 61470 |

**Table B2** Normal Standardized Distribution

(area under the curve between 0 and z)

| *z* | 0.00 | 0.01 | 0.02 | 0.03 | 0.04 | 0.05 | 0.06 | 0.07 | 0.08 | 0.09 |
|---|---|---|---|---|---|---|---|---|---|---|
| 0.0 | .0000 | .0040 | .0080 | .0120 | .0160 | .0199 | .0239 | .0279 | .0319 | .0359 |
| 0.1 | .0398 | .0438 | .0478 | .0517 | .0557 | .0596 | .0636 | .0675 | .0714 | .0753 |
| 0.2 | .0793 | .0832 | .0871 | .0910 | .0948 | .0987 | .1026 | .1064 | .1103 | .1141 |
| 0.3 | .1179 | .1217 | .1255 | .1293 | .1331 | .1368 | .1406 | .1443 | .1480 | .1517 |
| 0.4 | .1554 | .1591 | .1628 | .1664 | .1700 | .1736 | .1772 | .1808 | .1844 | .1879 |
| 0.5 | .1915 | .1950 | .1985 | .2019 | .2054 | .2088 | .2123 | .2157 | .2190 | .2224 |
| 0.6 | .2257 | .2291 | .2324 | .2357 | .2389 | .2422 | .2454 | .2486 | .2517 | .2549 |
| 0.7 | .2580 | .2611 | .2642 | .2673 | .2704 | .2734 | .2764 | .2794 | .2823 | .2852 |
| 0.8 | .2881 | .2910 | .2939 | .2967 | .2995 | .3023 | .3051 | .3078 | .3106 | .3133 |
| 0.9 | .3159 | .3186 | .3212 | .3238 | .3264 | .3289 | .3315 | .3340 | .3365 | .3389 |
| 1.0 | .3413 | .3438 | .3461 | .3485 | .3508 | .3531 | .3554 | .3577 | .3599 | .3621 |
| 1.1 | .3643 | .3665 | .3686 | .3708 | .3729 | .3749 | .3770 | .3790 | .3810 | .3830 |
| 1.2 | .3849 | .3869 | .3888 | .3907 | .3925 | .3944 | .3962 | .3980 | .3997 | .4015 |
| 1.3 | .4032 | .4049 | .4066 | .4082 | .4099 | .4115 | .4131 | .4147 | .4162 | .4177 |
| 1.4 | .4192 | .4207 | .4222 | .4236 | .4251 | .4265 | .4279 | .4292 | .4306 | .4319 |
| 1.5 | .4332 | .4345 | .4357 | .4370 | .4382 | .4394 | .4406 | .4418 | .4429 | .4441 |
| 1.6 | .4452 | .4463 | .4474 | .4484 | .4495 | .4505 | .4515 | .4525 | .4535 | .4545 |
| 1.7 | .4554 | .4564 | .4573 | .4582 | .4591 | .4599 | .4608 | .4616 | .4625 | .4633 |
| 1.8 | .4641 | .4649 | .4656 | .4664 | .4671 | .4678 | .4686 | .4693 | .4699 | .4706 |
| 1.9 | .4713 | .4719 | .4726 | .4732 | .4738 | .4744 | .4750 | .4756 | .4761 | .4767 |
| 2.0 | .4772 | .4778 | .4783 | .4788 | .4793 | .4798 | .4803 | .4808 | .4812 | .4817 |
| 2.1 | .4821 | .4826 | .4830 | .4834 | .4838 | .4842 | .4846 | .4850 | .4854 | .4857 |
| 2.2 | .4861 | .4864 | .4868 | .4871 | .4875 | .4878 | .4881 | .4884 | .4887 | .4890 |
| 2.3 | .4893 | .4896 | .4898 | .4901 | .4904 | .4906 | .4909 | .4911 | .4913 | .4916 |
| 2.4 | .4918 | .4920 | .4922 | .4925 | .4927 | .4929 | .4931 | .4932 | .4934 | .4936 |
| 2.5 | .4938 | .4940 | .4941 | .4943 | .4945 | .4946 | .4948 | .4949 | .4951 | .4952 |
| 2.6 | .4953 | .4955 | .4956 | .4957 | .4959 | .4960 | .4961 | .4962 | .4963 | .4964 |
| 2.7 | .4965 | .4966 | .4967 | .4968 | .4969 | .4970 | .4971 | .4972 | .4973 | .4974 |
| 2.8 | .4974 | .4975 | .4976 | .4977 | .4977 | .4978 | .4979 | .4979 | .4980 | .4981 |
| 2.9 | .4981 | .4982 | .4982 | .4983 | .4984 | .4984 | .4985 | .4985 | .4986 | .4986 |
| 3.0 | .4987 | .4987 | .4987 | .4988 | .4988 | .4989 | .4989 | .4989 | .4990 | .4990 |
| 3.1 | .4990 | .4991 | .4991 | .4991 | .4992 | .4992 | .4992 | .4992 | .4993 | .4993 |
| 3.2 | .4993 | .4993 | .4994 | .4994 | .4994 | .4994 | .4994 | .4995 | .4995 | .4995 |
| 3.3 | .4995 | .4995 | .4995 | .4996 | .4996 | .4996 | .4996 | .4996 | .4996 | .4997 |
| 3.4 | .4997 | .4997 | .4997 | .4997 | .4997 | .4997 | .4997 | .4997 | .4997 | .4998 |
| 3.5 | .4998 | .4998 | .4998 | .4998 | .4998 | .4998 | .4998 | .4998 | .4998 | .4998 |
| 3.6 | .4998 | .4998 | .4999 | .4999 | .4999 | .4999 | .4999 | .4999 | .4999 | .4999 |

This table was created using Microsoft® Excel 2002 using function command NORMSDIST(*value*)-0.5.

**Table B3** K-Values for Calculating Tolerance Limits (two-tailed)

| | 90% Confidence | | | 95% Confidence | | | 99% Confidence | | |
|---|---|---|---|---|---|---|---|---|---|
| n | 95% | 99% | 99.9% | 95% | 99% | 99.9% | 95% | 99% | 99.9% |
| 2 | 18.22 | 23.42 | 29.36 | 36.52 | 46.94 | 58.84 | 182.7 | 234.9 | 294.4 |
| 3 | 6.823 | 8.819 | 11.10 | 9.789 | 12.64 | 15.92 | 22.13 | 28.58 | 35.98 |
| 4 | 4.913 | 6.372 | 8.046 | 6.341 | 8.221 | 10.38 | 11.12 | 14.41 | 18.18 |
| 5 | 4.142 | 5.387 | 6.816 | 5.077 | 6.598 | 8.345 | 7.870 | 10.22 | 12.92 |
| 6 | 3.723 | 4.850 | 6.146 | 4.422 | 5.758 | 7.294 | 6.373 | 8.292 | 10.50 |
| 7 | 3.456 | 4.508 | 5.720 | 4.020 | 5.241 | 6.647 | 5.520 | 7.191 | 9.114 |
| 8 | 3.270 | 4.271 | 5.423 | 3.746 | 4.889 | 6.206 | 4.968 | 6.479 | 8.220 |
| 9 | 3.132 | 4.094 | 5.203 | 3.546 | 4.633 | 5.885 | 4.581 | 5.980 | 7.593 |
| 10 | 3.026 | 3.958 | 5.033 | 3.393 | 4.437 | 5.640 | 4.292 | 5.610 | 7.127 |
| 12 | 2.871 | 3.759 | 4.785 | 3.175 | 4.156 | 5.287 | 3.896 | 5.096 | 6.481 |
| 15 | 2.720 | 3.565 | 4.541 | 2.965 | 3.885 | 4.949 | 3.529 | 4.621 | 5.883 |
| 18 | 2.620 | 3.436 | 4.380 | 2.828 | 3.709 | 4.727 | 3.297 | 4.321 | 5.505 |
| 20 | 2.570 | 3.372 | 4.299 | 2.760 | 3.621 | 4.616 | 3.184 | 4.175 | 5.321 |
| 25 | 2.479 | 3.254 | 4.151 | 2.638 | 3.462 | 4.416 | 2.984 | 3.915 | 4.993 |
| 30 | 2.417 | 3.173 | 4.050 | 2.555 | 3.355 | 4.281 | 2.851 | 3.742 | 4.775 |
| 35 | 2.371 | 3.114 | 3.975 | 2.495 | 3.276 | 4.182 | 2.756 | 3.618 | 4.618 |
| 40 | 2.336 | 3.069 | 3.918 | 2.448 | 3.216 | 4.105 | 2.684 | 3.524 | 4.499 |
| 50 | 2.285 | 3.003 | 3.834 | 2.382 | 3.129 | 3.995 | 2.580 | 3.390 | 4.328 |
| 60 | 2.250 | 2.956 | 3.775 | 2.335 | 3.068 | 3.918 | 2.509 | 3.297 | 4.210 |
| 80 | 2.203 | 2.895 | 3.697 | 2.274 | 2.988 | 3.816 | 2.416 | 3.175 | 4.055 |
| 100 | 2.172 | 2.855 | 3.646 | 2.234 | 2.936 | 3.750 | 2.357 | 3.098 | 3.956 |
| 120 | 2.151 | 2.826 | 3.610 | 2.206 | 2.899 | 3.703 | 2.315 | 3.043 | 3.887 |
| 150 | 2.128 | 2.796 | 3.572 | 2.176 | 2.859 | 3.652 | 2.271 | 2.985 | 3.812 |
| 200 | 2.102 | 2.763 | 3.529 | 2.143 | 2.816 | 3.598 | 2.223 | 2.921 | 3.732 |
| 300 | 2.073 | 2.725 | 3.481 | 2.106 | 2.767 | 3.535 | 2.169 | 2.850 | 3.641 |
| 400 | 2.057 | 2.703 | 3.453 | 2.084 | 2.739 | 3.499 | 2.138 | 2.810 | 3.589 |
| 500 | 2.046 | 2.689 | 3.435 | 2.070 | 2.721 | 3.476 | 2.117 | 2.783 | 3.555 |
| 1000 | 2.019 | 2.654 | 3.390 | 2.036 | 2.676 | 3.418 | 2.068 | 2.718 | 3.473 |
| ∞ | 1.960 | 2.576 | 3.291 | 1.960 | 2.576 | 3.291 | 1.960 | 2.576 | 3.291 |

Modified from: Odeh, R.E. and Owen, D.B. (1980). *Tables for Normal Tolerance Limits, Sampling Plans, and Screening*, Marcel Dekker, Inc., New York, pp. 90-93 and 98-105. Reproduced with permission of the publisher.

**Table B4** K-Values for Calculating Tolerance Limits (one-tailed)

| | 90% Confidence | | | 95% Confidence | | | 99% Confidence | | |
|---|---|---|---|---|---|---|---|---|---|
| n | 95% | 99% | 99.9% | 95% | 99% | 99.9% | 95% | 99% | 99.9% |
| 2 | 13.09 | 18.50 | 24.58 | 26.26 | 37.09 | 49.28 | 131.4 | 185.6 | 246.6 |
| 3 | 5.311 | 7.340 | 9.651 | 7.656 | 10.55 | 13.86 | 17.37 | 23.90 | 31.35 |
| 4 | 3.957 | 5.438 | 7.129 | 5.144 | 7.042 | 9.214 | 9.083 | 12.39 | 16.18 |
| 5 | 3.400 | 4.666 | 6.111 | 4.203 | 5.741 | 7.502 | 6.578 | 8.939 | 11.65 |
| 6 | 3.092 | 4.243 | 5.556 | 3.708 | 5.062 | 6.612 | 5.406 | 7.335 | 9.550 |
| 7 | 2.894 | 3.972 | 5.202 | 3.399 | 4.642 | 6.063 | 4.728 | 6.412 | 8.346 |
| 8 | 2.754 | 3.783 | 4.955 | 3.187 | 4.354 | 5.688 | 4.285 | 5.812 | 7.564 |
| 9 | 2.650 | 3.641 | 4.771 | 3.031 | 4.143 | 5.413 | 3.972 | 5.389 | 7.014 |
| 10 | 2.568 | 3.532 | 4.629 | 2.911 | 3.981 | 5.203 | 3.738 | 5.074 | 6.605 |
| 12 | 2.448 | 3.371 | 4.420 | 2.736 | 3.747 | 4.900 | 3.410 | 4.633 | 6.035 |
| 15 | 2.329 | 3.212 | 4.215 | 2.566 | 3.520 | 4.607 | 3.102 | 4.222 | 5.504 |
| 18 | 2.249 | 3.105 | 4.078 | 2.453 | 3.370 | 4.415 | 2.905 | 3.960 | 5.167 |
| 20 | 2.208 | 3.052 | 4.009 | 2.396 | 3.295 | 4.318 | 2.808 | 3.832 | 5.001 |
| 25 | 2.132 | 2.952 | 3.882 | 2.292 | 3.158 | 4.142 | 2.633 | 3.601 | 4.706 |
| 30 | 2.080 | 2.884 | 3.794 | 2.220 | 3.064 | 4.022 | 2.515 | 3.447 | 4.508 |
| 35 | 2.041 | 2.833 | 3.729 | 2.167 | 2.995 | 3.934 | 2.430 | 3.334 | 4.364 |
| 40 | 2.010 | 2.793 | 3.679 | 2.125 | 2.941 | 3.865 | 2.364 | 3.249 | 4.255 |
| 50 | 1.965 | 2.735 | 3.605 | 2.065 | 2.862 | 3.766 | 2.269 | 3.125 | 4.097 |
| 60 | 1.933 | 2.694 | 3.552 | 2.022 | 2.807 | 3.695 | 2.202 | 3.038 | 3.987 |
| 80 | 1.890 | 2.638 | 3.482 | 1.964 | 2.733 | 3.601 | 2.114 | 2.924 | 3.842 |
| 100 | 1.861 | 2.601 | 3.435 | 1.927 | 2.684 | 3.539 | 2.056 | 2.850 | 3.748 |
| 120 | 1.841 | 2.574 | 3.402 | 1.899 | 2.649 | 3.495 | 2.015 | 2.797 | 3.682 |
| 150 | 1.818 | 2.546 | 3.366 | 1.870 | 2.611 | 3.448 | 1.971 | 2.740 | 3.610 |
| 200 | 1.793 | 2.514 | 3.326 | 1.837 | 2.570 | 3.395 | 1.923 | 2.679 | 3.532 |
| 300 | 1.765 | 2.477 | 3.280 | 1.800 | 2.522 | 3.335 | 1.868 | 2.608 | 3.443 |
| 400 | 1.748 | 2.456 | 3.253 | 1.778 | 2.494 | 3.300 | 1.836 | 2.567 | 3.392 |
| 500 | 1.736 | 2.442 | 3.235 | 1.763 | 2.475 | 3.277 | 1.814 | 2.540 | 3.358 |
| 1000 | 1.697 | 2.392 | 3.172 | 1.727 | 2.430 | 3.220 | 1.740 | 2.446 | 3.240 |
| ∞ | 1.645 | 2.326 | 3.090 | 1.645 | 2.326 | 3.090 | 1.645 | 2.326 | 3.090 |

Modified from: Odeh, R.E. and Owen, D.B. (1980). *Tables for Normal Tolerance Limits, Sampling Plans, and Screening*, Marcel Dekker, Inc., New York, pp. 22-25 and 98-107. Reproduced with permission of the publisher.

**Table B5** Student t-Distribution (1 - α/2)

| d.f. | $t_{.80}$ | $t_{.90}$ | $t_{.95}$ | $t_{.975}$ | $t_{.99}$ | $t_{.995}$ | $t_{.9975}$ | $t_{.9995}$ |
|---|---|---|---|---|---|---|---|---|
| 1 | 0.7265 | 3.0777 | 6.3137 | 12.706 | 31.821 | 63.656 | 127.32 | 636.58 |
| 2 | 0.6172 | 1.8856 | 2.9200 | 4.3027 | 6.9645 | 9.9250 | 14.089 | 31.600 |
| 3 | 0.5844 | 1.6377 | 2.3534 | 3.1824 | 4.5407 | 5.8408 | 7.4532 | 12.924 |
| 4 | 0.5686 | 1.5332 | 2.1318 | 2.7765 | 3.7469 | 4.6041 | 5.5975 | 8.6101 |
| 5 | 0.5594 | 1.4759 | 2.0150 | 2.5706 | 3.3649 | 4.0321 | 4.7733 | 6.8685 |
| 6 | 0.5534 | 1.4398 | 1.9432 | 2.4469 | 3.1427 | 3.7074 | 4.3168 | 5.9587 |
| 7 | 0.5491 | 1.4149 | 1.8946 | 2.3646 | 2.9979 | 3.4995 | 4.0294 | 5.4081 |
| 8 | 0.5459 | 1.3968 | 1.8595 | 2.3060 | 2.8965 | 3.3554 | 3.8325 | 5.0414 |
| 9 | 0.5435 | 1.3830 | 1.8331 | 2.2622 | 2.8214 | 3.2498 | 3.6896 | 4.7809 |
| 10 | 0.5415 | 1.3722 | 1.8125 | 2.2281 | 2.7638 | 3.1693 | 3.5814 | 4.5868 |
| 11 | 0.5399 | 1.3634 | 1.7959 | 2.2010 | 2.7181 | 3.1058 | 3.4966 | 4.4369 |
| 12 | 0.5386 | 1.3562 | 1.7823 | 2.1788 | 2.6810 | 3.0545 | 3.4284 | 4.3178 |
| 13 | 0.5375 | 1.3502 | 1.7709 | 2.1604 | 2.6503 | 3.0123 | 3.3725 | 4.2209 |
| 14 | 0.5366 | 1.3450 | 1.7613 | 2.1448 | 2.6245 | 2.9768 | 3.3257 | 4.1403 |
| 15 | 0.5357 | 1.3406 | 1.7531 | 2.1315 | 2.6025 | 2.9467 | 3.2860 | 4.0728 |
| 16 | 0.5350 | 1.3368 | 1.7459 | 2.1199 | 2.5835 | 2.9208 | 3.2520 | 4.0149 |
| 17 | 0.5344 | 1.3334 | 1.7396 | 2.1098 | 2.5669 | 2.8982 | 3.2224 | 3.9651 |
| 18 | 0.5338 | 1.3304 | 1.7341 | 2.1009 | 2.5524 | 2.8784 | 3.1966 | 3.9217 |
| 19 | 0.5333 | 1.3277 | 1.7291 | 2.0930 | 2.5395 | 2.8609 | 3.1737 | 3.8833 |
| 20 | 0.5329 | 1.3253 | 1.7247 | 2.0860 | 2.5280 | 2.8453 | 3.1534 | 3.8496 |
| 21 | 0.5325 | 1.3232 | 1.7207 | 2.0796 | 2.5176 | 2.8314 | 3.1352 | 3.8193 |
| 22 | 0.5321 | 1.3212 | 1.7171 | 2.0739 | 2.5083 | 2.8188 | 3.1188 | 3.7922 |
| 23 | 0.5317 | 1.3195 | 1.7139 | 2.0687 | 2.4999 | 2.8073 | 3.1040 | 3.7676 |
| 24 | 0.5314 | 1.3178 | 1.7109 | 2.0639 | 2.4922 | 2.7970 | 3.0905 | 3.7454 |
| 25 | 0.5312 | 1.3163 | 1.7081 | 2.0595 | 2.4851 | 2.7874 | 3.0782 | 3.7251 |
| 30 | 0.5300 | 1.3104 | 1.6973 | 2.0423 | 2.4573 | 2.7500 | 3.0298 | 3.6460 |
| 40 | 0.5286 | 1.3031 | 1.6839 | 2.0211 | 2.4233 | 2.7045 | 2.9712 | 3.5510 |
| 50 | 0.5278 | 1.2987 | 1.6759 | 2.0086 | 2.4033 | 2.6778 | 2.9370 | 3.4960 |
| 60 | 0.5272 | 1.2958 | 1.6706 | 2.0003 | 2.3901 | 2.6603 | 2.9146 | 3.4602 |
| 80 | 0.5265 | 1.2922 | 1.6641 | 1.9901 | 2.3739 | 2.6387 | 2.8870 | 3.4164 |
| 100 | 0.5261 | 1.2901 | 1.6602 | 1.9840 | 2.3642 | 2.6259 | 2.8707 | 3.3905 |
| 120 | 0.5258 | 1.2886 | 1.6576 | 1.9799 | 2.3578 | 2.6174 | 2.8599 | 3.3734 |
| 160 | 0.5254 | 1.2869 | 1.6544 | 1.9749 | 2.3499 | 2.6069 | 2.8465 | 3.3523 |
| 200 | 0.5252 | 1.2858 | 1.6525 | 1.9719 | 2.3451 | 2.6006 | 2.8385 | 3.3398 |
| ∞ | 0.5244 | 1.2816 | 1.6450 | 1.9602 | 2.3267 | 2.5763 | 2.8076 | 3.2915 |

This table was created using Microsoft® Excel 2002, function command INV(alpha,df).

**Table B6** Comparison of One-Tailed vs. Two-Tailed t-Distributions

| df | 95% Confidence | | 99% Confidence | |
|---|---|---|---|---|
| | Two-Tailed ($\alpha/2$) | One-Tailed ($\alpha$) | Two-Tailed ($\alpha/2$) | One-Tailed ($\alpha$) |
| 1 | 12.706 | 6.314 | 63.657 | 31.821 |
| 2 | 4.302 | 2.920 | 9.924 | 6.985 |
| 3 | 3.182 | 2.353 | 5.840 | 4.541 |
| 4 | 2.776 | 2.131 | 4.604 | 3.747 |
| 5 | 2.570 | 2.015 | 4.032 | 3.365 |
| 6 | 2.446 | 1.943 | 3.707 | 3.143 |
| 7 | 2.364 | 1.894 | 3.499 | 2.998 |
| 8 | 2.306 | 1.859 | 3.355 | 2.896 |
| 9 | 2.262 | 1.833 | 3.249 | 2.821 |
| 10 | 2.228 | 1.812 | 3.169 | 2.764 |
| 11 | 2.201 | 1.795 | 3.105 | 2.718 |
| 12 | 2.178 | 1.782 | 3.054 | 2.681 |
| 13 | 2.160 | 1.770 | 3.012 | 2.650 |
| 14 | 2.144 | 1.761 | 2.976 | 2.624 |
| 15 | 2.131 | 1.753 | 2.946 | 2.602 |
| 20 | 2.086 | 1.724 | 2.845 | 2.528 |
| 25 | 2.059 | 1.708 | 2.787 | 2.485 |
| 30 | 2.042 | 1.697 | 2.750 | 2.457 |
| 40 | 2.021 | 1.683 | 2.704 | 2.423 |
| 50 | 2.008 | 1.675 | 2.677 | 2.403 |
| 60 | 2.000 | 1.670 | 2.660 | 2.390 |
| 80 | 1.990 | 1.664 | 2.638 | 2.374 |
| 100 | 1.984 | 1.660 | 2.626 | 2.364 |
| 120 | 1.979 | 1.657 | 2.617 | 2.358 |
| 160 | 1.974 | 1.654 | 2.607 | 2.350 |
| 200 | 1.971 | 1.652 | 2.600 | 2.345 |
| $\infty$ | 1.960 | 1.645 | 2.576 | 2.326 |

This table was created using Microsoft® Excel 2002, function command INV(alpha,df).

**Table B7** Analysis of Variance F-Distribution

| $\nu_1$ | $\nu_2$ | $F_{.80}$ | $F_{.90}$ | $F_{.95}$ | $F_{.975}$ | $F_{.99}$ | $F_{.999}$ | $F_{.9999}$ |
|---|---|---|---|---|---|---|---|---|
| | 1 | 9.4722 | 39.864 | 161.45 | 647.79 | 4052.2 | $4 \times 10^5$ | $4 \times 10^7$ |
| | 2 | 3.5556 | 8.5263 | 18.513 | 38.506 | 98.502 | 998.38 | $1 \times 10^4$ |
| | 3 | 2.6822 | 5.5383 | 10.128 | 17.443 | 34.116 | 167.06 | 784.17 |
| | 4 | 2.3507 | 4.5448 | 7.7086 | 12.218 | 21.198 | 74.127 | 241.68 |
| | 5 | 2.1782 | 4.0604 | 6.6079 | 10.007 | 16.258 | 47.177 | 124.80 |
| | 6 | 2.0729 | 3.7760 | 5.9874 | 8.8131 | 13.745 | 35.507 | 82.422 |
| | 7 | 2.0020 | 3.5894 | 5.5915 | 8.0727 | 12.246 | 29.246 | 62.166 |
| | 8 | 1.9511 | 3.4579 | 5.3176 | 7.5709 | 11.259 | 25.415 | 50.699 |
| | 9 | 1.9128 | 3.3603 | 5.1174 | 7.2093 | 10.562 | 22.857 | 43.481 |
| | 10 | 1.8829 | 3.2850 | 4.9646 | 6.9367 | 10.044 | 21.038 | 38.592 |
| | 11 | 1.8589 | 3.2252 | 4.8443 | 6.7241 | 9.6461 | 19.687 | 35.041 |
| | 12 | 1.8393 | 3.1766 | 4.7472 | 6.5538 | 9.3303 | 18.645 | 32.422 |
| | 13 | 1.8230 | 3.1362 | 4.6672 | 6.4143 | 9.0738 | 17.815 | 30.384 |
| 1 | 14 | 1.8091 | 3.1022 | 4.6001 | 6.2979 | 8.8617 | 17.142 | 28.755 |
| | 15 | 1.7972 | 3.0732 | 4.5431 | 6.1995 | 8.6832 | 16.587 | 27.445 |
| | 16 | 1.7869 | 3.0481 | 4.4940 | 6.1151 | 8.5309 | 16.120 | 26.368 |
| | 17 | 1.7779 | 3.0262 | 4.4513 | 6.0420 | 8.3998 | 15.722 | 25.437 |
| | 18 | 1.7699 | 3.0070 | 4.4139 | 5.9781 | 8.2855 | 15.380 | 24.651 |
| | 19 | 1.7629 | 2.9899 | 4.3808 | 5.9216 | 8.1850 | 15.081 | 23.982 |
| | 20 | 1.7565 | 2.9747 | 4.3513 | 5.8715 | 8.0960 | 14.819 | 23.399 |
| | 22 | 1.7457 | 2.9486 | 4.3009 | 5.7863 | 7.9453 | 14.381 | 22.439 |
| | 24 | 1.7367 | 2.9271 | 4.2597 | 5.7166 | 7.8229 | 14.028 | 21.653 |
| | 26 | 1.7292 | 2.9091 | 4.2252 | 5.6586 | 7.7213 | 13.739 | 21.042 |
| | 30 | 1.7172 | 2.8807 | 4.1709 | 5.5675 | 7.5624 | 13.293 | 20.096 |
| | 35 | 1.7062 | 2.8547 | 4.1213 | 5.4848 | 7.4191 | 12.897 | 19.267 |
| | 40 | 1.6980 | 2.8353 | 4.0847 | 5.4239 | 7.3142 | 12.609 | 18.670 |
| | 45 | 1.6917 | 2.8205 | 4.0566 | 5.3773 | 7.2339 | 12.393 | 18.219 |
| | 50 | 1.6867 | 2.8087 | 4.0343 | 5.3403 | 7.1706 | 12.222 | 17.884 |
| | 60 | 1.6792 | 2.7911 | 4.0012 | 5.2856 | 7.0771 | 11.973 | 17.375 |
| | 90 | 1.6668 | 2.7621 | 3.9469 | 5.1962 | 6.9251 | 11.573 | 16.589 |
| | 120 | 1.6606 | 2.7478 | 3.9201 | 5.1523 | 6.8509 | 11.380 | 16.204 |
| | 240 | 1.6515 | 2.7266 | 3.8805 | 5.0875 | 6.7416 | 11.099 | 15.658 |
| | ∞ | 1.6423 | 2.7053 | 3.8415 | 5.0239 | 6.6349 | 10.828 | 15.134 |

continued

**Table B7** Analysis of Variance F-Distribution (continued)

| $\nu_1$ | $\nu_2$ | $F_{.80}$ | $F_{.90}$ | $F_{.95}$ | $F_{.975}$ | $F_{.99}$ | $F_{.999}$ | $F_{.9999}$ |
|---|---|---|---|---|---|---|---|---|
| | 2 | 4.000 | 9.000 | 19.00 | 39.00 | 99.00 | 998.8 | $1 \times 10^4$ |
| | 3 | 2.886 | 5.462 | 9.552 | 16.04 | 30.82 | 148.5 | 694.8 |
| | 4 | 2.472 | 4.325 | 6.944 | 10.65 | 18.00 | 61.25 | 197.9 |
| | 5 | 2.259 | 3.780 | 5.786 | 8.434 | 13.27 | 37.12 | 97.09 |
| | 6 | 2.130 | 3.463 | 5.143 | 7.260 | 10.92 | 27.00 | 61.58 |
| | 8 | 1.981 | 3.113 | 4.459 | 6.059 | 8.649 | 18.49 | 35.97 |
| 2 | 10 | 1.899 | 2.924 | 4.103 | 5.456 | 7.559 | 14.90 | 26.54 |
| | 12 | 1.846 | 2.807 | 3.885 | 5.096 | 6.927 | 12.97 | 21.86 |
| | 15 | 1.795 | 2.695 | 3.682 | 4.765 | 6.359 | 11.34 | 18.10 |
| | 20 | 1.746 | 2.589 | 3.493 | 4.461 | 5.849 | 9.953 | 15.12 |
| | 24 | 1.722 | 2.538 | 3.403 | 4.319 | 5.614 | 9.340 | 13.85 |
| | 30 | 1.699 | 2.489 | 3.316 | 4.182 | 5.390 | 8.773 | 12.72 |
| | 40 | 1.676 | 2.440 | 3.232 | 4.051 | 5.178 | 8.251 | 11.70 |
| | 60 | 1.653 | 2.393 | 3.150 | 3.925 | 4.977 | 7.768 | 10.78 |
| | 120 | 1.631 | 2.347 | 3.072 | 3.805 | 4.787 | 7.321 | 9.954 |
| | ∞ | 1.609 | 2.303 | 2.996 | 3.689 | 4.605 | 6.908 | 9.211 |
| | 2 | 4.1563 | 9.1618 | 19.164 | 39.166 | 99.164 | 999.31 | $1 \times 10^4$ |
| | 3 | 2.9359 | 5.3908 | 9.2766 | 15.439 | 29.457 | 141.10 | 659.38 |
| | 4 | 2.4847 | 4.1909 | 6.5914 | 9.9792 | 16.694 | 56.170 | 181.14 |
| | 5 | 2.2530 | 3.6195 | 5.4094 | 7.7636 | 12.060 | 33.200 | 86.380 |
| | 6 | 2.1126 | 3.2888 | 4.7571 | 6.5988 | 9.7796 | 23.705 | 53.667 |
| | 8 | 1.9513 | 2.9238 | 4.0662 | 5.4160 | 7.5910 | 15.829 | 30.443 |
| 3 | 10 | 1.8614 | 2.7277 | 3.7083 | 4.8256 | 6.5523 | 12.553 | 22.032 |
| | 12 | 1.8042 | 2.6055 | 3.4903 | 4.4742 | 5.9525 | 10.805 | 17.899 |
| | 15 | 1.7490 | 2.4898 | 3.2874 | 4.1528 | 5.4170 | 9.3351 | 14.639 |
| | 20 | 1.6958 | 2.3801 | 3.0984 | 3.8587 | 4.9382 | 8.0981 | 12.049 |
| | 24 | 1.6699 | 2.3274 | 3.0088 | 3.7211 | 4.7181 | 7.5543 | 10.965 |
| | 30 | 1.6445 | 2.2761 | 2.9223 | 3.5893 | 4.5097 | 7.0545 | 9.9972 |
| | 40 | 1.6195 | 2.2261 | 2.8387 | 3.4633 | 4.3126 | 6.5947 | 9.1277 |
| | 60 | 1.5950 | 2.1774 | 2.7581 | 3.3425 | 4.1259 | 6.1714 | 8.3528 |
| | 120 | 1.5709 | 2.1300 | 2.6802 | 3.2269 | 3.9491 | 5.7812 | 7.6579 |
| | ∞ | 1.5472 | 2.0838 | 2.6049 | 3.1162 | 3.7816 | 5.4220 | 7.0359 |

Continued

**Table B7** Analysis of Variance F-Distribution (continued)

| $\nu_1$ | $\nu_2$ | $F_{.80}$ | $F_{.90}$ | $F_{.95}$ | $F_{.975}$ | $F_{.99}$ | $F_{.999}$ | $F_{.9999}$ |
|---|---|---|---|---|---|---|---|---|
| 4 | 2 | 4.2361 | 9.2434 | 19.247 | 39.248 | 99.251 | 999.31 | $1 \times 10^4$ |
| | 3 | 2.9555 | 5.3427 | 9.1172 | 15.101 | 28.710 | 137.08 | 640.75 |
| | 4 | 2.4826 | 4.1072 | 6.3882 | 9.6045 | 15.977 | 53.435 | 171.83 |
| | 5 | 2.2397 | 3.5202 | 5.1922 | 7.3879 | 11.392 | 31.083 | 80.559 |
| | 6 | 2.0924 | 3.1808 | 4.5337 | 6.2271 | 9.1484 | 21.922 | 49.418 |
| | 8 | 1.9230 | 2.8064 | 3.8379 | 5.0526 | 7.0061 | 14.392 | 27.474 |
| | 10 | 1.8286 | 2.6053 | 3.4780 | 4.4683 | 5.9944 | 11.283 | 19.631 |
| | 12 | 1.7684 | 2.4801 | 3.2592 | 4.1212 | 5.4119 | 9.6334 | 15.789 |
| | 15 | 1.7103 | 2.3614 | 3.0556 | 3.8043 | 4.8932 | 8.2528 | 12.777 |
| | 20 | 1.6543 | 2.2489 | 2.8661 | 3.5147 | 4.4307 | 7.0959 | 10.419 |
| | 24 | 1.6269 | 2.1949 | 2.7763 | 3.3794 | 4.2185 | 6.5893 | 9.4224 |
| | 30 | 1.6001 | 2.1422 | 2.6896 | 3.2499 | 4.0179 | 6.1245 | 8.5420 |
| | 40 | 1.5737 | 2.0909 | 2.6060 | 3.1261 | 3.8283 | 5.6980 | 7.7598 |
| | 60 | 1.5478 | 2.0410 | 2.5252 | 3.0077 | 3.6491 | 5.3069 | 7.0577 |
| | 120 | 1.5222 | 1.9923 | 2.4472 | 2.8943 | 3.4795 | 4.9472 | 6.4356 |
| | ∞ | 1.4972 | 1.9449 | 2.3719 | 2.7858 | 3.3192 | 4.6166 | 5.8790 |
| 5 | 2 | 4.2844 | 9.2926 | 19.296 | 39.298 | 99.302 | 999.31 | $1 \times 10^4$ |
| | 3 | 2.9652 | 5.3091 | 9.0134 | 14.885 | 28.237 | 134.58 | 627.71 |
| | 4 | 2.4780 | 4.0506 | 6.2561 | 9.3645 | 15.522 | 51.718 | 166.24 |
| | 5 | 2.2275 | 3.4530 | 5.0503 | 7.1464 | 10.967 | 29.751 | 76.834 |
| | 6 | 2.0755 | 3.1075 | 4.3874 | 5.9875 | 8.7459 | 20.802 | 46.741 |
| | 8 | 1.9005 | 2.7264 | 3.6875 | 4.8173 | 6.6318 | 13.484 | 25.640 |
| | 10 | 1.8027 | 2.5216 | 3.3258 | 4.2361 | 5.6364 | 10.481 | 18.132 |
| | 12 | 1.7403 | 2.3940 | 3.1059 | 3.8911 | 5.0644 | 8.8921 | 14.465 |
| | 15 | 1.6801 | 2.2730 | 2.9013 | 3.5764 | 4.5556 | 7.5670 | 11.627 |
| | 20 | 1.6218 | 2.1582 | 2.7109 | 3.2891 | 4.1027 | 6.4606 | 9.3860 |
| | 24 | 1.5933 | 2.1030 | 2.6207 | 3.1548 | 3.8951 | 5.9767 | 8.4547 |
| | 30 | 1.5654 | 2.0492 | 2.5336 | 3.0265 | 3.6990 | 5.5338 | 7.6325 |
| | 40 | 1.5379 | 1.9968 | 2.4495 | 2.9037 | 3.5138 | 5.1282 | 6.8976 |
| | 60 | 1.5108 | 1.9457 | 2.3683 | 2.7863 | 3.3389 | 4.7567 | 6.2464 |
| | 120 | 1.4841 | 1.8959 | 2.2899 | 2.6740 | 3.1735 | 4.4156 | 5.6662 |
| | ∞ | 1.4579 | 1.8473 | 2.2141 | 2.5665 | 3.0172 | 4.1030 | 5.1477 |

continued

**Table B7** Analysis of Variance F-Distribution (continued)

| $\nu_1$ | $\nu_2$ | $F_{.80}$ | $F_{.90}$ | $F_{.95}$ | $F_{.975}$ | $F_{.99}$ | $F_{.999}$ | $F_{.9999}$ |
|---|---|---|---|---|---|---|---|---|
| | 2 | 4.3168 | 9.3255 | 19.329 | 39.331 | 99.331 | 999.31 | $1 \times 10^4$ |
| | 3 | 2.9707 | 5.2847 | 8.9407 | 14.735 | 27.911 | 132.83 | 620.26 |
| | 4 | 2.4733 | 4.0097 | 6.1631 | 9.1973 | 15.207 | 50.524 | 162.05 |
| | 5 | 2.2174 | 3.4045 | 4.9503 | 6.9777 | 10.672 | 28.835 | 74.506 |
| | 6 | 2.0619 | 3.0546 | 4.2839 | 5.8197 | 8.4660 | 20.031 | 44.936 |
| | 8 | 1.8826 | 2.6683 | 3.5806 | 4.6517 | 6.3707 | 12.858 | 24.360 |
| 6 | 10 | 1.7823 | 2.4606 | 3.2172 | 4.0721 | 5.3858 | 9.9262 | 17.084 |
| | 12 | 1.7182 | 2.3310 | 2.9961 | 3.7283 | 4.8205 | 8.3783 | 13.562 |
| | 15 | 1.6561 | 2.2081 | 2.7905 | 3.4147 | 4.3183 | 7.0913 | 10.819 |
| | 20 | 1.5960 | 2.0913 | 2.5990 | 3.1283 | 3.8714 | 6.0186 | 8.6802 |
| | 24 | 1.5667 | 2.0351 | 2.5082 | 2.9946 | 3.6667 | 5.5506 | 7.7926 |
| | 30 | 1.5378 | 1.9803 | 2.4205 | 2.8667 | 3.4735 | 5.1223 | 6.9995 |
| | 40 | 1.5093 | 1.9269 | 2.3359 | 2.7444 | 3.2910 | 4.7307 | 6.3010 |
| | 60 | 1.4813 | 1.8747 | 2.2541 | 2.6274 | 3.1187 | 4.3719 | 5.6825 |
| | 120 | 1.4536 | 1.8238 | 2.1750 | 2.5154 | 2.9559 | 4.0436 | 5.1332 |
| | ∞ | 1.4263 | 1.7741 | 2.0986 | 2.4082 | 2.8020 | 3.7430 | 4.6421 |
| | 2 | 4.3401 | 9.3491 | 19.353 | 39.356 | 99.357 | 999.31 | $1 \times 10^4$ |
| | 3 | 2.9741 | 5.2662 | 8.8867 | 14.624 | 27.671 | 131.61 | 614.67 |
| | 4 | 2.4691 | 3.9790 | 6.0942 | 9.0741 | 14.976 | 49.651 | 159.26 |
| | 5 | 2.2090 | 3.3679 | 4.8759 | 6.8530 | 10.456 | 28.165 | 72.643 |
| | 6 | 2.0508 | 3.0145 | 4.2067 | 5.6955 | 8.2600 | 19.463 | 43.539 |
| | 8 | 1.8682 | 2.6241 | 3.5005 | 4.5285 | 6.1776 | 12.398 | 23.429 |
| 7 | 10 | 1.7658 | 2.4140 | 3.1355 | 3.9498 | 5.2001 | 9.5170 | 16.327 |
| | 12 | 1.7003 | 2.2828 | 2.9134 | 3.6065 | 4.6395 | 8.0008 | 12.893 |
| | 15 | 1.6368 | 2.1582 | 2.7066 | 3.2934 | 4.1416 | 6.7412 | 10.230 |
| | 20 | 1.5752 | 2.0397 | 2.5140 | 3.0074 | 3.6987 | 5.6921 | 8.1563 |
| | 24 | 1.5451 | 1.9826 | 2.4226 | 2.8738 | 3.4959 | 5.2351 | 7.2978 |
| | 30 | 1.5154 | 1.9269 | 2.3343 | 2.7460 | 3.3045 | 4.8171 | 6.5374 |
| | 40 | 1.4861 | 1.8725 | 2.2490 | 2.6238 | 3.1238 | 4.4356 | 5.8644 |
| | 60 | 1.4572 | 1.8194 | 2.1665 | 2.5068 | 2.9530 | 4.0864 | 5.2678 |
| | 120 | 1.4287 | 1.7675 | 2.0868 | 2.3948 | 2.7918 | 3.7669 | 4.7385 |
| | ∞ | 1.4005 | 1.7167 | 2.0096 | 2.2875 | 2.6393 | 3.4745 | 4.2673 |

continued

**Table B7** Analysis of Variance F-Distribution (continued)

| $\nu_1$ | $\nu_2$ | $F_{.80}$ | $F_{.90}$ | $F_{.95}$ | $F_{.975}$ | $F_{.99}$ | $F_{.999}$ | $F_{.9999}$ |
|---|---|---|---|---|---|---|---|---|
| | 5 | 2.2021 | 3.3393 | 4.8183 | 6.7572 | 10.289 | 27.649 | 71.246 |
| | 10 | 1.7523 | 2.3771 | 3.0717 | 3.8549 | 5.0567 | 9.2041 | 15.745 |
| | 15 | 1.6209 | 2.1185 | 2.6408 | 3.1987 | 4.0044 | 6.4706 | 9.7789 |
| | 20 | 1.5580 | 1.9985 | 2.4471 | 2.9128 | 3.5644 | 5.4401 | 7.7562 |
| 8 | 30 | 1.4968 | 1.8841 | 2.2662 | 2.6513 | 3.1726 | 4.5816 | 6.1809 |
| | 40 | 1.4668 | 1.8289 | 2.1802 | 2.5289 | 2.9930 | 4.2071 | 5.5261 |
| | 60 | 1.4371 | 1.7748 | 2.0970 | 2.4117 | 2.8233 | 3.8649 | 4.9477 |
| | 120 | 1.4078 | 1.7220 | 2.0164 | 2.2994 | 2.6629 | 3.5518 | 4.4329 |
| | ∞ | 1.3788 | 1.6702 | 1.9384 | 2.1918 | 2.5113 | 3.2655 | 3.9781 |
| | 5 | 2.1963 | 3.3163 | 4.7725 | 6.6810 | 10.158 | 27.241 | 70.082 |
| | 10 | 1.7411 | 2.3473 | 3.0204 | 3.7790 | 4.9424 | 8.9558 | 15.280 |
| | 15 | 1.6076 | 2.0862 | 2.5876 | 3.1227 | 3.8948 | 6.2560 | 9.4224 |
| | 20 | 1.5436 | 1.9649 | 2.3928 | 2.8365 | 3.4567 | 5.2391 | 7.4397 |
| 9 | 30 | 1.4812 | 1.8490 | 2.2107 | 2.5746 | 3.0665 | 4.3929 | 5.8972 |
| | 40 | 1.4505 | 1.7929 | 2.1240 | 2.4519 | 2.8876 | 4.0243 | 5.2569 |
| | 60 | 1.4201 | 1.7380 | 2.0401 | 2.3344 | 2.7185 | 3.6873 | 4.6912 |
| | 120 | 1.3901 | 1.6842 | 1.9588 | 2.2217 | 2.5586 | 3.3792 | 4.1910 |
| | ∞ | 1.3602 | 1.6315 | 1.8799 | 2.1136 | 2.4073 | 3.0975 | 3.7471 |
| | 5 | 2.1914 | 3.2974 | 4.7351 | 6.6192 | 10.051 | 26.914 | 69.267 |
| | 10 | 1.7316 | 2.3226 | 2.9782 | 3.7168 | 4.8491 | 8.7539 | 14.901 |
| | 15 | 1.5964 | 2.0593 | 2.5437 | 3.0602 | 3.8049 | 6.0809 | 9.1313 |
| | 20 | 1.5313 | 1.9367 | 2.3479 | 2.7737 | 3.3682 | 5.0754 | 7.1814 |
| 10 | 30 | 1.4678 | 1.8195 | 2.1646 | 2.5112 | 2.9791 | 4.2387 | 5.6643 |
| | 40 | 1.4365 | 1.7627 | 2.0773 | 2.3882 | 2.8005 | 3.8744 | 5.0350 |
| | 60 | 1.4055 | 1.7070 | 1.9926 | 2.2702 | 2.6318 | 3.5416 | 4.4820 |
| | 120 | 1.3748 | 1.6524 | 1.9105 | 2.1570 | 2.4721 | 3.2371 | 3.9909 |
| | ∞ | 1.3442 | 1.5987 | 1.8307 | 2.0483 | 2.3209 | 2.9588 | 3.5561 |

continued

**Table B7** Analysis of Variance F-Distribution (continued)

| $\nu_1$ | $\nu_2$ | $F_{.80}$ | $F_{.90}$ | $F_{.95}$ | $F_{.975}$ | $F_{.99}$ | $F_{.999}$ | $F_{.9999}$ |
|---|---|---|---|---|---|---|---|---|
| | 5 | 2.1835 | 3.2682 | 4.6777 | 6.5245 | 9.8883 | 26.419 | 67.987 |
| | 10 | 1.7164 | 2.2841 | 2.9130 | 3.6210 | 4.7058 | 8.4456 | 14.334 |
| | 15 | 1.5782 | 2.0171 | 2.4753 | 2.9633 | 3.6662 | 5.8121 | 8.6875 |
| | 20 | 1.5115 | 1.8924 | 2.2776 | 2.6758 | 3.2311 | 4.8231 | 6.7812 |
| 12 | 30 | 1.4461 | 1.7727 | 2.0921 | 2.4120 | 2.8431 | 4.0006 | 5.3078 |
| | 40 | 1.4137 | 1.7146 | 2.0035 | 2.2882 | 2.6648 | 3.6425 | 4.6966 |
| | 60 | 1.3816 | 1.6574 | 1.9174 | 2.1692 | 2.4961 | 3.3153 | 4.1582 |
| | 120 | 1.3496 | 1.6012 | 1.8337 | 2.0548 | 2.3363 | 3.0161 | 3.6816 |
| | ∞ | 1.3177 | 1.5458 | 1.7522 | 1.9447 | 2.1847 | 2.7425 | 3.2614 |
| | 5 | 2.1751 | 3.2380 | 4.6188 | 6.4277 | 9.7223 | 25.910 | 66.590 |
| | 10 | 1.7000 | 2.2435 | 2.8450 | 3.5217 | 4.5582 | 8.1291 | 13.752 |
| | 15 | 1.5584 | 1.9722 | 2.4034 | 2.8621 | 3.5222 | 5.5352 | 8.2291 |
| | 20 | 1.4897 | 1.8449 | 2.2033 | 2.5731 | 3.0880 | 4.5616 | 6.3737 |
| 15 | 30 | 1.4220 | 1.7223 | 2.0148 | 2.3072 | 2.7002 | 3.7528 | 4.9386 |
| | 40 | 1.3883 | 1.6624 | 1.9245 | 2.1819 | 2.5216 | 3.4004 | 4.3456 |
| | 60 | 1.3547 | 1.6034 | 1.8364 | 2.0613 | 2.3523 | 3.0782 | 3.8217 |
| | 120 | 1.3211 | 1.5450 | 1.7505 | 1.9450 | 2.1915 | 2.7833 | 3.3597 |
| | ∞ | 1.2874 | 1.4871 | 1.6664 | 1.8326 | 2.0385 | 2.5132 | 2.9504 |
| | 5 | 2.1660 | 3.2067 | 4.5581 | 6.3285 | 9.5527 | 25.393 | 65.193 |
| | 10 | 1.6823 | 2.2007 | 2.7740 | 3.4185 | 4.4054 | 7.8035 | 13.155 |
| | 15 | 1.5367 | 1.9243 | 2.3275 | 2.7559 | 3.3719 | 5.2487 | 7.7562 |
| | 20 | 1.4656 | 1.7938 | 2.1242 | 2.4645 | 2.9377 | 4.2901 | 5.9517 |
| 20 | 30 | 1.3949 | 1.6673 | 1.9317 | 2.1952 | 2.5487 | 3.4927 | 4.5547 |
| | 40 | 1.3596 | 1.6052 | 1.8389 | 2.0677 | 2.3689 | 3.1450 | 3.9763 |
| | 60 | 1.3241 | 1.5435 | 1.7480 | 1.9445 | 2.1978 | 2.8265 | 3.4688 |
| | 120 | 1.2882 | 1.4821 | 1.6587 | 1.8249 | 2.0346 | 2.5344 | 3.0177 |
| | ∞ | 1.2519 | 1.4206 | 1.5705 | 1.7085 | 1.8783 | 2.2658 | 2.6193 |

This table was created using Microsoft® Excel 2002, function command FINV(alpha,df1,df2).

**Table B8** Upper Percentage Points of the $F_{max}$ Statistic

| | | K = number of variances | | | | | | | | | | |
|---|---|---|---|---|---|---|---|---|---|---|---|---|
| n-1 | α | 2 | 3 | 4 | 5 | 6 | 7 | 8 | 9 | 10 | 11 | 12 |
| 4 | .05 | 9.60 | 15.5 | 20.6 | 25.2 | 29.5 | 33.6 | 37.5 | 41.4 | 44.6 | 48.0 | 51.4 |
| | .01 | 23.2 | 37 | 49 | 59 | 69 | 79 | 89 | 97 | 106 | 113 | 120 |
| 5 | .05 | 7.15 | 10.8 | 13.7 | 16.3 | 18.7 | 20.8 | 22.9 | 24.7 | 26.5 | 28.2 | 29.9 |
| | .01 | 14.9 | 22 | 28 | 33 | 38 | 42 | 46 | 50 | 54 | 57 | 60 |
| 6 | .05 | 5.82 | 8.38 | 10.4 | 12.1 | 13.7 | 15.0 | 16.3 | 17.5 | 18.6 | 19.7 | 20.7 |
| | .01 | 11.1 | 15.5 | 19.1 | 22 | 25 | 27 | 30 | 32 | 34 | 36 | 37 |
| 7 | .05 | 4.99 | 6.94 | 8.44 | 9.70 | 10.8 | 11.8 | 12.7 | 13.5 | 14.3 | 15.1 | 15.8 |
| | .01 | 8.89 | 12.1 | 14.5 | 16.5 | 18.4 | 20 | 22 | 23 | 24 | 26 | 27 |
| 8 | .05 | 4.43 | 6.00 | 7.18 | 8.12 | 9.03 | 9.78 | 10.5 | 11.1 | 11.7 | 12.2 | 12.7 |
| | .01 | 7.50 | 9.9 | 11.7 | 13.2 | 14.5 | 15.8 | 16.9 | 17.9 | 18.9 | 19.8 | 21 |
| 9 | .05 | 4.03 | 5.34 | 6.31 | 7.11 | 7.80 | 8.41 | 8.95 | 9.45 | 9.91 | 10.3 | 10.7 |
| | .01 | 6.54 | 8.5 | 9.9 | 11.1 | 12.1 | 13.1 | 13.9 | 14.7 | 15.3 | 16.0 | 16.6 |
| 10 | .05 | 3.72 | 4.85 | 5.67 | 6.34 | 6.92 | 7.42 | 7.87 | 8.28 | 8.66 | 9.01 | 9.34 |
| | .01 | 5.85 | 7.4 | 8.6 | 9.6 | 10.4 | 11.1 | 11.8 | 12.4 | 12.9 | 13.4 | 13.9 |
| 12 | .05 | 3.28 | 4.16 | 4.79 | 5.30 | 5.72 | 6.09 | 6.42 | 6.72 | 7.00 | 7.25 | 7.48 |
| | .01 | 4.91 | 6.1 | 6.9 | 7.6 | 8.2 | 8.7 | 9.1 | 9.5 | 9.9 | 10.2 | 10.6 |
| 15 | .05 | 2.86 | 3.54 | 4.01 | 4.37 | 4.68 | 4.95 | 5.19 | 5.40 | 5.59 | 5.77 | 5.93 |
| | .05 | 4.07 | 4.9 | 5.5 | 6.0 | 6.4 | 6.7 | 7.1 | 7.3 | 7.5 | 7.8 | 8.0 |
| 20 | .05 | 2.46 | 2.95 | 3.29 | 3.54 | 3.76 | 3.94 | 4.10 | 4.24 | 4.37 | 4.49 | 4.59 |
| | .01 | 3.32 | 3.8 | 4.3 | 4.6 | 4.9 | 5.1 | 5.3 | 5.5 | 5.6 | 5.8 | 5.9 |
| 30 | .05 | 2.07 | 2.40 | 2.61 | 2.78 | 2.91 | 3.02 | 3.12 | 3.21 | 3.29 | 3.36 | 3.39 |
| | .01 | 2.63 | 3.0 | 3.3 | 3.4 | 3.6 | 3.7 | 3.8 | 3.9 | 4.0 | 4.1 | 4.2 |
| 60 | .05 | 1.67 | 1.85 | 1.96 | 2.04 | 2.11 | 2.17 | 2.22 | 2.26 | 2.30 | 2.33 | 2.36 |
| | .01 | 1.96 | 2.2 | 2.3 | 2.4 | 2.4 | 2.5 | 2.5 | 2.6 | 2.6 | 2.7 | 2.7 |
| ∞ | .05 | 1.00 | 1.00 | 1.00 | 1.00 | 1.00 | 1.00 | 1.00 | 1.00 | 1.00 | 1.00 | 1.00 |
| | .01 | 1.00 | 1.00 | 1.00 | 1.00 | 1.00 | 1.00 | 1.00 | 1.00 | 1.00 | 1.00 | 1.00 |

Modified from: Pearson, E.S. and Hartley, H.O. (1970). *Biometrika Tables for Statisticians*, Vol 1 (Table 31), Biometrika Trustees at the University Press, Cambridge, London. Reproduced with permission of the Biometrika Trustees.

**Table B9** Upper Percentage Points of the Cochran C Test for Homogeneity of Variance

| | | k = levels of independent variable | | | | | | | | |
|---|---|---|---|---|---|---|---|---|---|---|
| n-1 | α | 2 | 3 | 4 | 5 | 6 | 7 | 8 | 9 | 10 |
| 1 | .05 | .999 | .967 | .907 | .841 | .781 | .727 | .680 | .639 | .602 |
| | .01 | .999 | .993 | .968 | .928 | .883 | .838 | .795 | .754 | .718 |
| 2 | .05 | .975 | .871 | .768 | .684 | .616 | .561 | .516 | .478 | .445 |
| | .01 | .995 | .942 | .864 | .789 | .722 | .664 | .615 | .573 | .536 |
| 3 | .05 | .939 | .798 | .684 | .598 | .532 | .480 | .438 | .403 | .373 |
| | .01 | .979 | .883 | .781 | .696 | .626 | .569 | .521 | .481 | .447 |
| 4 | .05 | .906 | .746 | .629 | .544 | .480 | .431 | .391 | .358 | .331 |
| | .01 | .959 | .834 | .721 | .633 | .564 | .508 | .463 | .425 | .393 |
| 5 | .05 | .877 | .707 | .590 | .507 | .445 | .397 | .360 | .329 | .303 |
| | .01 | .937 | .793 | .676 | .588 | .520 | .466 | .423 | .387 | .357 |
| 6 | .05 | .853 | .677 | .560 | .478 | .418 | .373 | .336 | .307 | .282 |
| | .01 | .917 | .761 | .641 | .553 | .487 | .435 | .393 | .359 | .331 |
| 7 | .05 | .833 | .653 | .537 | .456 | .398 | .354 | .319 | .290 | .267 |
| | .01 | .899 | .734 | .613 | .526 | .461 | .411 | .370 | .338 | .311 |
| 8 | .05 | .816 | .633 | .518 | .439 | .382 | .338 | .304 | .277 | .254 |
| | .01 | .882 | .711 | .590 | .504 | .440 | .391 | .352 | .321 | .295 |
| 9 | .05 | .801 | .617 | .502 | .424 | .368 | .326 | .293 | .266 | .244 |
| | .05 | .867 | .691 | .570 | .485 | .423 | .375 | .337 | .307 | .281 |
| 16 | .05 | .734 | .547 | .437 | .364 | .314 | .276 | .246 | .223 | .203 |
| | .01 | .795 | .606 | .488 | .409 | .353 | .311 | .278 | .251 | .230 |
| 36 | .05 | .660 | .475 | .372 | .307 | .261 | .228 | .202 | .182 | .166 |
| | .01 | .707 | .515 | .406 | .335 | .286 | .249 | .221 | .199 | .181 |
| 144 | .05 | .581 | .403 | .309 | .251 | .212 | .183 | .162 | .145 | .131 |
| | .01 | .606 | .423 | .325 | .264 | .223 | .193 | .170 | .152 | .138 |

Modified from: Eisenhart, C., Hastay, M.W., and Wallis W.A., eds. (1947). *Techniques of Statistical Analysis* (Tables 15.1 and 15.2), McGraw-Hill Book Company, New York. Reproduced with permission of the publisher.

**Table B10** Percentage Point of the Studentized Range (q)

| df | α | k (or p) | | | | | | | | |
|---|---|---|---|---|---|---|---|---|---|---|
| | | 2 | 3 | 4 | 5 | 6 | 7 | 8 | 9 | 10 |
| 10 | .05 | 3.15 | 3.88 | 4.33 | 4.65 | 4.91 | 5.12 | 5.30 | 5.46 | 5.60 |
| | .01 | 4.48 | 5.27 | 5.77 | 6.14 | 6.43 | 6.67 | 6.87 | 7.05 | 7.21 |
| 12 | .05 | 3.08 | 3.77 | 4.20 | 4.51 | 4.75 | 4.95 | 5.12 | 5.27 | 5.39 |
| | .01 | 4.32 | 5.05 | 5.50 | 5.84 | 6.10 | 6.32 | 6.51 | 6.67 | 6.81 |
| 14 | .05 | 3.03 | 3.70 | 4.11 | 4.41 | 4.64 | 4.83 | 4.99 | 5.13 | 5.25 |
| | .01 | 4.21 | 4.89 | 5.32 | 5.63 | 5.88 | 6.08 | 6.26 | 6.41 | 6.54 |
| 16 | .05 | 3.00 | 3.65 | 4.05 | 4.33 | 4.56 | 4.74 | 4.90 | 5.03 | 5.15 |
| | .01 | 4.13 | 4.79 | 5.19 | 5.49 | 5.72 | 5.92 | 6.08 | 6.22 | 6.35 |
| 18 | .05 | 2.97 | 3.61 | 4.00 | 4.28 | 4.49 | 4.67 | 4.82 | 4.96 | 5.07 |
| | .01 | 4.07 | 4.70 | 5.09 | 5.38 | 5.60 | 5.79 | 5.94 | 6.08 | 6.20 |
| 20 | .05 | 2.95 | 3.58 | 3.96 | 4.23 | 4.45 | 4.62 | 4.77 | 4.90 | 5.01 |
| | .01 | 4.02 | 4.64 | 5.02 | 5.29 | 5.51 | 5.69 | 5.84 | 5.97 | 6.09 |
| 24 | .05 | 2.92 | 3.53 | 3.90 | 4.17 | 4.37 | 4.54 | 4.68 | 4.81 | 4.92 |
| | .01 | 3.96 | 4.55 | 4.91 | 5.17 | 5.37 | 5.54 | 5.69 | 5.81 | 5.92 |
| 30 | .05 | 2.89 | 3.49 | 3.85 | 4.10 | 4.30 | 4.46 | 4.60 | 4.72 | 4.82 |
| | .01 | 3.89 | 4.45 | 4.80 | 5.05 | 5.24 | 5.40 | 5.54 | 5.65 | 5.76 |
| 40 | .05 | 2.86 | 3.44 | 3.79 | 4.04 | 4.23 | 4.39 | 4.52 | 4.63 | 4.73 |
| | .01 | 3.82 | 4.37 | 4.70 | 4.93 | 5.11 | 5.26 | 5.39 | 5.50 | 5.60 |
| 60 | .05 | 2.83 | 3.40 | 3.74 | 3.98 | 4.16 | 4.31 | 4.44 | 4.55 | 4.65 |
| | .01 | 3.76 | 4.28 | 4.59 | 4.82 | 4.99 | 5.13 | 5.25 | 5.36 | 5.45 |
| 120 | .05 | 2.80 | 3.36 | 3.68 | 3.92 | 4.10 | 4.24 | 4.36 | 4.47 | 4.56 |
| | .01 | 3.70 | 4.20 | 4.50 | 4.71 | 4.87 | 5.01 | 5.12 | 5.21 | 5.30 |
| ∞ | .05 | 2.77 | 3.31 | 3.63 | 3.86 | 4.03 | 4.17 | 4.29 | 4.39 | 4.47 |
| | .01 | 3.64 | 4.12 | 4.40 | 4.60 | 4.76 | 4.88 | 4.99 | 5.08 | 5.16 |

Modified from: Pearson, E.S. and Hartley, H.O. (1970). *Biometrika Tables for Statisticians*, Vol 1 (Table 29), Biometrika Trustees at the University Press, Cambridge, London. Reproduced with permission of the Biometrika Trustees.

**Table B11** Percentage Points of the Dunn Multiple Comparisons

| Number of Comparisons (C) | α | (N - K) degrees of freedom | | | | | | | | |
|---|---|---|---|---|---|---|---|---|---|---|
| | | 10 | 15 | 20 | 24 | 30 | 40 | 60 | 120 | ∞ |
| 2 | .05 | 2.64 | 2.49 | 2.42 | 2.39 | 2.36 | 3.33 | 2.30 | 2.27 | 2.24 |
| | .01 | 3.58 | 3.29 | 3.16 | 3.09 | 3.03 | 2.97 | 2.92 | 2.86 | 2.81 |
| 3 | .05 | 2.87 | 2.69 | 2.61 | 2.58 | 2.54 | 2.50 | 2.47 | 2.43 | 2.39 |
| | .01 | 3.83 | 3.48 | 3.33 | 3.26 | 3.19 | 3.12 | 3.06 | 2.99 | 2.94 |
| 4 | .05 | 3.04 | 2.84 | 2.75 | 2.70 | 2.66 | 2.62 | 2.58 | 2.54 | 2.50 |
| | .01 | 4.01 | 3.62 | 3.46 | 3.38 | 3.30 | 3.23 | 3.16 | 3.09 | 3.02 |
| 5 | .05 | 3.17 | 2.95 | 2.85 | 2.80 | 2.75 | 2.71 | 2.66 | 2.62 | 2.58 |
| | .01 | 4.15 | 3.74 | 3.55 | 3.47 | 3.39 | 3.31 | 3.24 | 3.16 | 3.09 |
| 6 | .05 | 3.28 | 3.04 | 2.93 | 2.88 | 2.83 | 2.78 | 2.73 | 2.68 | 2.64 |
| | .01 | 4.27 | 3.82 | 3.63 | 3.54 | 3.46 | 3.38 | 3.30 | 3.22 | 3.15 |
| 7 | .05 | 3.37 | 3.11 | 3.00 | 2.94 | 2.89 | 2.84 | 2.79 | 2.74 | 2.69 |
| | .01 | 4.37 | 3.90 | 3.70 | 3.61 | 3.52 | 3.43 | 3.34 | 3.27 | 3.19 |
| 8 | .05 | 3.45 | 3.18 | 3.06 | 3.00 | 2.94 | 2.89 | 2.84 | 2.79 | 2.74 |
| | .01 | 4.45 | 3.97 | 3.76 | 3.66 | 3.57 | 3.48 | 3.39 | 3.31 | 3.23 |
| 9 | .05 | 3.52 | 3.24 | 3.11 | 3.05 | 2.99 | 2.93 | 2.88 | 2.83 | 2.77 |
| | .01 | 4.53 | 4.02 | 3.80 | 3.70 | 3.61 | 3.51 | 3.42 | 3.34 | 3.26 |
| 10 | .05 | 3.58 | 3.29 | 3.16 | 3.09 | 3.03 | 2.97 | 2.92 | 2.86 | 2.81 |
| | .01 | 4.59 | 4.07 | 3.85 | 3.74 | 3.65 | 3.55 | 3.46 | 3.37 | 3.29 |
| 15 | .05 | 3.83 | 3.48 | 3.33 | 3.26 | 3.19 | 3.12 | 3.06 | 2.99 | 2.94 |
| | .01 | 4.86 | 4.29 | 4.03 | 3.91 | 3.80 | 3.70 | 3.59 | 3.50 | 3.40 |
| 20 | .05 | 4.01 | 3.62 | 3.46 | 3.38 | 3.30 | 3.23 | 3.16 | 3.09 | 3.02 |
| | .01 | 5.06 | 4.42 | 4.15 | 4.04 | 3.90 | 3.79 | 3.69 | 3.58 | 3.48 |
| 30 | .05 | 4.27 | 3.82 | 3.63 | 3.54 | 3.46 | 3.38 | 3.30 | 3.22 | 3.15 |
| | .01 | 5.33 | 4.61 | 4.33 | 4.2 | 4.13 | 3.93 | 3.81 | 3.69 | 3.59 |

Modified from: Dunn, O.J. (1961). "Multiple Comparisons Among Means," *Journal of the American Statistical Association*, 56:62-64. Reproduced with permission of the American Statistical Association.

**Table B12** Critical Values of q for the Two-Tailed Dunnett's Test

| N-k df | α | number of means with the range from the control inclusive ($p$) | | | | | | | | |
|---|---|---|---|---|---|---|---|---|---|---|
| | | 2 | 3 | 4 | 5 | 6 | 7 | 8 | 9 | 10 |
| 10 | .05 | 2.23 | 2.57 | 2.81 | 2.97 | 3.11 | 3.21 | 3.31 | 3.39 | 3.46 |
| | .01 | 3.17 | 3.53 | 3.78 | 3.95 | 4.01 | 4.21 | 4.31 | 4.40 | 4.47 |
| 12 | .05 | 2.18 | 2.50 | 2.72 | 2.88 | 3.00 | 3.10 | 3.18 | 3.25 | 3.32 |
| | .01 | 3.05 | 3.39 | 3.61 | 3.76 | 3.89 | 3.99 | 4.08 | 4.15 | 4.22 |
| 14 | .05 | 2.14 | 2.46 | 2.67 | 2.81 | 2.93 | 3.02 | 3.10 | 3.17 | 3.23 |
| | .01 | 2.98 | 3.29 | 3.49 | 3.64 | 3.75 | 3.84 | 3.92 | 3.99 | 4.05 |
| 16 | .05 | 2.12 | 2.42 | 2.63 | 2.77 | 2.88 | 2.96 | 3.04 | 3.10 | 3.16 |
| | .01 | 2.92 | 3.22 | 3.41 | 3.55 | 3.65 | 3.74 | 3.82 | 3.88 | 3.93 |
| 18 | .05 | 2.10 | 2.40 | 2.59 | 2.73 | 2.84 | 2.92 | 2.99 | 3.05 | 3.11 |
| | .01 | 2.88 | 3.17 | 3.35 | 3.48 | 3.58 | 3.67 | 3.74 | 3.80 | 3.85 |
| 20 | .05 | 2.09 | 2.38 | 2.57 | 2.70 | 2.81 | 2.89 | 2.96 | 3.02 | 3.07 |
| | .01 | 2.85 | 3.13 | 3.31 | 3.43 | 3.53 | 3.61 | 3.67 | 3.73 | 3.78 |
| 24 | .05 | 2.06 | 2.35 | 2.53 | 2.66 | 2.76 | 2.84 | 2.91 | 2.96 | 3.01 |
| | .01 | 2.80 | 3.07 | 3.24 | 3.36 | 3.45 | 3.52 | 3.58 | 3.64 | 3.69 |
| 30 | .05 | 2.04 | 2.32 | 2.50 | 2.62 | 2.72 | 2.79 | 2.86 | 2.91 | 2.96 |
| | .01 | 2.75 | 3.01 | 3.17 | 3.28 | 3.37 | 3.44 | 3.50 | 3.55 | 3.59 |
| 40 | .05 | 2.02 | 2.29 | 2.47 | 2.58 | 2.67 | 2.75 | 2.81 | 2.86 | 2.90 |
| | .01 | 2.70 | 2.95 | 3.10 | 3.21 | 3.29 | 3.36 | 3.41 | 3.46 | 3.50 |
| 60 | .05 | 2.00 | 2.27 | 2.43 | 2.55 | 2.63 | 2.70 | 2.76 | 2.81 | 2.85 |
| | .01 | 2.66 | 2.90 | 3.04 | 3.14 | 3.22 | 3.28 | 3.33 | 3.38 | 3.42 |
| 120 | .05 | 1.98 | 2.24 | 2.40 | 2.51 | 2.59 | 2.66 | 2.71 | 2.76 | 2.80 |
| | .01 | 2.62 | 2.84 | 2.98 | 3.08 | 3.15 | 3.21 | 3.25 | 3.30 | 3.33 |
| ∞ | .05 | 1.96 | 2.21 | 2.37 | 2.47 | 2.55 | 2.62 | 2.67 | 2.71 | 2.75 |
| | .01 | 2.58 | 2.79 | 2.92 | 3.01 | 3.08 | 3.14 | 3.18 | 3.22 | 3.25 |

Modified from: Dunnett, C.W. (1955) "A multiple comparison procedure for comparing several treatments with a control," *Journal of the American Statistical Association*, 50:1119-1120. Reprinted with permission from *The Journal of the American Statistical Association*. 

**Table B13** Critical Values of q for the One-Tailed Dunnett's Test

| N-k | | number of means with the range from the control inclusive (p) | | | | | | | | |
|---|---|---|---|---|---|---|---|---|---|---|
| df | α | 2 | 3 | 4 | 5 | 6 | 7 | 8 | 9 | 10 |
| 10 | .05 | 1.81 | 2.15 | 2.34 | 2.47 | 2.56 | 2.64 | 2.70 | 2.76 | 2.81 |
| | .01 | 2.76 | 3.11 | 3.31 | 3.45 | 3.56 | 3.64 | 3.71 | 3.78 | 3.83 |
| 12 | .05 | 1.78 | 2.11 | 2.29 | 2.41 | 2.50 | 2.58 | 2.64 | 2.69 | 2.74 |
| | .01 | 2.68 | 3.01 | 3.19 | 3.32 | 3.42 | 3.50 | 3.56 | 3.62 | 3.67 |
| 14 | .05 | 1.76 | 2.08 | 2.25 | 2.37 | 2.46 | 2.53 | 2.59 | 2.64 | 2.69 |
| | .01 | 2.62 | 2.94 | 3.11 | 3.23 | 3.32 | 3.40 | 3.46 | 3.51 | 3.56 |
| 16 | .05 | 1.75 | 2.06 | 2.23 | 2.34 | 2.43 | 2.50 | 2.56 | 2.61 | 2.65 |
| | .01 | 2.58 | 2.88 | 3.05 | 3.17 | 3.26 | 3.33 | 3.39 | 3.44 | 3.48 |
| 18 | .05 | 1.73 | 2.04 | 2.21 | 2.32 | 2.41 | 2.48 | 2.53 | 2.58 | 2.62 |
| | .01 | 2.55 | 2.84 | 3.01 | 3.12 | 3.21 | 3.27 | 3.33 | 3.38 | 3.42 |
| 20 | .05 | 1.72 | 2.03 | 2.19 | 2.30 | 2.39 | 2.46 | 2.51 | 2.56 | 2.60 |
| | .01 | 2.53 | 2.81 | 2.97 | 3.08 | 3.17 | 3.23 | 3.29 | 3.34 | 3.38 |
| 24 | .05 | 1.71 | 2.01 | 2.17 | 2.28 | 2.36 | 2.43 | 2.48 | 2.53 | 2.57 |
| | .01 | 2.49 | 2.77 | 2.92 | 3.03 | 3.11 | 3.17 | 3.22 | 3.27 | 3.31 |
| 30 | .05 | 1.70 | 1.99 | 2.15 | 2.25 | 2.33 | 2.40 | 2.45 | 2.50 | 2.54 |
| | .01 | 2.46 | 2.72 | 2.87 | 2.97 | 3.05 | 3.11 | 3.16 | 3.21 | 3.24 |
| 40 | .05 | 1.68 | 1.97 | 2.13 | 2.23 | 2.31 | 2.37 | 2.42 | 2.47 | 2.51 |
| | .01 | 2.42 | 2.68 | 2.82 | 2.92 | 2.99 | 3.05 | 3.10 | 3.14 | 3.18 |
| 60 | .05 | 1.67 | 1.95 | 2.10 | 2.21 | 2.28 | 2.35 | 2.39 | 2.44 | 2.48 |
| | .01 | 2.39 | 2.64 | 2.78 | 2.87 | 2.94 | 3.00 | 3.04 | 3.08 | 3.12 |
| 120 | .05 | 1.66 | 1.93 | 2.08 | 2.18 | 2.26 | 2.32 | 2.37 | 2.41 | 2.45 |
| | .01 | 2.36 | 2.60 | 2.73 | 2.82 | 2.89 | 2.94 | 2.99 | 3.03 | 3.06 |
| ∞ | .05 | 1.64 | 1.92 | 2.06 | 2.16 | 2.23 | 2.29 | 2.34 | 2.38 | 2.42 |
| | .01 | 2.33 | 2.56 | 2.68 | 2.77 | 2.84 | 2.89 | 2.93 | 2.97 | 3.00 |

Modified from: Dunnett, C.W. (1955) "A multiple comparison procedure for comparing several treatments with a control," *Journal of the American Statistical Association*, 50:1117-1118. Reprinted with permission from *The Journal of the American Statistical Association*. 

**Table B14** Values of $r$ at Different Levels of Significance

| d.f. | .01 | .05 | .01 | .001 |
|---|---|---|---|---|
| 1 | .988 | .997 | .999 | 1.00 |
| 2 | .900 | .950 | .990 | .999 |
| 3 | .805 | .878 | .959 | .991 |
| 4 | .730 | .811 | .917 | .974 |
| 5 | .669 | .755 | .875 | .951 |
| 6 | .622 | .707 | .834 | .925 |
| 7 | .582 | .666 | .798 | .898 |
| 8 | .549 | .632 | .765 | .872 |
| 9 | .521 | .602 | .735 | .847 |
| 10 | .497 | .576 | .708 | .823 |
| 11 | .476 | .553 | .684 | .801 |
| 12 | .458 | .532 | .661 | .780 |
| 13 | .441 | .514 | .641 | .760 |
| 14 | .426 | .497 | .623 | .742 |
| 15 | .412 | .482 | .606 | .725 |
| 16 | .400 | .468 | .590 | .708 |
| 17 | .389 | .456 | .575 | .693 |
| 18 | .378 | .444 | .561 | .679 |
| 19 | .369 | .433 | .549 | .665 |
| 20 | .360 | .423 | .537 | .652 |
| 25 | .323 | .381 | .487 | .597 |
| 30 | .296 | .349 | .449 | .554 |
| 35 | .275 | .325 | .418 | .519 |
| 40 | .257 | .304 | .393 | .490 |
| 50 | .231 | .273 | .354 | .443 |
| 60 | .211 | .250 | .325 | .408 |
| 80 | .183 | .217 | .283 | .357 |
| 100 | .164 | .195 | .254 | .321 |
| 150 | .134 | .159 | .208 | .264 |
| 200 | .116 | .138 | .181 | .230 |

Modified from: Pearson, E.S. and Hartley, H.O. (1970). *Biometrika Tables for Statisticians*, Vol 1 (Table 13), Biometrika Trustees at the University Press, Cambridge, London. Reproduced with permission of the Biometrika Trustees.

**Table B15** Chi Square Distribution

| d.f. | α=.10 | .05 | .025 | .01 | .005 | .001 | .0001 |
|---|---|---|---|---|---|---|---|
| 1 | 2.7055 | 3.8415 | 5.0239 | 6.6349 | 7.8794 | 10.827 | 15.134 |
| 2 | 4.6052 | 5.9915 | 7.3778 | 9.2104 | 10.597 | 13.815 | 18.425 |
| 3 | 6.2514 | 7.8147 | 9.3484 | 11.345 | 12.838 | 16.266 | 21.104 |
| 4 | 7.7794 | 9.4877 | 11.143 | 13.277 | 14.860 | 18.466 | 23.506 |
| 5 | 9.2363 | 11.070 | 12.832 | 15.086 | 16.750 | 20.515 | 25.751 |
| 6 | 10.645 | 12.592 | 14.449 | 16.812 | 18.548 | 22.457 | 27.853 |
| 7 | 12.017 | 14.067 | 16.013 | 18.475 | 20.278 | 24.321 | 29.881 |
| 8 | 13.362 | 15.507 | 17.535 | 20.090 | 21.955 | 26.124 | 31.827 |
| 9 | 14.684 | 16.919 | 19.023 | 21.666 | 23.589 | 27.877 | 33.725 |
| 10 | 15.987 | 18.307 | 20.483 | 23.209 | 25.188 | 29.588 | 35.557 |
| 11 | 17.275 | 19.675 | 21.920 | 24.725 | 26.757 | 31.264 | 37.365 |
| 12 | 18.549 | 21.026 | 23.337 | 26.217 | 28.300 | 32.909 | 39.131 |
| 13 | 19.812 | 22.362 | 24.736 | 27.688 | 29.819 | 34.527 | 40.873 |
| 14 | 21.064 | 23.685 | 26.119 | 29.141 | 31.319 | 36.124 | 42.575 |
| 15 | 22.307 | 24.996 | 27.488 | 30.578 | 32.801 | 37.698 | 44.260 |
| 16 | 23.542 | 26.296 | 28.845 | 32.000 | 34.267 | 39.252 | 45.926 |
| 17 | 24.769 | 27.587 | 30.191 | 33.409 | 35.718 | 40.791 | 47.559 |
| 18 | 25.989 | 28.869 | 31.526 | 34.805 | 37.156 | 42.312 | 49.185 |
| 19 | 27.204 | 30.144 | 32.852 | 36.191 | 38.582 | 43.819 | 50.787 |
| 20 | 28.412 | 31.410 | 34.170 | 37.566 | 39.997 | 45.314 | 52.383 |
| 21 | 29.615 | 32.671 | 35.479 | 38.932 | 41.401 | 46.796 | 53.960 |
| 22 | 30.813 | 33.924 | 36.781 | 40.289 | 42.796 | 48.268 | 55.524 |
| 23 | 32.007 | 35.172 | 38.076 | 41.638 | 44.181 | 49.728 | 57.067 |
| 24 | 33.196 | 36.415 | 39.364 | 42.980 | 45.558 | 51.179 | 58.607 |
| 25 | 34.382 | 37.652 | 40.646 | 44.314 | 46.928 | 52.619 | 60.136 |

This table was created using Microsoft® Excel 2002, function command CHIINV(alpha,df).

**Table B16.** Critical Values for Kolmogorov Goodness-of-Fit Test ($\alpha = 0.05$)

| n | One-Tailed Test | Two-Tailed Test |
|---|---|---|
| 1 | 0.950 | 0.975 |
| 2 | 0.776 | 0.842 |
| 3 | 0.636 | 0.708 |
| 4 | 0.565 | 0.624 |
| 5 | 0.509 | 0.563 |
| 6 | 0.468 | 0.519 |
| 7 | 0.436 | 0.483 |
| 8 | 0.410 | 0.454 |
| 9 | 0.387 | 0.430 |
| 10 | 0.369 | 0.409 |
| 11 | 0.352 | 0.391 |
| 12 | 0.338 | 0.375 |
| 13 | 0.325 | 0.361 |
| 14 | 0.314 | 0.349 |
| 15 | 0.304 | 0.338 |
| 16 | 0.295 | 0.327 |
| 17 | 0.286 | 0.318 |
| 18 | 0.279 | 0.309 |
| 19 | 0.271 | 0.301 |
| 20 | 0.265 | 0.294 |
| 25 | 0.238 | 0.264 |
| 30 | 0.218 | 0.242 |
| 35 | 0.202 | 0.224 |
| 40 | 0.189 | 0.210 |
| Approximation for >40 | $1.22/\sqrt{n}$ | $1.36/\sqrt{n}$ |

From: Miller L.H. (1956). "Table of Percentage Points of Kolmogorov Statistics" *Journal of the American Statistical Association* 51:111-121. Reprinted with permission from *The Journal of the American Statistical Association*. 

**Table B17.** Critical Values for Smirnov Test Statistic ($\alpha = 0.05$)

| n | One-Tailed Test | Two-Tailed Test |
|---|---|---|
| 3 | 2/3 | ... |
| 4 | 3/4 | 3/4 |
| 5 | 3/5 | 4/5 |
| 6 | 4/6 | 4/6 |
| 7 | 4/7 | 5/7 |
| 8 | 4/8 | 5/8 |
| 9 | 5/9 | 5/9 |
| 10 | 5/10 | 6/10 |
| 11 | 5/11 | 6/11 |
| 12 | 5/12 | 6/12 |
| 13 | 6/13 | 6/13 |
| 14 | 6/14 | 7/14 |
| 15 | 6/15 | 7/15 |
| 16 | 6/16 | 7/16 |
| 17 | 7/17 | 7/17 |
| 18 | 7/18 | 8/18 |
| 19 | 7/19 | 8/19 |
| 20 | 7/20 | 8/20 |
| 25 | 8/25 | 9/25 |
| 30 | 9/30 | 10/30 |
| 35 | 10/35 | 11/35 |
| 40 | 10/40 | 12/40 |
| Approximation for >40 | $1.73/\sqrt{n}$ | $1.92/\sqrt{n}$ |

Modified from: Birnbaum, Z.W. and Hall, R.A. (1960). "Small-Sample Distribution for Multiple Sample Statistics of the Smirnov Type," *Annals of Mathematical Statistics* 31:710-720. Permission to reprint was granted by the Institute of Mathematical Statistics.

**Table B18.** Critical Values for the Runs Test ($\alpha = 0.05$)

Reject $H_0$ if $r$ is < Lower or > Upper Limits

| $n_1$ | $n_2$ | Lower | Upper | $n_1$ | $n_2$ | Lower | Upper |
|---|---|---|---|---|---|---|---|
| 6 | 6 | 4 | 10 | 11 | 16 | 9 | 19 |
| | 7-8 | 4 | 11 | | 17-18 | 10 | 19 |
| | 9-12 | 5 | 12 | | 19-20 | 10 | 20 |
| | 13-18 | 6 | 13 | 12 | 12 | 8 | 18 |
| | 19-20 | 7 | 13 | | 13 | 9 | 18 |
| 7 | 7 | 4 | 12 | | 14 | 9 | 19 |
| | 8 | 5 | 12 | | 15 | 9 | 20 |
| | 9 | 5 | 13 | | 16-18 | 10 | 20 |
| | 10-12 | 6 | 13 | | 19-20 | 11 | 21 |
| | 13-14 | 6 | 14 | 13 | 13 | 9 | 19 |
| | 15 | 7 | 14 | | 14 | 10 | 19 |
| | 16-20 | 7 | 15 | | 15-16 | 10 | 20 |
| 8 | 8 | 5 | 13 | | 17-18 | 11 | 21 |
| | 9 | 6 | 13 | | 19-20 | 11 | 22 |
| | 10-11 | 6 | 14 | 14 | 14 | 10 | 20 |
| | 12-15 | 7 | 15 | | 15-16 | 10 | 21 |
| | 16 | 7 | 16 | | 17-18 | 11 | 22 |
| | 17-20 | 8 | 16 | | 19 | 12 | 22 |
| 9 | 9 | 6 | 14 | | 20 | 12 | 23 |
| | 10 | 6 | 15 | 15 | 15 | 11 | 21 |
| | 11-12 | 7 | 15 | | 16 | 11 | 22 |
| | 13 | 7 | 16 | | 17 | 12 | 22 |
| | 14 | 8 | 16 | | 18-19 | 12 | 23 |
| | 15 | 8 | 17 | | 20 | 13 | 24 |
| | 18-20 | 9 | 17 | 16 | 16 | 12 | 22 |
| 10 | 10 | 7 | 15 | | 17 | 12 | 23 |
| | 11 | 7 | 16 | | 18 | 12 | 24 |
| | 12 | 8 | 16 | | 19-20 | 13 | 24 |
| | 13-15 | 8 | 17 | 17 | 17 | 12 | 24 |
| | 16-18 | 9 | 18 | | 18 | 13 | 24 |
| | 19 | 9 | 19 | | 19-20 | 13 | 25 |
| | 20 | 10 | 19 | 18 | 18 | 13 | 25 |
| 11 | 11 | 8 | 16 | | 19 | 14 | 25 |
| | 12 | 8 | 17 | | 20 | 14 | 26 |
| | 13 | 8 | 18 | 19 | 19-20 | 14 | 26 |
| | 14-15 | 9 | 18 | 20 | 20 | 15 | 27 |

Where $n_1$ is the small number of observations and $n_2$ is the larger

Modified from: Swed, F.S. and Eisenbar C. (1943). "Tables for Testing Randomness of Grouping in a Sequence of Alternatives," *Annals of Mathematical Statistics* 14:84-86. Permission to reprint was granted by the Institute of Mathematical Statistics.

**Table B19.** Critical Values for $T_I$ Range Test ($\alpha = 0.05$)

| n | One-Tailed Test | | Two-Tailed Test | |
|---|---|---|---|---|
| | $\alpha = 0.05$ | $\alpha = 0.01$ | $\alpha = 0.05$ | $\alpha = 0.01$ |
| 2 | 3.157 | 15.910 | 6.353 | 31.828 |
| 3 | 0.885 | 2.111 | 1.304 | 3.008 |
| 4 | 0.529 | 1.023 | 0.717 | 1.316 |
| 5 | 0.388 | 0.685 | 0.507 | 0.843 |
| 6 | 0.312 | 0.523 | 0.399 | 0.628 |
| 7 | 0.263 | 0.429 | 0.333 | 0.507 |
| 8 | 0.230 | 0.366 | 0.288 | 0.429 |
| 9 | 0.205 | 0.322 | 0.255 | 0.374 |
| 10 | 0.186 | 0.288 | 0.230 | 0.333 |
| 11 | 0.170 | 0.262 | 0.210 | 0.302 |
| 12 | 0.158 | 0.241 | 0.194 | 0.277 |
| 13 | 0.147 | 0.224 | 0.181 | 0.256 |
| 14 | 0.138 | 0.209 | 0.170 | 0.239 |
| 15 | 0.131 | 0.197 | 0.160 | 0.224 |
| 16 | 0.124 | 0.186 | 0.151 | 0.212 |
| 17 | 0.118 | 0.177 | 0.144 | 0.201 |
| 18 | 0.113 | 0.168 | 0.137 | 0.191 |
| 19 | 0.108 | 0.161 | 0.131 | 0.182 |
| 20 | 0.104 | 0.154 | 0.126 | 0.175 |

Modified from: Lord, E. (1947). “The Use of Range in Place of Standard Deviation in the t-test.” *Biometrika* 34:66. Reproduced with permission of the Biometrika Trustees.

**Table B20.** Critical Values for the $F_R$ Test for Dispersion

| $w_1$ = / $w_2$ | 2 | 3 | 4 | 5 | 6 | 7 | 8 | 9 | 10 |
|---|---|---|---|---|---|---|---|---|---|
| 2 | 12.66 | 19.23 | 25.64 | 27.78 | 29.41 | 31.25 | 32.26 | 33.33 | 35.71 |
| 3 | 3.23 | 4.35 | 5.00 | 5.56 | 6.25 | 6.67 | 7.14 | 7.14 | 7.69 |
| 4 | 2.00 | 2.70 | 3.13 | 3.45 | 3.70 | 3.85 | 4.00 | 4.17 | 4.35 |
| 5 | 1.61 | 2.04 | 2.38 | 2.50 | 2.78 | 2.86 | 3.03 | 3.13 | 3.23 |
| 6 | 1.35 | 1.75 | 2.00 | 2.17 | 2.33 | 2.44 | 2.50 | 2.63 | 2.70 |
| 7 | 1.25 | 1.56 | 1.75 | 1.92 | 2.04 | 2.13 | 2.22 | 2.27 | 2.33 |
| 8 | 1.16 | 1.43 | 1.61 | 1.75 | 1.85 | 1.96 | 2.00 | 2.08 | 2.13 |
| 9 | 1.10 | 1.33 | 1.49 | 1.64 | 1.72 | 1.82 | 1.89 | 1.92 | 1.96 |
| 10 | 1.05 | 1.25 | 1.43 | 1.43 | 1.64 | 1.70 | 1.75 | 1.82 | 1.85 |

Modified from: Link, R.F. (1950). "The Sampling Distribution of the Ratio of Two Ranges from Independent Samples," *Annals of Mathematical Statistics* 21 112-116. (These represent 1/*R*-values in original table to account for ratios >1). Permission to reprint was granted by the Institute of Mathematical Statistics.

**Table B21** Critical Values for Grubbs' Test (One-Sided Test for T)

| | α | | | |
|---|---|---|---|---|
| n | 0.1% | 0.5% | 1% | 5% |
| 3 | 1.155 | 1.155 | 1.155 | 1.153 |
| 4 | 1.499 | 1.496 | 1.492 | 1.463 |
| 5 | 1.780 | 1.764 | 1.749 | 1.672 |
| 6 | 2.011 | 1.973 | 1.944 | 1.822 |
| 7 | 2.201 | 2.139 | 2.097 | 1.938 |
| 8 | 2.358 | 2.274 | 2.221 | 2.032 |
| 9 | 2.492 | 2.387 | 2.323 | 2.110 |
| 10 | 2.606 | 2.482 | 2.410 | 2.176 |
| 11 | 2.705 | 2.564 | 2.485 | 2.234 |
| 12 | 2.791 | 2.636 | 2.550 | 2.285 |
| 13 | 2.867 | 2.699 | 2.607 | 2.331 |
| 14 | 2.935 | 2.755 | 2.659 | 2.371 |
| 15 | 2.997 | 2.806 | 2.705 | 2.409 |
| 16 | 3.052 | 2.852 | 2.747 | 2.443 |
| 17 | 3.103 | 2.894 | 2.785 | 2.475 |
| 18 | 3.149 | 2.932 | 2.821 | 2.504 |
| 19 | 3.191 | 2.968 | 2.854 | 2.532 |
| 20 | 3.230 | 3.001 | 2.884 | 2.557 |
| 21 | 3.266 | 3.031 | 2.912 | 2.580 |
| 22 | 3.300 | 3.060 | 2.939 | 2.603 |
| 23 | 3.332 | 3.087 | 2.963 | 2.624 |
| 24 | 3.362 | 3.112 | 2.987 | 2.644 |
| 25 | 3.389 | 3.135 | 3.009 | 2.663 |
| 30 | 3.507 | 3.236 | 3.103 | 2.745 |
| 35 | 3.599 | 3.316 | 3.178 | 2.811 |
| 40 | 3.673 | 3.381 | 3.240 | 2.866 |
| 45 | 3.736 | 3.435 | 3.292 | 2.914 |
| 50 | 3.789 | 3.483 | 3.336 | 2.956 |

Modified from: Grubbs, F.E. and Beck, G. (1972). "Extension of Sample Size and Percentage Points for Significance Tests of Outlying Observations," *Technometrics*, 14:847-54. Reproduced with permission of the American Statistical Association.

**Table B22** Values for Use in Dixon Test for Outlier ($\alpha$)

| Statistic | n | 0.5% | 1% | 5% |
|---|---|---|---|---|
| | 3 | .994 | .988 | .941 |
| | 4 | .926 | .889 | .765 |
| $\tau_{10}$ | 5 | .821 | .780 | .642 |
| | 6 | .740 | .698 | .560 |
| | 7 | .680 | .637 | .507 |
| | 8 | .725 | .683 | .554 |
| $\tau_{11}$ | 9 | .677 | .635 | .512 |
| | 10 | .639 | .597 | .477 |
| | 11 | .713 | .679 | .576 |
| $\tau_{21}$ | 12 | .675 | .642 | .546 |
| | 13 | .649 | .615 | .521 |
| | 14 | .674 | .641 | .546 |
| | 15 | .647 | .616 | .525 |
| | 16 | .624 | .595 | .507 |
| $\tau_{22}$ | 17 | .605 | .577 | .490 |
| | 18 | .589 | .561 | .475 |
| | 19 | .575 | .547 | .462 |
| | 20 | .562 | .535 | .450 |
| | 21 | .551 | .524 | .440 |
| | 22 | .541 | .514 | .430 |
| | 23 | .532 | .505 | .421 |
| | 24 | .524 | .497 | .413 |
| | 25 | .516 | .489 | .406 |

From: Dixon, W.J. and Massey, F.J. (1983). *Introduction to Statistical Analysis* (Table A-8e), McGraw-Hill Book Company, New York. Reproduced with permission of the publisher.

# Index